T0192881

CRC Biostatistics Series

Chapman & Hall/CRC Biostatistics Series
Shein-Chung Chow, Duke University School of Medicine
Byron Jones, Novartis Pharma AG
Jen-pei Liu, National Taiwan University
Karl E. Peace, Georgia Southern University
Bruce W. Turnbull, Cornell University

For more information about this series, please visit: www.crcpress.com/go/biostats

Analysis of Incidence Rates

Peter Cummings

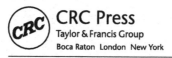

CRC Press
Taylor & Francis Group
Boca Raton London New York

CRC Press is an imprint of the
Taylor & Francis Group, an **informa** business

A CHAPMAN & HALL BOOK

CRC Press
Taylor & Francis Group
6000 Broken Sound Parkway NW, Suite 300
Boca Raton, FL 33487-2742

First issued in paperback 2020

ISBN 13: 978-0-367-73066-6 (pbk)
ISBN 13: 978-0-367-15206-2 (hbk)

Library of Congress Cataloging-in-Publication Data

Names: Cummings, Peter (Epidemiologist), author.
Title: Analysis of incidence rates / Peter Cummings.
Description: Boca Raton : CRC Press, Taylor & Francis Group, 2019.
Identifiers: LCCN 2018054753| ISBN 9780367152062 (hardback : alk. paper) | ISBN 9780429055713 (ebook)
Subjects: LCSH: Correlation (Statistics) | Multivariate analysis. | Regression analysis. |
Mathematical statistics. | Probabilities.
Classification: LCC QA278.2 .C86 2019 | DDC 519.5/36–dc23
LC record available at https://lccn.loc.gov/2018054753

Visit the Taylor & Francis Web site at
www.taylorandfrancis.com

and the CRC Press Web site at
www.crcpress.com

Contents

Preface

There are many books about linear regression (for mean differences), logistic regression (odds ratios), and the Cox proportional hazards model (hazard ratios). There are several fine books about count models, which are often used for the analysis of incidence rates (counts of new events divided by person-time). In 1987, Breslow and Day published *Statistical Methods in Cancer Research, Volume II: The Design and Analysis of Cohort Studies*, an excellent discussion of rate standardization, Poisson regression, and other methods for incidence rates (Breslow and Day 1987). Their book was cutting-edge when published and it is still in print and worth reading. In the last three decades there have been advances in computing power, software, and methods. My goal was to pull some of that material together in one place. I hoped to create a book that clarifies what incidence rates are, reviews their advantages and limitations, promotes understanding of analytic methods, provides practical suggestions for analyses, and points out problems and pitfalls.

I was a physician for 20 years and then became an epidemiologist. Therefore, some jargon and most examples in this book come from the biomedical field. The book is perhaps most suitable for the field of biostatistics. But the methods described should be useful for the disciplines of sociology, criminology, psychology, economics, and education. The book is aimed at researchers in any discipline who would like to analyze incidence rates. The orientation is toward practical issues of analysis regarding rate ratios and differences. Special attention was given to problems that recur in published papers. I tried to keep mathematical notation and statistical terminology to a minimum. The language and notation is not as statistically sophisticated as that in the book by Breslow and Day (Breslow and Day 1987). This has advantages and disadvantages. For those not used to some of this terminology, my hope was to make the discussion more accessible, but some may miss conventional notation and wording to which they are accustomed.

Writing this book involved decisions about what to include and what to omit. The first half of the book discusses fundamental ideas about rates, with an emphasis on topics not covered by other textbooks. The second half of the book is about extensions or modifications of the Poisson regression model. The last chapter compares Poisson regression with the Cox hazards model. I focused on methods most useful for incidence rates, so count data models of less relevance were ignored.

I find it useful to think about problems with simulated data. By creating data in which the association of interest is known, an analytic method can be tested to see whether it can correctly estimate that association. If the method fails, the goal is to understand why. Simulated data examples are common in this book, but other examples use real data.

All the analyses in the book were created using Stata statistical software. In the text I have put Stata commands in boldface, to distinguish them from other words. For example, the word Poisson describes a regression method, but **poisson** is a Stata command used to carry out Poisson regression. I have created files of Stata software commands that produce the data, calculations, tables, and figures for each chapter. Many details about Stata commands will be found in these files. Anyone seeking to use the methods described in the text can consult these online resources. The data and command files for each chapter are in a directory for that chapter. There is a text file that lists each file of statistical commands and briefly describes its contents. For example, if you want to see how I used Stata to produce exact P-values and confidence intervals for Chapter 4, go to the directory called "chap4data" and open the text file called "masterchap4.txt." Scroll down through that file until you find the description of "exact.do", which says "This file shows how we can compute exact CIs using poisson probability functions ..." Using a plain text editor, open the file called "exact.do" to read the commands

I used. Or run the file in Stata to see the commands and produce the output. Or open the file called "exact.log" in a text editor to see the commands and the output. You can modify command files to produce new analyses or adopt commands you like for your own work. This material can be found at https://sites.google.com/a/uw.edu/ratefiles.

For some publicly available mortality, traffic crash, and census data I omitted detailed citations. These data can be accessed from the Web sites of the Centers for Disease Control, the National Center for Health Statistics, the National Highway Transportation Safety Administration, and the U.S. Census Bureau. Stata publishes extensive manuals about every command in the software package and advice on many topics regarding data manipulation and analyses. Paper copies of these manuals are no longer available, but all the material is part of the Stata software package. These help files and other discussions are superb. They are clearly written, make extensive use of examples, and are sometimes even humorous. I decided not to give citations to this material, as there would be so many, but I urge you to read Stata's discussion of any command that you use.

A few words of thanks are warranted. I owe a debt to Noel Weiss, Thomas Koepsell, Beth Mueller, Bruce Psaty, and others at the University of Washington for the training they gave me in epidemiology. Barbara McKnight taught me about cohort study methods, including Poisson and Cox regression. She responded to several queries I had regarding the book. Fred Rivara, a past Director of the Harborview Injury Prevention and Research Center in Seattle, gave me my first job as an epidemiologist and became a friend and mentor. I was fortunate to have these people as teachers and later as colleagues. I thank Sander Greenland of UCLA, who generously answered questions I emailed to him while writing the book.

I thank both Noel Weiss and my friend Bart O'Brien for encouraging me to finish the book. Bart convinced me to plow ahead when I had doubts. This book would not exist without the support and encouragement from my wife Roberta.

I have tried to be clear and avoid mistakes. I apologize for any confusion or errors that remain.

Peter Cummings
Bishop, California
peterc@uw.edu

Author

Peter Cummings MD, MPH is Emeritus Professor of Epidemiology, School of Public Health, University of Washington, Seattle, Washington. His primary research interest has been in studies related to injuries, particularly car crashes. He has published articles about the use of case-control and matched-cohort methods for the study of injuries. He has over 100 publications in peer-reviewed journals.

Do Storks Bring Babies?

Incidence rates are ratios: counts of new (incident) events divided by person-time. Ratios can create difficulties in regression (Kronmal 1993), including analyses of rates. This chapter introduces this topic, which will be revisited later in Chapter 11, section 4. Problems with ratios in regression have been known for over a century but are still found in published studies.

1.1 KARL PEARSON AND SPURIOUS CORRELATION

Karl Pearson (1857–1936) made important contributions to statistics. The Pearson correlation coefficient is named for him. (Sadly, some of his work was devoted to his belief that humankind could be improved by eradicating "inferior races.") In 1897 he published a short paper (Pearson 1897) titled "Mathematical Contributions to the Theory of Evolution – On a Form of Spurious Correlation which May Arise when Indices Are Used in the Measurements of Organs." Pearson noted that if the values of three variables, x, y, and z, were selected randomly from a distribution, then on average we expect no correlation of x with y, x with z, or y with z. But if we divide both x and y by z, the ratios x/z and y/z will be correlated. He called this a "spurious" relationship.

To demonstrate what Pearson described, a pseudo-random number generator for uniform distributions was used to create hypothetical data for 30 geographic areas (Table 1.1). One variable was the count of area deaths during the year 2002, another the number of violins counted in the area on July 1, 2002, and the third was the number of area residents on July 1, 2002, which we will assume is a reasonable estimate of the person-years lived by people in each region during 2002.

Perhaps squeaky violin-playing promotes high blood pressure, which may increase mortality. Alternatively, soothing violin music may reduce blood pressure and the mortality rate. The Pearson correlation coefficient between the count of deaths and count of violins is only .12. Because both sets of counts were picked at random, this coefficient differs from zero only because we used a finite set of data. When I used the same pseudo-random method to create 3 million records, instead of 30, the coefficient was –.0005, essentially zero.

A researcher might be concerned that regions with more person-years during 2002 could have both more deaths and more violins. We can divide each count of deaths by that area's person-years, and multiply this by 1000, to create a mortality rate per 1000 person-years, which ranges from 0.45 to 13.33 in these data. Some researchers might also divide the violin count by person-years, to estimate the violin to person-time ratio, which ranges from .02 to 4.28. The correlation coefficient for these two ratios, mortality per 1000 person-years and violins per person-year, is an impressive .60.

Instead of estimating a correlation coefficient, we can analyze the violin data with linear regression. If the count of deaths is the outcome and the only explanatory (independent) variable is the number of violins, we can use linear regression to estimate that for each additional 100 violins in a region, the number of deaths increased by 0.12 (95% CI –0.26, 0.50). The standard error for this estimate is large, 0.19, the 95% CI is wide and includes an estimate of zero (no association), and the P-value for this association is also large, .52. At best this is weak evidence for any relationship between violins and death.

TABLE 1.1   Hypothetical data for 30 geographic regions: the number of deaths during 2002, the number of violins counted on July 1, 2002, and the number of people counted on July 1, which serves as an estimate of person-years during that year. Data from a pseudo-random number generator with draws from the range 0 to 200 for deaths, 0 to 20,000 for violins, and 0 to 100,000 for person-years. All numbers rounded to the nearest integer. Also shown are the mortality rate (deaths per 1000 person-years) and the violin-ratio (number of violins/person-years).

DEATHS	VIOLINS	PERSON-YEARS	MORTALITY RATE PER 1000 PERSON-YEARS	VIOLINS PER PERSON-YEAR
117	14788	32100	3.6449	0.461
86	1717	71369	1.2050	0.024
82	1569	71146	1.1526	0.022
44	18062	67077	0.6560	0.269
52	16696	3901	13.3299	4.280
116	5010	56689	2.0463	0.088
20	8411	7862	2.5439	1.070
149	15376	34110	4.3682	0.451
194	18569	65531	2.9604	0.283
26	2483	29893	0.8698	0.083
149	6661	72499	2.0552	0.092
43	5338	42827	1.0040	0.125
31	1133	56595	0.5478	0.020
57	14467	64045	0.8900	0.226
95	16316	23174	4.0994	0.704
46	6092	29361	1.5667	0.207
168	17427	21029	7.9890	0.829
176	1623	18590	9.4675	0.087
46	6341	10008	4.5963	0.634
42	5562	55753	0.7533	0.100
198	6495	17248	11.4796	0.377
72	5501	10724	6.7139	0.513
127	2731	34201	3.7133	0.080
67	10904	49027	1.3666	0.222
111	8181	67646	1.6409	0.121
114	3044	12628	9.0276	0.241
89	8489	81955	1.0860	0.104
20	6145	39794	0.5026	0.154
21	10945	46830	0.4484	0.234
154	3286	49625	3.1033	0.066

But if the outcome is the mortality rate, and the explanatory variable is the violin to person-years ratio, the linear regression output estimates that for each 1 unit increase in the violin ratio, the mortality rate increased by 2.73 deaths/1000 person-years with a 95% CI of 1.34 to 4.12, and a p-value < .001 for this association. This "spurious" result might lead some to advocate for the destruction of violins.

1.2 JERZY NEYMAN, STORKS, AND BABIES

Jerzy Neyman (1894–1981) is credited with introducing confidence intervals and he worked with Egon Pearson (Karl Pearson's son) on the theory of hypothesis testing (Royall 1997, Salsburg 2001). In 1947 Neyman gave a talk (later published as a book section [Neyman 1952]) in Berkeley, California, for which he created data regarding women, storks, and babies for 54 counties (Table 1.2). Neyman claimed, tongue-in-check, that the data had been collected by a friend. In these data, the number of babies increases as the number of storks increases and as the number of women increases (Figure 1.1). The number of storks also increases as the number of women increases, and Neyman's imaginary friend worried that any estimated association between storks and babies should account for the fact that counties with more babies and more storks also had more women. The friend therefore divided the number of babies by the number of women to estimate a birth rate per 10,000 women (per some unstated unit of time) and also estimated a stork ratio, the number of storks per 10,000 women. The birth rate increases with an increasing stork ratio, leading Neyman's friend to conclude that "… although there is no evidence of storks actually bringing babies, there is overwhelming evidence that, by some mysterious process, they influence the birth rate!" Here is linear regression output supporting this conclusion and the relationships in Figure 1.1.

TABLE 1.2 Data for 54 counties showing the number of women, storks, babies, the stork ratio (storks/10,000 women), and the birth rate (babies/10,000 women per unit of time). Data are from an imaginary friend of Jerzy Neyman's.

COUNTY	WOMEN	STORKS	BABIES	STORK RATIO	BIRTH RATE
1	10000	2	10	2	10
2	10000	2	15	2	15
3	10000	2	20	2	20
4	10000	3	10	3	10
5	10000	3	15	3	15
6	10000	3	20	3	20
7	10000	4	10	4	10
8	10000	4	15	4	15
9	10000	4	20	4	20
10	20000	4	15	2	7.5
11	20000	4	20	2	10
12	20000	4	25	2	13
13	20000	5	15	2.5	7.5
14	20000	5	20	2.5	10
15	20000	5	25	2.5	13
16	20000	6	15	3	7.5
17	20000	6	20	3	10
18	20000	6	25	3	13
19	30000	5	20	1.7	6.7
20	30000	5	25	1.7	8.3
21	30000	5	30	1.7	10
22	30000	6	20	2	6.7

(Continued)

TABLE 1.2   (Cont.)

COUNTY	WOMEN	STORKS	BABIES	STORK RATIO	BIRTH RATE
23	30000	6	25	2	8.3
24	30000	6	30	2	10
25	30000	7	20	2.3	6.7
26	30000	7	25	2.3	8.3
27	30000	7	30	2.3	10
28	40000	6	25	1.5	6.3
29	40000	6	30	1.5	7.5
30	40000	6	35	1.5	8.8
31	40000	7	25	1.8	6.3
32	40000	7	30	1.8	7.5
33	40000	7	35	1.8	8.8
34	40000	8	25	2	6.3
35	40000	8	30	2	7.5
36	40000	8	35	2	8.8
37	50000	7	30	1.4	6
38	50000	7	35	1.4	7
39	50000	7	40	1.4	8
40	50000	8	30	1.6	6
41	50000	8	35	1.6	7
42	50000	8	40	1.6	8
43	50000	9	30	1.8	6
44	50000	9	35	1.8	7
45	50000	9	40	1.8	8
46	60000	8	35	1.3	5.8
47	60000	8	40	1.3	6.7
48	60000	8	45	1.3	7.5
49	60000	9	35	1.5	5.8
50	60000	9	40	1.5	6.7
51	60000	9	45	1.5	7.5
52	60000	10	35	1.7	5.8
53	60000	10	40	1.7	6.7
54	60000	10	45	1.7	7.5

Data from Neyman, Jerzy. 1952. On a most powerful method of discovering statistical regularities. In *Lectures and Conferences on Mathematical Statistics and Probability*. Washington, DC: U.S. Department of Agriculture.

```
. regress babies storks, noheader
-----------------------------------------------------------------------
  babies |     Coef.  Std. Err.       t    P>|t|     [95% Conf. Interval]
-------- +-------------------------------------------------------------
  storks |  3.658537  .3475116    10.53    0.000     2.961204    4.35587
   _cons |  4.329268  2.322529     1.86    0.068    -.3312264   8.989763
-----------------------------------------------------------------------
```

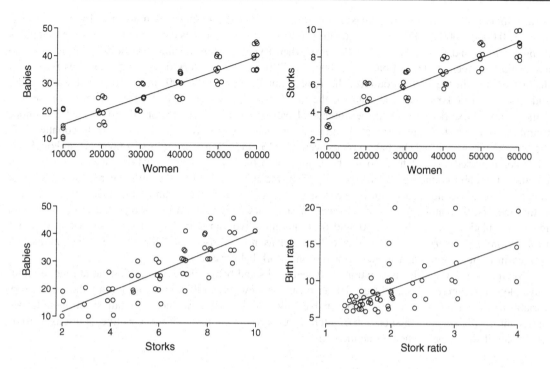

FIGURE 1.1 Scatterplots from the Table 1.2 data collected by a "friend" of Jerzy Neyman from 54 counties. Random jitter was used so that identical points would not overlap entirely. A linear regression line was fitted to each plot.

This output says that for each 1 stork increment in the count of storks, the count of babies increased by 3.7. Next we see that for each 1 point increase in the stork ratio (which ranges from 1.3 to 4.0) the birth rate per 10,000 women climbed by 3.3. Remarkable storks!

```
. regress birthrate storkratio, noheader
```

birthrate	Coef.	Std. Err.	t	P>|t|	[95% Conf. Interval]
storkratio	3.268316	.5674763	5.76	0.000	2.129592	4.407041
_cons	2.356049	1.228442	1.92	0.061	-.1090002	4.821099

Before funding further stork research, let us consider one more regression model:

```
. regress babies storks women, noheader
```

babies	Coef.	Std. Err.	t	P>|t|	[95% Conf. Interval]
storks	2.72e-15	.6618516	0.00	1.000	-1.328723	1.328723
women	.0005	.0000827	6.04	0.000	.0003339	.0006661
_cons	10	2.020958	4.95	0.000	5.942757	14.05724

In this model, a 1 unit increase in stork count increased the number of newborns by a minuscule amount: 0.00000000000000272. This quantity differs from zero only because computers store quantities in binary form and this results in small errors when trying to store decimal fractions. Why is there no association between storks and babies in this model? In Neyman's stork data, the 54 counties fell into 6 distinct groups; in the first 9 counties, the female population was 10,000, in the next 9 it was 20,000, and so on, up to 60,000. Look at data for the first 9 counties, which all had 10,000 women. In the first 3 the number of storks was 2 and the number of babies was either 10, 15, or 20. In the next 3 counties (numbers 4–6) the stork number was 3 and again the baby counts were 10, 15, and 20. In counties 7–9, the stork count was 4 and the baby counts were 10, 15, and 20. So in the first 9 counties, although the stork count varied from 2 to 3 to 4, the counts of babies showed no variation; in each group of 3 counties, the baby count was 10 in the 1st, 15 in the next, and 20 in the 3rd, regardless of the stork count. So there was no association between stork counts (or stork ratios) and baby counts (or birth rate) within the first 9 counties. The same absence of any stork-baby relationship is repeated in counties with female populations of 20, 30, 40, 50, and 60 thousand. Given no stork-baby association *within* counties *with identical numbers of women*, it should come as no surprise that adjustment for the number of women in a linear regression model removed any stork-baby association.

Neyman argued that the associations between storks and babies were not spurious at all; the relationships plotted in Figure 1.1 are all true. The error, in his view, lay in thinking that dividing the explanatory variable (storks) and the outcome variable (babies) by a third variable (women) will adjust for the influence of that third variable on the association of interest. As Neyman put it, "… if the adjective 'spurious' is to be used at all, it should be applied to the method …"

1.3 IS POISSON REGRESSION THE SOLUTION TO THE STORK PROBLEM?

Poisson regression is often used for the analysis of rates; indeed, Poisson regression and related count regression methods are the main analytic methods discussed in this book. In Poisson regression the outcome is a count (of babies in this example), the explanatory variable is the count of storks in each region, and the person-time that generated the counts for each region is used as an offset; time is converted to a logarithm and treated as a regression term with a coefficient fixed at 1. Details about this appear in later chapters, but let us apply this method now:

```
. poisson babies storks, irr nolog exp(women)

Poisson regression                              Number of obs   =        54
                                                LR chi2(1)      =     52.75
                                                Prob > chi2     =    0.0000
Log likelihood = -165.35755                     Pseudo R2       =    0.1376
------------------------------------------------------------------------------
    babies |        IRR   Std. Err.      z    P>|z|     [95% Conf. Interval]
---------+--------------------------------------------------------------------
    storks |   .9041434   .0123298    -7.39   0.000     .8802975    .9286352
    women  | (exposure)
------------------------------------------------------------------------------
```

In this model, the incidence rate ratio (IRR) for the storks term is 0.90. This means that for every 1 stork increase in the stork count, the county birth rate ratio was 0.90 compared with what it was in a county without that increase. The birth rate declined by 100% x (1 − .90) = 10% for each increment of 1 in the count of storks.

What is going on here? First it appeared that storks might be bringing babies. Then linear regression with adjustment for the number of women in each county suggested storks had nothing to do with babies. But Poisson regression suggests that the birth rate falls when more storks are present. Before you call the Audubon Society, be assured that we will return to these data in Chapter 14.

1.4 FURTHER READING

The problems described in this chapter are a few of the difficulties that may arise when ratios are used in regression. An excellent review can be found in Kronmal (1993); this review is heavy with mathematical notation, but the issues are explained in clear English. An exchange of letters about Kronmal's paper is illuminating and fun (Kronmal 1995, McShane 1995, Nevill and Holder 1995). Kronmal covered several topics. For example, use of a ratio term in regression, such as body mass index (BMI, the ratio of weight to height-squared), is not likely to adequately adjust for possible confounding by weight and height. The same topic is discussed by others (Michels, Greenland, and Rosner 1998). Firebaugh and Gibbs (1985) shed light on the use of ratios on both sides of a regression equation. Sankrithi, Emanuel, and van Belle (1991) note that several studies reported that as the number of physicians increased in an area, the infant mortality rate increased. Sankrithi et al. argue that this finding is related to the use of ratios in regression and that an alternative modeling approach leads to the opposite finding.

The topic of ratios in regression has been studied for over a century with repeated warnings about pitfalls (Fisher and van Belle 1993 pp390–391). Despite these admonitions, some investigators still use ratio terms in regression analyses. In studies of regional variations in rates, it is common to see a regression model with the rate as the outcome and explanatory variables which are counts divided by the population size; for example, the number of unemployed persons divided by the population size may be used in the regression variable. Is this a source of problems?

We will return to the stork and ratio problem later. Hopefully this discussion has made you curious about what will follow.

Risks and Rates

2

2.1 WHAT IS A RATE?

The word rate is used in many ways. Most rates are counts divided by a denominator. But the choice of numerator and denominator affects both interpretation and method of analysis. The word rate is often applied to proportions; a count divided by another count. I will give little attention to rates that are proportions and after this chapter I will try not to call these rates. This book is mostly about event rates; counts of new events divided by person-time. In the epidemiology literature these are called *incidence rates* meaning that the numerator is a count of incident (new) events. This book will discuss incidence rates for events that are nonrecurrent, such as death, first onset of prostate cancer, or first time in prison, and rates of recurrent events, such as the number of falls, asthma attacks, or bankruptcies experienced by individuals.

2.2 CLOSED AND OPEN POPULATIONS

Rates are measures of event frequency. If someone says there were 400 homicides, it is natural for us to wonder what population experienced these events, how large was the population, and when did the events occur. It is useful to distinguish between closed and open populations (Greenland and Rothman 2008d pp36–39, Weiss and Koepsell 2014 pp17–19).

A closed population is one in which all members are identified at the same time or something close to that ideal. Once all members are known, no new persons can join the population. Members can leave the population only when the planned observation period is over or they have the outcome of interest to the study. All people who graduated from Yale University in May 2008 may be considered members of a closed population. Another example is a clinical study in which everyone is enrolled on the same day and all are followed for a short period to some endpoint, without any lost to follow-up. The persons who boarded the *Titanic* on April 10, 1912, may be considered a closed population that was followed to the early morning of April 15, when some died and others survived as the ship sank.

In an open population, people can join and leave at different times. The population of Nashville, Tennessee, is open; people can become residents through birth or immigration, and they can leave through death and emigration. This definition could be refined. To be a Nashville resident, must you have a residential address? What about a student from Ohio who attends Vanderbilt University most of the year? What about a homeless person who sleeps on the streets of Nashville at night? What about a tourist staying in a Nashville hotel? What about someone who lives in the suburb of Oak Hill but is in the Nashville city jail for 30 days? Depending on our purpose, we might answer these questions differently.

Members of the Kaiser Permanente Health Plan in California are an open population, as people can enroll and disenroll. Employees of Wal-Mart are an open population. The students in the 11th grade at James A. Garfield High School in Seattle, Washington, are an open population; that population will change completely every year (unless a student is held back), some students may enter or leave during the school year, and the population will be reduced to zero for part of the summer.

At first blush people in a clinical trial with death as the outcome might seem to be members of a closed population. But a trial may not enroll all subjects on the same day. Subjects are often enrolled over a period of time, even over several years. Some subjects may be lost to observation for reasons other than death; for example, they may move without leaving information about their new address or they may refuse further participation. The key feature of a closed population is that the original members are a known group; but if many vanish during follow-up, the distinction between closed and open populations becomes blurred.

Closed and open populations can differ in ways that affect a research study. For example, in a closed population, average age must increase with the passage of time. In an open population of 11th grade students, average age may change little over time. In a geographic region with many young immigrants, average age could decrease over time.

2.3 MEASURES OF TIME

For a population we can define several measures of time. Three measures of time are relevant to most studies. Age (time since birth) at the moment each person becomes a member of the study population, calendar time (the date of enrollment and date of each outcome event), and follow-up time (outcome time minus enrollment time). If everyone was enrolled at the same moment, enrollment time is the same for all study subjects so the three time variables are not independent; for example, if two people have the same follow-up time, they also have the same outcome calendar date. Similarly, if two people had the same age at enrollment and the same follow-up time, they must have had the same age at the time of their outcomes. In an open population, these three measures of time can be distinguished; two people with the same follow-up time and the same age at enrollment need not have the same outcome or enrollment date.

We can separate out the influence of all three of these time measures if we have the necessary information about age, length of follow-up, and calendar time (either enrollment time or outcome time). Imagine a study in which we wish to assess the frequency of seizures. The outcome of interest is the count of new seizure events. If we know the age (time since birth) at which each person enters the study population, then we can estimate how age is related to seizure frequency. Length of follow-up data allows us to estimate how seizure frequency changes as time passes. Subjects may be enrolled over a long interval of calendar time; if this is known, we can estimate independently of age or follow-up time, whether calendar time (enrollment date) has a relationship with seizure occurrence. This could occur, for example, if the treatment of seizures changes over calendar time.

Additional time scales are often important: for example, knowledge of the time period during which a person took a certain medication, or when they drank alcohol versus abstaining, or when a person was employed or not.

2.4 NUMERATORS FOR RATES: COUNTS

The numerator of a rate is a count, a non-negative whole number. A rate numerator can be 0, but not -2. Counts are integers, not fractions. Counts cannot be subdivided; a count of 3 is possible, but not a count of 3.4.

Epidemiologists distinguish between two types of counts: *prevalent* cases (existing things at one point in time) and *incident* cases (new things that arise over some period of time). Prevalent cases are persons with a given condition at a single *moment* in time, regardless of when the condition may have first appeared or how long it may be expected to last. Prevalent conditions can be habits or behaviors, such as being a smoker. They might be characteristics, such as being obese or having a high school education. Most commonly in epidemiology, the counted prevalent conditions are diseases, including acute (short duration) diseases, such as pneumonia, or chronic diseases, such as diabetes. When prevalent conditions are used as rate numerators, the resulting rates are prevalence rates. In veterinary epidemiology, a prevalent case might be a cow with bovine spongiform encephalopathy (mad-cow disease). In economics, a prevalent case may be a currently unemployed person who is seeking a job; the count of job-seeking unemployed people is the numerator for the unemployment rate. In other applications, inanimate objects may be counted, such as the number of pickup trucks in the current fleet of vehicles on the road or the number of large companies that are unionized.

In contrast, *incident* cases are persons with a *new* condition in some *interval* of time; new onset of smoking, new onset of diabetes, a new breast cancer diagnosis, or new unemployment. The word *incident* is used in epidemiology as a synonym for *new*; an incident case is a new case. This jargon is not ideal, as it is easy to confuse "incident," the adjective that means new, with "incident," the noun that refers to the new condition onset or new event. Incident cases must be counted over a time interval during which people, or animals, or things, can transition from lacking to having the new condition. Incident cases can be animals with a new condition. Incident cases can also be events such as a car crash; several people may be involved in a single crash.

Incident cases can be counts of events that recur for individuals. For example, a person can fall multiple times. We might have counts of new falls for individuals. Or we might know only the total number of falls in a population of individuals over a given period of time (say the number of falls in a nursing home with 200 residents over 3 months), but not know how many each individual experienced. Many health-related events can recur; fractures, asthma attacks, urinary infections, rhinitis (the common cold), seizures, heroin overdose, and alcoholic intoxication. Being overweight could be a recurrent event, if someone gains weight, then loses weight, then gains weight again. Economic events can recur, such as unemployment, promotion, or bankruptcy. A person can have multiple arrests.

In many studies it is the first event that is of most interest for research about the causes of the event. For example, a study of factors related to the risk of myocardial infarction (heart attack) might study only the first occurrence of infarction. This approach would avoid dealing with variations in treatment that might affect the occurrence of a second infarction among persons who survive their first. In a study of the causes of breast cancer, a case might be defined by the onset of the first breast cancer. While some women may later develop cancer in the other breast, including them in the analysis may add a level of complexity, because factors that cause a first breast cancer and factors that cause repeated breast cancer may differ. Studying only the first event will simplify the analysis. For example, an analysis of recurrent myocardial infarctions would have to account for the drop-outs that will inevitably occur due to death with the first infarction.

For some outcomes that can recur, it may be useful to examine all events, including those after the first. For example, to study an intervention designed to prevent falls in the elderly, we might study all falls over some time interval. Including all falls will tend to increase statistical power, compared with an analysis of the same subjects limited to their first fall only; given the costs of study enrollment and the intervention, including all falls could increase study efficiency. We might justify the decision to study all falls on the grounds that we are interested in reducing the occurrence of all falls, not just the first. Including all falls might allow us to study whether any effect of the intervention persists after the first fall. Using all falls as the outcome may be easier to defend if we believe that the occurrence of additional falls is not greatly affected by a history of previous falls. Furthermore, a study truly limited to first falls only is not really possible, because any adult who enrolls in the study will already have a history of prior falls.

2.5 NUMERATORS THAT MAY BE MISTAKEN FOR COUNTS

Incidence rates have count numerators that cannot be subdivided. Being pregnant is a discrete prevalent condition and the onset of pregnancy is a discrete new (incident) event; someone cannot be a little bit pregnant. Rounded quantities can be confused with counts. The distinction between discrete counts and continuous quantities that are rounded to integers is important, because treating continuous quantities as discrete counts can result in analyses with incorrect estimates of statistical precision (variances, P-values, and confidence intervals (CI)). Count outcomes and incidence rates are often analyzed by methods that rely upon the Poisson distribution, a distribution for discrete non-negative integers such as 0, 1, 2, and so on. These counts are incorporated into the formulae for statistical precision (see Chapters 4 and 9).

Imagine 10 children who sold lemonade during a summer day. Rounded to the nearest dollar, 4 children had zero earnings, 3 each made 1 dollar, and 3 made 2 dollars. We will treat dollars per child-day as an incidence rate and use Poisson regression to estimate the average earnings per 1 child-day. Using dollars as the outcome, the average was $0.9 per child-day with a P-value (for a test against $1/child-day) of 0.8 and a 95% CI of $0.47 to $1.7. If we convert the outcomes to dimes, 4 children made 0 dimes, 3 made 10, and the best entrepreneurs made 20 dimes. Applying Poisson regression to dimes as the outcome, the average was 9 per child-day, equivalent to $0.9. But the P-value shrinks to <.001 (this has become a test against a null hypothesis of 1 dime per child-day) and the 95% CI is $0.73 to $1.1. Two things are happening here; changing the numerator units changes the reference for the null-hypothesis test and also changes the precision of the test. The gory details that explain these differences between dollars and dimes are described in Chapters 4, 9, and 13.

The moral is that we should not treat rounded units as if they were indivisible counts. When they appear in the numerator of a ratio, that ratio should not be called an incidence rate. As long as we are aware that a numerator quantity, such as hospital days or dollars, is not a discrete count, we can take special steps, described in Chapter 13, to obtain approximately correct estimates of statistical precision for these ratios. Examples of quantities that we can count, but that are continuous rather than discrete, include time, monetary units (dollars, pennies, rupees), speed, distance, area, volume, weight, height, temperature, brightness, and pressure. An interest rate, expressed as the amount of money owed per amount of money-time, is not an incidence rate because the numerator is not a count.

2.6 PREVALENCE PROPORTIONS

If we count the number of persons who are blind in a community at some moment in time, this count of prevalent cases may be useful. It might help us estimate how many people need services such as seeing-eye dogs or recorded books. We could compare this count with counts of other prevalent conditions in the same community. If we wished to know whether blindness was more or less prevalent compared with another community, we will want to account for any difference in the size of their populations. We can calculate a prevalence proportion, also called prevalence or prevalence rate, for each community; the count of persons with blindness at some point in time divided by the count of persons in the community at the same time. A prevalence proportion is one count divided by another count; it has no units and ranges from 0 to 1. Unlike an incidence rate, a prevalence proportion counts existing conditions, not new events, and is an estimate for a particular point in time. Realistically we cannot count all the prevalent cases at exactly one moment in time, but we can try to do this within a small window of time.

In the field of economics, the unemployment rate is a prevalence proportion. It is the count of unemployed persons who wish to work, divided by a count of all people who wish to work, whether employed or not, typically estimated for a given month.

2.7 DENOMINATORS FOR RATES: COUNT DENOMINATORS FOR INCIDENCE PROPORTIONS (RISKS)

Imagine that we follow 10,000 women for 3 years, all age 50 years at the start of follow-up, and all without current or past breast cancer. If 100 women in this closed population develop incident (new) breast cancer, the occurrence of events can be described as a proportion: the count of new events divided by the count of the original number of women being followed: 100/10,000 = .01, or 1%. This has been called a cumulative incidence rate or an attack rate. This proportion has also been called the cumulative incidence; unfortunately, that term has another meaning. We will use the term incidence proportion, which reminds us that this is a proportion.

Observed incidence proportion is an estimate of average risk; the risk or probability of breast cancer during a specific interval of time for the average person in the population. The incidence proportion ranges from 0 to 1. Incidence proportions are meaningless without relating them to a time interval. A woman may have a risk of developing breast cancer during the next 3 years equal to .01, but her risk of developing breast cancer in the next day is much less and her risk of developing breast cancer in the next 20 years is much greater. Incidence proportions are customarily considered to have no units; they are a count of people with the outcome divided by the count of people under surveillance. As we followed 10,000 women for 3 years to estimate the incidence proportion, the proportion is the number of women with new breast cancer *over 3 years of time* after age 50 years, divided by the original number of women; so the risk is .01 *over 3 years* after age 50 years. In this book we will follow the usual practice of treating risks as having no units, but the reader should keep in mind that risks only have a clear meaning when related to a time period.

In a closed study with an inevitable outcome, incidence proportion will eventually reach 1, as everyone has the outcome. The outcome of death, for example, will eventually occur for everyone in a closed population, so the risk is 1.0 if follow-up is sufficiently long.

Incidence proportion estimates average risk over an interval. The incidence proportion will be 100/10,000 regardless of whether all the incident cases arose during the first week of follow-up, the last week, or were evenly distributed over the 3 years. A lot is known about the occurrence of breast cancer, so we can reasonably expect new cases to arise in a fairly regular manner over the 3 year interval, with some increase in risk as the women age from their 50th birthday to one day younger than their 53rd birthday. If we divide the follow-up time into three separate 1-year intervals, the incidence proportion will be smallest in the first year, greatest in the last. An assumption of fairly constant average incidence proportion (risk) would not be correct for many outcomes. If we followed 50-year-old women for 20 years, the incidence proportion with breast cancer would be much larger in the last year of follow-up compared with the first, because the incidence of breast cancer increases considerably from age 50 to age 69 years.

The count of persons who die of a disease divided by the number who acquire the disease is an incidence proportion. This proportion has been called case fatality, case fatality rate, case fatality ratio, and case fatality risk (Greenland and Rothman 2008d p41, Kelly and Cowling 2013, Weiss and Koepsell 2014 pp37–38). This is not an incidence rate and to emphasize that it is a proportion that ranges from 0 to 1, we could call it the case fatality proportion. An even better term, but further removed from popular usage, might be fatality proportion. People enter the population to be followed when they are newly diagnosed with a potentially lethal illness, such as cholera, and they are followed until they die (the new, incident, event) or recover. The case fatality proportion is the count of deaths divided by the original number of cases of new illness over the follow-up time interval.

Sometimes the length of follow-up is so short and the brevity of the illness so well known, that the case-fatality proportion is presented without stating the actual follow-up time. But some time interval is always used in practice. Even for a disease with a short duration, the incidence of death may vary considerably with time. For example, after a car crash, about 50% of the deaths occur at the scene, 90% within the first 24 hours, 99% within the first 10 days, and nearly all the rest prior to 30 days. This variation might be important for some studies. Imagine that we wished to compare hospitals regarding their case-fatality proportions for victims of motor-vehicle crashes. If some hospitals receive most patients soon after a crash, while other hospitals receive most crash victims much later after a crash, the case-fatality proportions will tend to be lower in the latter group of hospitals, because many with the worst injuries died before they reached the hospital. For chronic conditions that are invariably fatal, the case fatality proportion until all deaths have occurred may not be of much interest as it will equal 1 if follow-up is sufficiently long.

Estimates of incidence proportion disregard deaths from other diseases during follow-up. Outcomes that remove study subjects from observation, typically through death, are called competing risks. In the hypothetical population of women followed for breast cancer, some may die of lung cancer the day before their 51st birthday; some of these women might have developed breast cancer during the last 2 years of follow-up, but we cannot observe this because the women died. These women will be counted in the denominator of the incidence proportion, but the numerator will underestimate the number of breast cancer cases that would have been observed if we could have followed all women for 3 years. Because of competing risks, estimates of incidence proportion (risk) may be too small. For women age 50 years followed for 3 years, the problem of competing risks may not be great. But following women age 75 years for 3 years would involve losing a substantial proportion to other causes of death. If competing risks are common the incidence proportion may be hard to estimate; instead, we are estimating a conditional risk, the risk of the outcome during follow-up conditional on not dying due to some other competing cause of death.

When we try to estimate an incidence proportion, difficulties may arise if some people are not followed for the entire planned period. Not only may some women die due to competing risks, but some may refuse further surveillance and others may be lost to follow-up because they moved and we cannot locate them. These problems will usually become more common with longer follow-up periods. If we estimate risk by dividing the outcome event count by the original number of study subjects, risk may be biased downward because we failed to count outcomes among those who did not undergo surveillance for the full 3 years.

Incidence proportion takes no notice of the decline in person-time at risk that necessarily occurs during the follow-up period as the first outcome occurs, even in the absence of competing risks or drop-outs. Once a woman develops her first breast cancer, she is no longer at risk for another first breast cancer. The incidence proportion of .01 is not based on follow-up of 10,000 women free of breast cancer for 3 years; 10,000 is the number free of breast cancer at the start of follow-up, but that number declines as cases of breast cancer arise.

Incidence proportions are not rates. The analytic methods for proportions (which range from 0 to 1) and incidence rates (which range from 0 to infinity) are different. The interpretation of the results is also different. Using the word rate for statistics that are proportions causes unnecessary confusion. Unfortunately, this usage is common. For example, researchers refer to a response rate to describe the proportion of contacted subjects who answered questions. In other situations, the word rate may be ambiguous; if we are following a group of subjects over time, the term drop-out rate could mean a proportion (count of drop-outs/count of original population) or an incidence rate (count of drop-out events divided by person-time at risk for drop-out).

2.8 DENOMINATORS FOR RATES: PERSON-TIME FOR INCIDENCE RATES

Incidence rates use person-time in the denominator. In the year 2000, the state of Nevada had an estimated mid-year resident population of 1,998,257. It is unlikely that there were actually 1,998,257 Nevada residents on every day, or even on any particular day, in 2000. Rather, 1,998,257 is an estimate of the number of Nevada residents near the middle of that year. The Bureau of the Census publishes estimates for April 1 and July 1 of each year (U.S. Census Bureau 2012). The count of residents can be used as an estimate of the number of *person-years* lived by Nevada residents during 2000, assuming that the movements in and out of Nevada were distributed evenly over the year. Not every moment of this person-time was lived in Nevada; someone with a Las Vegas address in 2000 is counted as a Nevada resident for the entire year, even if they took a 1-week vacation in Hawaii. Nevada is an open population, with people moving in and out of the state, being born, and dying, during 2000. Someone who moved into the state at 12:01 am on January 2, 2000, and resided there for the rest of the year, contributed 365/366 person-years, as 2000 was a leap-year. (A common practice is to disregard which years are leap-years and to treat all years as having 365.25 days.) Someone who moved to Nevada on March 15, 2000, and who died 6 months later, contributed 0.5 person-years. The millions of out-of-state visitors to Nevada casinos are not included in this estimate.

Census estimates cannot tally the actual person-year contributions of each person. Instead, they estimate a mid-year count that approximates the person-years. The mid-year estimate accounts for the growth or decrease in the population during the year, under the assumption that change is roughly constant over the year. If 10% of Nevada's population left the state in September 2000, the mid-year estimate of person-time would be too large; if we knew about this exodus, we could adjust for it. The Bureau of the Census actually did this for some estimates to account for the evacuation of people from New Orleans after Hurricane Katrina in 2005 (National Cancer Institute). But for Nevada's population in 2000, it is plausible that births, deaths, immigration, and emigration occurred in an approximately regular manner over the year.

According to death certificates, the underlying cause of death for 872 Nevada residents was cerebrovascular disease (stroke and related conditions) in 2000. Therefore, the mortality rate due to stroke in that year was 872/1,998,257 = 0.000436 strokes *per person-year*. This is often reported as 43.6 deaths per 100,000 person-years in mortality tables. Using 100,000 person-years is just a convention which may make it easier to read tables of mortality data and to compare mortality over different populations. By using the same units of person-time, it is easier to compare tabulated rates for deaths due to different conditions. We can express this same incidence rate as 0.0436 stroke deaths per person-century or 0.0000000008297 deaths per person-minute. We can use any person-time units that suit us; seconds, months, or millennia.

Sometimes a mortality incidence rate is reported as a rate per 100,000 or a rate per 100,000 persons. This is imprecise wording is potentially misleading, as the incidence rate can be mistaken for an incidence proportion, a count of deaths divided by the number of people. It is clearer to report incidence rates as counts per person-time. During the 5-year period from 2000 through 2004, the state of Nevada recorded 4,819 deaths due to cerebrovascular disease (stroke and related conditions). The mid-year state population was estimated as 1,998,257 in 2000 and increased to 2,329,960 in 2004. The total number of person-years lived by Nevada residents during this 5-year period was 10,829,329. There were *not* 10,829,329 different residents in Nevada during these 5 years; the number of people who were residents for all or some of this time was probably closer to 3 million. The mortality incidence rate due to stroke was 4819/10,829,329 = 44.5 stroke deaths per 100,000 person-years, not 44.5 deaths per 100,000 persons.

The use of person-time may not be intuitive. While incidence proportions range from 0 to 1, incidence rates range from 0 to infinity. They can be much larger or smaller than 1, depending upon the ratio of events to person-time and the units chosen for time. Is a mortality incidence rate of 28.2 per person-year possible? Obviously, a single person followed for a year cannot die 28 times. This is a rate of 2,820,429 deaths per 100,000 person-years. Can anything be this lethal? This rate is indeed possible; it is the approximate mortality incidence rate suffered by Union and Confederate troops at Antietam on September 17, 1862. About 6400 soldiers died out of about 82,881 who were in the battle area: 365.25 × 6400 deaths/82,881 person-days = 28.2 deaths per person-year. (The number involved in actual combat may have been smaller than 82,881, which would make the incidence rate even higher for those who fought. Probably not all the deaths were on the first day, which would make the rate somewhat lower if we widen the person-time window to an interval that would include 99% of the deaths.)

For mortality rates the mid-year population count is typically used as an approximation of the total person-years for that year and region. But for many studies, actual person-time can be used. In a cohort study or clinical trial, it is common to know time from entry to exit from the study population to the nearest day. For example, in studies of the populations of some large health maintenance organizations, such as Kaiser Permanente in California, enrollment periods in the health plan are recorded to the day in computerized files. In studies of occupational diseases, worker time at a particular job position is often available in company records. Researchers in Denmark (Hviid et al. 2003) wished to study whether receiving a vaccine containing thimerosal, a mercury containing compound, was related to the later diagnosis of autism. They linked birth, vaccination, and diagnostic records for all 467,540 children born in Denmark from January 1, 1990, through December 31, 1996. Follow-up ended on December 31, 2000. Among children who received a vaccine with thimerosal, the incidence of new autism was 104/1,220,006 person-years = 8.5 per 100,000 person-years, compared with 303/1,660,159 person-years = 18.3 among children who received the same vaccine without thimerosal: incidence rate ratio 0.47. After adjustment for calendar period and other factors, the incidence rate of autism was still less among those given thimerosal: incidence rate ratio 0.85.

The denominator of an incidence rate is not merely a measure of time; it is a measure of time for some person or thing; person-years, woman-years, child-years, elephant-years, or aircraft-years might be the denominator for an incidence rate.

Sometimes the denominator of an incidence rate is described as the *person-time at risk* for an outcome. For death from any cause, this is always accurate; as long as we are alive, we are at risk for death. However, some rates may reasonably use person-time that includes persons not at risk for the outcome. The rate of death due to uterine cancer may be reported using person-time for the entire U.S. population, even though men are not at risk for cancer of the uterus. Including all person-time in the rate denominator makes it easy to compare the impact of uterine cancer (which affects women only), prostate cancer (which affects men only), and lung cancer (which affects all), on population health. Another term for the rate denominator is observed person-time or person-time under observation. The words "at risk" may be better interpreted as meaning free of the disease or other outcome of interest; an incidence rate for a nonrecurrent outcome is calculated using the person-time of all those who have not yet had the outcome, including some with zero risk. Regardless of the terminology used, everyone is best served if the meaning of the rate denominator is clear.

Some women have a hysterectomy for reasons other than cancer and those women are no longer at risk for cancer of the uterus. The National Center for Health Statistics does not report person-time for women with a uterus only. To study how the incidence of uterine cancer death changed over time, we might use uterine cancer rates per 100,000 women-years among women 50 years and older; this assessment includes change in cancer rates partly related to changes in hysterectomy incidence for noncancerous disease. If we wanted to estimate changes in uterine cancer mortality aside from any change related to hysterectomy incidence, then some special adjustment to the total women-time denominator would be desirable.

In a closed population, the incidence rate for an inevitable outcome, such as death, does not approach 1.0, but approaches a quantity that varies according to how quickly death comes to the studied population. The more quickly death arrives, the greater the incidence rate. Once all are dead, the rate (deaths/person-time) is the inverse of the average survival time (person-time/deaths) (Greenland and Rothman 2008d p37).

2.9 RATE NUMERATORS AND DENOMINATORS FOR RECURRENT EVENTS

Rate numerators can be counts of recurrent events. Imagine a study of ten patients with epilepsy to estimate their seizure frequency while on a new medication. During a month of follow-up, 30 seizures occurred. Even though all persons had the same follow-up time, an incidence proportion makes no sense, because the count of seizures divided by the number of persons exceeds one. The results are easily summarized by an incidence rate; 30/10 = 3 seizures per person-month.

Most seizures are short in duration, so it is reasonable to count all person-time during the 1 month of follow-up. But if the recurrent outcome has a duration of more than a few hours, and if during that time a new event is not possible or cannot be identified, then we may wish to omit from the denominator the person-time during which each subject was not at risk for a new event because they currently have the outcome. For example, if the recurrent event is an episode of genital herpes or a urinary infection, there will be a period of a few days during which another episode cannot occur or cannot be recognized. The current episode has to resolve before a new one can be identified. If the outcome is being sent to prison, a new episode of being imprisoned cannot begin until the person is released from the current episode. Similarly, a new pregnancy cannot occur while a woman is pregnant. In all these examples, if we wish to study factors that may be related to the outcome occurrence, we may wish to omit intervals of person-time during which a new outcome is not possible.

2.10 RATE DENOMINATORS OTHER THAN PERSON-TIME

Not all incidence rates have person-time in the denominator. In the study of traffic crashes, it is common to use rates of crashes per mile driven; vehicle-travel-distance, rather than person-time, is the denominator. Different rate denominators tell different stories. The rate of all deaths in motor vehicle crashes per person-year is a measure of the influence of driving on public health. But we may wish to examine the rate of all crash deaths (or just driver death, as all cars have one driver) per vehicle-mile driven, which is one measure of the danger of driving.

We could use only *some* person-time as a rate denominator. For example, to study drowning among boaters, we might use only person-time spent while boating. In effect, that is what we are doing when we sample only boaters for a study of boating and alcohol use; we are sampling from person-time spent as a boater. In occupational epidemiology, the person-time of interest could be the time some spent in a particular occupation that potentially exposed them to an acute injury. In veterinary epidemiology, the denominator for a rate might be parakeet-time or cow-time.

The denominator may use area or volume (Haight 1967). Agricultural studies can use ears of corn per acre as an outcome. Bacteriologists can study the count of bacteria per area on an agar plate, or per gram of soil, or per milliliter of fluid. A retailer may use the number of purchases per store per day. In these examples, the incidence rate is the ratio of discrete counts to some continuous measure of area, space, weight, volume, or store-time.

2.11 DIFFERENT INCIDENCE RATES TELL DIFFERENT STORIES

Using different denominators for incidence rates can be instructive. For the outcome of being a driver of a passenger vehicle involved in a fatal crash in 1990 (Table 2.1), the rate per vehicle-miles per year was 11.5 for drivers 75 years and older, somewhat greater than the rate of 9.2 for the youngest drivers (16–19 years) (Insurance Institute for Highway Safety 1992). Many older persons are aware that their night vision is failing and their reflexes slower, so they cut back on their driving. Some give up their driving license. Consequently, the rate of being a driver in a fatal crash was 2.2 per person-year for the oldest group, similar to the rate of 2.0 for persons 40–44, and less than half that of teenagers. To better understand the story behind a rate, it may help to separately examine the numerator and denominator. Average miles driven per year in 1990 was 7,079 for teenagers 16–19 years, 11,400 miles for persons in their 40–44, and only 3,055 miles for persons 75 years and older.

TABLE 2.1 Incidence rates for being the driver of a passenger vehicle in a crash in which someone died. U.S. data, 1990.

	AGE GROUP (YEARS)		
RATE DENOMINATOR	*16–19*	*40–44*	*75 AND OLDER*
100 million vehicle-mile-years	9.2	1.8	11.5
10,000 licensed-driver years	6.6	2.1	3.6
10,000 person-years	4.6	2.0	2.2

Data from Insurance Institute for Highway Safety 1992. Crashes, fatal crashes per mile. *Status Report* 27 (11):1–7.

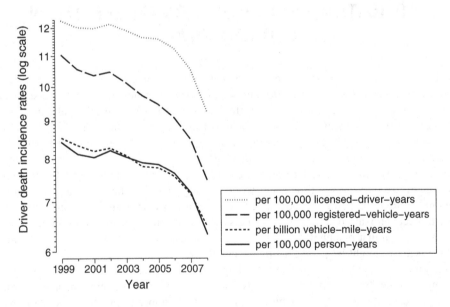

FIGURE 2.1 Driver mortality rates in the United States during 1999–2008, using four denominators: deaths per licensed-driver-years, per registered-vehicle-years, per vehicle-mile-years, and per person-years.

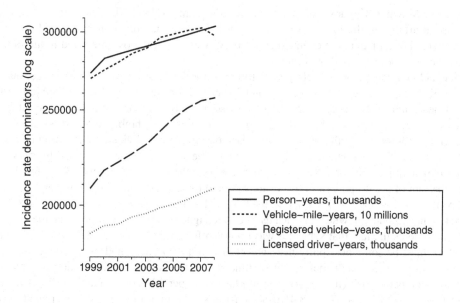

FIGURE 2.2 Estimates of licensed-driver-years, registered-vehicle-years, vehicle-mile-years, and person-years for the United States during 1999–2008.

During the 10-year interval from 1999 through 2008, driver deaths in traffic crashes declined in the United States (Figure 2.1), regardless of the denominator used; deaths per licensed driver-years, per registered-vehicle-years, per miles-driven-years, and per person-years all decreased over time. Between 2007 and 2008 the decrease was particular steep. It has been suggested that this sharper decrease may be related to the economic recession that started in 2007 and deepened in 2008. Some evidence for this exists, as miles driven actually decreased in 2008 (Figure 2.2). While the decrease in miles of driving does not explain all of the decline in the four mortality rates, it may account for the sharp downturn of these rates in the last year of the data. It is possible to formally test whether the decrease in rates from 2007 to 2008 is greater than what we might expect based on the previous 9 years of data. We could use the first 9 years of data to estimate, for example, an expected rate per person-year for 2008, and then compare the expected change in rates to the observed change in rates, and repeat this comparison after adjustment for the change in miles-driven-years.

Not only is it worth examining rate denominators, but it is often useful to examine rate numerators. To understand the size of a health problem, we will often want to know not just the rate, but the counts in the numerator.

For rates of recurrent events, it may be wise to collect and report data about how events are distributed among study subjects; are there a few subjects with many events or many subjects with few events? This information would be important in studies of falls among the elderly or flare-ups of genital herpes.

2.12 POTENTIAL ADVANTAGES OF INCIDENCE RATES COMPARED WITH INCIDENCE PROPORTIONS (RISKS)

In college, I decided to study medicine and told a physician mentor that I wanted to "save lives" and "prevent death." The physician pointed out that we cannot prevent death, we can only postpone it. The economist John Maynard Keynes (Keynes) acknowledged this truism: "The long run is a misleading guide to current affairs. In the long run we are all dead." More than one comic has said "No one gets out of life alive." For an inevitable event, such as death, we are often most interested in the time to that outcome, which can be expressed as a rate.

Imagine a closed population of eight people followed for the outcome of death due to coronary artery disease over 52 weeks (Figure 2.3). Subjects 1 and 2 survived for the entire 52 weeks. Subjects 3 through 6 died of a heart attack due to coronary artery disease at 5, 10, 30, and 48 weeks. Subject 7 refused further follow-up after 2 weeks. Subject 8 was struck and killed by lightning at 50 weeks. The incidence proportion (risk) was $4/8 = .5$, the count of coronary disease deaths divided by the original number of population members. This estimate is a weighted average; the sum of the outcomes (1 if the person dies, 0 if they survive) multiplied by the weights (which are all 1 as everyone is "followed" for 52 weeks), divided by the sum of the weights (8 in this example): sum (outcomes × weights)/sum(weights) = $(1 \times 1 + 1 \times 1 + 1 \times 1 + 1 \times 1 + 0 \times 1 + 0 \times 1 + 0 \times 1 + 0 \times 1)/(1 + 1 + 1 + 1 + 1 + 1 + 1 + 1) = 4/8 = .5$. This estimate takes no account of when the deaths occurred, ignores our ignorance about the outcome for subject 7, and ignores the fact that subject 8 was observed for only 50 weeks. The risk of .5 is surely too small, as there must be some possibility that subjects 7 and 8 could have had the outcome.

The incidence rate of death makes use of time to infarction death, time to dropout, and time to death due to a competing risk (lightning). The mortality rate per 10 person-years = $(10 \times 4 \times 52)/(52 + 52 + 5 + 10 + 30 + 48 + 2 + 50) = 8.4/10$-person-years. The mortality rate is a weighted average of each person's rate with outcomes coded as 1 (death from infarction) or 0, and weights equal to each subject's follow-up time. For a person followed for all 52 weeks and did not die, their weight is 52 (weeks) and their rate is 0/52 person-weeks. So the rate per 10 person-years, expressed as a weighted average, is $10 \times 52 \times [(52 \times 0/52) + (52 \times 0/52) + (5 \times 1/5) + (10 \times 1/10) + (30 \times 1/30) + (48 \times 1/48) + (2 \times 0/2) + (50 \times 0/50)]/(52 + 52 + 5 + 10 + 30 + 48 + 2 + 50) = 8.4/10$ person-years. All observed time is used to estimate the rate. The dropout of subject 7 is assumed to be unrelated to that person's

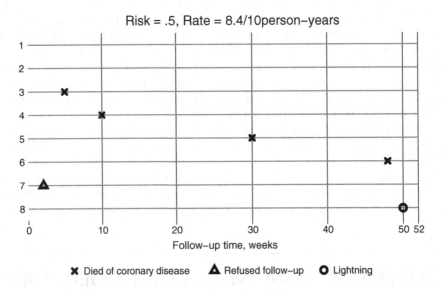

FIGURE 2.3 Information for 8 people followed for the outcome of death due to coronary artery disease over 52 weeks. Subjects 1 and 2 survived for the entire 52 weeks. Subjects 3 through 6 died of a heart attack due to coronary artery disease at 5, 10, 30, and 48 weeks. Subject 7 refused further follow-up after 2 weeks. Subject 8 was struck and killed by lightning at 50 weeks.

risk of coronary disease; this assumption may not be true, but it is weaker than the assumption of survival for 50 more weeks used to estimate the mortality risk. We know little about subject 7, who was followed for only 2 weeks, compared with subject 8, who did not have an infarction for 50 weeks; the calculation of the rate accounts for this difference in our knowledge, as subject 7 gets a weight of only 2 weeks, compared with 50 weeks for subject 8. The rate estimate assumes that being hit by lightning is unrelated to the risk of a heart attack; this seems reasonable. If subject 8 had died of a stroke, however, the assumption that the loss of 2 weeks of observation was unrelated to the risk of coronary disease death would be implausible, as both coronary disease and stroke deaths share causal factors such as high blood pressure, high cholesterol, and a history of smoking. To summarize, a rate may make better use of available information about observed time compared with a risk. And in this example, the rate estimate, compared with the risk estimate, uses weaker assumptions for its validity.

Imagine four closed populations, each with five subjects, all the same age, followed for 10 years for the outcome of death (Figure 2.4). Each population consists of persons with a new onset disease (numbered 1 through 4) and we wish to estimate mortality for each disease. For diseases 1 and 2, the 10-year mortality incidence proportions are the same, .6. But death occurs much earlier with disease 1 (after just 1 year for 3 subjects) compared with disease 2 (after 9 years for 3 subjects); the mortality rates, 1.30 per 10 person-years for disease 1 and 0.64 per 10 person-years for disease 2, reflect these differences in time to death. Similarly, diseases 3 and 4 both have mortality proportions of 1 after 10 years, but disease 4 has a much larger mortality rate (20 per 10 person-years) compared with disease 3 (1.30 per 10 person-years), because average survival for disease 4 is just 0.5 years and average survival with disease 3 is 7.7 years.

Rates are useful in situations where information about risks is unavailable. For example, by combining information from death statistics and census estimates, we can estimate mortality rates for populations. Finally, rates are useful estimates when events are recurrent.

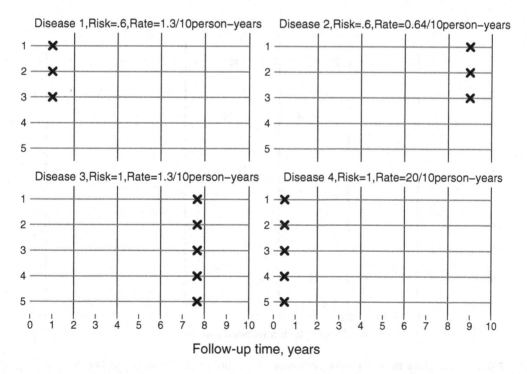

FIGURE 2.4 Survival information for four groups of five patients followed for 10 years. Each group has a different disease. Death is indicated by an X.

2.13 POTENTIAL ADVANTAGES OF INCIDENCE PROPORTIONS (RISKS) COMPARED WITH INCIDENCE RATES

In a closed population we can often estimate both risks and rates. Sometimes risks may have clearer or more useful interpretations. Atrial fibrillation is an irregular heart rhythm which is often fast and uncomfortable. Five hypothetical patients come to your emergency department with new atrial fibrillation and to fix this you administer Drug A intravenously for up to 30 minutes (Figure 2.5). All patients reverted to normal rhythm within 30 minutes, an incidence proportion of 1. The rate of conversion to normal rhythm for Drug A was $60 \times 5/(22 + 27 + 21 + 24 + 25) = 2.5$ conversion events per person-hour. For the next five patients who present with this problem you decide to use newer Drug B. The rate for Drug B was superior, $60 \times 3/(3 + 4 + 2 + 30 + 30) = 2.6$ conversions to normal rhythm per person-hour, but the incidence proportion for conversion was only .6. If Drug B works, it does so quickly, but Drug A yielded a greater overall proportion with normal rhythm after 30 minutes. For the average patient, all other things being equal (cost, side effects) Drug A produced a better result. In this example, a comparison based upon risks (incidence proportion), rather than rates, may be preferred.

As previously mentioned, most deaths after a traffic occur quickly, nearly all within 30 days. The National Highway Safety Administration collects data for crashes with a death within 30 days. Investigators have used these data to estimate the association of seat belt wearing with death. Time to death is usually known. Should these studies use risk of death or rate of death for the outcome? If someone survives to reach a hospital but still dies within 3 or 4 weeks, they will likely spend that time in great pain, often on

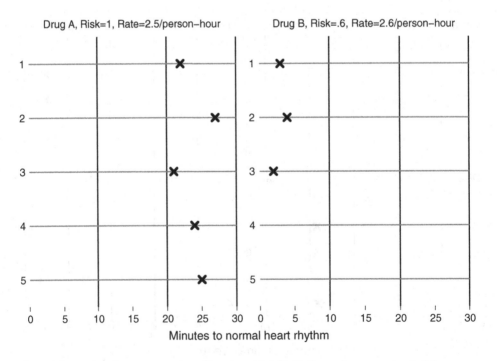

FIGURE 2.5 Information for ten people with new atrial fibrillation who were treated in an emergency department with an intravenous infusion of old Drug A or new Drug B. Treatment lasted up to 30 minutes. Time of conversion to normal heart rhythm is shown with an X.

a ventilator in an intensive care unit. If seat belts reduce injury severity enough to postpone death, but not enough to prevent death within 30 days, then the rate of death would be less among those wearing belts, but the few additional days of life would be spent in misery, or while comatose, with no survival benefit at 30 days. These studies, therefore, have all used risk of death within 30 days as the outcome.

For some purposes, the choice between risk and rate estimates may be of no importance. Both statistics can help us understand and describe event occurrence. A researcher comfortable with both these measures can use one or both as needed.

2.14 LIMITATIONS OF RISKS AND RATES

No single statistic, neither a risk nor a rate, can capture all we may wish to know about incidence. Figure 2.4 showed that identical risk estimates may describe very different outcome situations. It is preferable to have disease 2 compared with 1, or disease 4 compared with 3; the risks alone fail to describe the incident outcomes adequately because they fail to account for the time to each outcome. Similarly, diseases 1 and 3 had the same incidence rate, 1.30 per 10 person-years, but disease 1 had 3 early deaths and 2 long-term survivors, whereas everyone lives past 7 years with disease 3 and no one lives to 8 years. One remedy for these shortcomings of both risks and rates is to describe how outcomes are distributed in time. Sometimes the use of shorter time intervals may reveal more detail. An incidence rate of 1 new event per 30 person-years can be produced by 30 persons who are followed for 1 year or 1 person followed for 30 years. It will be important to distinguish between these two patterns of outcome occurrence.

2.15 RADIOACTIVE DECAY: AN EXAMPLE OF EXPONENTIAL DECLINE

If an event rate is constant in a closed population, the number of population members without the outcome will decrease linearly on the log scale. This is exponential decay; the event count will decrease exponentially over time and the survival times to each event will increase exponentially. Radioactive decay offers an ideal example of how a constant rate produces an exponential decrease in population size.

Imagine you live in Moab, Utah, and your daughter is a honor student at Grand County High School. She wants to win at the science fair by purifying uranium-238 (238 U) from the tailings of a local uranium mine. Working in your garage, she purifies 1 milligram of 238 U. She plans to exhibit this speck of material with a Geiger counter which counts the alpha particles (2 protons, 2 neutrons) from 238 U decay. The counts per second will be displayed on a laptop computer.

How many alpha particles will your daughter's computer count per second, on average? The half-life of 238 U is 4.468 billion years; this is the time at which, on average, half the original atoms remain and the other half have decayed by emitting an alpha-particle. We can convert a "1/2 – life" to a "1/e – life" by dividing by ln(2); e is the constant 2.71828, the base of natural logarithms. At the "1/e – life" time an average of 1/2.71828 = 36.8% of the atoms remain. This "1/e – life time" has a useful meaning; it is the average life-span of a 238 U atom prior to decay. If we invert this 1/e – life time (ln(2)/4.468 billion years) we get a tiny fraction, 1.551×10^{-10} alpha-particles (or atoms) per atom per year, which is a rate: the average number of decay events per atom per year.

You may recall from high-school that Avogadro's number is 6.02×10^{23} and the atomic weight of 238 U is 238.03. We can convert years to seconds by multiplying 365.25 (average days per year, including leap years) × 24 × 60 × 60 seconds. Therefore, the initial decay rate should be:

[Decay rate per atom per year] × [number of atoms in 1 milligram]/[seconds in 1 year]

$= [\ln(2)/(4.468 \times 10^9)] \times [.001 \times 6.02 \times 10^{23}/238.03]/[365.25 \times 24 \times 60 \times 60]$

$= 12.43$ alpha particles per milligram per second

The rate of uranium atom decay events (a sort of atomic mortality), 12.43 alpha particles per milligram-second, is an incidence rate; the count of atom deaths divided by the amount of U 238 (expressed as a mass) per second. Just as with person-years, the denominator of the rate uses a measure of time for something, in this case time for a unit of mass, rather than time for a person. For a radioactive gas, the decay rate can be given per volume of gas at a given pressure.

All atoms of 238 U are identical, as best anyone can tell, and all have the same risk of decay by alpha emission in the next moment in time. Unlike people, atoms do not seem to age; their risk of decay does not change as time passes. In any second of time, a discrete number of alpha particles will be emitted, signaling the death of 238 U atoms. This count will be a non-negative integer: 0 or 6 or 12 or 17. Initially the *average* count will be 12.43 per second. No matter how much time passes, the average decay incidence rate will be 12.43 per milligram-second. The mean count of alpha particles per second will not be constant but will gradually decrease as the number of remaining atoms, and therefore the remaining mass in milligrams, decreases. After 4.468 billion years, only half the original atoms will remain, so the remaining mass will be 0.5 milligrams and the mean count per second will be 6.215

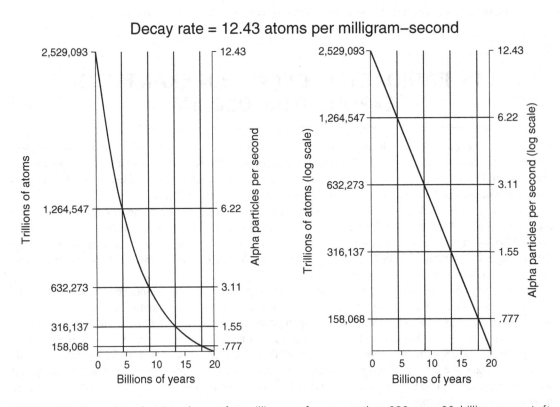

FIGURE 2.6 Two plots showing decay of a milligram of pure uranium-238 over 20 billion years. Left vertical-axis shows the number of remaining atoms and the right vertical-axis shows the number of alpha particles emitted per second. The plot on the right uses a logarithmic scale for the vertical-axis.

alpha particles per second. Given a constant incidence rate of atomic decay, the number of atoms remaining at any time t can be expressed as

$$N_t = N_0 \times e^{-\lambda t} \tag{Ex.2.1}$$

where N_t is the number of atoms at time t, N_0 is the initial number of atoms at time 0, e is the constant 2.718 (the base of natural logarithms), and λ (the Greek letter lambda) is a symbol commonly used for the decay constant. In epidemiology, we call λ the incidence rate, so the expression may be written as $N_t = N_0 \times e^{-\text{rate} \times t}$. If the science fair at Grand County High School lasts for 20 billion years, the average count of alpha particles and the count of remaining atoms of 238 U will decrease by half with every half-life of 4.468 billion years (Figure 2.6). After 1 half-life the number of remaining atoms will be 50% of the original number, after 2 half-lives it will be 25%, and after 3 half-lives it will be 12.5%. Plotting the remaining count of atoms, or the count of emitted alpha-particles, on the log scale will produce a straight line. With exponential decay, plotting the alpha-particle count on the log scale corresponds to plotting on a ratio or multiplicative scale. If we take the natural logarithm of both sides of Expression 2.1, we can rearrange the terms in several useful ways:

$$\ln(N_t) = \ln(N_0 \, e^{-\text{rate} \times t}) = \ln(N_0) - \text{rate} \times t \tag{Ex.2.2}$$

$$\ln(N_t) - \ln(N_0) = \ln(N_t/N_0) = \ln(1 - \text{risk}) = -\text{rate} \times t \tag{Ex.2.3}$$

$$\ln(N_0/N_t) = \text{rate} \times t \tag{Ex.2.4}$$

$$\ln(N_{t1}/N_{t2}) = \text{rate} \times (t_2 - t_1) \tag{Ex.2.5}$$

$$N_0 - N_t = N_0(1 - e^{-\text{rate} \times t}) = \text{new events (alpha particles emitted) up to time } t \tag{Ex.2.6}$$

$$\text{Total atom} - \text{time to time } t = N_0(1 - e^{-\text{rate} \times t})/\text{rate} \tag{Ex.2.7}$$

The expressions above all show that a linear change in time (shown on the horizontal axis of Figure 2.6) corresponds to a linear change in the logarithm of the ratio of the number of atoms or the size of a population (shown on the vertical axis of Figure 2.6). If initial time is time 0 and final time is 3 half-lives (13.404 billion years), because each half-life reduces the population by 1/2, the final population of atoms will be $(1/2)^3$, or 1/8th of the original population.

These equations show the relationship between risks and rates. The decay constant is the incidence rate: the number of atomic deaths per unit of time. The proportion of atoms still surviving at time t is N_t/N_0, the survival proportion. Therefore $1 - N_t/N_0$ is the incidence proportion, the risk of atomic death (decay) from the start of follow-up to time t. So we can write:

$$\ln(1 - \text{risk}) = -\text{rate per 1 time unit} \times (\text{elapsed time}) \tag{Ex.2.8}$$

$$\text{risk at time } t = 1 - e^{-\text{rate} \times t} \tag{Ex.2.9}$$

$$\text{rate} = -\ln(1 - \text{risk})/\text{time} \tag{Ex.2.10}$$

The example of radioactive decay illustrates properties of a constant incidence rate in a closed population with no competing risks and an inevitable, nonrecurrent outcome.

2.16 THE RELEVANCE OF EXPONENTIAL DECAY TO HUMAN POPULATIONS

Unlike atoms, humans do not all have the same risk of death when observation starts. Their risk varies with initial age, exposure history, and genetic background. Truly exponential decline of a population (a steady rate) may never actually occur in a closed population of humans followed to death. The rate of death cannot remain constant because the population is aging (unlike uranium atoms) and this will increase the rate, especially for populations of older adults.

But if events are uncommon, a rate may be roughly constant. If we divide calendar time into short intervals, so that outcomes are uncommon within those intervals, it may be reasonable to assume a rate is constant within those intervals. Mortality data is often grouped by region and year. Within these categories, deaths are usually sufficiently rare that we can think of the events as arising from a constant rate that produces exponential decay. In analyses we can stratify on factors that influence rates, including time, and produce strata within which the rate is approximately constant. For example, while the rate of death may increase over time for a closed population, if we stratify on categories of age the rate within age strata may change little. In an open population, with young people entering as older ones leave, a rate may be approximately constant.

2.17 RELATIONSHIPS BETWEEN RATES, RISKS, AND HAZARDS

When a risk is small (say .2 or less), the risks and rates for an inevitable, nonrecurrent event in a closed population are approximately related by these expressions:

$$\text{incidence proportion} \approx \text{incidence rate} \times \text{time} \tag{Ex.2.11}$$

$$\text{incidence proportion}/\text{time} \approx \text{incidence rate} \tag{Ex.2.12}$$

Imagine the outcome event is death, population size is 1000, and the risk for death over 1 year of follow-up is 0.1. If outcome events occur at a steady rate, the incidence rate is approximately (Expression 2.12) 0.1/(1 year) = 0.1 deaths per person-year. The actual incidence rate (Expression 2.10) is $-\ln(1 - \text{risk})/\text{time} = -\ln(1 - .1)/1$ year = 0.105 deaths per person-year, close to the result from Expression 2.12. When risks are less than .1, incidence rates and incidence proportions (risks), when expressed using the same time units, are close to one another (Figure 2.7). When risk is .2, the rate is 0.22 and when risk is .3, the rate is 0.36. Expressions 2.11 and 2.12 are less useful approximations once risk is larger than .2.

Rates can be expressed using any unit of time, so a comparison of rates and risks can be misleading unless care is taken to be sure that both measures use the same time scale. If the incidence proportion is based on follow-up of 2.5 years, then the rates should be expressed as events per 2.5 person-years. You could multiply the rate by 40,000, to get the rate per 100,000 person-years. But you would then have to multiply the risk by 40,000, which might create a "risk" that is greater than 1, which is not possible. The comparison between this new "risk" and the rate per 100,000 person-years can still be made, but it is easier to understand what is being compared if the risk is left unchanged and the rate denominator is a quantity of person-time equal to the follow-up time used for the risk.

In the example used earlier, why is the rate 0.105 per 1 person-year when the risk is .1 for 1 year of follow-up? Larger risks for the same followed population, compared with smaller risks, have a larger

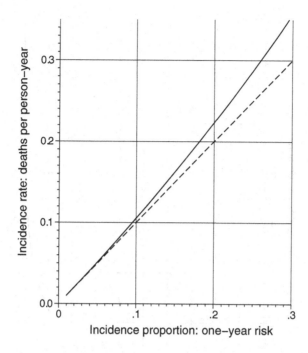

FIGURE 2.7 Plot of 1-year risk versus rate per person-year (solid line), for a closed population with a constant risk and rate. The dashed line shows the line of equality for reference.

numerator for the incidence proportion (the count of outcome events), but the denominator of the proportion is not affected; the denominator is the number of subjects at the start of follow-up, regardless of the size of the risk. For larger risks, the incidence rate will be larger still, because increasing risk increases the number of outcome events and also shrinks the person-time denominator for the incidence rate, by removing more people from the pool still at risk for the outcome. Higher risk means only a larger numerator for the incidence proportion, but higher risk means both a larger numerator and a smaller person-time denominator for the incidence rate.

If the 1-year incidence proportion is .1 in a closed population of 1000, then 100 people will be dead by the end of the first year. The rate numerator is therefore 100. The 900 survivors contribute a total of 900 person-years to the incidence rate denominator. If this is a closed homogenous population with a constant rate of death throughout the year (assume a year equals 365 days), then the 100 deaths will be *nearly* evenly distributed over the year; the first person will die after 3.65 days, contributing 3.65 days to the denominator. The next person contributes 2 × 3.65 days, and so on. The total number of days contributed by those who died adds up to 3.65 + 2 × 3.65 + 3 × 3.65 ... = 18,432.5 days = 50.5 years. So the rate is 100/(900 + 50.5) = 100/950.5 person-years = .105 deaths per person-year.

The method used to estimate the person-time in the denominator in the preceding paragraph is only approximate. If the incidence rate were truly constant, the deaths would be closer together early in follow-up when more subjects were alive, but more spread out later in follow-up, as the population shrinks. The exponential formula accounts for this; the correct rate to several decimals is $-\ln(1-.1)/1$ year $= 0.10536052$, so the person-years total for the denominator is the count of deaths/rate $= 100/0.10536052 = 949.12216$ years, instead of the 950.5 from the approximate method.

For larger values of the 1-year risk of death, the denominator person-time necessarily becomes smaller and consequently the incidence rate will deviate more from the risk (Figure 2.8). As the rate increases toward infinity, the incidence proportion (risk) approaches, but never quite reaches, 1. For example, if the rate of death is 8/person-year, the risk of death after 1 year of follow-up is .99966454.

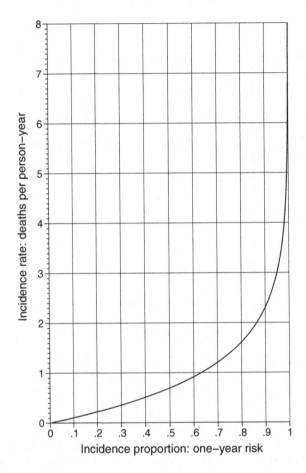

FIGURE 2.8   Plot of 1-year risk versus rate per person-year, for a closed population with a constant risk and rate for an inevitable nonrecurrent outcome, such as death.

In a finite population of humans or uranium atoms, the incidence proportion will eventually reach 1; everyone will die and all uranium atoms will decay.

Expressions 2.11 and 2.12 are approximately correct when the incidence proportion is .2 or less. In theory we can always force this to be true if we examine sufficiently short time intervals. For example, the same range of rates (.01 to 8) that was used in Figure 2.8 can be divided by 52.1429, the number of weeks in a year of 365 days; the rates for 1 week of follow-up range from 0.0001918 to 0.1534245 and the corresponding risks range from .0001918 to .1422345. Expressions 2.1 and 2.2 work fairly well within this range (Figure 2.7). Thus, when expressed using the same units of time, the risk after time t and the rate per person-t, will closely approximate each other when the risk is small over the interval t. Since t can usually be made arbitrarily small, the approximate formulae can often be used.

There is a relationship between analyses that use rates and analyses using Kaplan-Meier methods, Cox proportional hazard regression, or other survival analysis methods. These methods all deal with observation time, time to a new event, and are used to analyze cohort study data. All of these methods often have to deal with problems related to incomplete observation time that may arise because of refusal to continue as a study participant, loss to follow-up, the occurrence of a competing outcome event, or the planned cessation of the study. In addition, these methods can deal with different entry times in which some subjects come under observation later than others.

Survival analysis methods such as the Cox model estimate what are called hazards: the hazard for an outcome is the potential per unit time for the event to occur in the next *instant* given survival up to a given time. The hazard is an incidence rate with an infinitesimal amount of time in the denominator. In survival analysis, the hazard of the outcome can be estimated for each small window of time from the previous event to the next event. If we estimate the incidence rate for an outcome using intervals of time that are so small that they each include only a single outcome event, then in each time window the incidence rate multiplied by the time of the interval will be approximately equal to the incidence proportion (risk) of the outcome in that same time interval. So incidence rate × time interval ≈ risk ≈ hazard within small intervals of time. Alternatively, the incidence rate is the ratio of average risk during a small period of time divided by the time period, for small intervals of elapsed time. This is equivalent to the definition of a hazard.

2.18 FURTHER READING

Several textbooks have excellent discussions regarding incidence rates. The paperbacks by Gordis (2009) and Rothman (2012) are short and well written. More details can be found in the textbook by Weiss and Koepsell (2014). Advanced discussions are in Rothman, Greenland, and Lash (2008c) and an older, but informative, book by Breslow and Day (1987).

Rate Ratios and Differences

3

3.1 ESTIMATED ASSOCIATIONS AND CAUSAL EFFECTS

Rates are useful for description. But researchers are often interested in estimating associations between an exposure and an outcome. Sometimes it is convenient to do this using a rate ratio or a rate difference.

Epidemiologists use *exposure* to mean a factor or characteristic that may be related to an outcome. For example, if the outcome is lung cancer, the exposure of interest might be a history of smoking, perhaps expressed as pack-years. If the outcome is death in a car crash, the exposure might be wearing a seat belt, compared with not wearing one. Equivalent terms for exposure include independent variable, explanatory variable, or predictor. Exposure also has another meaning; the person-time denominator of a rate is sometimes called the *exposure time*. Stata software for rate regression requires that the person-time be entered into the model using a command option called **exposure**. This usage refers to the amount of time during which a person was exposed to the risk of the outcome under study. To avoid confusion, I will not use "exposure" in this way; instead, I will specify that the rate denominator is person-time or some other continuous variable.

Researchers often estimate an *association* to quantify a possibly causal relationship between an exposure (a treatment, habit, characteristic) and an outcome (death, illness, or a continuous measure such as blood pressure or weight). Statistics used to quantify associations include ratios of risks, rates, hazards, means, and odds, or differences in risks, rates, or means.

Sometimes a rate ratio or difference is estimated without any presumption that this will approximate a causal effect. A ratio or difference could be used to compare the 2007 rate of cancer in Nevada (173 per 100,000 person-years) with the rate in neighboring Utah (99) (CDC WONDER). It is not likely that merely living in Nevada causes cancer, compared with living in Utah. These rates differ because smoking, drinking alcohol, and other cancer-causing behaviors are more common in Nevada compared with Utah. Associations sometimes provide useful descriptive information, without any inference that the association is causal.

If an estimated association is thought to be causal, it describes the *effect* of exposure on the outcome. The causal effect of exposure for studied subjects is usually the average outcome if all were exposed (or at some exposure level) compared with the average outcome if all were not exposed (or at a different level of exposure) (Morgan and Winship 2007a, Greenland, Rothman, and Lash 2008b). The effect for the exposed only or the effect for those not exposed can also be estimated. Most clinical trials estimate the causal effect averaged across the characteristics of all study subjects. Most observational studies, in which exposure is not assigned randomly, estimate causal effects conditional on the covariates used for adjustment.

To infer that an estimated association is a causal effect depends on judgment not only about the biases that may afflict a particular study (confounding, measurement error, and selection bias), but judgments about results from other studies and possible causal (biological, psychological, economic) mechanisms. It is rare that an estimated association can be judged to be a causal effect based on the results of a single study (Weiss 2001, Cummings 2007b). Willingness to make judgments about causality vary from one researcher to the next. I will usually use the word *association* to refer to an estimate that may or may not be causal and will reserve the word *effect* to refer to causal effects.

3.2 SOURCES OF BIAS IN ESTIMATES OF CAUSAL EFFECT

An estimated association may be biased from the true causal effect for many reasons. Potential sources of bias are named and classified somewhat differently by different disciplines. Epidemiologists often group biases into three categories: confounding bias, selection bias, and measurement error. I will briefly describe each of these to introduce terminology that will be used in this book.

Confounding bias

To estimate the effect of seat belt use on the risk of death, we could compare the proportions of restrained and unrestrained occupants who died in crashes. But this may be a biased estimate of belt effects if those belted and unbelted *differ* on other *factors related to death*. Factors that might produce this bias include vehicle features (model, weight), crash attributes (force due to deceleration, distance to a trauma center), and occupant characteristics (age, seat position). This type of bias is called confounding and these factors are called confounders. Several methods can be used to reduce confounding. One method is restriction; if risk of death differs by sex, we can eliminate confounding by sex by restricting the study population to women. Statistical adjustment creates estimates that compare women with women and men with men and then combines these estimates. This can be done using stratified Mantel-Haenszel methods or regression methods that adjust for sex. We could match each belted woman to a unbelted woman, each belted man to an unbelted man, and create estimates using these matched sets. Restriction, adjustment, and matching can also be done using propensity scores. Each method tries to compare belted and unbelted subjects who are similar with respect to confounding variables. Failure to adequately account for an important confounding factor, measured or unmeasured, can produce bias.

Selection bias

Imagine exercise reduces mortality and we wish to estimate how much mortality is reduced by exercise done when not at work. We will study this among workers at Widget International. Based on how much each worker exercises away from work, we classify them as a fitness buff or a couch potato. Then we follow workers to the outcome of death. Slinging widgets all day is hard work, but the pay is good, so fit workers stay on the job and remain in our study. But couch potatoes often find themselves exhausted and sore, so many quit work and are lost to follow-up. The couch potatoes who quit most often are the ones who exercised the least and who were therefore most likely to die. This means that among the couch potatoes who remain in our study, mortality will be less than what we would have found with complete follow-up. This will bias our estimate of the exercise-mortality association by reducing the mortality difference between the fitness buffs and the couch potatoes. Selection bias may arise if inclusion in the study is related both to the exposure and the outcome of interest. This bias cannot be fixed by adjustment in regression or other statistical methods.

Measurement error

If the exposure and outcome are measured with error, this may bias estimates of association. If the exposure or outcome is binary, errors in measurement are often called misclassification, meaning that we misclassify an exposed person as not exposed (or vice versa) or we misclassify someone with the disease outcome as not diseased (or vice versa).

Randomized controlled trials have the advantage that randomization, will, on average, create groups of subjects who are similar regarding not only measured confounding variables, but also *similar regarding variables that we cannot measure or have not even considered*. Thus, any comparison should, *on average*, be free of confounding bias. In any particular trial, of course, especially a small trial, confounding bias could be present. Selection bias can arise due to dropouts. Measurement error can also bias a randomized trial. For example, the outcome might be a pain score reported by trial subjects. If some patients deduce which arm of the trial they are in (treatment versus placebo), this might influence their reports of pain.

3.3 ESTIMATION VERSUS PREDICTION

Sometimes statistical models are used to develop estimates that can be used for prediction (Stiell and Wells 1999, Altman and Royston 2000, Stiell 2001, Pepe 2003, Royston and Sauerbrei 2008, Royston et al. 2009, Steyerberg 2009). In developing a prediction model, the analyst typically selects from many variables to develop a model that can be used for decision making, research, or other prognostic purposes. Prediction modeling involves methods distinct from the estimation of associations. For example, a variable might be useful in a prediction model even though it has no causal effect on the outcome. Variables in a prediction model might be biased estimates of causal effects, but that would be of little concern if they serve well as predictors. We judge prediction models by their ability to predict, using measurements such as sensitivity, specificity, and area under the receiver operating curve. In prediction model development, the model is often developed in one population and then evaluated in a second population.

This book is primarily about estimating associations using incidence rates, which is somewhat different from the goal of prediction. In estimating associations, we are often interested in how one or a few exposure variables may be related to the outcome of interest. Other variables are of interest only to the extent that they may be confounders of the associations of primary interest. Some analysts refer to potential confounders as nuisance variables, the idea being that we are only interested in these variables for their ability to remove confounding bias.

3.4 RATIOS AND DIFFERENCES FOR RISKS AND RATES

For risks and incidence rates we can use either differences or ratios to estimate associations. Risk and rate ratios both range from 0 to infinity, with no association indicated by a value of 1, which is sometimes called the "null" value, meaning the value that is true if a "null" hypothesis of no association is true. Neither ratio has units. Risk differences range from −1 to +1; no difference is indicated by zero and the difference has no units. Incidence rate differences vary from minus infinity to plus infinity, with no difference marked by 0. Rate differences *have* units: events per person-time.

Rate differences are sometimes called absolute differences or effects, whereas rate ratios are sometimes called relative rates or relative effects. This terminology can be confusing, as both a difference and a ratio are "relative" to something; either one rate is divided by the other or one rate is subtracted from the other. I will try to avoid the ambiguous word "relative."

3.5 RELATIONSHIPS BETWEEN MEASURES OF ASSOCIATION IN A CLOSED POPULATION

As described in Chapter 2, as outcome risk increases in a closed population, the size of the incidence rate will increase faster than the size of the incidence proportion, because increasing risk increases the rate numerator *and* shrinks the rate denominator. This divergence of incidence rate from incidence proportion is made easily apparent when the rate is expressed as events per 1 unit of person-time, using a unit equal to the follow-up time used to estimate the incidence proportion.

If the outcome event is sufficiently uncommon over the observation interval, compared with the size of the observed population, then the incidence proportion will be small and the incidence rate will be close to the incidence proportion because the population still under observation will not shrink much as outcomes occur. A rare outcome will only have a minimal impact on the person-time denominator of an incidence rate. If the original closed population has size N_0, the count of those without the outcome (survivors) at time t is N_t, and all are followed to time t, then risk $= (N_0 - N_t)/N_0$ and rate $= (N_0 - N_t)/$total person-time to time t. If the count of survivors is close to N_0, which will be true if the outcome is rare, then total person-time accumulated to time t will be close to $N_0 \times t$, so the rate will be close to $(N_0 - N_t)/(N_0 \times t)$ which is equal to $(N_0 - N_t)/N_0$ per t units of person-time.

Likewise, the odds of the outcome will be similar to the incidence proportion when outcomes are rare, as the outcome odds are the incidence proportion/(1 − incidence proportion) and if the incidence proportion is small, 1 − incidence proportion will be close to 1. Because of these relationships, if outcomes are rare (say less than 10% for a closed population), then

risk ratio ≈ rate ratio ≈ odds ratio

These claims should be qualified a bit; they apply to crude (unadjusted) ratios. Even when the outcome is rare as a fraction of all study participants, the odds ratio could still be substantially further from 1 than the risk ratio if adjustment was made for a potential confounding variable and both the following are true in some levels of that variable: (a) the outcomes are not rare, and (b) a noteworthy proportion of all outcomes occur within those levels (Greenland 1987b, Cummings 2009b). This caution also applies to the adjusted rate ratio, which will not approximate the risk ratio if outcomes are common in any noteworthy stratum of the variable used for adjustment.

The risk, rate, and odds ratios will all equal 1 if exposure has no effect on average outcome risk and there are no sources of bias. If exposure does affect average risk, the 3 ratios will tend to diverge as events are more common and as the risk ratio (or any of the ratios) is further from 1. If exposure affects average risk and subjects are followed until all have the outcome, the final risk ratio will be 1, but the final incidence rate ratio will not be 1, because those at greater risk for the outcome will have their outcomes sooner on average. If all in a closed population are followed to death, the rate ratio that compares exposed to unexposed persons will equal the average survival time among the unexposed divided by the average survival among the exposed.

When the risk ratio is greater than 1, the order of these ratios (Greenland, Rothman, and Lash 2008b p61, Greenland and Rothman 2008b p250) will usually be

1 < risk ratio < rate ratio < odds ratio

and for risk ratios less than 1 the order will be reversed

1 > risk ratio > rate ratio > odds ratio.

If differences are expressed in the same units (events per amount of time equal to the follow-up time for a closed population) then these relationships will usually be true:

0 < risk difference < rate difference < odds difference
0 > risk difference > rate difference > odds difference

3.6 THE HYPOTHETICAL TEXCO STUDY

Consider a hypothetical closed cohort study of exposure to X, The Exposure to X COhort (TEXCO) study. Subjects were exposed or not exposed to X, a harmful chemical. The incidence rate of death per person-year was 0.1 for those unexposed and was five times greater, 0.5, for those exposed (Figures 3.1 and 3.2, Table 3.1).

To eliminate confounding bias from this example, the average risk for death, aside from exposure to X, should be the same for those exposed and unexposed. But for this example we will go further and require that subjects have *identical* risks for death aside from exposure. Because of this uniformity, the survival times for each exposure group will follow an exponential distribution, just as the uranium atoms discussed in Chapter 2. (In later chapters we will see what happens when risk of death varies from one subject to the next.)

The exposed and unexposed cohorts, initially equal in size, were followed for 10 years. In the first year of follow-up, the rate of death among those unexposed was 0.1 per 1 person-year. The risk of death in the first year is shown as .1, which appears to be identical with the rate per 1 person-year after 1 year (first row of Table 3.1). The risk is actually a bit smaller than the rate, .09516, but it is shown as .1 because of rounding. As we expect from the discussion in Chapter 2, the risk is smaller than the rate,

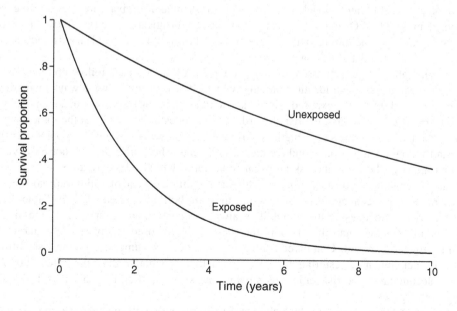

FIGURE 3.1 Survival of persons exposed and unexposed to substance X in a closed population: hypothetical TEXCO study. Mortality rate 0.1 per person-year if unexposed, 0.5 if exposed.

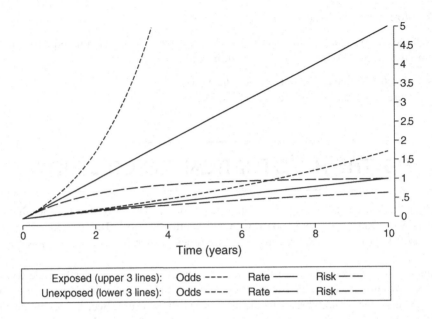

FIGURE 3.2 Data for the hypothetical TEXCO study, a closed population followed for 10 years (Table 3.1). Risks, rates, and odds are shown for exposed and unexposed subjects. The statistic for each time includes data from all prior times. Risks and odds are for the *risk or odds during T years*, where T is the number of follow-up years. Rates are for *deaths per T years of person-time*. Odds greater than 5 are omitted.

but the two are fairly close until the risk is >.1. For the exposed subjects, row 1 of Table 3.1 shows a risk of .39 and rate of 0.5. The odds are always larger than the risks and the rates.

The hazard for an outcome is the instantaneous rate for that outcome in the next small moment of time; it is the rate at time t, for a time interval that approaches 0. Hazard ratios are most often estimated by the Cox proportional hazards model. When rates are constant and survival times follow an exponential distribution, as in the TEXCO study, the hazards and rates are identical, as are their ratios. To save space, the constant hazards and the hazard ratios of 5.0 are not shown in Table 3.1. Hazards and hazard ratios will be discussed in more detail in Chapter 25.

The rates in Table 3.1 are expressed as rates per T person-years for each follow-up time. The rate per T person-years gets bigger by an identical amount with each year of follow-up, always increasing by 0.1 for the unexposed and 0.5 for the exposed. Since the rate of death is constant over time, then in any interval of time (say from 0.7 to 1.7 years), the risk, hazard, rate, and odds of death will be the same as they are in any other interval of time of the same length (say from 4.2 to 5.2 years). At any time point during follow-up, if we start follow-up at that point and we pick a sufficiently short time interval, not only will the rate ratios and hazard ratios be 5, but the risk ratios and odds ratios will also be close to 5.

The rates change by a constant amount with each additional year of follow-up, so the rate ratio and hazard ratio do not change during follow-up; they are both always equal to 5 (Table 3.1, Figure 3.3). But the risk ratio does change, and it is always smaller than 5. In year 1, the risk for the unexposed is a bit smaller than the rate and the risk for the exposed is smaller, by a larger amount, than the rate for the exposed. Compared with the rate ratio, the numerator of the risk ratio shrinks more than its denominator, resulting in a risk ratio that is smaller than the rate ratio. As more person-time accumulates, the risk ratio gets smaller and smaller; after 10 years it is 1.57 and it will eventually converge to 1.

The odds of death are equal to the risk/(1-risk), so the odds will always be larger than the risk. For a short time interval, where the risk is small, the denominator of the odds ratio will be close to 1

TABLE 3.1 Data for the hypothetical TEXCO study, a closed population followed for 10 years. Subjects were exposed or not exposed to harmful substance X. Survival proportions are in Figure 3.1. Risks, rates, and odds are shown for exposed and unexposed subjects, as well as ratios of risks, rates, and odds, and differences in risks and rates. Outcomes of those exposed are compared with those unexposed. Each statistic was estimated after 1, 2, 3, 4, 5, and 10 years of follow-up. The statistic for each year includes data from all prior years. Risks and risk differences are for the *risk during T years*, where T is the number of follow-up years. Rates and rate differences are for *deaths per T years of person-time*. These denominators facilitate comparison of risks, rates and their differences across *rows*. Because risks, rates and their differences have different units from one year to the next, comparisons within columns are difficult.

YEAR	RISKS		RATES		ODDS		RATIOS			DIFFERENCES	
	UNEXPOSED	EXPOSED	UNEXPOSED	EXPOSED	UNEXPOSED	EXPOSED	RISK RATIO	RATE RATIO	ODDS RATIO	RISK DIFFERENCE	RATE DIFFERENCE
1	.10	.39	0.1	0.5	0.11	0.65	4.13	5.00	6.2	.30	0.40
2	.18	.63	0.2	1.0	0.22	1.72	3.49	5.00	7.8	.45	0.80
3	.26	.78	0.3	1.5	0.35	3.48	3.00	5.00	10.0	.52	1.20
4	.33	.86	0.4	2.0	0.49	6.39	2.62	5.00	13.0	.53	1.60
5	.39	.92	0.5	2.5	0.65	11.18	2.33	5.00	17.2	.52	2.00
10	.63	.99	1.0	5.0	1.72	147.41	1.57	5.00	85.8	.36	4.00

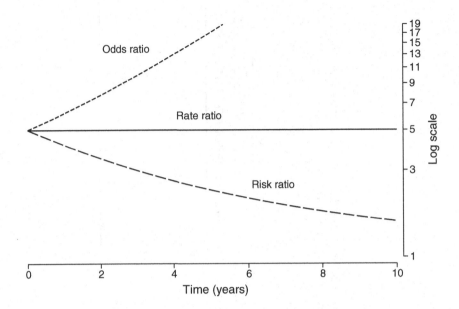

FIGURE 3.3 Data for the hypothetical TEXCO study of a closed population followed for 10 years (Table 3.1, Figures 3.1 and 3.2). Risk ratios, rate ratios, and odds ratios are shown comparing exposed with unexposed subjects. Odds ratios greater than 19 are omitted. Y axis on log scale.

and the odds and risks will be similar, resulting in risk, odds, and rate ratios that all close to 5. But as time passes and more deaths occur, the risk to time T becomes larger and the odds becomes larger still (Figure 3.2). Because this increase in the odds, compared with the risk, is greater for greater risks, the odds ratio comparing the exposed with those not exposed will become larger over time. As time passes, the risk ratio converges toward 1, the odds ratio moves toward infinity, and the rate ratio remains 5. These relations support our earlier claim that when rates are approximately constant, if the risk ratio is greater than 1, then 1 < risk ratio < rate ratio < odds ratio.

The rate difference is larger than the risk difference (Table 3.1) when the rate difference uses time units equal to the follow-up time used for the risk difference. Over time the difference in rates per T person-years becomes larger. But if we always express rates using the same denominator units, such as rate per 1 person-year, the rate difference will always be 0.4 (Figure 3.4). The risk difference, which first becomes larger, starts to shrink after year 4 because the risk in the exposed has started to bump up against its upper limit of 1. Eventually the risk difference will shrink to 0, as both risks approach 1.

If we followed subjects long enough, eventually all would die, resulting in incidence proportions (risks) of 1 for both groups, a risk ratio of 1.0, and a risk difference of 0. The odds ratio would be undefined once all are dead in either group, as the odds is equal to the incidence proportion divided by 1 minus the incidence proportion; once all are dead, this would mean dividing 1 by zero, which is undefined. The rate ratio, however, would be greater than one, even after all are dead, reflecting the fact that death came more swiftly for the exposed. The rate ratio would equal the average survival time of those unexposed divided by the average survival time of those exposed.

We can summarize some of these relationships by considering person-time. If the outcome is rare (say < 10% in a closed population) during some interval of time, then person-time changes little during that interval and risks, rates, and odds will all approximate each other. Consequently, their ratios will be similar and their differences will be similar. To estimate risks, we use counts of persons at the start of the study and ignore the timing of the outcomes. Since odds are equal to risk/(1-risk), the same is true of odds. Rates account for the time to each outcome by adjusting the person-time denominator. So long as the person-time denominator changes little, risks, rates, and odds will all be similar.

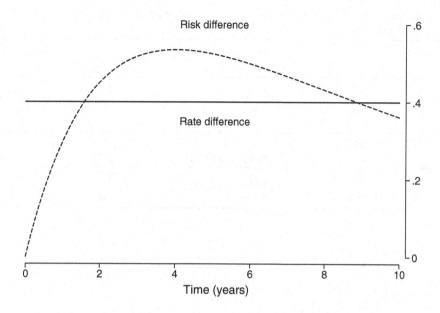

FIGURE 3.4 Data for the hypothetical TEXCO study, a closed population followed for 10 years (Table 3.1, Figures 3.1–3.3). Risk differences and rate differences are shown here. Rates were expressed as the count of deaths per 1 person-year; rate difference is constant at 0.4 deaths per 1 person-year.

All estimates of association share a common weakness; they can change over time. In the example in Table 3.1, there are no changes with time in the rate ratios, and the future risks, rates, and odds are the same at each moment in time. But in real data, there could be important changes and estimates of association based on 4 years of follow-up might differ from those after 8 years (Hernán 2010). If that were the case, we might want to know why and may wish to estimate associations for different intervals. A single statistic may not reveal all we may wish to know about an association.

3.7 BREAKING THE RULES: ARMY DATA FOR COMPANIES A AND B

In the hypothetical TEXCO study, both rates and risks were constant in any short window of time. The rule that 1 < risk ratio < rate ratio < odds ratio was true in the TEXCO data, where survival times followed an exponential distribution. This rule will usually be true if events are not common, even if rates do vary over time, as the risk, rate, and odds tend to be similar when events are rare. But if survival times are very different from an exponential distribution, meaning that the event rate varies over time, and if events are common, the rule regarding the order of these ratios may not be true.

Imagine 200 soldiers in Company A who are sent to a combat area. In less than 3 months, 99 were killed (Table 3.2, Figure 3.5); the initial rate of death was 3 per 1 person-year. The decimated Company A was then withdrawn from the front and followed to 2.7 years, with no further deaths: a mortality rate of 0 for nearly 2.5 years. Company B was sent to an area where the mortality rate from combat and disease was 0.3 per 1 person-year; after 2.7 years they are sent home, after suffering 110 deaths. If we compare Company A with B, the risk of death by 2.7 years was lower in Company A: risk ratio 0.9.

TABLE 3.2 Hypothetical data for Companies A and B, both followed for 2.7 years (see Figure 3.5). Rates are incidence rates per 1 person-year.

COMPANY	DIED N	TOTAL N (%)	RISK	RISK RATIO
A	99	200	.495	0.9
B	110	200	.550	

COMPANY	DIED N	PERSON-YEARS	RATE	RATE RATIO
A	99	282.7	.350	1.18
B	110	371.4	.296	

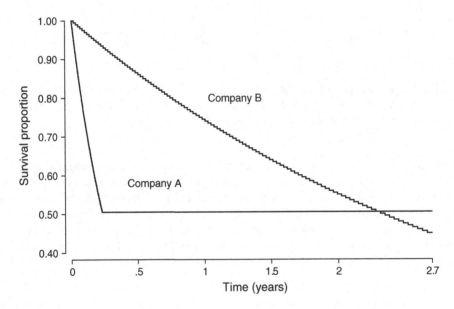

FIGURE 3.5 Kaplan-Meier survival plots for soldiers in Company A and Company B. Both groups were followed for 2.7 years.

But the rate of death was greater in Company A, with a rate ratio of 1.18. Both these ratio statistics are correct, but they tell different stories about these data. Which is best?

If you were a soldier, would you prefer to serve in Company A or B? This is a choice between two bad situations. You might reason that Company A is the preferred choice; although death may come quickly, your time in combat will be less than 3 months, your survival probability would be greater over the 2.7 years, and you might have many more years of life to enjoy after that interval. Being in Company B means 2.7 years spent in combat with a high risk of death, and less chance of being alive at the end of follow-up. So perhaps the risk ratio is your preferred statistic as it indicates that being in Company A is the better choice.

But imagine that the people in Figure 3.5 are not soldiers, but octogenarians in an assisted living facility with a loving staff and tasty food. Those in "Company B" all die peacefully in their sleep and they are in good health up until the time of death. Those in "Company A" undergo a painful surgical procedure that has a very high initial rate of death, followed by nearly 2.5 years of death-free survival, although much of that time is spent recovering from the operation. Some might feel that being in "Company B" is preferable, as persons in that group get to live more person-time: 371 person-years over the 2.7-year interval, versus only 283 years in the surgical group. Furthermore, their person-time is spent in relative comfort. And they are so old that survival for 2.7 years may not be paramount. So perhaps the rate ratio may be preferable for this comparison.

In these data, the risk ratio and rate ratios are in opposite directions. Whether one or the other is preferred may depend not on statistical considerations, but on the quality of life among the living and preferences that may differ from one person to the next. If risks (or rates) are not roughly constant over time and outcomes are common, a single summary estimate may not adequately describe the association of interest.

3.8 RELATIONSHIPS BETWEEN ODDS RATIOS, RISK RATIOS, AND RATE RATIOS IN CASE-CONTROL STUDIES

In 1926 a report identified lower fertility as a risk factor for breast cancer (Lane-Claypon 1926). Some consider this to be the first case-control study (Paneth, Susser, and Susser 2004, Morabia 2010, Press and Pharoah 2010). A few more case-control studies appeared prior to 1950 (Holcomb 1938, Cummings, Koepsell, and Roberts 2001, Paneth, Susser, and Susser 2004, Morabia 2010). In these studies, the investigators reasoned that if an exposure is causally related to a disease outcome, then a history of that exposure should be more common among those with the outcomes (cases) compared with persons without that outcome (controls).

Not until 1951 was it realized that when the outcome is rare in the population from which the cases and controls were sampled, the odds ratio for disease in the case-control study subjects, comparing those exposed with those not exposed, will approximate the risk ratio in the original larger population (Cornfield 1951). Imagine a cohort study in which 100,000 subjects are exposed to X and an equal number are not exposed (Table 3.3). After a year of follow-up, the cumulative incidence (risk) of death was .003 among those exposed and .001 among those not exposed: risk ratio = .003/.001 = 3.000.

TABLE 3.3 Hypothetical data for a cohort study and a case-control study of exposure X and the outcome of death. Follow-up was for 1 year.

EXPOSED TO X	DIED N	SURVIVED N	TOTAL N	RISK	RISK RATIO	ODDS	ODDS RATIO
Cohort study:							
Yes	A 300	B 99,700	100,000	.003000	3.000	.003009	3.006
No	C 100	D 99,900	100,000	.001000	1.000	.001001	1.000
Total	400	199,600	200,000				
Case-control study:							
Yes	A' 300 x .9 = 270	B' 99700 x .01 = 997	1267	.213102	2.579	.270812	3.006
No	C' 100 x .9 = 90	D' 99900 x .01 = 999	1089	.082645	1.000	.090090	1.000
Total	360	1996	2356				

Because the risk of death was small in both groups, the odds ratio for death is close to the risk ratio: odds ratio = [.003/(1 − .003)]/[.001/(1 − .001)] = 3.006. This cohort study might be expensive, as we would have to ascertain both the exposure status and outcomes of 200,000 persons.

A case-control design would be more efficient. We might first try to ascertain the exposure histories of those who died, the cases. Imagine we were only able to sample 90% of the cases, but sampling was not related to exposure status, so the prevalence of exposure among the dead was the same in both the cohort study and the case-control study: $A/(A + C) = .9 \times A/[(.9 \times A) + (.9 \times C)] = A'/(A' + C') = .75$ (see notation in Table 3.3). For the case-control study, we sampled only 1% of the survivors (controls); again, our sampling method resulted in an exposure prevalence that is the same for both the cohort study and the case-control study: $B/(B + D) = B'/(B' + D') = .4995$. The estimates of exposure related risk in the 2356 case-control subjects are now biased away from 0 compared with the original cohort: .21 for the exposed compared with .003, .08 for the unexposed compared with .001. Because the degree of bias in the risk ratios varies with exposure status, the risk ratio of 2.579 is biased compared with the true risk ratio of 3.0. The odds are also biased away from 0, but they are equally biased on a ratio scale, so the odds ratio for disease in the case-control sample is the same as that in the cohort study:

$$
\begin{aligned}
\text{Cohort study odds ratio} &= (A/B)/(C/D) \\
&= (.9 \times A/.01 \times B)/(.9 \times C/.01 \times D) \\
&= (A'/B')/(C'/D') \\
&= \text{case} - \text{control odds ratio} \\
&= 3.006 \\
&\approx 3.000 \\
&= \text{cohort study risk ratio}
\end{aligned}
$$

The case-control study in Table 3.3 selected controls from those who were not cases at the end of follow-up. This is sometimes called a cumulative case-control design. In this design, the cohort study odds ratio and the case-control odds ratio will be the same, aside from sampling variation, regardless of whether the outcome is rare or not. For example, at the end of the 2-year interval for the TEXCO data in Table 3.1, 41% of the study subjects were dead. The cohort study odds ratio was 7.8. If we sampled just a fraction of the cases and controls at the end of year 2, without regard to their exposure status, then aside from sampling variation the case-control odds ratio would also be 7.8. Neither of these estimates is a useful approximation of the risk ratio of 3.5 at 2 years. For both a cohort study and a cumulative case-control study, the odds ratio will only approximate the risk ratio when the outcome is sufficiently *rare*, say a cumulative proportion less than 0.1. As stated earlier, if the association is adjusted, the outcome also must be rare in all noteworthy strata of the adjusting variables.

A case-control study can also sample controls from the source population *at the time that each case arises*. This is called density sampling, incidence density sampling, or risk-set sampling. When this method is used, the odds ratio can estimate the rate ratio without any assumption that the outcome is rare.

The TEXCO study (Table 3.1 and Figures 3.1–3.4) can be used to illustrate incidence density sampling. In that study, the rate ratio was always 5.0. During follow-up the outcome was so common that the risk ratio soon fell below 5 and the odds ratio increased to more than 5. Recall that in any time interval, the risks, rates, and odds were the same as in any other interval of the same length. If an interval is sufficiently short, the outcome would be rare enough that the risk, rate, and odds ratios should all be approximately the same, or about 5.0. So as each person dies (and thereby becomes a case), if we quickly sample a control (or perhaps several controls), from among the survivors at about the same time, we will have a miniature case-control study in a small window of time, with a rare outcome. If we do this as each case arises and retain each case and the controls selected at that time as matched sets, we can summarize the odds ratios across all these matched sets. Because each of these odds ratios will be for a rare outcome (just one case in a small window of time), the summary odds ratio for the entire cohort should be 5, the same as the rate ratio.

A simulated example can demonstrate density sampling. The TEXCO data were created for 10,000 subjects exposed to X and 10,000 unexposed. The mortality rate among the exposed was a constant 0.5 deaths per person-year and deaths followed an exponential decay process. The first death among the exposed occurred after an interval (Expression 2.5) of $\ln(10,000/9,999)/0.5 = .0002$ years or 0.07 days. At the time of that death, the computer randomly sampled 4 controls from the 19,999 subjects who were still alive: 9,999 exposed and 10,000 unexposed subjects. These controls should, on average, have an exposure prevalence of about 50%. With the next death, 4 more controls were sampled from the remaining 19,998 living subjects. And so on. Exposed subjects died more quickly, so over time the prevalence of exposure declined among those who remained alive (Figure 3.6). The results were analyzed using conditional logistic regression with each matched set consisting of one case and four randomly selected controls who were alive when the death occurred. The odds ratio after one simulation was 5.04, which is the same, aside from sampling error, as the cohort study rate ratio of 5.0. No rare disease assumption was needed. In this design, a person can be sampled as a control more than once and they can be sampled as both a control and later as a case. But once someone is a case, they can no longer be sampled as a control. Similarly, in a cohort study with a nonrecurrent outcome, once a person has the outcome they no longer contribute person-time.

In the TEXCO study, since the rates of death were constant, differing only according to exposure status, the formulae for exponential decay (Chapter 2) can be used to estimate the count of exposed and unexposed persons at each point in time. If we start with 10,000 exposed subjects, the number remaining alive at time T (Expression 2.1) will be $N_{ex} = 10,000 \times e^{(-.5 \times t)}$. For the unexposed count, N_{unex}, the formula is the same, except .1 is substituted for .5. The prevalence of exposure among the living (potential controls) at each point in time is $N_{ex}/(N_{ex} + N_{unex})$ and the prevalence of exposure for the next new case at each time is $5 \times N_{ex}/((5 \times N_{ex}) + N_{unex})$. The number 5, the rate ratio, enters into the formulae for the exposure prevalence of the next case, because an exposed person is 5 times more likely to become a case than one unexposed, at each time. These formulae were used to create Figure 3.6. At

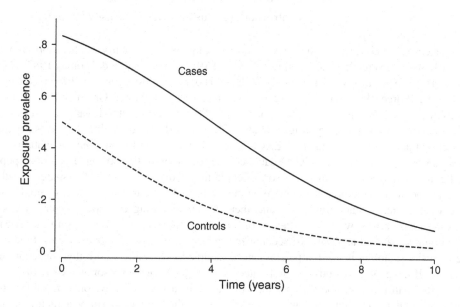

FIGURE 3.6 Plot showing changes over time in prevalence of exposure to X among the cases and potential controls in the TEXCO study.

time 0, the exposure prevalence of the first case is 5 x 10,000/((5 x 10,000) + 10,000) = 50,000/60,000 = .83333. The exposure prevalence for the first control is 10,000/(10,000+10,000) = 0.5. Therefore the odds ratio for exposure, comparing cases and controls, is (.8333/(1 − .8333)/(.5/(1 − .5)) = 5, which is equal to the rate ratio. If we carry out the calculations at time equal to 5 years, the prevalence is .4036 for a case and .1192 for a control; again, the odds ratio for exposure is .4036/(1−.4036)/(.1192/(1 − .1192)) = 5. The odds ratio for exposure comparing cases to controls ($(A'/C')/(B'/D')$ in Table 3.3) is equal to the odds ratio for the outcome comparing those exposed to those not exposed ($(A'/B')/(C'/D')$). Since the odds ratio for exposure is constant at all times T in Figure 3.6, the odds ratio for the outcome must also be constant, at 5.

Finally, we can show more directly why the cohort rate ratio is equal to the case-control odds ratio when incidence density sampling is used. The rate of death among the exposed is the count of the exposed dead divided by the total person-time prior to death accumulated by the exposed: $Cases_{ex}/T_{ex}$. Similarly, the rate among the unexposed is $Cases_{unex}/T_{unex}$. The person-time denominator is created by study subjects prior to having the outcome; in a sense, the person-time is accumulated by controls only; once a person has the outcome in a cohort study (becomes a case in a case-control study), they no longer contribute person-time. In a case-control study, we can obtain both the numerator counts ($Cases_{ex}$ and $Cases_{unex}$) or at least a fraction of these counts, but not the person-time accumulated prior to the outcome. We need counts of people which can correctly substitute for the person-time denominators used in rates. By using incidence density sampling, the ratio of $Controls_{ex}/Controls_{unex}$ should be equal to the ratio of T_{ex}/T_{unex} in the cohort population. If 25% of the person-time in the cohort study is generated by exposed people, then 25% of the controls should be exposed. We may only sample a fraction of the controls, but so long as sampling is unrelated to exposure status (equivalent to saying there is no selection bias), the ratio of exposed to unexposed controls should be equal to the ratio of exposed to unexposed person-time. Then, without any rare disease assumption, we can write:

$$
\begin{aligned}
\text{Cohort study odds ratio} &= (Cases_{ex}/T_{ex})/(Cases_{unex}/T_{unex}) \\
&= (Cases_{ex}/Cases_{unex})/(T_{ex}/T_{unex}) \\
&= (Cases_{ex}/Cases_{unex})/(Controls_{ex}/Controls_{unex}) \\
&= (Cases_{ex}/Controls_{ex})/(Cases_{unex}/Controls_{unex}) \\
&= \text{case} - \text{control odds ratio using incidence density sampling}
\end{aligned}
$$

Early papers that described incidence density sampling for case-control studies appeared in 1976 (Miettinen 1976), 1978 (Prentice and Breslow 1978) and 1982 (Greenland and Thomas 1982). Additional discussions can be found in several papers (Greenland, Thomas, and Morgenstern 1986b, Rodrigues and Kirkwood 1990, Pearce 1993, Knol et al. 2008) and textbooks (Rothman, Greenland, and Lash 2008a p124–125, Greenland 2008b p430–431, Rothman 2012 p90–94). This method was used to estimate rate ratios in a study of anti-inflammatory drugs and atrial fibrillation (Schmidt et al. 2011). This design can be used for a closed population, such as the TEXCO study (Table 3.1) or for an open population.

Exposure prevalence varied in TEXCO data because the exposed died sooner. In an open population, exposure frequency may vary for many reasons. People may move in or out of the source population or exposure may be more common in some time intervals and less in others. For example, smoking prevalence in the United States increased and then decreased during the 20th century. By sampling controls as each case arises, we sample the exposure history from all noncase person-time as each case occurs. By doing a matched analysis, we account for changes in exposure frequency over time.

When density sampling is used, a person can be sampled as a control more than once and they can later be a case. If the goal is to study the first outcome only, then once a person is a case, they no longer contribute further information about exposure. Similarly, in a cohort study, once a subject becomes a case they no longer contribute person-time. However, if the goal is to study a recurrent outcome, a person could be a case at more than one point in time.

Case-control study design is not the focus of this book, but for the sake of completeness, the case-cohort design should be mentioned. In this design controls are sampled from all initial study subjects, regardless of whether or not they later become a case. The resulting odds ratio will then estimate the risk ratio without any rare disease assumption (Wacholder 1991, Rothman, Greenland, and Lash 2008a pp123–124, Rothman 2012 pp96–98).

3.9 SYMMETRY OF MEASURES OF ASSOCIATION

If we estimate the association between a dichotomous exposure X (X = 1 means exposed and X = 0 means unexposed) and a dichotomous outcome Y (Y = 1 means death and Y = 0 means survival), the 4 ratio (risk, odds, rate, hazard) and 2 difference (risk, rate) measures of association described above are all symmetrical if X is recoded so that exposed = 0 and unexposed = 1. By symmetrical, I mean that the ratio estimate for the association of exposed, compared with unexposed, with the outcome Y is the inverse of the association for unexposed, compared with exposed. For the risk and rate difference, symmetry means that only the direction of any difference will be reversed (the sign for the difference will change) if we reverse the comparison regarding exposure X.

Only the odds ratio and the risk difference are symmetrical with regard to the outcome Y. Imagine that we always compare those exposed (X = 1) with those unexposed (X = 0). Then the odds ratio for the outcome of death (Y = 1) will be the reciprocal of the odds ratio for the outcome of survival. The risk difference for the outcome Y = 1 will equal to the risk difference for the outcome Y = 0, but the sign of the difference will change.

The risk ratio for an association is not symmetric with regard to the coding of the outcome variable Y. Except when the risk ratio is equal to 1, the risk ratio comparing the exposed and unexposed for the outcome Y = 1 (the ratio of incidence proportions) will not be the inverse of the risk ratio comparing the exposed and unexposed for the outcome Y = 0 (the ratio of the survival proportions). When outcomes are rare, the survival proportions for both the exposed and unexposed groups will be close to 1. This means the risk ratio for the survival proportions will necessarily be close to 1 and therefore not of much interest when outcomes are rare.

For rate ratios, rate differences, and hazard ratios, symmetry with regard to the outcome is not usually of interest. These three measures of association all deal with person-time to a new, incident, event. Event-free time is used by these association estimates, as a measure of all person-time during which the new event of interest (Y = 1) might have occurred. While the survivor function can be plotted, there is usually no reason to estimate survival ratios or differences. If all members of the population are diseased at the start of follow-up, then the outcome of interest might be the new (incident) onset of a return to health; a health rate or health hazard ratio, or a health rate difference, could be computed.

3.10 CONVERGENCE PROBLEMS FOR ESTIMATING ASSOCIATIONS

For ratios of odds, risk, or rates, and differences in risks or rates, estimation of crude (unadjusted) associations is usually straightforward, requiring only simple calculations. But regression models based on maximum likelihood and some other methods typically use algorithms which must converge to a solution in a series of steps. Problems with convergence may arise when a variable is a perfect or nearly-perfect predictor of the outcome. Additional problems afflict the estimation of risk ratios and risk differences, because risks are bounded by 0 and 1, unlike odds or rates. Because of these convergence problems, several methods have been developed to estimate risk ratios or differences when convergence is difficult (Greenland and Holland 1991, Joffe and Greenland 1995, Altman, Deeks, and Sackett 1998, Robbins, Chao, and Fonseca 2002, McNutt et al. 2003, Greenland 2004, Zou 2004, Carter, Lipsitz, and Tilley 2005, Blizzard and Hosmer 2006, Lumley, Kronmal, and Ma 2006, Localio, Margolis, and Berlin 2007, Deddens and Petersen 2008, Cummings 2009a, 2009b, Kleinman and Norton 2009, Savu, Liu, and Yasui 2010). Since rates have no upper bounds, the estimation of rate ratios and differences is less likely to encounter convergence difficulties.

3.11 SOME HISTORY REGARDING THE CHOICE BETWEEN RATIOS AND DIFFERENCES

Ratio measures of association predominate in the biomedical literature. Studies which use ratios of odds or hazards are common, whereas estimated differences in odds are never presented and differences in hazards are rarely shown. Ratios of risks or rates are common compared with differences for these measures. Reliance on ratio measures may stem in part from early debates about whether the association of smoking with increased rates of lung cancer was causal. Studies reporting an association between smoking and lung cancer started appearing in 1950 (Doll and Hill 1950, Schrek et al. 1950, Wynder and Graham 1950). By 1964, 29 case-control studies and 7 prospective cohort studies had reported that smoking was associated with an increased risk or rate of lung cancer (Hill 1965). In that year the U.S. Public Health Service issued a 387 page report which reviewed evidence regarding smoking and lung cancer and concluded that the observed association was causal (Public Health Service 1964).

Critics of a causal relationship between smoking and lung cancer, including the renowned statistician Sir Ronald A. Fisher (1958a, 1958b, Kluger 1996 p248–250), pointed out that association does not prove causation. Epidemiologists knew that not all associations were causal and during this era they struggled (as they still do) to develop criteria to help judge whether an association is causal. One proposed criterion was specificity: an observed association was said to be more plausibly causal if the putative risk factor was associated with only one specific disease outcome and less likely to be causal if the risk factor was associated with several diverse outcomes. This specificity standard was proposed as early as 1959 (Yerushalmy and Palmer 1959). The criterion of specificity was quickly criticized by some researchers (Sartwell 1960), but at the time of the early smoking debates, specificity was thought to be a useful criterion for causality by others (Yerushalmy and Palmer 1959, Lilienfeld 1959b, Hill 1965), including the authors of Smoking and Health (1964). In retrospect, it seems surprising that specificity was so readily adopted as a test of causation. Many exposures can cause several disease outcomes; for example, frequent drinking of alcohol is thought to cause heart disease (alcohol cardiomyopathy), brain disease (Wernicke's encephalopathy), liver disease (cirrhosis), and traffic crashes.

Those who thought that smoking caused lung cancer, but who also felt specificity was a criterion for causal inference, were in a bind, as cohort studies suggested associations between smoking and many disease outcomes. In 1958, Hammond and Horn reported results from a cohort study that followed 187,783 men from 1952 to 1955, an interval of about 3.7 years (Hammond and Horn 1958a, 1958b). The men were age 50 to 69 at study entry and 11,870 died during follow-up. Deaths were more common among the smokers, but 52% of the excess deaths were attributed to heart disease and only 14% to lung cancer. The authors reported several associations; a few are in Table 3.4. Smoking was associated with *all* the outcomes in the table.

One of the most vociferous critics of the smoking studies was Joseph Berkson, a statistician at the prestigious Mayo Clinic in Rochester, Minnesota (Kluger 1996). Berkson pounced (Berkson 1958, 1960,

TABLE 3.4 Deaths, rates, rate ratios and rate differences from a cohort study of smoking and nonsmoking men followed from 1952 to 1955. Ratios and differences compare smokers with nonsmokers. Rates are per 100,000 person-years. Rates for nonsmokers are directly standardized to the age distribution of the smokers. Results are shown for a few of the disease outcomes reported in the original paper.

DISEASE	SMOKERS		NONSMOKERS		RATE RATIO	RATE DIFFERENCE
	DEATHS	RATE	DEATHS	RATE		
Genitourinary cancer	218	57	49	32	1.8	25
Cancer of mouth, larynx, esophagus	91	24	6	5	5.0	19
Lung cancer	400	104	15	10	10.7	94
Other lung disease	231	61	30	21	2.9	40
Coronary artery disease	3361	879	709	516	1.7	363

Data from Hammond, E. C., and D. Horn. 1958b. Smoking and death rates; report on forty-four months of follow-up of 187,783 men. II. Death rates by cause. *J Am Med Assoc* 166 (11):1294–1308.

1963) on the results reported by Hammond and Horn (1958a, 1958b) and by Doll and Hill (1956). Berkson argued that the nonspecific association of smoking with so many diseases (Table 3.4) cast doubt on any causal relationship. In these cohort studies smoking was more strongly associated with coronary artery disease (rate difference 363) than with lung cancer (rate difference 94) using the rate difference measure. A causal link with coronary disease seemed implausible to Berkson and he argued that since the studies had found a larger association of smoking with heart disease on a difference scale, this meant that the smaller rate difference between smoking and lung cancer was "spurious." He wrote that

> … when an investigation set up to test the theory … that smoking causes lung cancer, turns out to indicate that smoking causes … a whole gamut of disease, inevitably it raises the suspicion that something is amiss. It is as though, in investigating a drug that previously had been indicated to relieve the common cold, the drug was found … to cure pneumonia, cancer, and many other diseases. A scientist would say "There must be something wrong with this method of investigation."

> *(Berkson 1958)*

Even some who believed that smoking did cause lung cancer found the results in Table 3.4 puzzling. How could cigarettes cause heart disease or genitourinary cancer? If specificity of association supported causal inference, how should Table 3.4 be interpreted? One approach was to argue that causal associations should be assessed on a ratio scale (Lilienfeld 1959b). In 1959, Cornfield and five other influential researchers reviewed the evidence regarding smoking and lung cancer (Cornfield et al. 1959). They rejected specificity of association as a criterion for causality. But in response to Berkson's claim (Berkson 1958) that rate differences were superior to rate ratios, Cornfield and colleagues argued that causal inference should rely on rate ratios:

> Both the absolute [difference] and the relative [ratio] measures serve a purpose. The relative [ratio] measure is helpful in … appraising the possible noncausal nature of an agent having an apparent effect … The absolute [difference] measure would be important in appraising the public health significance of an effect known to be causal.

On a ratio scale, the rate of lung cancer was about tenfold greater among smokers compared with nonsmokers (Table 3.4). Cornfield et al. (1959) showed mathematically that if all of this increase is not causal, but due entirely to a binary confounding factor, then the confounder must be at least ten times more prevalent among smokers than nonsmokers. This information seemed useful to the researchers, as Fisher claimed that some psychological factor explained smoking's relationship with lung cancer. One attempt to find this alleged factor reported that a "neurotic trait" was more common among smokers, but the prevalence ratio of this trait among smokers compared with nonsmokers was only 2.6, too small to account for all of the smoking – lung cancer risk ratio of 10 (Lilienfeld 1959a). Cornfield et al. (1959) made the further claim that the rate difference could not be used in a similar way to judge the possible confounding influence of a binary exposure. But, as explained by Poole (2010), this claim is mistaken. In the study by Hammond and Horn (1958b), the rate of coronary death for smokers was 879 per 100,000 person-years and average follow-up was 44 months. Using Expression 2.9, we can convert rates from Table 3.4 to approximate risks, assuming deaths were exponentially distributed and competing risks had little influence: risk = 1 – exp(–rate per 1 person-year x time in years). The risk of coronary death for a smoker was $1 - \exp(-(879/100{,}000) \times (44/12)) = .032$, and the risk for nonsmokers, using the standardized rate of 516 per 100,000 person-years, was .019, for a risk difference of .013. Poole (2010) showed that if a confounding factor is to fully account for an observed noncausal association, in this case a risk difference of .013, the prevalence of the confounder in the smokers must be greater than in the nonsmokers by at least .013. But in Lilienfeld's study (Lilienfeld 1959a) the prevalence difference was less, although not by much, .012.

Cornfield et al. (1959) gave two additional arguments in favor of ratios, but these were also flawed. Details about the history of this argument and the mathematical reasoning involved, are in an excellent paper by Poole (2010). Today the criterion of specificity is rarely invoked to support causal inference, expect in special circumstances (Weiss 2002, Rothman et al. 2008 pp27–28, Weiss and Koepsell 2014 pp161). But the argument that ratios are best for causal inference and differences best for public health decisions still appears in some form in several textbooks (Hennekens and Buring 1987 pp93–95, Lilienfeld and Stolley 1994 pp200,263, Kelsey et al. 1996 p37, MacMahon and Trichopoulos 1996 pp226–227, Gordis 2009 pp155,176, Weiss and Koepsell 2014 pp159,169). This distinction seems fuzzy to me. All of the associations in Table 3.4 are probably causal to some degree. Rate differences seem useful for both causal inference and for decision making. Rates can be compared on a ratio or difference scale, or both, for several purposes. Whether one or the other is preferred should depend on something other than the arguments that Cornfield and colleagues offered in 1959 (Cornfield et al. 1959).

Circular reasoning may have played a role in these arguments (Rothman et al. 2008 p27). Berkson (1958) recognized that the rates in Table 3.4 implied that smoking was related to many disease outcomes. Because he felt strongly that smoking could not cause all these diseases, he concluded that case-control and cohort study methods could not be trusted. Cornfield et al. (1959) believed that smoking was a cause of lung cancer and thought their case looked stronger when ratios were used, so they devised arguments supporting the use of ratios over differences for causal inference.

3.12 OTHER INFLUENCES ON THE CHOICE BETWEEN USE OF RATIOS OR DIFFERENCES

In many epidemiological studies, the decision to use a ratio as the measure of association stems from the fact that epidemiologists often study binary outcomes, such as death or disease, and the textbooks that teach these methods emphasize ratio measures because these are easily estimated by the regression models used. In addition, some study designs lend themselves to ratio measures. For example, case-control studies are typically analyzed using logistic regression, which estimates the odds ratio for the outcome. There is no regression model for differences in odds and even if there were the results would have no clear interpretation in a case-control study. Having learned one method for estimating a binary association, it is not surprising that epidemiologists might then use logistic regression and estimate odds ratios for the outcomes of a cohort study, even though a difference in risks or rates could be estimated.

Even though adjusted rate differences can be estimated in most cohort studies, this approach is often given little discussion in textbooks. Epidemiologists usually use Poisson regression to analyze rates, and the examples of Poisson regression found in textbooks almost always estimate rate ratios, not rate differences.

Rate differences are more often estimated in the econometrics and sociology literature. In econometrics and sociology, it is common to use linear regression to estimate how various factors are associated with continuous outcomes, such as income, education, or IQ. Not surprisingly, linear regression is sometimes used to estimate differences in rates.

In short, researchers may sometimes choose between ratios or differences out of habit or because they have learned tools that can estimate one of these more easily than the other, and not from a conscious decision that one of these measures is preferred over the other. In later chapters I will show how both rate ratios and rate differences can usually be estimated.

3.13 THE DATA MAY SOMETIMES BE USED TO CHOOSE BETWEEN A RATIO OR A DIFFERENCE

In many studies, the choice between estimating a rate ratio or a rate difference may not matter. It may often be possible, when two groups are compared, to present the rates or adjusted rates for both groups; this seems like good practice when it can be done. The choice of then estimating a rate difference or ratio may be immaterial. In some studies, it may be possible to estimate both, which presents readers with two summaries of the data. This might be useful, for example, for future meta-analysts, who might prefer one scale over the other (Deeks 2002).

Sometimes the data may influence the choice between a ratio or difference summary. Imagine that we have conducted a randomized controlled trial of new drug X intended to prevent bad health outcome event Y (Table 3.5). Among those who received drug X the incidence rate of Y was (100 + 20)/(2000 + 2000 person-days) = 120/4000 person-days = 3 Y events per 100 person-days in the treated group. The event incidence rate was (200 + 40)/(2000 + 2000 person-days) = 6 Y events per 100 person-days in the control group. Comparing those taking drug X with those given a placebo, the rate ratio was 0.5. The rate difference was 3–6 = –3 events per 100 person-days. But among the untreated, the rates of Y were 10/2 = 5 times greater for men than for women. In this trial, drug X had the same multiplicative effect on the event rate for men and women, so the rate ratio was 0.5 in both

TABLE 3.5 Hypothetical data for a harmful health outcome event Y and person-days in a trial of drug X that is intended to prevent outcome Y. The size of the association varies with sex on the rate difference scale, but not on the rate ratio scale.

	MALES		FEMALES	
	DRUG X	PLACEBO	DRUG X	PLACEBO
Y events	100	200	20	40
Person-days	2000	2000	2000	2000
Incidence rate per 100 person-days	5.0	10.0	1.0	2.0
Rate ratio (drug X/placebo)	0.5		0.5	
Rate ratio for all	0.5			
Rate difference per 100 person-days (drug X minus placebo)	–5.0		–1.0	
Rate difference per 100 person-days for all	–3.0			

groups. But on the rate difference scale, the effect of drug X was greater for men (−5.0 events per 100 person-days) than for women (−1.0).

In this example (Table 3.5) the size of the association of drug X with the outcome *varies* by sex on the difference scale but not on a ratio scale. Some epidemiologists call this *effect modification*; the effect of drug X on the outcome Y is modified by sex on the difference scale. In meta-analysis, it common to call this *heterogeneity* of effect; in Table 3.5, the effect is homogeneous on the ratio scale, but heterogeneous on the difference scale. Heterogeneity of an estimated association can be identified by using an interaction term in a regression model, so this variation is often described as an *interaction* between sex and drug X. In the clinical trial literature, investigation of heterogeneity of treatment effect on the outcome is often called *subgroup analysis*. Regardless of the terminology used, Table 3.5 illustrates that if there is an association between exposure X and outcome Y and if the outcome rate when not exposed varies between 2 or more groups, absence of effect modification on the multiplicative scale implies that there must be effect modification on the additive scale. The reverse is also true. When we say that the association of X with Y varies with the level of an effect-modifier Z, we should be clear about the scale we are using, as the variation may depend on the whether we are summarizing on a ratio or difference scale.

Although the rate difference is sometimes touted as the best measure for public health decisions, the rate difference of −3 in Table 3.5 is not very helpful. This average does not apply to men or to women. It is the average for a population that is half female, but for any other population it is inaccurate. The rate ratio, however, applies to both men and women, or men and women in combination, and therefore it may be a better summary of the association in Table 3.5. Alternatively, one could present separate rate difference estimates for men and women.

The opposite may be true: there may be variation of the association on the ratio scale, but not on the difference scale. In Table 3.6, the rate ratio for the association of drug X with event Y is 0.9 for men, 0.5 for women. The rate difference is −1 per 100 person-days for both sexes. The rate ratio of 0.833 in Table 3.6 does not apply to men or women.

Effect modification can occur on both the additive and multiplicative scales. In Table 3.6, changing the count of Y events for males on drug X to 150 would produce a rate ratio of 0.75 for men and a rate difference of −2.5 for men, both different from the rate ratio of 0.5 for women and the rate difference − 1 for women.

Variation in the risk or rate for an outcome when not exposed is ubiquitous. For this reason, summarizing associations on a rate ratio scale may often be a better fit to the data, as in Table 3.5, compared with a summary on the difference scale. Imagine that we did a study in a population where

TABLE 3.6 Hypothetical data for harmful health outcome event Y and person-days in a trial of drug X that is intended to prevent Y. The size of the association varies on the rate ratio scale, but not on the rate difference scale.

	MALES		FEMALES	
	DRUG X	PLACEBO	DRUG X	PLACEBO
Y events	180	200	20	40
Person-days	2000	2000	2000	2000
Incidence rate per 100 person-days	9.0	10.0	1.0	2.0
Rate ratio (drug X/placebo)	0.9		0.5	
Rate ratio for all	0.833			
Rate difference per 100 person-days (drug X minus placebo)	−1.0		−1.0	
Rate difference per 100 person-days for all	−1.0			

the outcome event rate under no exposure was 1 per 10,000 person-years. Imagine our study found that those exposed had an incidence rate of 3 per 10,000 person-years: the exposure-related rate ratio is therefore 3 and the rate difference +2 per 10,000 person-years. What do we expect the incidence rates under exposure to be if we study the same exposure in a population with an incidence rate under no exposure of 5 per 10,000 person-years? Our intuitive response may be to expect an exposure incidence rate of 5 x 3 = 15, not 5 + 2 = 7, per 10,000 person-years. If the incidence under no exposure is 25, we expect an incidence under exposure closer to 3 x 25 = 75 than to 25 + 2 = 27. Our gut response is to feel that it is not likely, as incidence when not exposed moves from 1 to 5 to 25, that the causal effect of exposure will be to add 2 to the incidence rate per 10,000 person-years. I cannot think of any exposures that work that way. In defense of this intuition, Deeks and colleagues summarized data from 551 different meta-analyses of clinical trials with binary outcomes (Deeks 2002). They reported that heterogeneity (variation) in effects between trials was usually less using a ratio measure (risk or odds ratio) compared with a risk difference measure, although there were a few exceptions to this general finding. I acknowledge that an argument based upon intuition is weak and my view is surely influenced by training and habits.

To summarize, the choice between estimating a rate difference and a rate ratio will depend upon (1) what we want to know; (2) whether we think exposure may influence the outcome on a ratio or difference scale; (3) the study design used; (4) perhaps the estimating method we use; (5) relationships discovered in the data after they are collected; and (6) perhaps other considerations. In this book, when the method and data allow it, I will show how to estimate both rate differences and ratios.

The Poisson Distribution 4

The *Los Angeles Times* ran this headline on December 10, 2012: "Highway deaths at lowest level since 1949; bike, truck fatalities rise." The article noted that in 2011, compared with 2010, "… bicycle deaths rose 8.7% to 677", from 623. These numbers were for bicyclist deaths in collisions with a motor vehicle, which account for most bicycle-related deaths. Some increase in deaths might be related to population growth. The population was 308,745,538 in 2010 and 311,591,917 in 2011, an increase of only 0.9%. The rate of fatal bicycle crashes was 309.7 per million person-years in 2010 and 311.6 per million person-years in 2011, a 7.7% jump.

When we study finite samples taken from a large population, we expect to find variation in any statistic from one sample to the next. This is sometimes called "chance" or "random" or "sampling" variation. But there is only one United States of America, only one year 2010, and only one year 2011, and the bicyclist mortality rates were for the entire country in each year. So how could sampling variation arise? If some process produces a constant rate of mortality among bicyclists over a long time interval, we might expect the observed rate to vary in shorter time intervals, such as a week or a year (Chiang 1961). We can think of the 2010 and 2011 mortality rates as samples from a large amount of person-time spanning many years. Is the mortality rate increase from 2010 to 2011 more than expected from sampling variation alone? To answer that question, we need to know how much variation we should expect if a constant rate was present. How are counts of deaths distributed in short intervals of time if the incidence rate is constant over a long time interval?

We need some way to describe the expected distribution of counts so that we can compare this with the observed distribution of the counts. With an expected distribution, we can estimate statistics such as the spread of the counts or rates (variance and standard deviation (SD)), confidence intervals (CI) for counts, rates, rate ratios, or rate differences, and P-values for comparisons of rates. The first distribution to be described for counts is the Poisson distribution, the focus of this chapter. At the end of the chapter we will return to the bicycle mortality rates and formally address whether the observed rate increase might be greater than expected from random variation alone.

4.1 ALPHA PARTICLE RADIATION

At the start of the 20th century Ernest Rutherford described the exponential nature of radioactive decay (Chapter 2) while working at McGill University in Montreal. In 1907 he took over the physics department at the University of Manchester where he worked with Hans Geiger, co-inventor of the Geiger counter. In 1910 Rutherford and Geiger published (Rutherford, Geiger, and Bateman 1910) a short paper called "The probability variations in the distribution of α particles." Radioactive atoms decay at a constant rate, but the time at which the next atom ejects an alpha particle (a helium nucleus of two protons and two neutrons) varies, so in short intervals of time, the count of emitted alpha particles varies. The authors wrote

> It is of importance to settle whether these variations in distribution [of alpha particle counts in short time intervals] are in agreement with the law of probability, i.e., whether the distribution of alpha particles on an average is that to be anticipated if the alpha particles are expelled at random …

For this experiment they used polonium, which has a short half-life of 138 days. To count emitted alpha particles, polonium was placed near a zinc sulphide screen which could be observed through a microscope. When an alpha particle hit the screen, a flash of light could be seen and this was recorded on a moving tape by pressing a switch; 10,097 flashes were tediously counted over 5 days. The rapid decay meant that many flashes could be counted in a short period, but the dwindling polonium source had to be moved closer to the phosphor screen each day to keep the mean flash rate constant. The recorded tape was divided into 2608 intervals of 1/8th minute and the number of intervals with alpha particle counts of 0, 1, 2, 3, ... 14 was listed in the paper. There were 57 intervals with no emitted particles, 525 with 3 alpha ejections, and only 1 interval with 14 ejected particles (Table 4.1).

To determine whether the observed variations in alpha particle counts are what might be expected from "random" variations around a constant rate of decay, the authors needed to know how the counts should be distributed if the time to each alpha expulsion was truly random. They turned to Harry Bateman, an English mathematician in Manchester. (Bateman would later move to the U.S. and teach at Bryn Mawr, Johns Hopkins, and the California Institute of Technology.) Bateman worked out the mathematics of the expected distribution. In a short appendix to the paper by Rutherford and Geiger (Rutherford, Geiger, and Bateman 1910), Bateman showed that the probability that an interval would have an alpha particle count equal to n is given by:

$$(\text{Probability of count } n = (\text{rate} \times \text{time})^n \times e^{(-\text{rate} \times \text{time})}/n! \tag{Ex.4.1}$$

TABLE 4.1   Observed number of 1/8th minute time intervals according to the count of alpha particle emissions in each interval. The probabilities and predicted number of time intervals are from a Poisson distribution with a rate of 10,097 alpha emissions per 2608 time intervals = 3.871549 alpha emissions per 1/8th minute interval.

COUNT OF ALPHA PARTICLES EMITTED	NUMBER OF TIME INTERVALS OBSERVED FOR EACH COUNT OF ALPHA PARTICLES	PROBABILITY OF EACH NUMBER GIVEN THE MEAN RATE	NUMBER OF TIME INTERVALS PREDICTED
0	57	.020826	54
1	203	.080629	210
2	383	.156080	407
3	525	.201424	525
4	532	.194955	508
5	408	.150956	394
6	273	.097406	254
7	139	.053873	141
8	45	.026071	68
9	27	.011215	29
10	10	.004342	11
11	4	.001528	4
12	0	.000493	1
13	1	.000147	0
14	1	.000041	0

Data from Rutherford, E., H. Geiger, and H. Bateman. 1910. The probability variations in the distribution of α particles. *Phil Mag J Sci* 20:698–707. In the 1910 publication, a few of the predicted counts were in error. The paper predicted 140 intervals with 7 alpha particles, 4 intervals with 13 particles, and 1 interval with 14 particles; the correct values are 141, 0, and 0.

The rate in Expression 4.1 is the constant mean incidence rate of alpha particle ejections. We do not know the true rate, but in the experiment the observed estimate of this rate was 10,097 alpha particles/2608 1/8th minute time intervals = 3.87 particles per 1/8th of a minute (Table 4.1). Since over 10,000 alpha particles were counted, this mean count should be a good approximation of the mean count that would be observed over an infinite number of intervals. The symbol e is the base of natural logarithms, 2.718 (to 3 decimals). The symbol n in Expression 4.1 is a positive integer, including 0, and is the expected count of alpha particles in any short interval, 1/8 minute in this example. The symbol n! indicates the factorial of n, the product of n multiplied by all integers smaller than n: 4! = 4 x 3 x 2 x 1. The factorial for both 0 and 1 is 1. Using values of n = 0, 1, 2, … , 14, we can use Bateman's formula to estimate the probability that an interval will have 0, 1, … , 14 alpha particles, given a constant rate of 3.87 (Table 4.1). Calculations for 0, 2, and 5 alpha particles are shown below. The rate is rounded to 3.87 for this presentation, but more precision was used for the actual calculations, to avoid rounding errors:

$$P_0 = 3.87^0 \times \text{exponential}(-3.87)/0! = 1 \times \text{exponential}(-3.87)/1 = .020826$$

$$P_2 = 3.87^2 \times \text{exponential}(-3.87)/2! = 3.87^2 \times \text{exponential}(-3.87)/(2 \times 1) = .156080$$

$$P_5 = 3.87^5 \times \text{exponential}(-3.87)/5!$$
$$= 3.87^5 \times \text{exponential}(-3.87)/(5 \times 4 \times 3 \times 2 \times 1) = .150956$$

Instead of these calculations, Stata's statistical functions for the Poisson distribution can be used: **poisson, poissonp,** and **poissontail.** Also useful are the inverse functions: **invpoisson, invpoissontail.** For example, to get the probability for a count of 5, we can use the **poissonp(m,k)** function and insert the mean count (10,097/2608) in place of m and the number 5 in place of k, as follows:

```
display poissonp(10097/2608,5)
.15095594
```

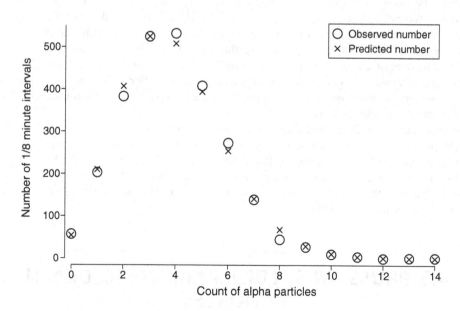

FIGURE 4.1 Observed and predicted number of 1/8 minute time intervals according to the count of alpha particle emissions in each interval. Predicted numbers from a Poisson distribution with a mean rate of 3.87 alpha particle emissions per 1/8th minute. Data from Rutherford, E., H. Geiger, and H. Bateman 1910. The probability variations in the distribution of α particles. *Phil Mag J Sci* 20:698–707.

To get the expected (predicted) number of intervals for each count from 0 to 14, the probabilities from the formula were multiplied by the number of intervals, 2608, and rounded to the nearest integer. The observed and predicted numbers are pleasingly close (Table 4.1, Figure 4.1). Rutherford and Geiger (Rutherford, Geiger, and Bateman 1910) wrote, "As far as the experiments have gone, there is no evidence that the variation in number of α particles from interval to interval is greater than would be expected in a random distribution."

4.2 THE POISSON DISTRIBUTION

Bateman's expression for the distribution of counts was clever. But we do not call this Bateman's distribution because, unknown to Bateman, the same formula was published in 1837 by the Frenchman Siméon Denis Poisson. Stephen Stigler, a historian of statistics, notes that Poisson devoted only a single page in all his work to this distribution and he never applied it to data (Stigler 1982, 1986 p182–183). Some authors (Newbold 1927) credit Abraham De Moivre with the first description of this distribution in 1718. Stigler says that De Moivre presented an equation for probability = .5 and n = 3, but never wrote the more general Expression 4.1, so assigning credit to Poisson seems fair (Stigler 1982).

There were others who independently rediscovered the Poisson distribution (Haight 1967 p114). The mathematician and astronomer Simon Newcomb derived the distribution and used it to estimate the probability that a square degree of the sky would contain 0, 1, 2, ..., or 6 stars visible to the eye, publishing his results in 1860 (Newcomb 1860, Stigler 1982).

A random process for a continuous variable is described by the Normal (Gaussian) distribution with its bell-shaped curve. Counts are not continuous and are always positive. Their distribution around a mean count is not symmetrical, because one end of the distribution is bounded by 0. The distribution for a mean count is not symmetric but has a shorter tail toward smaller counts and a longer tail toward larger counts. For small mean counts, the distribution is very asymmetrical, with many 0's, a small number of 1's, and only a few higher counts (Figure 4.2). For example, if the expected mean count in a time interval (or an area of space or unit of volume) is 0.01, the probability that an observed interval will have a count of 0 is .9900, the probability that the count will be 1 is .0099 (nearly .01), the probability of a count of 2 is .00005, and the probability of a count of 3 is only .0000002. This means that when a rate is small, only counts of 0 and 1 are likely to arise. For binary outcomes, such as death or survival, we can treat the observed outcomes as if they came from a Poisson distribution if the outcome events are sufficiently rare.

If the mean count is 0.2, the probability of a count of 2 increases to .02 (Figure 4.2). If the mean count is .5, the probability of a 0 count is only .61 and the probability for a count of 2 is .08. One in a hundred intervals will have a count of 3. If the mean count is 1, the probability of a 0 count is .37, equal to that for a count of 1. When the mean count is greater than 1, the most likely count is greater than 0 and by the time the mean count is 10, the distribution of the counts looks nearly symmetric; the probability of a 0 count is only .00005.

4.3 PRUSSIAN SOLDIERS KICKED TO DEATH BY HORSES

Simon Newcomb's use of the Poisson distribution to describe how stars were grouped received little notice (Newcomb 1860, Stigler 1982). But a 1898 publication by Ladislaus von Bortkewitsch (1898)

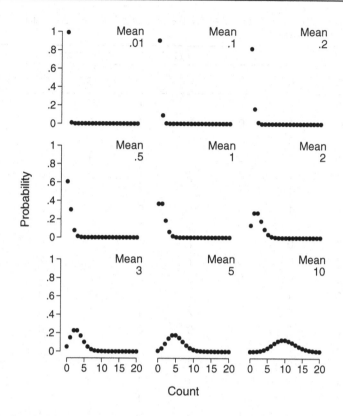

FIGURE 4.2 Predicted probabilities that counts from 0 to 20 will be observed in a short time interval when the mean count per interval takes values of 0.01, 0.1, 0.2, 0.5, 1, 2, 3, 5, and 10. Predictions are from the Poisson distribution, Expression 4.1.

attracted attention and helped disseminate knowledge about the Poisson distribution (Newbold 1927, Haight 1967 p114–120). Von Bortkiewicz showed predicted and observed counts for several sets of data. His best-known example used data regarding deaths due to horse kicks in 14 Prussian military units during the 20 years from 1875 to 1894 (von Bortkewitsch 1898 p24, Winsor 1947, Quine and Seneta 1987). Of the 14 military corps, 10 were similar regarding the number of cavalry squadrons and therefore they might share a common rate of mortality from kicks by horses. In the 10 similar corps, there were 122 deaths for a rate of 122/per 200 corps-years = 0.61 deaths per corps-year (Table 4.2). Using this mean count, 0.61, the observed and fitted number of corps-years with 0, 1, 2, 3, 4, and 5 deaths were remarkably similar (Table 4.3). The probabilities for each count are similar to those for a mean count of 0.5 in Figure 4.2.

4.4 VARIANCES, STANDARD DEVIATIONS, AND STANDARD ERRORS FOR COUNTS AND RATES

The mean rate was 122/200 = 0.61 deaths per 1 corps-year in the horse-kick data (Table 4.2). There are several ways to describe variation in a sample of counts. One useful statistic is the variance, the difference between each measurement and the mean measurement, squaring each of those quantities, summing them,

TABLE 4.2   Observed number of soldiers killed by the kick of a horse in ten similar Prussian military corps during the years 1875 through 1894.

| YEAR | | | | | CORPS NUMBER | | | | | |
	II	III	IV	V	VII	VIII	IX	X	XIV	XV
1875	0	0	0	0	1	1	0	0	1	0
1876	0	0	1	0	0	0	0	0	1	1
1877	0	0	0	0	1	0	0	1	2	0
1878	2	1	1	0	0	0	0	1	1	0
1879	0	1	1	2	0	1	0	0	1	0
1880	2	1	1	1	0	0	2	1	3	0
1881	0	2	1	0	1	0	1	0	0	0
1882	0	0	0	0	0	1	1	2	4	1
1883	1	2	0	1	1	0	1	0	0	0
1884	1	0	0	0	1	0	0	2	1	1
1885	0	0	0	0	0	0	2	0	0	1
1886	0	0	1	1	0	0	1	0	3	0
1887	2	1	0	0	2	1	1	0	2	0
1888	1	0	0	1	0	0	0	0	1	0
1889	1	1	0	1	0	0	1	2	0	2
1890	0	2	0	1	2	0	2	1	2	2
1891	0	1	1	1	1	1	0	3	1	0
1892	2	0	1	1	0	1	1	0	1	0
1893	0	0	0	1	2	0	0	1	0	0
1894	0	0	0	0	0	1	0	1	0	0

Data from von Bortkewitsch, Ladislaus. 1898. *Das Gesetz der Kleinen Zahlen*. Leipzig: Druck und Verlag von B. G. Teubner.

TABLE 4.3   Observed number of corps-years in Prussian military units with counts of 0 to 5 soldiers who were killed by the kick of a horse.

COUNT OF DEATHS DUE TO HORSE KICKS	NUMBER OF CORPS-YEARS OBSERVED FOR EACH COUNT OF DEATHS	NUMBER OF CORPS YEARS PREDICTED FOR EACH COUNT OF DEATHS
0	109	108.7
1	65	66.3
2	22	20.2
3	3	4.1
4	1	0.6
5	0	0.1

Data from von Bortkewitsch, Ladislaus. 1898. *Das Gesetz der Kleinen Zahlen*. Leipzig: Druck und Verlag von B. G. Teubner.

and then dividing by the number of measurements in the sample. The formula for the variance of x is in Expression 4.2, where the subscript i indexes each measurement, mean(x) is the mean, and n is the number of observations.

$$(\text{Variance} = [\text{Sum}(x_i - \text{mean}(x))^2]/n \qquad\qquad (\text{Ex.4.2})$$

In many textbooks the variance formula is given as $[\text{sum}(x_i - \text{mean}(x))^2]/(n-1)$; division is by $n-1$, not n. In a large sample, the difference between these formulae will be trivial. If we have data for the entire population of interest, then division by n can be justified. But we usually study a finite sample from a population and for statistical testing we want to account both for the variation in the population and the variation due to sampling; this leads us to divide by n minus the degrees of freedom, or $n-1$. A clear discussion is in Armitage et al. (2002 pp40–42, 147–150).

For the 200 counts in Table 4.2,

$$\begin{aligned}
\text{variance} &= [109 \times (0-.61)^2 + 65 \times (1-.61)^2 + 22 \times (2-.61)^2 + 3 \times (3-.61)^2 + 1 \times (4-.61)^2]/(200) \\
&= 121.58/200 \\
&= 0.6079
\end{aligned}$$

The number 121.58 in the second line of these calculations is close to the observed count of 122 and the variance of 0.6079 is close to the estimated mean count of 0.61. These similarities are not coincidental. When data fit a Poisson distribution, the variance of the mean count is equal to the mean count. If we use C to represent the total count and n to indicate the number of observations, the mean count is C/n and the variance is also C/n. If we know the mean count, we know its variance without carrying out any calculations, provided that the data are from a Poisson distribution. As we have already shown (Table 4.3), the horse-kick data closely fit a Poisson distribution and the estimated variance of 0.6079 confirms this. The SD is the square root of the variance = $\sqrt{.61} = 0.781$.

The mean count of 0.61 deaths arose from 200 corps-years; this mean is also an incidence rate, 0.61 deaths per corps-year. If we use C to indicate the total count and T to indicate the amount of person-time in the denominator for a rate, then C/T is an incidence rate. The number of deaths was 122 and the corps-year time was 200, so the incidence rate was 0.61 per corps-year. The variance for this rate (Table 4.4) is the rate/person-time = $C/T^2 = 122/200^2 = .00305$ (Keyfitz 1966, Breslow and Day 1987 p59). If we multiply the numerator and denominator of this rate by 100, we can express the rate as 61 deaths per 100 corps-years. We should be careful in calculations of variance, SD, and SE, to use the actual count and then rescale the result.

What if we knew that 122 deaths occurred among Prussian military units over a 20-year period, but we did not know the number of corps involved? That would make the mean count 122/20, or 6.1 deaths per year for the entire group of 20 corps. The variance for this mean count would then be 6.1, if we assume the data came from a process that generated a Poisson distribution; all we have done is multiply both the mean count and its variance by 10. If we use the actual data with the counts for each of the 20 years, the variance using Expression 4.2 is 8.1, bigger than the assumed variance of 6.1, but not wildly different. In fact, a formal test that the counts for the 20 years are from a Poisson distribution does not reject that hypothesis; these tests will be discussed in later chapters. With only 20 observations the calculated variance might be 8.1 even if the process producing the deaths is really Poisson; in a small sample the observed data are not likely to precisely fit the expected distribution.

When we estimate a mean count or an incidence rate, we can describe how precisely we know the mean or the rate by using the standard error (SE). We use SEs for the calculation of CIs. For a mean count the SE = $\sqrt{(C/n^2)}$ = (SD of the mean count)/$\sqrt{n}$ and for an incidence rate the SE = $\sqrt{(C/T^2)}$. So if we know that 122 deaths occurred in 200 corps-years, the mean rate is 122/200 = 0.61 per corps-year, the variance of the rate is 0.00305, the SD is 0.055, and the SE = .055. See Table 4.4 for these formulae and more.

For most of the quantities in Table 4.4, the SD and SE are identical. How can this be? When we estimate the variance and SD of the mean of a continuous variable, we use Expression 4.2. To estimate

TABLE 4.4 Formulae for the variance, standard deviation (SD), and standard error (SE) of counts, rates, rate differences, and the natural log (ln) of these quantities (used for ratio estimates), assuming that the counts were produced from a Poisson distribution. See footnote for definitions of abbreviations. The delta-method approximation for variance of ln(x) is variance(x)/(mean x)^2. Ln(C/constant) = ln(C) − ln(constant), so for constants such as n or T the variance of ln(C/constant) equals the variance of ln(C).

NUMBER	QUANTITY	VARIANCE	STANDARD DEVIATION	STANDARD ERROR
	Formulae for each quantity; used for calculation of differences			
1	Total count = C	C	$\sqrt{C}$	$\sqrt{C}$
2	Mean count = C/n	C/n	$\sqrt{(C/n)}$	$\sqrt{((C/n)/n)}$ $= (C/n)/\sqrt{C}$
3	Count difference $= C_1 - C_2$	$C_1 + C_2$	$\sqrt{(C_1 + C_2)}$	$\sqrt{(C_1 + C_2)}$
4	Incidence rate $= C/T$	C/T^2 $= \text{rate}/T$	$\sqrt{(C/T^2)}$ $= \sqrt{(\text{rate}/T)}$	$\sqrt{(C/T^2)}$ $= \sqrt{(\text{rate}/T)}$ $= \sqrt{(C)}/T$ $= (C/T)/\sqrt{C}$
5	Incidence rate difference $= C_1/T_1 - C_2/T_2$	$(C_1/T_1^2) + (C_2/T_2^2)$ $= \text{rate}_1/T_1 + \text{rate}_2/T_2$	$\sqrt{((C_1/T_1^2) + (C_2/T_2^2))}$ $= \sqrt{(\text{rate}_1/T_1 + \text{rate}_2/T_2)}$	$\sqrt{((C_1/T_1)/T_1 + (C_2/T_2)/T_2)}$ $= \sqrt{((C_1/T_1^2) + (C_2/T_2^2))}$ $= \sqrt{(\text{rate}_1/T_1 + \text{rate}_2/T_2)}$
	Formulae for the natural logarithm of each quantity; used for calculation of ratios			
6	Ln(count) = ln(C)	$1/C$	$\sqrt{(1/C)}$	$\sqrt{(1/C)}$
7	Ln(mean count) = ln(C/n)	$1/C$	$\sqrt{(1/C)}$	$\sqrt{(1/C)}$
8	Ln(count ratio) = ln(C_1/C_2)	$1/C_1 + 1/C_2$	$\sqrt{(1/C_1 + 1/C_2)}$	$\sqrt{(1/C_1 + 1/C_2)}$
9	Ln(incidence rate) = ln(C/T)	$1/C$	$\sqrt{(1/C)}$	$\sqrt{(1/C)}$
10	Ln(incidence rate ratio) = ln($\text{rate}_1/\text{rate}_2$) = ln(($C_1/T_1$)/($C_2/T_2$))	$1/C_1 + 1/C_2$	$\sqrt{(1/C_1 + 1/C_2)}$	$\sqrt{(1/C_1 + 1/C_2)}$
11	Ln(standardized mortality ratio) = ln(C_{obs}/C_{exp})	$1/C_{obs}$	$\sqrt{(1/C_{obs})}$	$\sqrt{(1/C_{obs})}$

Abbreviations: C = total count, n = number of observations, T = person-time, C_{obs} = observed count, C_{exp} = expected count. C/n is a mean count for a sample of counts; if n = 1, then C is both the total count and the mean count for one observation. C/T is a mean count based on person-time and is therefore an incidence rate.

the precision of the mean itself, we use the SE (also called the SE of the mean, or SE for the average) which is equal to SD/√n, where n is the number of measurements. This formula for the SE appears in many textbooks. This formula, number 2 in Table 4.4, is used for the SE of a mean count based upon several observations. But unlike the situation for a continuous variable, Table 4.4 has SD and SE formulae for single quantities, such as a single count or the ln of a single rate; here the SD and SE are identical. For a continuous variable we have no formula to estimate the precision of a single measurement.

4.5 AN EXAMPLE: MORTALITY FROM ALZHEIMER'S DISEASE

Let us apply these ideas to US mortality data. In 2009 there were 79,003 deaths in the US attributed to Alzheimer's disease (Kochanek et al. 2012). The estimated mid-year population was 307,006,550, so the crude mortality rate was .00025733 deaths per person-year due to Alzheimer's. Using the usual reporting format of the National Center for Health Statistics, the rate was 25.7 per 100,000 person-years. Provided we think the process that produced the deaths would produce counts with a Poisson distribution, the SE of this rate is √((79003/3070.006550)/3070.006550)) = 0.0916. Note that I used person-years in units of 100,000.

Deaths only occur once, so counts of 0 (no death) and 1 (one death) are the only possible counts for a person followed for one year. So why should we think these Alzheimer's mortality counts fit a Poisson distribution that allows counts of 2, 3, or 6? From Expression 4.1 we can estimate that if the mean rate is 0.00025733 from a closed population of 307,006,550, the probability that an observed count will be 0 is .9997427. The closed population size is not strictly true because we have an estimate of person-time from an open population, but this approximation is close enough. The probability that a count will be 1 is .00025727, which is equal to the observed rate of .00025733 for the first 7 digits after the decimal. If we add up these two probabilities, calculated to more precision than shown here, and subtract them from 1, the probability of a count of 2 or larger is .0000000331045; this can be estimated using Stata's **poissontail()** function. I multiplied these probabilities by the closed population size to get the predicted number for each count. The number of persons predicted not to die of Alzheimer's was 306,927,557.16, which is only 10.16 greater than the number who in fact did not die of Alzheimer's, 306,927,547. The number of predicted Alzheimer deaths was 78,982.67, about 20 less than the observed count of 79,003. The number predicted to die two or more times from Alzheimer's was 10.16, compared with 0 people who actually died more than once. When an outcome is sufficiently uncommon, we expect to observe only persons with and without the outcome, and hardly any with two or more outcomes, even if the outcome could occur more than once and a Poisson process produced the outcome counts. So even though death occurs only once, the observed counts of 0 and 1 for Alzheimer's death closely fit a Poisson distribution. Indeed, the total of all deaths is sufficiently rare compared with the size of the US population that we can treat US mortality rates as if they were from a Poisson distribution.

For anyone accustomed to estimating a variance for continuous data, where we need more than one observation and must use Expression 4.2, the idea that the variance of a rate or count can be determined from a single record may seem strange or even perverse. But many distributions make assumptions about the variance for a mean. Consider the binomial distribution: if the proportion with the outcome is equal to p and the total in the sample is n, the variance of p is assumed to be $p \times (1 - p)/n$. For continuous data we use the data to estimate the mean and use the data again to estimate the variance of quantities around the mean. But for discrete data, such as counts and proportions, or rates and risks, we often use the data to estimate the mean and then rely on distributional assumptions about the mean to estimate the variance. Because all we need is the mean rate or count to estimate a variance, we need minimal information for the analysis of rates, which can be advantageous. This can also be a problem, as it means we may be relying on distributional assumptions which are not true and which we sometimes cannot check. The same is true for the analysis of odds from logistic regression. Later in this book I will show how to test the assumption that the data are from a Poisson distribution and even relax this assumption. But the rest of this chapter will discuss methods that rely on this assumption.

4.6 LARGE SAMPLE P-VALUES FOR COUNTS, RATES, AND THEIR DIFFERENCES USING THE WALD STATISTIC

Three large-sample (approximate) methods for testing a hypothesis with a P-value are the Wald statistic, the score statistic, and the likelihood ratio (Garthwaite, Jolliffe, and Jones 2002 pp84–90, Greenland and Rothman 2008a pp225–231). Probably the most commonly of these is the Wald statistic, also called the standard score, Z-statistic, Normal score, or Z-score. The Wald statistic for a mean count or rate is the mean divided by its SE. This is a measure, in SE units, of how far the observed value is from the hypothesized null value, which is 0 for a difference in counts or rates. This hypothesis can be stated in 3 ways: (1) the hypothesis that the true, but unobserved, count or rate is 0; (2) the hypothesis that the difference between the observed count or rate and a count or rate of 0 is equal to 0; and (3) the hypothesis that the ratio of the observed count or rate to another count or rate is 1.

There were 56 deaths in Montana in 2010 attributed to cancer of the ovary (CDC WONDER). Is that count statistically different from 0? Assuming this count is from a Poisson process, the variance is 56, SD = $\sqrt{56}$ = 7.48, and the SE is equal to the SD because there is only 1 observation (Table 4.4, formula number 1). The Wald statistic is 56/7.48 = $\sqrt{56}$ = 7.48. We then compare 7.48 with the cumulative standard normal distribution. This assumes that if the observed count of 56 represents the true count, then if we could somehow sample the Montana population for 2010 an infinite number of times, the distribution of counts around the mean of 56 would be normal; counts of 55 and 57 would be pretty common, counts of 54 and 58 less common, and counts of 6 and 102 very rare. To put this another way, if a Poisson process generated the counts of ovarian cancer deaths, then over many samples, the mean would be 56 and the SD and SE around this mean would be 7.48. As we saw in Figure 4.2, once a mean count is about 10 or greater, the distribution of counts around the mean starts to look like a Normal distribution. A standard Normal distribution has a mean of 0, SD = 1, a symmetric bell-shaped appearance, and the area under the curve is taken to be equal to 1. The area under the curve is bunched toward 0; 68% of the area lies between z-values (SD units) of –1 to +1, 90% between values of –1.64 and +1.64, 95% between –1.96 and +1.96, and 99% between –2.58 and +2.58. A one-sided P-value is the area under the curve for all values greater than the absolute value of the observed Wald statistic; the two-sided P-value is twice that area. How much area is under the curve when the Wald statistic (Z) is 7.48; that is, 7.48 SDs greater than the mean of 0? The answer is a tiny .000000000000036. The two-sided P-value is twice this amount.

At first-glance a two-sided P-value may seem unjustified for a test that a count of 56 differs from 0. A one-sided P-value estimates the probability that the observed Wald statistic, 7.48, or an even larger Z-statistic would be observed if the true count was 0. A two-sided P-value would add in the probability that the Wald statistic was – 7.48 or smaller. But because counts cannot be negative, how could the Wald statistic be – 7.48? We compared the Montana population with an observed count of 56 to a hypothetical population with a true count of 0, and initially we might think of the comparison as 56–0 = 56. But we could frame the question in the opposite direction, comparing a hypothetical count of 0 with the observed count of 56: 0–56 = –56; then the Wald statistic is negative: –56/7.48 = – 7.48. So for a count *difference* the Wald statistic can be positive or negative, depending on whether the comparison of counts or rates produces a negative or positive difference. This symmetry justifies a two-sided hypothesis test. A two-sided P-value can also be justified by stating that the hypothesis is that two counts being compared are the same; the difference between two rates can be positive or negative.

For small counts the Wald statistic will not give us the correct P-value. Figure 4.2 shows us this method will not work well for small counts, because the assumption that counts will be distributed normally around a mean is not true for small counts. For counts of 1 or 3 the distribution around the mean value is not symmetric under the Poisson distribution.

The rate of death from ovarian cancer was 56 per 989,415 person-years in Montana in 2010 or 100,000 x 56/989,415 = 5.66 per 100,000 person-years. What is the P-value comparing this rate with a rate of 0? Following formula 4 in Table 4.4, the SE is 0.76. The Wald statistic is the rate/SE = 5.66/0.76 = 7.4. If the calculations are done with sufficient precision, the Wald statistic for the rate is 7.48, exactly what it was for the count alone. This is terrific news, because it means we can express rates in whatever time units we like: per 1 person-year, 100,000 person-years, person-centuries, or person-minutes. The choice of person-time units will have no impact on statistical hypothesis testing for rates, as long as the comparison is on a difference scale with a rate of zero. Confidence limits will look different in size because their units will change, but their width relative to the size of the rate will not be affected by the choice of person-time units. A corollary is that statistical uncertainty about a rate depends entirely upon the *numerator* of the rate. A rate based on many person-years will be just as precise, or imprecise, as a rate based on only a few person-years, *if the count numerators are the same*. Studying a large population does not necessarily make a rate precise; it is the count numerator, not the rate denominator, that determines precision. An additional corollary is that we should not rescale the count used for the rate numerator; if the count is 56, we should not convert this to a count of 5.6 or 560, because this will alter the size of statistical tests when we use Poisson methods. We should limit any rescaling to the rate denominator. To see why the Wald statistic did not change, despite converting the count to a rate per 100,000 person-years, examine the calculations below:

$$
\begin{aligned}
\text{Wald statistic} \;&=\; \text{Rate/SE of the rate} \\
&=\; (100,000 \times 56/989,415)/[(\sqrt{(100,000 \times 56/989,415)}/\sqrt{(989,415/100,000)}] \\
&=\; \sqrt{(989,415/100,000)} \times (100,000 \times 56/989,415)/\sqrt{(100,000 \times 56/989,415)} \\
&=\; \sqrt{(989,415/100,000)} \times (100,000 \times 56/989,415) \\
&=\; \sqrt{(989,415/100,000)} \times (100,000/989,415) \times \sqrt{56} \\
&=\; \sqrt{(989,415 \times 100,000/989,415 \times 100,000))} \times \sqrt{56} \\
&=\; \sqrt{56} \\
&=\; \text{count/SE of the count}
\end{aligned}
$$

We can use Wald statistics to compare the mortality rate due to ovarian cancer in Montana (5.66 per 100,000 person-years) with the ovarian cancer mortality rate in Texas in 2010. There were 934 ovarian cancer deaths in Texas (CDC WONDER) in 2010: rate = 10^5 x 934/25,145,561 = 3.71. The difference between the two rates is 5.66–3.71 = 1.96. To get a P-value, use formula 5 (Table 4.4) to compute the SE. To work on the scale of rates per 100,000 person-years, divide both person-year estimates by 100,000. The SE of the difference is then $\sqrt{(56/9.89415^2 + 934/251.45561^2)} = 0.766$, the Wald Z-statistic is 1.95/0.766 = 2.54, and the two-sided P-value is .011.

For any hypothesis test, the validity of the result assumes that our statistical model is correct and our estimates free of bias. That is not the case here. There are substantial differences in the age distributions of the populations of Montana and Texas and their age-adjusted rates are closer than their crude rates. Montana's crude mortality rate of 5.66 for ovarian cancer is not that different from the rate of 4.72 for the entire United States. I picked Texas for comparison because its crude rate was one of the lowest, making the contrast statistically significant; only Texas, Utah, Nevada, and the District of Columbia had crude ovarian cancer mortality rates less than 4 per 100,000 person-years in 2010.

You may never need to carry out the calculations shown above, because modern statistical software can do them for you. But having read this section, you will know that your software is relying on assumptions related to the Poisson distribution.

4.7 COMPARISONS OF RATES AS DIFFERENCES VERSUS RATIOS

I said above that changing the units for person-time has no influence on the Z-statistics, P-values, and CIs for a rate. Precision depends only on the count in the rate numerator. This is true when an observed rate is compared with a rate of zero or when two rates are compared using an additive or difference scale. But if we make comparisons on a ratio scale (ln rate scale) then the comparison of a single rate is usually with a null or baseline rate of *1 event per 1 unit of person-time*. For this comparison, a change in time units will change the statistics regarding statistical precision, because a comparison of the Montana ovarian cancer rate with a rate of 1 cancer per person-century is different from a comparison with a rate of 1 cancer per person-week. I will return to this idea in Chapter 9 when discussing baseline rates which are estimated by the constant or intercept term in Poisson regression. On the other hand, if we compare the rate in Montana with the rate in Texas on a ratio scale, a change that time units will have no influence on statistical tests of precision, because the same time units will be used for each population.

4.8 LARGE SAMPLE P-VALUES FOR COUNTS, RATES, AND THEIR DIFFERENCES USING THE SCORE STATISTIC

The large sample test statistic for the hypothesis that an observed count (C_{obs}) does not differ from a hypothetically true expected count (C_{exp}) has a simple form called the score statistic (Breslow and Day 1987 p68–69, Altman 1991 p246, Newman 2001 p255–258, Armitage, Berry, and Matthews 2002 p665, Greenland and Rothman 2008b p242). The score statistic tests the null hypothesis that there is no difference between two rates; it is a test that the rate difference is 0 and a test that the rate ratio is 1. The score test is typically used when C_{obs} is the event count from a small population and C_{exp} comes from the rate of a much larger population and is therefore larger and more precise compared with C_{obs}. C_{exp} is the count we expect (to observe) if the larger population's rate represents the true, unobserved rate, and this rate is applied to the person-time of the small population. Under the null hypothesis of no difference between the two population rates, our best estimate of the true value of C_{obs} is C_{exp} and assuming that the counts come from a Poisson process, we estimate that the SE of C_{obs} is $\sqrt{C_{exp}}$ (Table 4.4, formulae 1). The difference between the imprecise observed count and the more precise expected count is $C_{obs} - C_{exp}$, the expected difference under the null hypothesis is 0, and the SE for the observed count is $\sqrt{C_{exp}}$. The score statistic, a measure of how far the observed difference deviates from 0, is:

Score statistic $= (C_{obs} - C_{exp}) / \sqrt{C_{exp}}$ (Ex.4.3)

The size of the score statistic is compared with the Normal distribution; it is treated as a Z-statistic just like the Wald statistic. Some authors describe the score statistic as $(C_{obs} - C_{exp})^2/C_{exp}$, which can be compared with the chi-squared distribution for 1 degree of freedom. This is the usual chi-squared statistic that compares an observed cell frequency with the expected frequency under the null hypothesis. This comparison with the chi-squared distribution will produce exactly the same P-value as the comparison of expression 4.3 with the Normal distribution.

The score test cannot be calculated for an expected count of 0 and is unreliable for an expected count of 5 or less, because it assumes the distribution of counts is Normal. Once a count is less than about 5, the normality assumption does not fit a Poisson distribution (Figure 4.2). If C_{exp} is less than 5, small sample methods are preferred to the score statistic (Newman 2001 p 257, Greenland and Rothman 2008b p 243). Better formulae than the score statistic are available (Breslow and Day 1987 p69) and exact methods are available in software.

One variation on the score statistic is to use a continuity correction, subtracting .5 from the absolute value of the difference in the observed and expected counts (Breslow and Day 1987 p68):

Score statistic $= ($absolute value $(C_{obs} - C_{exp}) - .5) / \sqrt{C_{exp}}$ (Ex.4.4)

The continuity correction is used to estimate a P-value close to the P-value we would get if we used an exact test (Greenland and Rothman 2008a p232). Since modern software can provide exact P-values, Expression 4.4 is of little practical importance.

We can use the score statistic to compare the mortality rate from ovarian cancer in Montana with the rate in Texas. C_{obs} in Montana was 56. C_{exp} is the number of deaths we expect if the mortality rate in Texas was applied to the person-time of Montana: Cexp = (934/25,145,561) x 989,415 = 36.75. So the score test statistic is $(C_{obs} - C_{exp})/\sqrt{C_{exp}} = (56–36.75)/\sqrt{36.75} = 3.1753$. Software can tell us that .00075 is the proportion of the normal distribution that lies above a standard normal deviate, or Z-score, of 3.1753. Therefore, the one-sided P-value for the comparison of the Montana rate with the Texas rate is .00075 and the two-sided P-value is twice this amount, .0015.

4.9 LARGE SAMPLE CONFIDENCE INTERVALS FOR COUNTS, RATES, AND THEIR DIFFERENCES

A P-value for a hypothesis test conveys limited information. It fails to tell us the strength or direction of the estimated association (we need the estimated association for that) and the P-value gives us little feel for the precision of the estimated association. Confidence intervals provide some information about precision (Rothman 1978, Gardner and Altman 1986, Rothman 1986b, Altman and Bland 2004, Cummings and Koepsell 2010).

Using the SE to construct a CI is the Wald method and some version of this method is what statistical software will use to report CIs for tables of regression estimates. In Montana in 2010 the rate of death from ovarian cancer was 100,000 × 56/989,415 = 5.66 per 100,000 person-years and using formula 4 for Table 4.4, the SE of this rate was 0.76. To calculate the 95% confidence limits for this rate we use Expressions 4.5:

$$\text{Lower 95\% confidence limit} = \text{rate} - (z \text{ for } 1 - \text{alpha}/2) \times \text{SE}$$
$$= \text{rate} - 1.96 \times \text{SE}$$
$$= 5.66 - 1.96 \times 0.76$$
$$= 4.18 \qquad \text{(Ex.4.5)}$$
$$\text{Upper 95\% confidence limit} = \text{rate} + 1.96 \times \text{SE}$$
$$= 5.66 + 1.96 \times 0.76$$
$$= 7.14$$

Expression 4.5 assumes possible values of the rate have a distribution with the shape of the Normal curve but with a mean of 5.66 and SD of 0.76. For alpha = .05, the proportion of the standard normal distribution below a standard deviate of 1.96 is .025 and the proportion above z = 1.96 is also .025; the sum of these proportions is .05. Using the standard Normal distribution, which has mean 0 and SD = 1, − 1.96 corresponds to a P_{lower} level of alpha/2 = .025 and P_{upper} = 1 − alpha/2 = .975. While 95% CIs are commonly reported, we could pick alpha = .01 (99% CI) or alpha = .10 (90% CI) or any level of alpha. Using Expression 4.5, we can calculate CIs for an infinite number of alpha values; this creates two P-value function curves (Figure 4.3) which meet at an apex when alpha = 1 and which show how compatible any rate value may be with the observed rate (Poole 1987a, Sullivan and Foster 1990, Rothman, Greenland, and Lash 2008d p157–163, Cummings and Koepsell 2010). The P-value function curves for the crude ovarian cancer mortality rates in Montana and Texas show some overlap, but not a lot. Confidence intervals do not exclude any possible rate values (Poole 1987b), but they make it easy for us to see that true rates less than

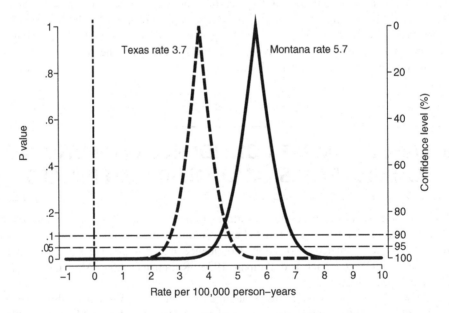

FIGURE 4.3 Wald method P-value function curves for the rates of death due to cancer of the ovary in Texas (3.7 per 100,000 person-years) and Montana (5.7) in 2010. The SE used comes from formula 4 in Table 4.4, which calculates on the difference scale. The vertical dashed line indicates the null rate of 0 and horizontal dashed lines indicate alpha levels of .1 and .05, corresponding to confidence levels of 90% and 95%.

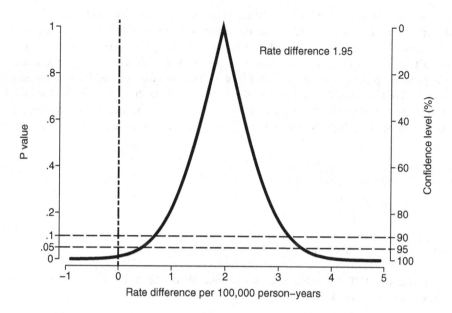

FIGURE 4.4   Wald method P-value function curves for the difference (Montana – Texas) in the rates of death due to cancer of the ovary in Texas (3.7 per 100,000 person-years) and Montana (5.7) in 2010. The SE used comes from formula 3 in Table 4.4, which calculates on the difference scale. The vertical dashed line indicates the null rate difference of 0 and horizontal dashed lines indicate alpha levels of .1 and .05, corresponding to confidence levels of 90% and 95%.

3 or greater than 8 seem unlikely for Montana, whereas a true rate of 3 would not be unlikely in Texas. Texas had more cancer deaths and so the P-value function curve for Texas is narrower than for Montana. Although articles typically report only one CI for each estimate, we can use that interval along with the rate estimate to visualize the entire P-value function for an infinite number of CIs; this gives us some appreciation for how likely other possible rates may be given the observed rate (Rothman 1978, Gardner and Altman 1986, Rothman 1986b, Altman and Bland 2004).

   We can use formula 5 in Table 4.4 to create P-value function curves for the difference between the rates in Texas and Montana (Figure 4.4). The difference in rates (Texas rate – Montana rate) is 1.95 per 100,000 person-years. The Wald 95% CI for this difference is 0.23 to 3.66.

4.10 LARGE SAMPLE P-VALUES FOR COUNTS, RATES, AND THEIR RATIOS

When we estimate rate ratios it is convenient to work with the logarithms of the rates. On the log scale the ratio of 2 rates can be treated as a linear expression: $\ln(\text{rate}_1/\text{rate}_2) = \ln(\text{rate}_1) - \ln(\text{rate}_2)$. Natural logarithms (ln values) based on the quantity $e \approx 2.718$ are used, so exponentiating (finding the antilog of) a quantity Q means calculating e^Q. On the log scale the null value for no difference is 0, which corresponds to a null value of 1 on the rate ratio scale: $\ln(1) = 0$, exponential$(0) = e^0 = 1$.

   The variance of the log of a count is not equal to the log of the variance of the count. Formulae for the approximate variance, SD, and SE of ln counts and ln rates (formulae 6–10 in

Table 4.4) are derived from the delta method (Hosmer, Lemeshow, and May 2008 p355–356, Greenland and Rothman 2008b p242). The delta-method approximation for variance of ln(x) is variance(x)/(mean x)2. Ln(C/constant) = ln(C) − ln(constant), so for constants such as n or T, the variance of ln(C/constant) equals the variance of ln(C). Note: where it says variance(x)/(mean x) 2, the 2 is a superscript, the x terms are the letter x. The variance of the ln of a single count C is 1/C, the SD is $\sqrt{(1/C)}$ and the SE is equal to the SD. For all the ln quantities in Table 4.4, the SD and SE are the same and person-time plays no role. Using C to indicate a count, Expressions 4.6 and 4.7 show the relationships between the SE (or SD) for a count and the SE for the ln of a count:

$$SE \ln(count) = (SE \, of \, count)/count$$
$$= (\sqrt{(C)})/C \qquad \qquad (Ex.4.6)$$
$$= (\sqrt{(1/C)}$$

$$SE \, count = count \times SE \ln(count) \qquad \qquad (Ex.4.7)$$

For a rate equal to C/T, the relationships between SE of the ln(rate) and the SE of the rate are shown in Expressions 4.8 and 4.9.

$$SE \ln(rate) = (SE \, of \, rate)/rate$$
$$= \sqrt{((C/T)/T)}/(C/T)$$
$$= \sqrt{(C/T)} \times \sqrt{T}/(C/T)$$
$$= \sqrt{T}/(\sqrt{C} \times \sqrt{(1/T)}) \qquad \qquad (Ex.4.8)$$
$$= \sqrt{T} \times \sqrt{(1/T)}/\sqrt{C}$$
$$= 1/\sqrt{C}$$
$$= \sqrt{(1/C)}$$

$$SE \, rate = rate \, x \, SE \ln(rate)$$
$$= C/T \times \sqrt{(1/C)} \qquad \qquad (Ex.4.9)$$
$$= \sqrt{(C/T^2)}$$

The delta method can be extended to ratios estimated on the ln scale:

$$SE \ln(rate \, ratio) = (SE \, of \, rate \, ratio)/(rate \, ratio) \qquad \qquad (Ex.4.10)$$

$$SE \, rate \, ratio = rate \, ratio \times SE \ln(rate \, ratio) \qquad \qquad (Ex.4.11)$$

The expressions here apply to other ratios estimated on the ln scale. For example, the SE of the ln(odds ratio) is equal to the SE of the odds ratio divided by the odds ratio. Anyone who uses logistic regression has seen tables of output that show coefficients for differences on the ln odds scale along with SEs, Z-statistics, P-values, and CIs. If the software is asked to report exponentiated coefficients instead, these are odds ratios and they are shown with SEs that are related to the SEs for the ln odds using the formulae above. The same is true for the hazard ratio.

The ratio of the mortality rate in Montana compared with Texas, on the log scale, is ln(56/989,415) − ln(934/25,145,561) = ln((56/989,415)/(934/25,145,561)) = .4212. The SE of the ln of the rate ratio (formula 10 in Table 4.4) is $\sqrt{(1/56 + 1/934)}$ = .1376. The Wald statistic is therefore .4212/.1376 = 3.062 and the two-sided P-value is .0022.

4.11 LARGE SAMPLE CONFIDENCE INTERVALS FOR RATIOS OF COUNTS AND RATES

Working on the ln scale, the formulae for the CI of a rate are derived by calculating the upper and lower confidence limits for the ln of the rate and then exponentiating those endpoints. For the Montana mortality rate, the calculations, based on formula 9 in Table 4.4, are:

$$
\begin{aligned}
\text{Lower 95\% confidence limit} &= \exp(\ln(\text{rate}) - (z \text{ for } 1 - \text{alpha}/2) \times \text{SE of ln rate}) \\
&= \exp(\ln(\text{rate}) - 1.96 \times \sqrt{1/C}) \\
&= \exp(\ln(56/9.89415) - 1.96 \times \sqrt{1/56}) \\
&= 4.36 \\
\text{Upper 95\% confidence limit} &= \exp(\ln(\text{rate}) + 1.96 \times \text{SE}) \\
&= 7.35
\end{aligned}
$$

(Ex.4.12)

Earlier we used formula 4 in Table 4.4 to calculate a 95% CI of 4.18 to 7.14, using methods for the rate difference. The new limits of 4.36, 7.35 are further from 0 and they are asymmetrical on the difference scale: rate − lower confidence limit = 5.66 − 4.36 = 1.30, whereas upper confidence limit − rate = 7.35 − 5.66 = 1.69. Which CI should we prefer? Counts and rates cannot be less than 0. If we use a CI calculated on the ln (ratio) scale, the lower bound of the CI cannot be less than 0, because the exponential of the ln of a rate will always be positive, no matter how small the rate. If we work on the difference scale, the lower bound of the CI could be negative. Working on the ln scale means the CI for a rate ratio will be asymmetric on the difference scale. On a ratio (multiplicative or ln) scale, the "distance" from 0 to 1 is the same as the "distance" from 1 to infinity. On a ratio scale, the CI of 4.36, 7.35 is symmetric: rate/lower CI limit = 5.66/4.36 = 1.3 = upper CI limit/rate = 7.35/5.66.

Using the ln scale for rates, I generated P-value functions for Montana and Texas mortality rates due to ovarian cancer (Figure 4.5). We can see several changes compared with Figure 4.3. The CIs for Texas are narrower, so a true rate of 3 seems less likely for Texas compared with Figure 4.3. There is now little overlap between the two sets of CIs; this reflects the fact that on the rate difference scale the P-value for the null hypothesis of no difference was .011, but on the rate ratio scale, the P-value for the null hypothesis that the rate ratio is 1 was smaller, .0022. Figure 4.6 shows the P-value function curves for the rate ratio comparing Montana with Texas using the ln scale (formula 10 in Table 4.4).

4.12 A CONSTANT RATE BASED ON MORE PERSON-TIME IS MORE PRECISE

Two populations may have the same rate, say .01 events per person-year, but if one rate comes from observation of only 100 person-years (event count = .01 x 100 = 1) and the second comes from 1 million person-years (event count .01 x 1,000,000 = 10,000), then all other things being equal, the second rate should be more precise. The variance for a mean count is equal to the mean count, the variance for a count of 1 is only 1, but the variance for a count of 10,000 is 10,000. Because the bigger count has a larger variance, in what sense is it more precise?

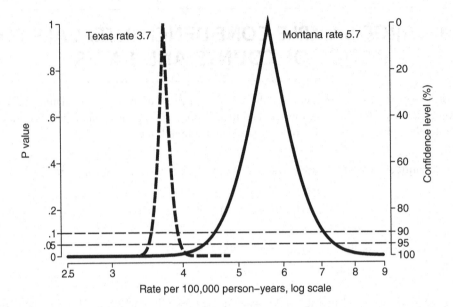

FIGURE 4.5 Wald method P-value function curves for the rates of death due to cancer of the ovary in Texas (3.7 per 100,000 person-years) and Montana (5.7) in 2010. The SE used comes from formula 9 in Table 4.4, which uses the log (ratio) scale. Horizontal dashed lines indicate alpha levels of .1 and .05, corresponding to confidence levels of 90% and 95%. The X-axis uses the log scale.

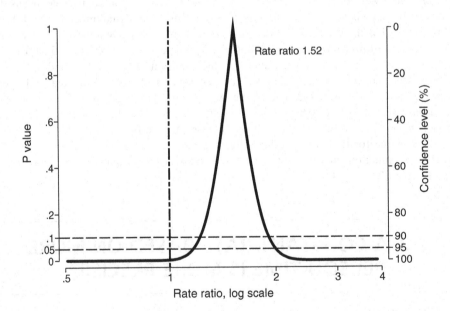

FIGURE 4.6 Wald method confidence interval function curves for the ratio (Montana/Texas) of the rates of death due to cancer of the ovary in Montana (5.7 per 100,000 person-years) and Texas (3.7) in 2010. The SE used comes from formula 10 in Table 4.4 for the log scale. The vertical dashed line indicates the null rate ratio of 1 and horizontal dashed lines indicate alpha levels of .1 and .05, corresponding to confidence levels of 90% and 95%. X-axis is on the log scale.

TABLE 4.5   Counts, person-time, rates, variance of the mean rate, SE of the mean rate, and the Z statistic for populations with the *same* event rate, 0.01 per 1 person-year, but increasing values of person-time.

EVENT COUNT	PERSON-TIME	RATE PER 1 PERSON-YEAR	VARIANCE[a]	SE[b]	Z[c]
1	100	0.01	0.0001	0.01	1
10	1000	0.01	0.00001	0.00316	3.16
100	10,000	0.01	0.000001	0.001	10
1000	100,000	0.01	0.0000001	0.00032	31.62
10,000	1,000,000	0.01	0.00000001	0.0001	100

[a] Variance of the mean rate (Table 4.4, formula 4) = SE^2 = Count/person-time^2
[b] SE of the mean rate (Table 4.4, formula 4) = $\sqrt{(\text{Count/person-time}^2)}$
[c] Z = (mean rate)/SE of mean rate = (Count/person-time)/$\sqrt{(\text{Count/person-time}^2)}$

To judge the precision of estimates with CIs, we use the formulae for the SE in Table 4.4. Formula 4 in that table shows that the SE of a mean rate is $\sqrt{(C/T^2)}$. For a constant rate, if the person-time is multiplied by X, the variance of the mean rate will be divided by X and the SE will be divided by $\sqrt{X}$. (Table 4.5). The variance of the mean rate is equal to the SE squared = C/T^2, so the variance for a constant rate shrinks as person-time increases; the shrinkage is proportional to the inverse of the ratio increase in the count. The Wald or Z-statistic, which is a large-sample method for estimating the P-value for a rate compared with a null rate of 0, is the ratio of the rate to its SE. As person-time increases for a constant rate, the size of the Z-statistic will increase multiplicatively with the square-root of the count. This is even easier to see if we use formula 9 in Table 4.4, where the SE is equal to $1/\sqrt{C}$.

4.13 EXACT METHODS

Exact P-values and CIs are not exact in the sense of being exactly correct. They are methods which can provide better P-values and confidence limits for small samples by avoiding the normality assumptions used by Wald or score tests. Exact methods have disadvantages: some are so computer intensive that solutions are not possible even in samples of modest size, some methods are not yet widely available in software, and exact methods do not yet exist for some problems. For counts and rates, exact methods can be divided into two categories: (1) tests that use the Poisson distribution (Expression 4.1) for a few simple quantities and (2) exact Poisson regression which uses permutation methods. I will discuss exact Poisson regression in Chapter 23 and focus here on how we can use knowledge of the Poisson distribution to estimate exact P-values and CIs.

In 1994, Rossing et al. reported evidence that treatment of infertility in women might be related to the outcome of cancer of the ovary (Rossing et al. 1994). In a cohort of 3837 women who were treated for infertility, 11 subsequently developed ovarian tumors. Using data about the rate of ovarian cancer in the much larger population of all women in the same geographic region, the authors estimated that 4.4 cases of cancer were expected. So C_{obs} was 11, C_{exp} 4.4, and the rate ratio was 11/4.4 = 2.5. Is this rate ratio significantly different from 1 using an alpha of .05? Assuming the counts arose from a Poisson process, we can use Expression 4.1: The one-sided probability that a count of 11 or more would be observed if the true count was 4.4, is given by summing Poisson probabilities for counts from 0 to 10 and subtracting these from 1:

$$P = 1 - (4.4^0 \times \exp(-4.4)/0! \times \exp(-4.4)/0!$$
$$+ \, 4.4^1 \times \exp(-4.4)/1! \times \exp(-4.4)/1!$$
$$+ \, 4.4^2 \times \exp(-4.4)/2! \times \exp(-4.4)/2!$$
$$+ \, 4.4^3 \times \exp(-4.4)/3! \times \exp(-4.4)/3!$$
$$+ \ldots$$
$$+ \, 4.4^{10} \times \exp(-4.4)/10! \times \exp(-4.4)/10!)$$
$$= .00569$$

In Stata you could just type:

```
di "1-sided exact P value for K>=11 = " poissontail(4.4,11)
1-sided exact P value for K>=11 = .00568824
```

The two-sided P-value is just twice the one-sided value: $2 \times 0.0569 = .011$. These are exact P-values, based upon the Poisson probability function. Given these *P*-values, it is not likely that sampling variation alone explains the observed rate ratio of 2.5. But biases such as measurement error and confounding (group differences in risk for cancer, aside from infertility treatment) could explain the observed difference.

With continuous data we can set alpha as the frequency with which we are willing to reject the null hypothesis when it is true. But we cannot do this precisely for discrete data, such as binary proportions or counts and rates. Because counts increase in integer steps, the P-values also increase in discrete jumps. Imagine that we plan to reject the null hypothesis of no association between infertility and the occurrence of an ovarian tumor if a P-value for this test is < .05. Given an expected count of 4.4, the exact two-sided P-value is .07 for a count of 9 and .03 for a count of 10. There is no way to get a two-sided P-value of .05. We can reject the null hypothesis using the P-value of .03, but that means that we expect to reject the null hypothesis in 3% of the samples. Exact methods may force us to use a P-value cutoff smaller or larger than alpha.

Another option is to use a mid-P-value, a P-value that includes an additional term for the probability of a count mid-way between the observed count and the next higher count (or next lower count if the counts are less than the mean). For our ovarian cancer example, this means calculating:

$$P = 1 - (4.4^0 \times \exp(-4.4)/0! \times \exp(-4.4)/0!$$
$$+ \, 4.4^1 \times \exp(-4.4)/1! \times \exp(-4.4)/1!$$
$$+ \ldots$$
$$+ \, 4.4^{10} \times \exp(-4.4)/10! \times \exp(-4.4)/10!$$
$$+ .5 \times (4.4^{11} \times \exp(-4.4)/11! \times \exp(-4.4)/11!)$$
$$= .00385$$

The two-sided mid-P-value is .0077, smaller than the exact P-value of .011.

Exact CIs can be constructed using the Poisson distribution. To estimate a lower bound for a 95% CI, we need to find the value of "lower" such that .025 is equal to the expression given here. We use the value .025 because 95% CI limits should include 95% of all possible estimates, omitting those in the lowest 2.5% of the distribution and those at or above 97.5% of the distribution.

$$.025 = 1 - (\text{lower}^0 \times \exp(-\text{lower})/0! \times \exp(-\text{lower})/0!$$
$$+ \text{lower}^1 \times \exp(-\text{lower})/1! \times \exp(-\text{lower})/1!$$
$$+ \text{lower}^2 \times \exp(-\text{lower})/2! \times \exp(-\text{lower})/2!$$
$$+ \text{lower}^3 \times \exp(-\text{lower})/3! \times \exp(-\text{lower})/3!$$
$$+ \ldots$$
$$+ \text{lower}^{10} \times \exp(-\text{lower})/10! \times \exp(-\text{lower})/10!)$$

To get the upper confidence limit, the following expression must be solved for "upper."

$$.025 = 1 - (\text{upper}^0 \times \exp(-\text{upper})/0! \times \exp(-\text{upper})/0!$$
$$+ \text{upper}^1 \times \exp(-\text{upper})/1! \times \exp(-\text{upper})/1!$$
$$+ \text{upper}^2 \times \exp(-\text{upper})/2! \times \exp(-\text{upper})/2!$$
$$+ \text{upper}^3 \times \exp(-\text{upper})/3! \times \exp(-\text{upper})/3!$$
$$+ \ldots$$
$$+ \text{upper}^{10} \times \exp(-\text{upper})/10! \times \exp(-\text{upper})/10!$$
$$+ \text{upper}^{11} \times \exp(-\text{upper})/11! \times \exp(-\text{upper})/11!$$

For the rate ratio of 2.5, the exact 95% CI is 1.25 to 4.47. Stata statistical software has several commands that quickly find this result. An exact CI for counts or rates or rate ratios has a limitation similar to that for exact P-values. The exact 95% CI may include (cover) the true count (or rate ratio) in 95% or *more* of repeated samples; this is called overcoverage. We may seek a 95% CI, but we may get a 96% or 98% CI. Some feel that overcoverage is desirable or at least acceptable. Others prefer a CI which will, *on average*, include the true value in 100 x (1 − alpha/2) % of the intervals, even if this interval may sometimes be too wide (overcoverage) and sometimes too small (undercoverage). Such an interval can be constructed using a method similar to that for mid-P-values. To get the lower limit for a mid-*P* 95% CI we need to solve the following for the value of "lower":

$$.025 = 1 - (\text{lower}^0 \times \exp(-\text{lower})/0! \times \exp(-\text{lower})/0!$$
$$+ \text{lower}^1 \times \exp(-\text{lower})/1! \times \exp(-\text{lower})/1!$$
$$+ \ldots$$
$$+ \text{lower}^{10} \times \exp(-\text{lower})/10! \times \exp(-\text{lower})/10!$$
$$+ .5 \times \text{lower}^{11} \times \exp(-\text{lower})/11! \times \exp(-\text{lower})/11!)$$

To get the upper mid-*P* 95% confidence limit, the following expression must be solved for "upper."

$$.025 = \text{upper}^0 \times \exp(-\text{upper})/0! \times \exp(-\text{upper})/0!$$
$$+ \text{upper}^1 \times \exp(-\text{upper})/1! \times \exp(-\text{upper})/1!$$
$$+ \ldots$$
$$+ \text{upper}^{10} \times \exp(-\text{upper})/10! \times \exp(-\text{upper})/10!$$
$$+ .5 \times \text{upper}^{11} \times \exp(-\text{upper})/11! \times \exp(-\text{upper})/11!$$

TABLE 4.6 Two-sided P values and 95% confidence intervals (CI) for an incidence rate ratio of 2.50 computed from an observed count of 11 and an expected count of 4.4: 11/4.4 = 2.50.

METHOD	TWO-SIDED P VALUE	95% CI
Wald ratio method	.0024	1.38, 4.51
Exact	.0114	1.25, 4.47
Mid-P exact	.0077	1.31, 4.35

The value of lower is 5.78 and upper is 19.12. These are mean counts, but we want to get lower and upper values for the rate ratio. We divide each of these values by the expected mean count of 4.4 to get 1.3 and 4.3 as the mid-*P* corrected 95% confidence limits for the rate ratio of 2.5.

For comparison, I calculated a P-value and 95% CI using the Wald ratio method (formula 11 in Table 4.4). The Wald method P-value is small compared with the exact values (Table 4.6), probably too small given the normality assumptions and the small counts. The Wald CI for the rate ratio is too narrow and shifted upward away from 1. The exact *P*-value is larger and the exact CI wider. The mid-P-value is smaller and its associated CI narrower compared with the exact values. There is debate regarding whether exact or mid-P statistics should be preferred. Those who prefer exact methods, which estimate P-values and CIs that are always as large and possibly larger (overcoverage) than demanded for the level of alpha, will also favor the use of continuity corrections when using approximate large sample methods. I have sometimes ignored continuity corrections in this chapter, giving attention instead to exact methods. Those who prefer statistics that provide correct *average* coverage, albeit sometimes with over- or undercoverage, will also prefer not to use continuity corrections. There is an interesting literature on this topic (Armitage, Berry, and Matthews 2002 p118–120,133–137, Greenland and Rothman 2008a p231–233).

As a practical matter, if the choice between exact (or continuity corrected) statistics and mid-P statistics (without continuity correction) influences interpretation of results, this suggests there is little data regarding the association or excessive devotion to statistical significance. I prefer estimation as a goal, use CIs to describe precision, and give less attention to P-values. Whether a CI for a rate ratio or difference just barely includes or excludes a null value is usually not of much interest. The study by Rossing et al exemplifies these issues (Rossing et al. 1994). Despite a 95% CI (1.25 to 4.47) that excluded 1 for the rate ratio relating infertility (or treatment for infertility) to ovarian tumors, the authors did not claim this association was causal and suggested that larger studies were needed. This is a difficult question to study because both the exposure (infertility treatment) and the outcome (ovarian cancer) are uncommon; whether there is any causal association between infertility treatment and ovarian cancer remains unsettled (Jensen et al. 2009, Braem et al. 2010, Siristatidis et al. 2013, Stewart et al. 2013).

4.14 WHAT IS A POISSON PROCESS?

I have repeatedly referred to a Poisson process that generates counts, but so far I have not defined a Poisson process. A Poisson process will, on average, produce counts with a Poisson distribution in intervals of time or units of area or volume. This definition is circular. I have already hinted at what is needed: a mechanism for producing counts at a constant rate over time.

One feature of a Poisson process is *independence* (Cook and Lawless 2007 p12,31–33, Winkelmann 2008 p11–13, Cameron and Trivedi 2013a p5–6). This means that the occurrence of each event does not influence the occurrence of other events. This is easy to imagine for radioactive decay. When an alpha particle is emitted, it flies off without influencing other atoms. Although an alpha particle could strike another atom, on the atomic scale atoms consist mostly of space, so this potential interaction can be ignored. The probability that an atom will decay in any time interval is unaffected by (independent of) what happens in other time intervals. After each event, the probability of a new event for those who remain in the population is unchanged.

In the study of human populations, it may be reasonable to think that many events are independent. It is doubtful that ovarian cancer in one woman will influence the occurrence of this disease in another. Deaths due to a kick by a horse are probably independent.

The assumption of independence may not be tenable for some outcomes. Consider an outbreak of measles; the probability that someone will get measles is influenced by the number of other persons who recently developed measles, the vaccination status of others, and the proximity of others. Consider deaths due to traffic crashes. In some sense these are not all independent, as sometimes a car can hit and kill several pedestrians, several people can die in the same vehicle, and vehicles can collide. Does this mean we cannot use Poisson methods to study year-to-year variations in traffic deaths? Not necessarily. The mechanisms that produce traffic-related deaths may sometimes generate a crash with several deaths. But most deaths in intervals of time will be independent of the deaths in other time periods; probably independent enough for Poisson methods. The property of independence means that recent events do not influence future events, which does not necessarily imply complete absence of any relationship between events. And later chapters will show that the assumption of independence can be relaxed.

There is another sense in which events might not be independent. Imagine that we count recurrent events that produce one or more fractures. If you fall and break two ribs and your wrist, we could count this as one fracture event. Over time one person can have several events that produce new fractures; I have had five! In 1980, I fractured an ankle while mountaineering and was in a cast and on crutches for a month. This probably lowered my risk of another fracture for a while, as I had to forgo skiing and mountain climbing for a few months. So one fracture event may have influenced the rate of future fracture events for some period. But does this violate the Poisson independence assumption a great deal? Perhaps not. The five fractures were spread over 74 years and in each instances activities were limited for only a month or two. While risk of a new fracture may have been reduced for a period, the reduction was probably minimal. It may be reasonable to study recurrent fracture events with Poisson methods.

For some recurrent events, we may wish to omit some person-time after each event; this idea was mentioned in Chapter 2. For example, imagine a study of urinary infections which may recur. While a subject has an active infection, they are probably not susceptible to a new one until they have recovered. Even if they are susceptible, we may not be able to recognize a new infection event. In this study, one could omit 2 weeks of person-time from the rate denominator after the onset of each infection.

If a mechanism is to produce counts with a Poisson distribution, the process must be *stationary* (Cook and Lawless 2007 pp12,31–33, Winkelmann 2008 pp11–13, Cameron and Trivedi 2013a pp5–6). This means that the rate or risk of a new event does not change from one time interval to the next. Furthermore, the average rate or risk of a new event is the same for all the study units, whether those units are people or cavalry corps. This property has been called homogeneity of risk (Greenland and Rothman 2008b p241).

The property of constant risk and the property of independence often overlap. For example, if a recent fracture influences the risk of a new fracture, the consequence is a change in risk from one time period to another; this violates both the independence property and the constant risk property.

The rate of fracture events in a short window of time probably changes little for most people. But fracture rates vary a great deal with age. Wrist fractures are common among young children who use skateboards and roller-skates. Wrist fractures are less common among aging epidemiologists who write research papers at their desks. With old age, the risk of hip fracture rises sharply (Fisher et al. 1991, Baron et al. 1996). Assuming a constant fracture rate for people of different ages would be unrealistic. We can deal with this variation by accounting for it. If we do an analysis that stratifies on age or adjusts finely enough for age, within each age group the assumption of similar risk may be reasonable. Earlier in this chapter I noted that the rates of ovarian cancer were not the same in Montana and Texas, but I noted the rates became more similar when we accounted for age differences between these states. The ovarian cancer rates I computed used person-time from the entire population. But the rate of ovarian cancer in men is 0. We can account for this heterogeneity by either adjusting for sex, or by limiting the rate comparison to women only. In short, we can often deal with violations of the stationary rate property by using stratification, adjustment, restriction, or matching. To use statistical jargon, we assume the rate is stationary *conditional* on the levels of the other variables in our model for the outcome.

Sometimes we are forced to do something else about violations of the assumption of constant rate for the outcome. Colleagues and I conducted a randomized controlled trial of an intervention intended to reduce falls among the elderly (Shumway-Cook et al. 2007). Within the intervention and control arms of the trial, there were large differences in the propensity of subjects to fall, differences that made untenable the assumption that the variance of the fall counts in each trial arm was equal to the mean count. We used modifications of the Poisson method to deal with this. Later chapters will describe modified Poisson methods that can be used for count data, or even continuous data, that are not from a Poisson process.

4.15 SIMULATED EXAMPLES

The properties that describe a process that generates counts with a Poisson distribution are simple: independence of events over time and a constant rate over time. Given these properties, the probability that an event will occur is proportional to the amount of time that passes. Mathematically, it can be shown that when these properties are present, the variance of a Poisson count is equal to the mean count. Here I describe a simulated example. I had a computer create a record for each of 10 million days. Each day had an identifying number. The computer then created 23 million events which were assigned at random to these days, using a pseudorandom number generator. The event rate was therefore a constant 2.3 per day. Assignment was independent of previous assignments; each day had an equal chance of receiving an event, regardless of whether it had already received 1 or more events. These characteristics describe a Poisson process.

Having done this, how close were the resulting counts to a Poisson distribution? The mean rate was exactly 2.3 events per day; that had to be true no matter how the computer distributed the 23 million events. Using Expression 4.2, the variance of the mean count was 2.3007, essentially the same as the predicted variance of 2.3 for a Poisson distribution. This nicely demonstrates that if events are generated by a Poisson process, then the variance will be equal to the mean count. The mean and variance are not equal because anyone made them equal, but because this is what happens when events occur randomly in time or space at a constant rate. I used Poisson's formula (Expression 4.1) to compute the predicted probabilities of counts from 0 to 14 and plotted these along with the observed distribution of counts across the 10 million days. The agreement was excellent (Figure 4.7).

A Poisson distribution can be created using dried beans and a checkerboard. I did this in high school, around 1958; I think the idea came from Scientific American magazine. Put a checkerboard with its 8 x 8 = 64 squares in the bottom of a cardboard box. Be sure there is little space between the outer margins of the squares and the walls of the box, so that each bean lands in a square and the square sizes are equal. Select 32 dry navy beans. Throw the beans into the box and count the number of squares with 0 beans, 1 bean, 2, and so on. After several dozen throws, these counts will begin to fit a Poisson distribution. In this example the mean count per square is 32/64 = 0.5 beans per square. This process can be simulated using software. I had the computer generate groups of 32 beans. Each bean was randomly assigned coordinates on the checkerboard by picking two random quantities from a uniform distribution that ranged from 0 to 8. If the first bean was assigned coordinates 4.1 and 2.5, then it was located in the 4th column and 2nd

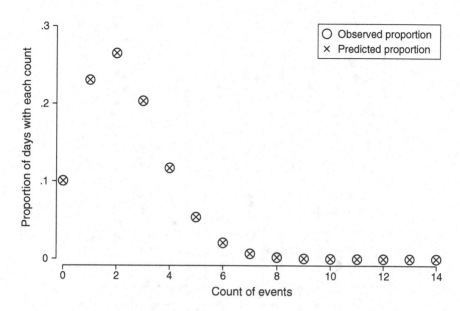

FIGURE 4.7   Observed proportions and predicted probabilities for counts 0 through 14 when there are 23 million events randomly distributed across 10 million day-long intervals. Observed proportions were from a single computer simulation in which events were distributed at a constant rate (stationary property) and without regard to how earlier events were assigned (independence property). Predicted probabilities were from the Poisson distribution for a rate of 2.3 events per day.

row of checkerboard squares starting from the square in the lower left corner. The assignment of each bean to a square was independent of the assignment of any other bean. The process (or rate) was stationary because 32 beans were thrown with each toss. The location of the imaginary beans on the imaginary checkerboard in the first four imaginary tosses is shown in Figure 4.8. The computer created 5000 sets of 32 beans and the proportion of the 64 squares with counts of 0 to 6 beans corresponded closely with the predictions from Expression 4.1 with rate set equal to 0.5 and time (area in this example) set to 1 (Table 4.7).

These simulations demonstrate the principles of a Poisson distribution. If the number of beans (and therefore the rate per square) varies from one throw to the next, the stationary principle is violated and the counts will not fit a Poisson distribution. If too many beans are used, they can crowd each other out of the squares, the independence principle will be violated and the distribution will not be Poisson.

4.16 WHAT IF THE DATA ARE NOT FROM A POISSON PROCESS? PART 1, OVERDISPERSION

The deaths by horse-kick per corps-year were distributed across the corps-year units with counts that were close to a Poisson distribution (Tables 4.2 and 4.3). These data could be generated by a Poisson process with a rate of 0.61 deaths per corps-year. Let us imagine that the number of deaths was 122, as in Tables 4.2 and 4.3, but they were distributed differently. During the years 1875–1879 the new rate of death is 2.44. Since there were 50 corps-years in that 5-year period, the expected number of

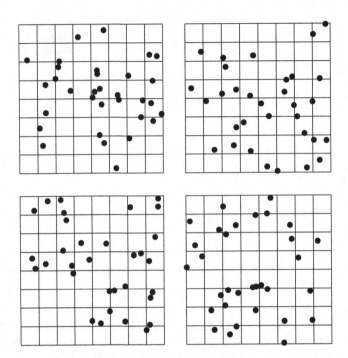

FIGURE 4.8   A computer program created data for imaginary beans thrown randomly onto an imaginary checkerboard with 64 squares. Sets of 32 beans were simulated and the beans were randomly assigned to locations on each checkerboard. The first four checkerboards are shown, each with 32 bean locations randomly selected by the computer.

TABLE 4.7   A computer program created data for beans thrown randomly onto a checkerboard with 64 squares. 5000 sets of 32 beans were simulated and the number of beans on each square was counted. The proportions of the squares with bean counts of 0 through 7 are shown in the table along with the proportions predicted by Expression 4.1 for a Poisson process with rate = 32/64 = 0.5. Bean counts greater than 7 are ignored because they would be so rare.

COUNT OF BEANS	PROPORTION OF SQUARES WITH EACH COUNT IN SIMULATED DATA	PREDICTED PROPORTIONS FROM POISSON FORMULA
0	.604137	.606531
1	.306613	.303265
2	.076016	.075816
3	.011747	.012636
4	.001334	.001580
5	.000141	.000158
6	.000013	.000013
7	.000000	.000001

deaths, on average, was 50 × 2.44 = 122. These were distributed so that 3 corps-years had 0 deaths, 12 had 1, 13 had 2, 10 had 3, 7 had 4, 4 had 5, and the one remaining corps-year had 6 deaths. These counts are (deliberately) close to those expected from a Poisson distribution with mean 2.44. Then from 1880 to 1894, imagine the horse-kick mortality rate fell to 0 and no further deaths occur. There are now more corps-years with counts of 0, 3, 4, 5, and 6 deaths and fewer corps-years with counts of 1 and 2, so compared with Table 4.3, the counts are more spread out or dispersed. The mean count (and rate) per corps-year is still 122/200 = 0.61, but the count variance from Expression 4.2 is 1.64, greater than the previously estimated variance of 0.61. If we use Poisson methods that assume the variance and mean are both 0.61, when the true variance is 1.64, we will get P-values that are too small and CIs that are too narrow. The wider spread in the counts, compared with a Poisson distribution with a mean of 0.61, is called overdispersion.

If the data are overdispersed, we can still use Poisson methods to estimate adjusted rate ratios or differences. Overdispersion will produce incorrect P-values and CIs, but if the model is correct and the study free of biases, the estimated size of the associations will be correct. In Chapter 13 I will show how correct P-values and CIs can still be produced using one of several methods that correct for the overdispersion in the data.

Overdispersion is not limited to Poisson methods. This can be a problem for logistic regression or any method that makes assumptions about the variance rather than estimating the variance from the data.

4.17 WHAT IF THE DATA ARE NOT FROM A POISSON PROCESS? PART 2, UNDERDISPERSION

Now imagine that in the Prussian military data there are 122 corps-years with 1 death and the other 78 corps-years have no deaths, so there are 78 counts of 0 and 122 counts of 1, with no counts of 2, 3, or 4. When the outcome is rare (Figure 4.2), a Poisson distribution may have counts of 0 and 1 with few or no higher counts. But if over half the corps-years have a death the outcome is not rare and these data are unlikely to arise from a Poisson process. With a mean count of 0.61, a Poisson process would likely produce some counts of 2 and 3 (Table 4.3). Instead the counts are bunched into a narrow range with 0s and 1s only; this is underdispersion. While the rate is still 0.61, the variance from Expression 4.2 is now 0.24, smaller than the expected variance of 0.61. If we use Poisson methods that fail to account for underdispersion we will get P-values that are too big, CIs that are too wide. Underdispersion would arise if outcome events are nonrecurrent (such as death) and events are not rare. There are methods for dealing with underdispersion and we can obtain approximately correct P-values and CIs as long as we recognize the underdispersion. In summary, many methods for counts and rates assume that the data were generated by a Poisson process and that the variance is therefore equal to the mean count or rate. But modified Poisson methods allow us to estimate P-values and CIs that relax this assumption about the variance.

4.18 MUST ANYTHING BE RARE?

It is not uncommon to find statements in the literature suggesting that Poisson regression is suited for the analysis of rare events. But if counts arise from a Poisson process, nothing need be rare. Poisson methods are often capable of handling common events, large counts, or large rates. But there are situations where some caution is needed.

First, if the outcome is binary, then Poisson methods that assume the mean and its variance are the same will correctly estimate variances only when the outcome is sufficiently rare that we expect few counts larger than 1 in our data based on the Poisson distribution. This will usually be true, for example, for mortality rates. I have already given a detailed example concerning mortality due to Alzheimer's disease. If counts of 2 or more are expected, but observed counts are never larger than 1, this signifies underdispersion. If the data consists of many records, there are methods for correcting the variance for this underdispersion. But for a single mortality rate these methods cannot be used. So if Poisson methods are used to estimate the precision of a single mortality rate, or to compare two summary mortality rates, estimated P-values and CIs may be too large if the outcome is common. On the other hand, a single mortality rate summarizes data across disparate groups which may experience different rates. So a single mortality rate, or a simple comparison of two summary rates, may be ignoring hidden overdispersion, meaning that estimated P-values and CIs may be too small. There is no solution to this conundrum; for a single summary rate (just one count and one denominator) or a few summary rates, the P-values and CIs from Poisson methods rest on the assumption that the variance and mean are the same. This assumption may be untrue in many instances.

Second, some derivations of the Poisson distribution start with the binomial distribution and show that the Poisson distribution will arise if the outcome is sufficiently rare that no more than one outcome is expected in any interval of time. This clever derivation was used by Poisson himself and appears elsewhere (Armitage, Berry, and Matthews 2002 pp71–74, Clayton and Hills 1993 p115). This derivation has the advantage of avoiding the calculus used by Bateman (1910). But the Poisson distribution can be derived without describing anything as rare and there is no absolute requirement that outcomes must be rare for us to use Poisson methods.

Third, imagine we study a closed population with a nonrecurrent outcome, such as death, and the rates for the outcome are constant among those exposed and not exposed. I described this situation for the TEXCO study in Chapter 3 (Table 3.1, Figures 3.1–3.4). In this situation, the hazard ratio and the rate ratio will be the same. To put this otherwise, if survival times follow an exponential distribution (a consequence of a constant rate), the rate and hazard ratios will agree. But if the rate varies over time, the hazard ratio and rate ratio will diverge as events become more common. By limiting the analysis to a time interval in which events are not common (say <10% of the original population has the event), the rate and hazard ratios will be similar. This will be discussed in Chapter 25 about hazard ratios and survival analysis.

Fourth, if person-time is ignored after the first outcome (i.e., the outcome is or is treated as nonrecurrent) and the outcome is common, rate ratios and rate differences usually will no longer have interpretations as estimates of an average causal effect, even in the absence of any bias (Greenland 1996). This problem arises because rates are not collapsible, a topic discussed in Chapter 8. I can put this another way: when a nonrecurrent outcome is sufficiently rare, using rates based on time to the first event will produce a rate ratio (or difference) that closely approximates the risk ratio (or difference) for the same outcome. These estimates have interpretations as average effects. But when the outcome is common, this agreement of rate and risk ratios will no longer be true, as described in Chapter 2, and because rates are not collapsible, rate ratios or differences will not estimate the average causal effect. This problem does not arise if rates are used to analyze recurrent events and all person-time is used; that is, person-time at risk does not end with the first event. Even if the events are not generated by a Poisson process, the only concern in that situation is that we may need to correct the Poisson variance for under or overdispersion.

There may be a historical reason for statements that the Poisson distribution is suitable for rare events. The monograph by von Bortkiewicz which presented the horse-kick data and spread knowledge about the Poisson distribution was titled "Das Gesetz der Kleinen Zahlen" which means "The Law of Small Numbers" in English (von Bortkewitsch 1898). Just what the author meant by this title has been debated in the literature, but he probably did not mean that the Poisson distribution applied *only* to small numbers; his "law" was something else (Winsor 1947, Haight 1967 pp118–119, Quine and Seneta

1987). Regardless of what von Bortkiewicz meant, the association of his title with the Poisson distribution may contribute to some claims that Poisson methods are suitable when outcomes are uncommon.

In summary, justification for the use of Poisson regression or other Poisson methods does not depend upon whether something is rare or not. But in some situations, the estimates from Poisson methods may have more defensible or useful interpretations if outcomes are uncommon.

4.19 BICYCLIST DEATHS IN 2010 AND 2011

As described at the start of this chapter, the mortality rate of bicyclists (who collided with vehicles) increased from 309.7 per million person-years in 2010 to 311.6 in 2011. Is this increase more than we might expect from one year to the next if a Poisson process with a constant rate produced bicyclist deaths in both years? Using large sample methods (Table 4.4, formulae 5 and 10), the rate difference comparing year 2011 with 2010 was 0.15 (95% CI − .07, +0.38) and the rate ratio was 1.08 (95% CI 0.97, 1.20). The exact confidence limits for the rate ratio were nearly the same, 0.96, 1.20. The two-sided P-value from a Wald test was 0.18 and the two-sided mid-P-value was the same. So the observed difference in rates was not inconsistent with year-to-year rate variations that we expect if the underlying rate is constant. More loosely, the observed change might be due to "chance." This does not mean the observed rate change can be entirely attributed to chance variation, but this is certainly possible. Nor does this mean we should have no concern about this problem. The best mortality rate would be zero and we would like to see a declining rate over time.

Criticism of Incidence Rates

5

Some authors have suggested that incidence rates have no useful interpretation or are so seriously flawed that they should not be used. Examining these criticisms can shed some light on the properties of rates.

5.1 FLORENCE NIGHTINGALE, WILLIAM FARR, AND HOSPITAL MORTALITY RATES. DEBATE IN 1864

Florence Nightingale (b.1820–d.1910) has been described as the founder of modern nursing. She also made contributions to medical statistics and was the first female member of the Royal Statistical Society (Wikipedia). The third edition of her book about hospital design, published in 1863, advocated for clean, spacious, well-ventilated wards (Nightingale 1863). To show that some hospitals might be healthier than others, she reproduced (Nightingale 1863 p3) part of a table from Britain's 1861 census report from the Registrar General (Registrar General 1863 p205), showing data for 24 London hospitals and 25 rural hospitals (Table 5.1). The table showed the count of inpatients on April 8, 1861, the count of deaths during 1861, and the mortality rate per 100 patient-years. Assuming the April 8 inpatient count represents the average daily amount of inpatient time in days, we can multiply that count by 365 to estimate inpatient-days for the entire year and divide by 365 to convert inpatient-days to inpatient-years. The mortality rate per 100 patient-years is 100 x (deaths in 1861)/(365 x (inpatients on April 8)/365) = 100 x deaths/(inpatients on April 8). The number of inpatients on April 8 was used because it was available: April 8 was the date of the census. The inpatient count was greater in winter and smaller in summer, so April 8 may be a good choice (Farr 1864b).

The hospital mortality rates in the table had the title "Mortality per Cent on Inmates" in both the Registrar General's report (Registrar General 1863 p205) and Nightingale's book (Nightingale 1863 p3). This usage of "per Cent" meant deaths "per 100," but failed to state that the units were patient-years. This use of per cent was common in that era; the Registrar General's report referred to event rates per unit of person-time, usually per person-year based upon the mid-year population estimate, as "annual mortality per 100," "death-rate per cent," or "rate per cent" in dozens of tables. Proportions were described as "proportion per cent." Throughout the report it is easy to distinguish rates based upon person-time from proportions, despite the use of "per cent" for both (Registrar General 1863). Nightingale understood that a mortality per cent of 90.84 was the same as a mortality rate of .9084 per 1 inpatient-year: "We have 24 London hospitals, affording a mortality of no less than 90.84 per cent, very nearly every [occupied] bed yielding a death in the course of a year" (Nightingale 1863 p4).

Nightingale thought clean air promoted health and that densely-populated industrial cities were unhealthy. In discussing the hospital mortality data she wrote:

TABLE 5.1   Hospital mortality rates in England in 1861.

HOSPITAL CATEGORY	NUMBER OF INPATIENTS ON APRIL 8, 1861	NUMBER OF DEATHS IN 1861	MORTALITY INCIDENCE RATE PER 100 PATIENT-YEARS
24 London hospitals	4214	3828	90.8
25 County and Provincial Hospitals	2248	886	39.4

Data from William Farr, published in Nightingale, Florence. 1863. *Notes on Hospitals*. 3rd ed. London: Longman, Green, Longman, Roberts, and Green. The original table labeled the last column "Mortality per Cent on Inmates."

> Here we have at once a hospital problem demanding solution. However the great differences in the death rates may be explained, it cannot be denied that the most unhealthy hospitals are those situated within the vast circuit of the metropolis ... and that by far the most healthy hospitals are those of the smaller country towns.
>
> *(Nightingale 1863 p4)*

She qualified her remarks by noting that patients in different hospitals could differ regarding age, type of illness, and illness severity (Nightingale 1863 p2). She seemed impressed by the mortality differences, but not confident that the differences necessarily reflected the sanitary conditions of the hospitals.

On January 30, 1864, the *Medical Times and Gazette* published an unsigned review of Nightingale's book (Anonymous 1864c). While favorable in its final paragraphs, most of the review was devoted to attacking the Registrar General's table of hospital mortality rates:

> In 1861, returns were obtained ... giving the number of inmates in each on April 8. The number of deaths registered in each Hospital during the year 1861 is also given. Our readers will hardly believe that on these two bases a percentage of mortality is struck. The inmates of a single day are balanced with the deaths of a whole year ... Surely it is the very essence of percentages ... that the figures dealt with should stand on one and the same bottom, and that deaths for one year should be compared with admissions or discharges for that period ... The problem as here put is exactly that so often asked of forward schoolboys – what is the quotient of a hundred apples divided by fifteen red herrings.

The reviewer did not understand the meaning of a mortality rate with a patient-time denominator and thought the percents were incidence proportions, a case fatality proportion with each "case" being a hospital admission.

An exchange of angry letters followed, much of the content snide and arrogant. Nightingale avoided this exchange, leaving her defense to her friend William Farr (b.1807–d.1883), a physician who worked for the Registrar-General, the English agency established in 1836 to collect health and population statistics. Farr promoted the use of incidence rates (Farr 1838, Susser and Adelstein 1975, Langmuir 1976, Eyler 2003, Gerstman 2003, Hill 2004) and he may have created the table that Nightingale used. In addition, in the same Registrar General's report, he contributed an appendix that discussed hospital mortality rates and presented a table showing how rates varied by hospital size (Farr 1863). Farr described the difference between incidence proportions and incidence rates in a paper in 1838; in that article he called proportions "mortality" and incidence rates "the force of mortality" (Farr 1838).

On February 13 a letter by Farr explained how a mortality rate was calculated, although his words " ... dividing the deaths in a given time by the lifetime ... " were not terribly clear (Farr 1864b). Farr also described how a hospital admission fatality proportion was calculated and presented data from 1839 showing that of 100 admitted patients, 9 died in London hospitals and 4 in country hospitals. The incidence proportion ratio comparing London with rural hospitals was 9/4 = 2.25 and the incidence rate ratio from Table 5.1 was 90.8/39.4 = 2.30; the choice of mortality statistic did not matter much. Unsigned comments from the editor also appeared on Feb 13; these had a civil tone (Editor 1864). The editor thought the different case-mix from one hospital to the next made it difficult to interpret mortality differences: "Any comparison which ignores the difference between the apple-cheeked farm-labourers who seek relief at Stoke Pogis (probably for rheumatism and sore legs), and the wizzened, red-herring-like mechanics of Soho or Southwark, who come into London Hospitals, is fallacious." On February 20 short letters from J. S. Bristowe (a physician) (Bristowe 1864b) and the anonymous reviewer (Anonymous 1864a) dumped fuel on the fire. Another letter from Farr on February 27 (Farr 1864a) quoted some of his remarks in the Registrar-General's Twenty-Fourth Report (Farr 1863) showing mortality incidence rates for a variety of institutions in 1861: mental institutions (11 deaths per 100 occupant-years), workhouses for the poor (19), and hospitals (57). He charged that unsanitary and crowded hospital conditions spread disease and killed patients and wrote that better hospital statistics were needed to study this problem. On April 30 Bristowe showed how admission fatality proportions (with admissions as the denominator) and mortality rates (with patient-time as the denominator) could be calculated (Bristowe 1864a). Bristowe understood the difference but argued that most readers would not. He felt that mortality rates greater than 100% would be misinterpreted and that rates based upon patient-time served no purpose.

Similar debates erupted in *The Lancet*, where Nightingale's book was reviewed on Feb 27 (Anonymous 1864b). An anonymous reviewer lauded the book but focused on the mortality differences between urban and rural hospitals. This reviewer understood how mortality rates were estimated and described them as

> … a mode of estimating mortality by the number of deaths which each [occupied] bed gives annually, and is a more equal and safe way of determining mortality than by estimating it per head from patients passing through the hospital, who stay for very varying periods.

The reviewer discussed the table of hospital mortality rates presented by Farr in the Registrar General's report (Farr 1863). The reviewer felt that differences in the patient populations might account for the rate differences and suggested that this should be studied by collecting data regarding the diagnoses of admitted patients. A letter on March 19 from T. Holmes (a surgeon) (Holmes 1864a) called Farr's statistics "utterly delusive." Holmes wrote that " … Farr is attempting to settle by statistics a question which mere figures are not sufficient to solve." Holmes wrote that he had visited most British hospitals and based on his observations " … the difference in mortality depends entirely (or almost entirely) on the difference in the severity of the cases under treatment … " A March 26 letter from Holmes (1864c) argued that Farr's rates were flawed because they failed to account for "the varying period of treatment at different hospitals." Holmes noted that a hospital could reduce its mortality incidence rate just by keeping patients for a longer period; he assumed that staying longer would not increase the likelihood of death. He described two hypothetical hospitals. The first treated only terminally ill cancer patients: 36 patients were admitted in a year, 6 died, and 30 patient-years of time are accumulated for a mortality rate of 100 × (6/30) = 20 per 100 patient-years. The second hospital treated trauma patients: 360 were admitted in a year, 26 died, and 30 patient-years of time are accumulated for a mortality rate of 87 per 100 patient-years. Holmes argued that since all the admitted cancer patients would die in the hospital, whereas most of the injury patients would survive, the rates were misleading. He refused to acknowledge or did not realize that these rates describe what we expect when we compare mortality due to an ultimately fatal but chronic condition with mortality due to an acute illness during which death or recovery will occur quickly.

On April 9, a rambling response from Farr discussed the Greek temples of Asclepius, hospitals in Paris, Prospero from The Tempest, and rudely declared "It is not my office to give any writer lessons in the first elements of statistical learning … " (Farr 1864c). He suggested, as he did in another letter (Farr 1864b), that it made little difference whether hospitals were compared using mortality incidence rates or mortality incidence proportions: " … the relative mortality is nearly the same by the two methods." He felt both methods could be used and said that he had recommended that approach to the "Lunacy Commissioners" who regulated insane asylums. In response to the example offered by Holmes regarding cancer patients, Farr gave one of his best arguments for incidence rates:

> … if the mortality in one cancer hospital is at the rate of 212 deaths to every 100 occupied beds, here is a basis of comparison with any other hospital *treating the same class of cases* [italics added]. But the usual method in such cases is to divide the annual deaths by the annual admissions; and what does that show? If the cases were all followed to their fatal termination, it would show almost invariably a mortality of 100 per cent, whatever the future lifetime of the patient might be. Yet under bad treatment cancer patients might live half as long as they live under skilful treatment; and this would be clearly shown in the doubling of the annual rate of mortality by the true method.

Holmes (1864b) and Bristowe (1864c) had the last word on April 16. Both were indignant and self-righteous. Holmes wrote that he could not understand Farr's remarks about rates; it is hard to tell if Holmes really did not understand or was so angry that he refused to acknowledge any explanation Farr might offer. Holmes even took a swipe at Nightingale:

> … I may perhaps be allowed to say about Miss Nightingale – that the good by which she has earned the love and gratitude of her countrymen and all the whole world was done by personal service and personal work in hospitals, not by summing up figures.

These letters reflect misunderstandings about mortality incidence rates. One reviewer did not understand what these were, and others who understood the calculations saw no utility in these statistics. In fairness to these critics, describing the rates as "mortality per cent" without units, while customary at the time, was not clear and William Farr's bombastic letters were unhelpful. The debate was muddled by the terminology of the era; today we distinguish between mortality incidence rates and admission fatality proportions, but in the letters both were called "death-rates."

Other issues clouded the debate. Nightingale and Farr suspected that crowded hospitals for the poor were spreading fatal febrile diseases, but transmission of infection was poorly understood in 1864. Ignaz Semmelweis's (b.1818–d.1865) advice about handwashing was still ignored. John Snow (b.1813–d.1858) stopped a London cholera epidemic in 1856 by convincing officials to remove the handle from the Broad Street water pump, but the concept that water could carry disease was not yet accepted. Joseph Lister's (b.1827–d.1912) studies of antiseptics would not be published until 1867. Louis Pasteur (b.1822–d.1895) and Robert Koch (b.1843–d.1910) were unknown in 1864. Many physicians resented suggestions that they might cause harm.

Most parties to this debate were concerned about the future location for St. Thomas' Hospital. This London institution was founded in the 12th century in Southwark (Wikipedia). Nightingale started her new nursing school there in 1860. The hospital was forced to move in 1862 and Holmes and Bristowe (who worked at St Thomas') prepared a report for the government regarding a new location. Farr feared that the hospital would be moved to the unhealthy air by the banks of the Thames in Stangate (Farr 1864c). The new hospital did indeed open in Stangate (Lambeth) in 1871, using designs based on Nightingale's suggestions. The arguments regarding the new location spilled over into the letters about mortality rates.

The letter writers had different views about the value of statistics. Farr and Nightingale thought better statistics would lead to better decisions which would improve health care (Vandenbroucke and Vandenbroucke-Grauls 1988). Holmes thought otherwise; "I believed medical men to be pretty well agreed that conclusions founded only on hospital death-rates, without further facts, were hardly worth examination" (Holmes 1864c). He preferred to rely upon his personal examination of hospitals (Holmes 1864a).

5.2 FLORENCE NIGHTINGALE, WILLIAM FARR, AND HOSPITAL MORTALITY RATES. DEBATE IN 1996–1997

In 1996 Iezzoni published an article titled "100 apples divided by 15 red herrings: a cautionary tale from the mid-19th century on comparing hospital mortality rates" (Iezzoni 1996a). The apple and herrings part of the title was from the 1864 review of Nightingale's book (Anonymous 1864c), in which the reviewer misunderstood the meaning of a mortality rate; unfortunately, Iezzoni made the same mistake. Iezzoni discussed incidence proportions and incidence rates and thought the two could be compared without concern for the units used. While discussing a mortality rate of 90.8 per 100 patient-years she wrote: " ... hospital mortality rates improved considerably when calculated as the annual number of deaths divided by the total number of inpatients treated during the year. By using this method, mortality rates in ... 14 London hospitals average 9.7%." Iezzoni thought that an incidence rate of 90.8 per 100 patient-years was somehow worse than an incidence proportion (more correctly, an admission-fatality proportion) of 9.7%. She failed to realize that the denominator of an incidence rate can change its units, so the mortality rate of 90.8 per 100 patient-years could have been expressed as 0.908 deaths per patient-year, a quantity that looks "smaller" than 9.7%.

As noted in Chapter 2 (Expressions 2.11, 2.12, and related discussion), a comparison of risks and rates will be misleading unless both use the same time scale. We do not know the number of admissions in 1861 for the hospitals in Table 5.1, but Farr said in a letter (Farr 1864b) that there were 9 deaths for every 100 admissions in a group of London hospitals; this agrees well with the incidence proportion of .097 that Iezzoni reported. Because the risk of death per admission is < .2, Expression 2.11 can be used: mortality incidence proportion of .09 per admission lasting X days is equal to the incidence rate of .908/ 365 patient-days × X days. So the average stay per admission was about 365 × .09/.908 = 36 days. The incidence proportion of .09 in 36 days should be compared with an incidence rate of .09 deaths/per 36 patient-days. Iezzoni further confused the discussion by not realizing that mortality per occupied bed per year was just another way of saying mortality per patient-year.

Iezzoni wrote: "Today, observers might view Farr and Nightingale as erring in their calculations or intentionally skewing statistics ... " This seems unfair. Farr's calculations were correct for incidence rates and Nightingale (1863 pp3–4), Holmes (1864c), and Bristowe (1864a) understood the calculations. Holmes and Bristowe thought the rate statistics were useless for comparison, but they did not dispute the arithmetic.

Two Dutch epidemiologists defended Farr and Nightingale in a letter that explained how incidence rates are calculated for hospital events (Vandenbroucke and Vandenbroucke-Grauls 1996). Iezzoni's reply conceded no mistakes and argued that only incidence proportions should be used to compare hospitals in public documents (Iezzoni 1996b). The two epidemiologists were not placated and wrote another letter (Vandenbroucke and Vandenbroucke-Grauls 1997). Iezzoni's response gave them no satisfaction, claiming that " ... deaths per 100 days in hospital ... would not make intuitive sense to the average reader" (Iezzoni 1997).

What statistic should be used to compare hospitals? When a comparison is made, hospitals with the worst outcomes may argue that their patients were the sickest. That could be true. We want to make comparisons that remove bias due to between-hospital differences in illness severity, patient age, inter-hospital transfers, and other factors that affect mortality. Granted that we can do better than the crude comparisons used by Farr, should we prefer incidence rates or proportions? For an event that may arise during the course of hospitalization with occurrence roughly proportional to the amount of time spent in the hospital, an incidence rate may be the best choice. Examples include hospital-acquired infections (Vandenbroucke and Vandenbroucke-Grauls 1988, Freeman 1996), medication errors, and falls. For an outcome such as death after admission for coronary artery bypass surgery, hip fracture, or pneumonia, the admission fatality incidence proportion seems reasonable to me. It may be ideal to calculate this statistic by following each admitted person to death or discharge, even if the final outcome of some persons admitted in one year may occur in the next year. An alternative is to count the deaths from January 1 to December 31 and divide by admissions during that same interval, even though some deaths may arise among persons admitted in the previous year and some deaths will not have occurred among persons admitted near the end of the year. Most admissions are short in acute care hospitals and if the admissions and discharges are in a steady state, omitting a few admissions from the denominator at the start of the year and omitting a few deaths from the numerator after the end of the year will tend to balance each other, reducing any error. An alternative that may be more precise is to calculate (deaths during the year)/(admissions in that year + inpatient count on January 1 – inpatient count on December 31); this method was used in the middle of the 19th century (Anonymous 1865).

As discussed in Chapter 2, a case-fatality incidence proportion, or an admission-fatality proportion, is not a risk. Strictly speaking risks involve a measure of time. Most hospital admissions are short, so this proportion can be treated as a risk; the admission-fatality proportion is approximately the risk that admitted patients will die in the next week or so before being discharged.

There are still many difficulties with efforts to fairly compare hospital performance. But I agree with William Farr's view that both rates and proportions may be useful statistics (Farr 1864a, 1864c).

5.3 CRITICISM OF RATES IN THE BRITISH MEDICAL JOURNAL IN 1995

In 1982 Riggs et al. (1982) described outcomes for postmenopausal women given different treatments for osteoporosis. Groups were compared using fracture incidence rates: counts of new fractures per 1000 years of follow-up time. Over the next decade several studies used fracture incidence rates as outcome measures (Palmieri et al. 1989, Pak, Sakhaee, and Zerwekh 1990, Riggs et al. 1990, Storm et al. 1990, Watts et al. 1990, Kleerekoper et al. 1991, Lufkin et al. 1992, Tilyard et al. 1992). Most of the studies examined the rate of new vertebral fractures, which are common in this population and can be identified by repeated x-ray studies.

In 1995 Windeler and Lange (1995) published an article in the *British Medical Journal* criticizing the use of fracture incidence rates. Their main concern was that counting two or more fractures from the same patient violated the assumption of independence that underlies many statistical tests.

If we use a statistical method that requires an assumption of independence and that assumption is not true, we can still estimate the ratio or difference of two rates, but estimates of the variance, confidence intervals (CI), and P-values will be wrong If the fracture rate is approximately the same for all study subjects, varies little during follow-up, and is not much changed by the occurrence of each fracture, then the counts of fractures in the population will follow a Poisson distribution with patients having 0, 1, 2, 3, or more fractures in any given period of time. A Poisson process generates events that are independent of each other in any small window of time; the probability of an event depends upon the constant rate and the length of the time interval (Cameron and Trivedi 2013a pp5–6). If a person has two or more fractures, this does not violate any assumption about independence for a Poisson process; indeed, if the mean rate is large enough, failure to find persons with two or more fractures would be evidence that the data were not from a Poisson process. Windeler and Lange knew this, but wrote that an assumption of a constant rate "is hardly ever justified in clinical medicine" (Windeler and Lange 1995). People do vary in their fracture risk (and therefore their fracture rate), but the trials considered here all selected patients thought to be at high risk for fractures. If the selection process was sufficiently refined a trial might have a population that was fairly homogeneous in risk for a fracture. The trial reports did not present details that would allow us to determine whether the rates were from a Poisson process.

Windeler and Lange (1995) discussed the possibility that the fracture rate could be constant and therefore follow a Poisson distribution within each patient, but the rate might vary between patients. In this situation they felt "no simple estimator is available ... to describe a group of patients." This situation, however, is described by the negative binomial distribution which assumes that each unit (person, geographic region, cavalry regiment) generates counts at a constant rate, but variation in the rates between units follows a gamma distribution (McCullagh and Nelder 1989 pp198–200). The use of the negative binomial distribution for counts and rates was described in articles and books prior to or during 1995 (Greenwood and Yule 1920, Fisher 1941, McCullagh and Nelder 1989 pp198–200, Glynn et al. 1993, Stukel et al. 1994, Gardner, Mulvey, and Shaw 1995, Levy, Vernick, and Howard 1995). Negative binomial regression models became available in GLIM software in 1992, in Stata in 1993, and in SAS in 1994 (Hilbe 2011 pp5–11). An osteoporosis study by Kleerekoper et al. (1991) mentioned that they used the negative binomial distribution for their power calculations.

Windeler and Lange (1995) went on to claim that no statistically valid analysis was possible if no assumption of a constant rate could be made. This ignored a growing literature regarding regression analysis of recurrent events (Zeger and Liang 1986, Lawless 1987, Thall 1988, Breslow and Clayton 1993). Variations in fracture rates that produce under- or overdispersion could be dealt with using robust variance estimators, bootstrap methods, and rerandomization methods. All of these will be discussed in Chapter 13.

Aside from their concerns about statistical methods, Windeler and Lange (1995) argued that a comparison of rates has no useful clinical interpretation. They expressed concern that a rate of 20 per 100 person-years might derive from 20 persons who each have 2 fractures during 10 years of observation or 1000 persons who were followed for 0.5 years during which 100 had a single fracture. Their calculations were correct, but it is not clear why these facts troubled them. When it is relevant, these two different situations can be described by presenting the rate numerator and denominator information with sufficient clarity.

Windeler and Lange (1995) wrote that " ... the fracture rates do not provide the information needed to decide about the application of a certain treatment to the individual patient." But if persons who receive treatment A have a fracture rate of 20 per 100 person-years and those who receive treatment B have a fracture rate of 10 per 100 years, why wouldn't this information be relevant to clinical decisions? When we do a randomized study of the association between a treatment and an outcome, we estimate the overall association. Whether that overall association is the effect we can expect in any individual will usually be unknown. The treatment may have no effect on the outcomes of some, harmful effects on others, and beneficial effects for the rest. If, in aggregate, benefit outweighs harm, the rate of the outcome will be less in the treated subjects and the treatment that produces this lower rate will be preferred by the next patient, unless we have specific reasons to think that this particular patient will not be benefited.

In 1996 the *British Medical Journal* published a rejoinder to Winderler and Lange. Glynn and Buring (1996) described how the negative binomial distribution could be applied to rates, gave an example of the generalized estimating equation (GEE) approach of Zeger and Liang (1986), and cited some of the literature about recurrent events. They gave examples of how the analysis of rates might add to knowledge. Their article helped disseminate knowledge about rate analysis, particularly the use of the negative binomial distribution.

Windeler and Lange (1995) were correct that an analysis of fracture rates might produce CIs that were too small if fracture rates between subjects varied more than expected under the Poisson distribution. It was reasonable for them to ask for information about the distribution of fracture counts. But their criticisms often ignored available statistical literature regarding the analysis of recurrent events. Perhaps their most useful contribution was to stimulate Glynn and Buring (1996) to publish their response.

5.4 CRITICISM OF INCIDENCE RATES IN 2009

In 2009 an article by Kraemer (2009) appeared with the provocative title: "Events per person-time (incidence rate): a misleading statistic?" Her article began with the general claim that the field of epidemiology often produces misleading studies and she suggested one reason for this problem is that epidemiologists sometimes use incidence rates. Kraemer focused her discussion on events that happen once, in which people are followed to that event and no further, so independence of events was not an issue in her article.

Several of Kraemer's concerns are valid, but unrelated to the use of incidence rates. For example, she pointed out that if subjects enter a study on different dates, their risk for the outcome may vary with entry date and failure to account for this might produce bias. This is true, but this is also true for studies that use risk ratios or odd ratios or risk differences. Failure to account properly for changes over calendar time, time since birth (age), time since an event (start of treatment, start of smoking, time since delivering a child), or other measures of time can produce bias (Greenland 1987c, Altman and Royston 1988). It is also true that if some subjects are lost to follow-up, bias may arise depending on the reasons for this attrition. But Kraemer endorsed Kaplan-Meier methods and the proportional hazards model, both of which can be biased due to attrition.

The heart of Kraemer's criticism of incidence rates lies in an example shown in her figures 1 and 2 and described on pages 1034–1035 of her paper. Using formulae in Kraemer's paper (where each formula for her Figure 2 says P', Kraemer meant P, the proportion of each population that can have the outcome after infinite time has passed), I recreated her example in Figure 5.1. In Group 1 the risk of the outcome increases quickly with time, but then tapers off and never exceeds 0.5. In Group 2 the outcome risk increases more slowly, but it will reach 0.9 if subjects are followed long enough. The top panel of Figure 5.1 shows the cumulative incidence (risk) for each group at time t up to 30 time units. Given these risks, the resulting incidence rate per time unit is shown in the middle panel of Figure 5.1 for each time up to 30 units. In Group 1, the rate is 0.1 initially but falls to 0.03 at time 30. In Group 2 the rate changes little over time, from 0.045 to 0.041. The risk and rate ratios, shown in the bottom panel of Figure 5.1, are not too far apart over the interval shown, but the risk ratio is 1 at time 15.0 and the rate ratio is 1 at time 17.8.

Kraemer noted that the risk ratio and the odds ratio are equal to 1 at time 15.0 when the two risk curves cross each other. At that point the cumulative incidence of death is the same in both groups. But since the incidence rate ratio is 1 at time 17.8, she declared that the incidence rate ratio "is uninterpretable." But this ratio has a ready interpretation; the rate ratio reflects the fact that events come more quickly in Group 1 and at 17.8 time units the ratio of cumulated events to cumulated event-free person-time is equal in both groups. The speed with which events occurred is used in the calculation of the rate ratio. The risk and odds ratios, however, compare the proportion that survive at each time, without any concern that the events came more quickly in one group compared with the other. The reasons for differences in cumulative incidence and incidence rate were discussed in Chapter 2 in relation to Figures 2.4 and 2.5.

Kraemer correctly points out that risks and rates do not estimate the same thing and risk and rate ratios may not agree. But because they do not always agree does not necessarily make one of these statistics superior to the other or either of them uninterpretable. If they differ, understanding the reason for any difference may provide useful knowledge. Kraemer is also correct in suggesting that when we estimate a rate ratio, we sometimes wish to interpret it as if it were a risk ratio. While that interpretation is not always correct, it may be close enough in many studies to be of use. Even in the extreme example that she gives (Figure 5.1), the risk and rate ratios do not differ greatly. At time 15, when the risk ratio is 1, the rate ratio is 1.1, and at time 17.8, when the rate ratio is 1, the risk ratio is 0.92; not terribly different. Kraemer implies that the odds ratio is useful because it also equals 1 at time 15. But in her example, the rate ratio approximates the risk ratio more closely than the odds ratio does at time units less than 10.4 or greater than 18.

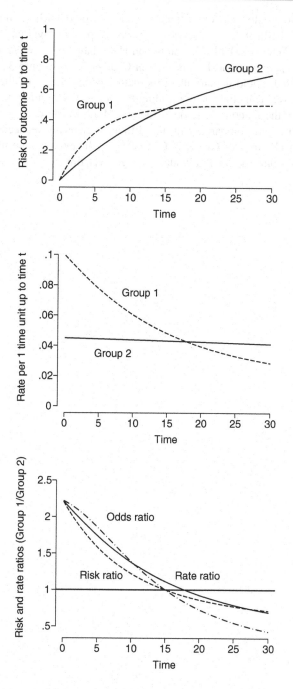

FIGURE 5.1 In Group 1 outcome risk (cumulative incidence) increases quickly but never exceeds 0.5. In Group 2 outcome risk increases more slowly but eventually reaches 0.9. The top panel shows the risks at each time t, the middle panel shows the incidence rates to time t, and the bottom panel shows the risk, rate, and odds ratios.

Any analysis of the data in Figure 5.1 would face difficulties. Because the hazards for the outcome are not proportional (i.e., the ratio of the instantaneous rates for the outcome changes throughout the study period and even changes direction), a Cox proportional hazards analysis, as usually performed, would not be suitable. No single ratio or difference statistic would fairly summarize a comparison of Groups 1 and 2 (Hernán 2010). A better analysis might be to plot survival curves (Hernán 2010) or to use the life expectancy difference (Dehbi, Royston, and Hackshaw 2017). Kraemer's example is similar to the Army data for Companies A and B described in Chapter 3 and Figure 3.5. Whether membership in Group 1 or 2 is preferred would depend upon the nature of the outcome, the costs or difficulties of being in one group or the other, feelings about trading the possibility of an earlier outcome for the hope of more time later without the outcome, and other factors. Modest differences between the risk and rate ratios may be a minor problem compared with the difficulty of trying to decide whether it would be better to be a member of Group 1 or Group 2. Chapter 25 will review some methods of analysis that may be used when rates or hazards for individuals change over time.

Stratified Analysis

Standardized Rates

6

Mortality due to drowning ranged from 2.4 to 5.2 per 100,000 person-years in Alaska during 2006–2010 (Table 6.1) (CDC WONDER). Alaska has a small population and the number of drownings fluctuated substantially from year to year. To describe the drowning rate in Alaska with more precision, we could summarize the rate over the entire 5-year interval. If we do this, we are essentially assuming that there is an underlying process or several processes that generate drowning deaths at a constant rate over the 5-year interval, and the observed yearly variations reflect what we loosely call chance. We may not truly believe this assumption, but we may still feel that a summary rate over 5-years is a better estimate of Alaska's drowning rate than a rate from just one of the years. A 5-year rate might be preferred if we want to compare Alaska's drowning rates with those of other states.

The numerator for the 5-year rate is the counts of deaths over five years and the rate denominator is 3,452,183 person-years, the sum of person-time for all five years: $100,000 \times 131/3,452,183 = 3.8$ drowning deaths per 100,000 person-years (Expression 6.1). We can get the same 5-year rate by calculating a weighted average of the rates using weights equal to the person-time estimate for each year. If we index each yearly observation with subscript i, use C for counts of deaths, and T for person-time, then

$$
\begin{aligned}
&5 - \text{year rate} \\
&= \text{sum}[C_i]/\text{sum}[T_i] \\
&= (21 + 27 + 29 + 17 + 37)/(675,302 + 680,300 + 687,455 + 698,895 + 710,231) \\
&= 131/3,452,183 \\
&= .0000379 \text{ per 1 person} - \text{year} \\
&= \text{sum}[(C_i/T_i) \times T_i]/\text{sum}[T_i] \\
&= \text{sum}[\text{rate}_i \times T_i]/\text{sum}[T_i] \\
&= \text{sum}[\text{rate}_i \times T_i/T]/\text{sum}[T_i/T]
\end{aligned}
$$

(Ex.6.1)

All of the expressions in Expression 6.1 produce the same rate. In the last line of Expression 6.1 the weights are equal to the proportion of total 5-year person-time in each year and the sum of those weights, $\text{sum}[T_i/T]$, is equal to 1.

The weighted average of the five yearly rates is a *standardized* rate, standardized to the distribution of Alaska-resident person-time in each of the 5 years. Any crude rate can be thought of as a standardized rate. For example, the drowning rate in Alaska in 2010 can be thought of as a weighted average of stratum-specific rates with strata for the age or sex distribution of Alaskans in that year and weights equal to the stratum-specific person-time (population) by age or sex in that year.

TABLE 6.1 Counts and rates of death due to drowning in Alaska, 2006–2010. Rates are per 100,000 person-years.

YEAR	DEATHS	MID-YEAR POPULATION	RATE
2006	21	675,302	3.11
2007	27	680,300	3.97
2008	29	687,455	4.22
2009	17	698,895	2.43
2010	37	710,231	5.21

Data from CDC WONDER. Compressed Mortality File. CDC WONDER Online Database. http://wonder.cdc.gov: Centers for Disease Control and Prevention, National Center for Health Statistics.

6.1 WHY STANDARDIZE?

Standardized rates are used to compare the rates of two or more populations while removing differences due to a potential confounding factor. The confounding factor could be population differences in the distribution of income or smoking. Because age is powerfully related to mortality and commonly available in data, standardization is often used to remove differences in rates due to different age distributions in the compared populations. It is also common to use standardization to remove rate differences related to sex, another variable often known. Standardization of mortality rates on sex is usually less important than age-standardization, as differences in the distribution of sex between populations is often small and variations in mortality related to sex are usually less than those related to age.

The use of standardization (weighted-averaging) of rates to remove confounding bias is computationally simple and came into use over two centuries ago. Indirect standardization was used in 1777 by Englishman William Dale and in 1786 by the German Johannes Tetens (Keiding 1987). Both men said that some life insurance societies were underfunded because observed deaths of beneficiaries were less common than expected deaths based on mortality rates of the general population. The beneficiaries were apparently healthier than the general population and both Dale and Tetens pointed out that this meant payments would be needed for a longer time than the fund actuaries had predicted using life expectancy data from the entire population. In 1844, Neison (1844, Keiding 1987 p5741) described both direct and indirect standardization. In 1859 William Farr (1859 pp174–176) used indirect standardization to compare mortality in London with mortality in a group of districts that he deemed to be healthy. These early examples of standardization used strata for age and sex.

6.2 EXTERNAL WEIGHTS FROM A STANDARD POPULATION: DIRECT STANDARDIZATION

Imagine we know the event rates for population A, such as the rate of cancer mortality among a cohort of workers exposed to a chemical, the rate of myocardial infarction in a geographic region, or the rate of hip fracture among members of a health plan. We may wish to know if these rates differ from rates in some other population B but have concern that populations A and B differ with regard to age. To remove most of any rate difference related to different population age distributions, we could calculate the incidence rates for population A within 10-year age groups and calculate a weighted average of those rates using the age distribution of population B. This is called direct standardization, with the person-time distribution of population B used as the standard. It is also called external standardization, as the weighted-average rate for population A uses person-time weights from population B, a population external to population A. The directly standardized rate for population A can then be compared with the crude rate of population B, which is already standardized to the person-time of population B (Expression 6.1).

Formulae for direct standardization can be written in several ways that are similar to Expression 6.1. We can use subscript i to index the strata, subscript A to indicate the exposed cohort, subscript S to indicate the standard population, T for person-time, and C for counts of events:

directly standardized rate for population A using standard population S

$$= sum[rate_{Ai} \times T_{Si}]/sum[T_{Si}]$$
$$= sum[rate_{Ai} \times T_{Si}]/T_S$$
$$= sum[rate_{Ai} \times T_{Si}/T_S]$$

(Ex.6.2)

The observed event count in population A can be expressed as:

observed total event count in population A

$$= C_A$$
$$= sum[C_{Ai}]$$
$$= sum[rate_{Ai} \times T_{Ai}]$$
$$= T_A \times sum[rate_{Ai} \times T_{Ai}]/T_A$$
$$= rate_A \times T_A$$

(Ex.6.3)

Expression 6.3 assumes that the person-time units are the same for both person-time and the rate.

We can define the expected count in population A, C_{Aexp}, as the total person-time from population A multiplied by the directly standardized rate from Expression 6.2. This is the count we expect from the total person-time in population A if the stratum-specific rates of population A are weighted using the person-time distribution of the standard population:

expected count in population A using standard population weights

$$= C_{Aexp}$$
$$= T_A \times sum[rate_{Ai} \times T_{Si}]/sum[T_{Si}]$$
$$= T_A \times sum[rate_{Ai} \times T_{Si}]/T_S$$
$$= (T_A/T_S) \times sum[rate_{Ai} \times T_{Si}]$$
$$= T_A \times sum[rate_{Ai} \times T_{Si}/T_S]$$

(Ex.6.4)

Using Expressions 6.2–6.4, we can describe a directly standardized rate in terms of the crude rate and the observed and expected counts in population A:

directly standardized rate for population A using standard population S

$$= sum[rate_{Ai} \times T_{Si}/T_S]$$
$$= T_A \times sum[rate_{Ai} \times T_{Si}/T_S]/T_A$$
$$= C_{Aexp}/T_A$$
$$= rate_A \times C_{Aexp}/rate_A \times T_A$$
$$= rate_A \times C_{Aexp}/C_A$$

(Ex.6.5)

It is common to see directly standardized rates in reports from public health agencies; the mortality of a population is often standardized to the population distribution of a much larger population. For example, in 2010 the mortality rate due to cancer was 124 per 100,000 person-years in Alaska (Table 6.2) (Murphy, Xu, and Kochanek 2013 Table 19). In the year 2000 the cancer-related mortality rate for the entire United States was 197 (CDC WONDER) (Table 6.3). Do these rates indicate that cold weather prevents cancer? Perhaps bears devour so many Alaskans that few live to the older ages at which most cancers occur? We can examine rates within age groups to see whether Alaska cancer mortality rates differed from those of the United States for people of similar ages. Stratification on age reveals that cancer mortality incidence rates increase with age, exceeding 1800 per 100,000 person-years for those 85 years and older in both Alaska and the United States (CDC WONDER). The United States in 2000 had an older age distribution compared with Alaska in 2010 (Figure 6.1, Tables 6.2 and 6.3); 8% of Alaskans and 12% of all Americans were 65 or older. As age was associated both with region (Alaskans were younger) and with cancer mortality (seniors died of cancer more often), age confounds the crude association of region with cancer mortality. The crude rate per 100,000 person-years for cancer deaths was lower in Alaska compared with the United States: rate difference = 124.5–196.5 = – 72 per 100,000 person-years, rate ratio = 124.5/196.5 = 0.63. This comparison of crude rates is misleading. In the older age strata where most cancer deaths occur, the ratio of the Alaska to U.S. rate was 0.73 for ages 45–54, 0.65 for ages 55–64, 0.81 for ages 65–74, 1.10 for ages 75–84 and 1.00 for age 85 and older; any weighted average of these rate ratios must be larger than 0.63.

Examining 11 age-specific rate ratios or differences is cumbersome. Direct standardization can be used to remove most confounding by age and create a single statistic to compare Alaska's cancer

TABLE 6.2   Age-categorized counts and rates of death due to cancer in Alaska and Florida, 2010. Rates are per 100,000 person-years.

AGE (YRS)	COUNT[a]	ALASKA PERSON-TIME	RATE	COUNT	FLORIDA PERSON-TIME	RATE	RATE RATIO[b]	RATE DIFFERENCE[c]
<1	1	10,828	9.2	2	208,724	1.0	9.64	+8.3
1–4	2	43,168	4.6	22	864,782	2.5	1.82	+2.1
5–14	1	101,703	1.0	29	2,211,102	1.3	0.75	–0.3
15–24	5	106,560	4.7	88	2,457,140	3.6	1.31	+1.1
25–34	9	103,125	8.7	196	2,289,545	8.6	1.02	+0.2
35–44	21	92,974	22.6	746	2,431,254	30.7	0.74	–8.1
45–54	103	111,026	92.8	3,282	2,741,493	119.7	0.77	–26.9
55–64	205	85,909	238.6	7,335	2,337,668	313.8	0.76	–75.1
65–74	233	35,350	659.1	10,734	1,727,940	621.2	1.06	+37.9
75–84	218	14,877	1465.3	11,795	1,097,537	1074.7	1.36	+390.7
85+	86	4,711	1825.5	7,238	434,125	1667.3	1.09	+158.3
All	884	710,231	124.5	41,467	18,801,310	220.6	0.56	–96.1

[a] The public files from CDC Wonder do not report counts for categories with fewer than 10 deaths because of privacy concerns. There were 18 deaths among Alaskans younger than age 35 years, but counts were not reported for age categories in that range. The missing counts were created so that the rates were roughly similar to those of Florida, with the constraint that there had to be at least one death in each Alaska age category.
[b] Rate ratio = Alaska rate/Florida rate.
[c] Rate difference = Alaska rate per 100,000 person-years – Florida rate per 100,000 person-years.
Data from CDC WONDER. Compressed Mortality File. CDC WONDER Online Database. http://wonder.cdc.gov: Centers for Disease Control and Prevention, National Center for Health Statistics.

TABLE 6.3   The United States 2000 standard population. Age-categorized estimates of the U.S. population in 2000 and weights representing the proportion of the population in each age category. The last column shows age-specific rates of death due to cancer in the United States during 2000.

AGE (YRS)	POPULATION ESTIMATES	WEIGHTS PROPORTIONAL TO POPULATION SIZE	CANCER MORTALITY RATES IN 2000 (PER 100,000 PERSON-YEARS)
<1	3,794,901	.01382	2.4175
1–4	15,191,619	.05532	2.7326
5–14	39,976,619	.14556	2.4685
15–24	38,076,743	.13865	4.3717
25–34	37,233,437	.13557	9.8166
35–44	44,659,185	.16261	36.5903
45–54	37,030,152	.13483	127.4857
55–64	23,961,506	.08725	366.6577
65–74	18,135,514	.06604	816.3293
75–84	12,314,793	.04484	1335.6249
85+	4,259,173	.01551	1819.4225
All	274,633,642	1.00000	196.5305*

* The crude rate of 196.5 was calculated using counts from death certificates and person-time from the census in 2000; this rate was directly standardized to the distribution of person-time from the census. If the age-specific rates of cancer in the table are directly standardized to the United States 2000 standard population, which comes from projections made prior to 2000, the result is a rate of 199.6.

Data from CDC WONDER. Compressed Mortality File. CDC WONDER Online Database. http://wonder.cdc.gov: Centers for Disease Control and Prevention, National Center for Health Statistics.

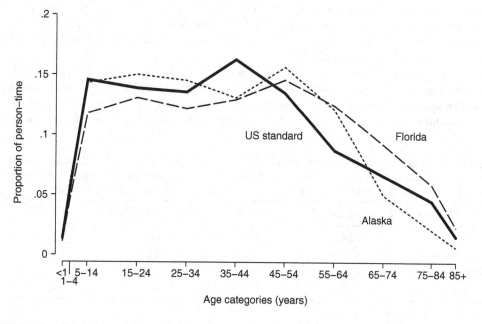

FIGURE 6.1   Age distribution of 3 populations using 11 categories of age: Florida in 2010, Alaska in 2010, and the 2000 U.S. standard.

mortality with U.S. cancer mortality. For many years the National Center for Health Statistics created age-standardized rates using the 1940 standard, a set of weights that described the age distribution of the United States in 1940. The 2000 U.S. standard is now used (Table 6.3) (Klein and Schoenborn 2001, Murphy, Xu, and Kochanek 2013 Table X). These weights are estimates, based on projections made in the 1990's, of the age-categorized U.S. population in the year 2000 (Anderson and Rosenberg 1998). The Bureau of the Census counted 281.4 million residents in the 2000 census, greater than the estimate of 274.6 million for the U.S. 2000 standard population (Table 6.3). But the age distributions of the projected U.S. 2000 standard and the year 2000 census were similar. The crude U.S. cancer mortality rate per 100,000 person-years in 2000 was 196.5 using the count of cancer deaths divided by the census population count in 2000. If weights from the U.S. 2000 standard population are used, created from projections prior to the 2000 census, the weighted-average is 199.6, close to the crude rate. Since a crude rate is a weighted average of stratum-specific rates, the rate of 196.5 is directly standardized to the *observed* age distribution of person-time in 2000 and the rate of 199.6 is directly standardized to the *projected* U.S. 2000 standard.

The directly age-standardized rate for Alaska is a weighted average of the age-stratified mortality rates from Alaska (Table 6.2) summarized with weights from the 2000 U.S. standard population. One can use weights equal to the person-time estimates (column 2 of Table 6.3) or equal to the proportion of person-time in each stratum of age (column 3 of Table 6.3). The directly standardized Alaska rate per 100,000 person-years is 177, larger than the crude Alaska rate of 124 (Table 6.4), because the U.S. 2000 standard population distribution gives more weight to the Alaska rates of the elderly compared with weights based on the Alaska age distribution. Most (61%) cancer deaths in Alaska occurred among persons 65 years and older. The crude Alaska rate is a weighted average of the age-specific Alaska rates, with weights from the Alaska age-categorized distribution of person-time in 2010. For the older age groups where cancer rates were highest, weights based upon Alaska's age distribution were smaller than weights from the U.S. 2000 standard: .050 versus .066 for ages 65–74, .021 versus .045 for ages 75–84, and .007 versus .016 for ages 85+ years. The directly standardized rate of cancer deaths per 100,000 person-years was still lower in Alaska compared with the United States, 176.9–199.6 = −23 per 100,000 person years, but this is less than the difference of −72 between the crude rates. Comparing the age-standardized Alaska cancer rate with the standardized U.S. rate, the rate ratio was 0.89, closer to 1 than the rate ratio of 0.63 of the crude rates. Most of the difference between the crude Alaska and U.S. cancer mortality rates in 2010 was due to differences in the age distributions of the two populations.

Direct standardization can minimize confounding by age, sex, calendar year, or any other characteristic that is measured with sufficient detail in the study population and the standard population. Public health agencies often publish tables of crude and standardized rates. A reader of these tables can readily assess how much of any crude difference between several populations or categories may be due

TABLE 6.4 Crude and age-standardized mortality rates for deaths due to cancer in Alaska and Florida, 2010. Rates are per 100,000 person-years. Rate ratios and rate differences are shown comparing Alaska with Florida according to the population distribution used for standardization of the Alaska and Florida rates.

STANDARD POPULATION	ALASKA RATE	FLORIDA RATE	RATE RATIO[a]	RATE DIFFERENCE[b]
None	124.5	220.6	0.56	−96.1
U.S. 2000 Standard	176.9	165.6	1.07	+11.3
Florida 2010	236.5	220.6	1.07	+15.9
Alaska 2010	124.5	127.3	0.98	−2.8

[a] Rate ratio = Alaska rate/Florida rate.
[b] Rate difference = Alaska rate per 100,000 person-years − Florida rate per 100,000 person-years.
Data from CDC WONDER. Compressed Mortality File. CDC WONDER Online Database. http://wonder.cdc.gov: Centers for Disease Control and Prevention, National Center for Health Statistics.

to confounding by the factors used for standardization. Risks, means, and other statistics can be standardized using similar methods.

Standardized rates are not rates for any actual population. The directly age-standardized rate of 177 is an estimate of what the overall cancer mortality rate would have been if the age-specific rates observed in Alaska in 2010 were applied to a population with the age distribution of the U.S. 2000 standard population. To describe the rate of events in a population or cohort, the crude rate is usually best. A standardized rate provides information useful for comparison with other populations.

If exposure can alter the distribution of the person-time used as the standardizing weights, then a standardized rate will not precisely estimate what would happen if the observed stratum rates were applied to another population. This could happen if the exposure were so powerfully related to the outcome that it would substantially reduce the population (person-time) estimates in some strata of the standard population. If living in Alaska is the exposure, the Alaska rates are not large enough for this to be an important concern. But if the Alaska rates were ten-fold greater, then standardizing Alaska rates to the U.S. 2000 standard would not correctly estimate what would have happened in the United States in 2000 under those rates, as cancer deaths would be so common that person-time in the U.S. 2000 population would have been reduced in the older age strata; the exposure would shrink the person-time in the rate denominators of the standard population (Greenland, Rothman, and Lash 2008b p68). This problem could be dealt with by accounting for the impact of large rates on person-time (Greenland and Rothman 2008c pp265–266).

As with any adjustment method, direct standardization may not remove all confounding if the categories used are not sufficiently narrow. For example, the standardized rate for Alaska cancer mortality was calculated by using a mortality rate of 659 for persons age 65–74 years (Table 6.2). But rates increased rapidly in the older age groups. It may be more realistic to think that the rate varied from about 500 at age 65 to 800 at age 74. Depending on how person-time was distributed within the age category of 65–74 years in Alaska and the U.S. standard, use of a 10-year age category may not remove all age-related confounding from the comparison of the two populations.

6.3 COMPARING DIRECTLY STANDARDIZED RATES

The ratio of two rates that are both directly standardized to the same population is called a standardized rate ratio (SRR) (Checkoway, Pearce, and Crawford-Brown 1989 p123, Porta 2008, Greenland, Rothman, and Lash 2008b pp67–68). It might be clearer to call this a ratio of directly standardized rates or a directly standardized rate ratio. Because the crude rate for a standard population S is itself a directly standardized rate based on the person-time weights of population S, the ratio of a directly standardized rate to the crude rate of the standard population is also a ratio of directly standardized rates. This ratio, in which the crude rate from the standard population is the denominator, has also been called the cumulative mortality figure (CMF). That name may have been coined (Yule 1934) by William Ogle, who succeeded William Farr as the Superintendent of Statistics in the Registrar-General Office of England and Wales, serving from 1880 to 1893. The term "cumulative mortality figure" has been used in many publications from the Registrar-General Office. Breslow and Day (1987 pp61–63) used this term in their 1987 book about the analysis of cohort studies. Many epidemiology textbooks (Kleinbaum, Kupper, and Morgenstern 1982, Kelsey, Thompson, and Evans 1986, Rothman, Greenland, and Lash 2008c, Weiss and Koepsell 2014) do not use "cumulative mortality figure" and that term has the disadvantage of not being particularly descriptive of what is meant.

In this chapter, I use SRR to mean the ratio of a directly standardized rate to the crude rate from the standard population. Some authors multiply the SRR (or CMF) by 100, but I will ignore that convention. The difference between two directly standardized rates is a directly standardized rate difference; there is no special term for this difference.

The ratio of two SRRs for two different populations standardized to the same standard population is simply the ratio of the two standardized rates. Using the notation from Expressions 6.2–6.5:

directly standardized rate ratio comparing population A with population B

$$
\begin{aligned}
&= SRR_A/SRR_B \\
&= ((sum[rate_{Ai} \times T_{Si}]/T_S)/rate_S)/((sum[rate_{Bi} \times T_{Si}]/T_S)/rate_S) \\
&= (sum[rate_{Ai} \times T_{Si}]/T_S)/(sum[rate_{Bi} \times T_{Si}]/T_S) \\
&= (sum[rate_{Ai} \times T_{Si}/T_S])/(sum[rate_{Bi} \times T_{Si}/T_S]) \\
&= (sum[(rate_{Ai}/rate_{Bi}) \times rate_{Bi} \times T_{Si}/T_S])/(sum[rate_{Bi} \times T_{Si}/T_S])
\end{aligned}
$$

(Ex.6.6)

The last line of Expression 6.6 shows that ratio of two SRRs is a weighted average of stratum-specific rate ratios ($rate_{Ai}/rate_{Bi}$). The weights are equal to the usual standardization weights (T_{Si}/T_S) multiplied by the stratum-specific rates in population B. If we think of population A as an exposed cohort and population B as an unexposed cohort, then the ratio of the SRRs for each cohort is a weighted average of the stratum rate ratios, with weights equal to the unexposed stratum rates multiplied by the person-time weights from the standard population (Greenland and Rothman 2008c p267).

The difference in two directly standardized rates is a weighted-average of the stratum rate differences using person-time weights from the standard population:

directly standardized rate difference comparing population A with population B

$$
\begin{aligned}
&= (sum[rate_{Ai} \times T_{Si}]/T_S) - (sum[rate_{Bi} \times T_{Si}]/T_S) \\
&= (sum[rate_{Ai} \times T_{Si}] - sum[rate_{Bi} \times T_{Si}])/T_S \\
&= (sum[(rate_{Ai} - rate_{Bi}) \times T_{Si}])/T_S
\end{aligned}
$$

(Ex.6.7)

If population B is the standard population, we can rearrange Expression 6.6 to simplify the computation of the SRR comparing population A with standard population S (Breslow and Day 1987 p63):

directly standardized rate for population A/crude rate for standard population S

$$
\begin{aligned}
&= SRR_A \\
&= (sum[rate_{Ai} \times T_{Si}]/T_S)/(sum[rate_{Si} \times T_{Si}]/T_S) \\
&= sum[rate_{Ai} \times T_{Si}]/sum[rate_{Si} \times T_{Si}] \\
&= sum[rate_{Ai} \times T_{Si}]/C_S
\end{aligned}
$$

(Ex.6.8)

Expression 6.8 can be rearranged to show that the SRR comparing population A with standard population S is a weighted average of the stratum-specific rate ratios with weights equal to stratum-specific event counts in population S (Breslow and Day 1987 p63):

directly standardized rate for population A/crude rate for population S

$$
\begin{aligned}
&= SRR_A \\
&= sum[rate_{Ai} \times T_{Si}]/C_S \\
&= sum[(rate_{Ai}/rate_{Si}) \times rate_{Si} \times T_{Si}]/C_S \\
&= sum[(rate_{Ai}/rate_{Si}) \times C_{Si}]/C_S \\
&= sum[(rate_{Ai}/rate_{Si}) \times C_{Si}]/sum[C_{Si}]
\end{aligned}
$$

(Ex.6.9)

Direct standardization can be used to compare the mortality rate from cancer in Alaska with the rate in Florida, both during 2010 (Tables 6.2 and 6.3). The crude rate in Alaska was 124, much smaller than the crude rate of 221 in Florida. If we directly age-standardize both of these rates using weights from the U.S. 2000 standard population, the directly standardized rate for Alaska is 177, slightly larger than the standardized rate of 166 for Florida. This can be done using Stata's **dstdize** command, applied below to the Alaska data only to compute the standardized rate for Alaska:

```
. dstdize count pop agecat, by(state) using(standard2000)
------------------------------------------------------------------------
-> state= 0
```

Stratum	Pop.	Cases	Unadjusted Pop. Dist.	Stratum Rate[s]	Std. Pop. Dst[P]	s*P
1	10828	1	0.015	0.0001	0.014	0.0000
1-4	43168	2	0.061	0.0000	0.055	0.0000
15-24	106560	5	0.150	0.0000	0.139	0.0000
25-34	103125	9	0.145	0.0001	0.136	0.0000
35-44	92974	21	0.131	0.0002	0.163	0.0000
45-54	111026	103	0.156	0.0009	0.135	0.0001
5-14	101703	1	0.143	0.0000	0.146	0.0000
55-64	85909	205	0.121	0.0024	0.087	0.0002
65-74	35350	233	0.050	0.0066	0.066	0.0004
75-84	14877	218	0.021	0.0147	0.045	0.0007
85+	4711	86	0.007	0.0183	0.016	0.0003

```
------------------------------------------------------------------------
Totals:    710231       884            Adjusted Cases:    1256.4
                                           Crude Rate:    0.0012
                                        Adjusted Rate:    0.0018
                          95% Conf. Interval:    [0.0016, 0.0019]
```

Summary of Study Populations:

state	N	Crude	Adj_Rate	Confidence Interval
0	710231	0.001245	0.001769	[0.001643, 0.001895]

In this output, the first column lists the age strata and the next 4 columns show person-time, deaths, the person-time proportions, and stratum rates for Alaska. The 2000 Standard population proportions (weights) are shown next and finally the Alaska rates multiplied by the standard population proportions (s x P). At the time this was written, this command has several limitations: (1) it requires that person-time be expressed as an integer, precluding expressing person-time in units of 100,000 person-years or other units; (2) it insists that the numerator count be less than the person-time quantity, which also restricts transformations of person-time; and (3) it reorders the standardizing strata according to their value labels, instead of the order of the strata in the data. Because of the first two limitations, most of the rates in the last column (s x P), are all zero to four places after the decimal, making the results less transparent.

The directly standardized Florida rate was much smaller (166) than the crude rate (221) because a greater fraction of Florida residents were seniors compared with the U.S. 2000 standard population (Figure 6.1). The old retirees of the Sunshine State received less weight in the age-standardized rate compared with their contribution to Florida's crude rate. The situation was reversed for Alaska, where the high cancer rates of the elderly contributed more to the standardized rate.

Rate comparisons are often more homogeneous on a ratio scale than a difference scale (Breslow and Day 1987 pp61–63). This is true when comparing Alaska with Florida (Table 6.2). The rate ratios among those older than 35 years, where the rates start to have some precision, fall into a fairly narrow range of 0.74 to 1.36. The rate differences, however, have a wide range from −75 to +391. To produce these rate ratios and differences, as well as other useful statistics, we can use Stata's **ir** command for stratified rate ratios or difference. In the output below weights equal to the stratum person-time of the 2000 Standard Population were used:

```
. ir count alaska pop2, by(agecat) standard(pop)
Age, 11 categori |     IRR       [95% Conf. Interval]      Weight
-----------------+------------------------------------------------
             1 |   9.63816     .1633664    185.14      3794901  (exact)
           1-4 |   1.821176    .2075938   7.408422     1.52e+07  (exact)
          5-14 |    .7496819   .0183554   4.521574     4.00e+07  (exact)
         15-24 |   1.310156    .4151356   3.174781     3.81e+07  (exact)
         25-34 |   1.019463    .459307    1.975306     3.72e+07  (exact)
         35-44 |    .7361211   .4529502   1.133598     4.47e+07  (exact)
         45-54 |    .7749275   .6306186    .9429465    3.70e+07  (exact)
         55-64 |    .7604977   .658696     .8738111    2.40e+07  (exact)
         65-74 |   1.061044    .927879    1.208177     1.81e+07  (exact)
         75-84 |   1.363523   1.187064    1.559078     1.23e+07  (exact)
           85+ |   1.094918    .8746952   1.354099      4259173  (exact)
-----------------+------------------------------------------------
         Crude |    .5643365   .5273743    .6032341              (exact)
  Standardized |   1.068419    .9938787   1.14855
```

6.4 CHOICE OF THE STANDARD INFLUENCES THE COMPARISON OF STANDARDIZED RATES

The size of a standardized rate, and differences or ratios based on standardized rates, will depend upon the choice of standard population (Doll and Cook 1967). If we compare Alaska with Florida using the Florida population as the standard, the rate difference is +15.9 per 100,000 person-years, but if we compare Alaska with Florida using the Alaska population as the standard, the rate difference is −2.8 (Table 6.4). While the choice of standard population alters the size of the Alaska-Florida comparison, the differences are not great in this example.

The choice of a standard population will not affect the directly-standardized comparison of two cohorts if the stratum-specific rates are the same in both cohorts; the rate ratio based upon the directly standardized rates will be 1 and the rate difference will be 0, regardless of the standard population used. If the stratum-specific rate ratios are the same across the standardization strata in two cohorts, but not equal to 1, then the choice of standard population will not affect comparison of the standardized rates using a rate ratio, but will affect a comparison using the rate difference, unless there is no variation in the rates over the strata. If the stratum-specific rate differences are the same across all the standardizing strata in two cohorts and not equal to 0, then the choice of standard population will not affect comparison of the standardized rates using the rate difference, but will affect a comparison using the rate ratio if the rates are not the same in all strata.

Because estimated associations can change depending on the choice of standard population, it may be more transparent to use standard populations that have been published or used often (Doll and Cook 1967, Breslow and Day 1987 pp56–57). Doing this may make it easier to compare results from different studies.

6.5 STANDARDIZED COMPARISONS VERSUS ADJUSTED COMPARISONS FROM VARIANCE-MINIMIZING METHODS

The fact that standardized comparisons can change in size depending upon the choice of the standard population might be considered a limitation of direct standardization. But the choice of comparison group will usually affect the size of any estimated association between an exposure and an outcome regardless of the method used. Standardization has the merit of making the choice of the standard explicit. With other methods the choice that was made is not as obvious (Rothman 2012 pp188–192).

Instead of standardization, we could compare the cancer mortality in Alaska with that in Florida, adjusted for age or some other factor, by using any of several statistical methods, including inverse-variance weighting, Mantel-Haenszel stratified analysis, iteratively reweighted least squares, or maximum likelihood. Details about these methods are in Chapter 7. If we think it is reasonable and useful to summarize the age-specific rate ratio or difference estimates as if they were from a single homogeneous process, we can use these methods to estimate a single Alaska versus Florida rate ratio or difference, adjusted for age. Under the assumption of homogeneity (also called uniformity of effect), these methods treat variation in the ratio or difference estimates by levels of some third factor, such as age, as if this was random variation around the true value. This homogeneity assumption underlies all these methods (Greenland and Rothman 2008c pp270–272). This assumption is not strictly true for the data in Table 6.2 and we may not necessarily believe this assumption, but we may still want a single age-adjusted estimate and these methods can provide this estimate.

The inverse-variance and Mantel-Haenszel methods treat each difference or ratio estimate at each level of a third characteristic as an estimate of the true difference or ratio. The stratum-specific estimates are summarized using a weighted average with weights representing the statistical precision of each estimate. Iteratively reweighted least squares and maximum likelihood do not actually create stratum-specific estimates, but in effect they summarize the data as if they had done this (Greenland and Rothman 2008c p271). By using statistical precision to weight each stratum-specific estimate, all these methods produce a summary rate difference or ratio that should have the smallest possible variance given the data used for the comparison. In statistical jargon, these methods are *efficient* in that they seek the most precise estimate possible given the data (Rothman 2012 pp189–191). These are sometimes called variance-minimizing methods or methods for pooling. The methods assume homogeneity across the strata. Unless the stratum-specific rate differences are all zero (and the rate ratios therefore all 1) the estimates will typically be more homogeneous on one scale compared with the other (Greenland and Rothman 2008c p277).

Inverse-variance weighting is easy to describe, so I will use it to illustrate what happens when a variance-minimizing method is used for comparing cancer mortality in Alaska with Florida. This method has also been called direct pooling, precision weighting, the Woolf method, and weighted least squares (Greenland and Rothman 2008c p271). The weights are the inverse of the variance of each rate difference or ratio. The variances are equal to the square of the standard error (SE) of the mean for row 5 (rate differences) or row 10 (rate ratios) in the last column of Table 4.4. Here are Stata commands that produce the pooled (inverse-variance) results for the rate ratio and rate difference, using population in units of 100,000 person-years and using the Alaska population as the standard. The standardized estimates are also reported:

```
. ir count alaska pop2, by(agecat) istandard pool
```

Age, 11 categori |	IRR	[95% Conf.	Interval]	Weight	
1 |	9.63816	.1633664	185.14	.10828	(exact)
1-4 |	1.821176	.2075938	7.408422	.43168	(exact)
5-14 |	.7496819	.0183554	4.521574	1.01703	(exact)
15-24 |	1.310156	.4151356	3.174781	1.0656	(exact)
25-34 |	1.019463	.459307	1.975306	1.03125	(exact)
35-44 |	.7361211	.4529502	1.133598	.92974	(exact)
45-54 |	.7749275	.6306186	.9429465	1.11026	(exact)
55-64 |	.7604977	.658696	.8738111	.85909	(exact)
65-74 |	1.061044	.927879	1.208177	.3535	(exact)
75-84 |	1.363523	1.187064	1.559078	.14877	(exact)
85+ |	1.094918	.8746952	1.354099	.04711	(exact)
Crude |	.5643365	.5273743	.6032341		(exact)
Pooled (direct) |	1.005856	.9409589	1.075229		
I. Standardized |	.9776556	.9144901	1.045184		

```
Test of homogeneity (direct)  chi2(10) =  49.92   Pr>chi2 = 0.0000
```

```
. ir count alaska pop2, by(agecat) istandard pool ird
```

Age, 11 categori |	IRD	[95% Conf.	Interval]	Weight
1 |	8.277113	-9.872422	26.42665	.10828
1-4 |	2.089068	-4.419313	8.597449	.43168
5-14 |	-.328308	-2.313692	1.657076	1.01703
15-24 |	1.110793	-3.069535	5.29112	1.0656
25-34 |	.1666198	-5.659688	5.992928	1.03125
35-44 |	-8.096794	-18.00497	1.811381	.92974
45-54 |	-26.94473	-45.32296	-8.566496	1.11026
55-64 |	-75.14965	-108.5949	-41.70443	.85909
65-74 |	37.92093	-47.52346	123.3653	.3535
75-84 |	390.6702	195.1872	586.1532	.14877
85+ |	158.253	-229.4737	545.9798	.04711
Crude |	-96.08723	-104.5623	-87.61215	
Pooled (direct) |	-.4022102	-2.021802	1.217382	
I. Standardized |	-2.844692	-11.16289	5.473506	

```
Test of homogeneity (direct)  chi2(10) =  48.29   Pr>chi2 = 0.0000
```

Comparing Alaska with Florida (Table 6.2 and output above), the inverse-variance rate ratio, summarized on the ln scale and then exponentiated, was 1.006, and the inverse-variance rate difference was −0.40 per 100,000 person-years. These estimated associations are in the opposite direction, but only to a trivial degree. Despite a lot of variation (heterogeneity) in the stratum estimates, the difference estimate is close to the null value of 0 and the ratio estimate close to the null value of 1.

The inverse-variance difference and ratio estimates were closest to the standardized estimates based on the 2010 Alaska population (Table 6.4). This was because the smaller counts and person-time from Alaska dominated in creating the size of the inverse-variance weights. Mantel-Haenszel methods and maximum likelihood methods will also produce estimates similar to these.

To summarize, variance-minimizing methods assume homogeneity of effect and produce summary estimates with the smallest variance given the data. Inverse-variance and Mantel-Haenszel methods pool stratum-specific ratio or difference estimates using stratum-specific weights that reflect the precision of each stratum estimate. In contrast, standardization requires no assumption about homogeneity, can use weights that are external to the data and explicit, applies the weights to the rates themselves prior to estimating the association of interest, and may be inefficient if large weights are given to strata with little data.

6.6 STRATIFIED ANALYSES

A stratified analysis estimates associations between an exposure and an outcome within levels of some third factor, such as age. Confounding due to the third factor can be reduced within each stratum if the stratifying categories are sufficiently narrow. Stratification also allows us to see whether the estimated association varies greatly from one level to the next, or whether the association seems to be approximately homogeneous across the levels used. The method can be extended to several factors if the data allow this.

In a standardized analysis of rate ratios or differences, the stratum-specific estimates of association are summarized using weights based upon person-time. When inverse-variance or Mantel-Haenszel methods are used, the weights reflect the statistical precision of each stratum estimate. Despite these differences, all stratified methods share a degree of transparency compared with regression methods. A stratified analysis allows us to see how much data are in each stratum, how estimates vary between strata, and how the stratified summary estimate differs from a summary estimate that ignores the stratification variable. Even if the final analysis may use a regression model, a preliminary stratified analysis will often provide useful insight.

6.7 VARIATIONS ON DIRECTLY STANDARDIZED RATES

Depending upon our goal, we may not wish to standardize rates using all available strata. For example, Doll and Cook (1967) argued that if the goal is to find etiologic clues by comparing rates of cancer between different populations, a truncated standardized rate might be best. For certain leukemias and nephroblastoma, comparisons could be limited to persons younger than 15 years, for osteogenic sarcoma and Hodgkin's Disease the upper age limit might be 44 years, and for other cancers an age-range of 35 to 64 years is a good choice. The strata to be summarized and the choice of summary weights might be determined in part by the purposes for which the standardized rates are intended.

To compare rates of cancer in Alaska and Florida, an argument could be made that the comparison should be limited to persons older than 35 or 45 years. Cancer death is rare among the young and the rate ratios and differences from the youngest age strata are statistically imprecise. Using the large amount of person-time contributed by those younger than 35 years adds little to the comparison and may promote confounding by age. Tables of standardized rates produced by the National Center for Health Statistics often include all ages to avoid making choices about which age groups to include for every rate shown. But the Center is aware of this issue and has produced several standard population tables for subgroups of age (Klein and Schoenborn 2001, Murphy, Xu, and Kochanek 2013 Tables X–XIII).

6.8 INTERNAL WEIGHTS FROM A POPULATION: INDIRECT STANDARDIZATION

A century ago it was common to see indirectly standardized rates in tables of mortality rates. In 1923, Wolfenden (1923) reviewed methods for both direct and indirect standardization of rates. Using Expressions 6.3–6.5, we can describe the directly standardized rate as:

directly standardized rate for population A using standard population S

$$
\begin{aligned}
&= \text{rate}_A \times C_{A\text{exp}}/C_A \\
&= \text{rate}_A \times (T_A \times \text{sum}[\text{rate}_{Ai} \times T_{Si}]/T_S)/\text{sum}[\text{rate}_{Ai} \times T_{Ai}] \\
&= \text{rate}_A \times (\text{sum}[\text{rate}_{Ai} \times T_{Si}]/T_S)/(\text{sum}[\text{rate}_{Ai} \times T_{Ai}]/T_A) \\
&= \text{rate}_A \times (\text{sum}[\text{rate}_{Ai} \times T_{Si}]/T_S) \times (T_A/\text{sum}[\text{rate}_{Ai} \times T_{Ai}])
\end{aligned}
$$

(Ex.6.10)

In these expressions the first term is the crude rate for population A. Wolfenden (1923) called the remaining terms the standardizing factor. All formulae for directly standardized rates, including those in Expression 6.10, require the use of the stratum-specific rates from population A. A century ago the calculations were done using pencil and paper, a cumbersome chore for hundreds of community populations. Workers in the English Registrar General's office realized that something *close* to the directly standardized rate could be obtained for most communities by using the stratum-specific rates of the standard population in place of the stratum-specific rates from population A. This substitution meant that:

directly standardized rate for population A using standard population S

$$
\begin{aligned}
&= \text{rate}_A \times (\text{sum}[\text{rate}_{Ai} \times T_{Si}]/T_S) \times (T_A/\text{sum}[\text{rate}_{Ai} \times T_{Ai}]) \\
&\approx \text{rate}_A \times (\text{sum}[\text{rate}_{Si} \times T_{Si}]/T_S) \times (T_A/\text{sum}[\text{rate}_{Si} \times T_{Ai}]) \\
&= \text{rate}_A \times \text{rate}_S \times T_A/\text{sum}[\text{rate}_{Si} \times T_{Ai}] \\
&= \text{indirectly standardized rate for population A using standard population S}
\end{aligned}
$$

(Ex.6.11)

The next to last line of Expression 6.11 simplifies the calculation. The crude rates for populations A and S are needed, but both are easy to calculate and are useful in their own right. The stratum specific rates from the standard population are needed, but these can be computed just once and then used repeatedly for each community. The stratum-specific person-time estimates for each community are needed; these may be readily available as counts from census data. Ease of computation made indirectly standardized rates popular before computers became available. Now computers make it easy to calculate directly standardized rates and so these have replaced indirectly standardized rates in government reports.

Expression 6.11 reveals a potential problem with indirect standardization. If the intent is to estimate the directly standardized rate, the indirectly standardized rate will not always do this. The direct and indirect methods may produce different results. Wolfenden (1923) was aware of this; "in all normal cases [the substitution] will clearly give very close results. The validity of this substitution, however – upon which … the indirect method is in effect founded – should be tested numerically prior to any extensive application …"

The last part of the next to last line in Expression 6.11 is $T_A/\text{sum}[\text{rate}_{Si} \times T_{Ai}]$. This quantity is the reciprocal of the rate that would arise in population A if the stratum-specific rates of the standard population were applied to the person-time of population A. This means that the standardizing weights used by the indirect method come from population A, not the standard population. These are sometimes called internal weights in contrast to the external weights used by direction standardization. Because the standardizing weights will vary from one population to the next, comparison of indirectly standardized rates may still be confounded by the variables, such as age, used for standardization.

The indirectly standardized rate of cancer mortality in Alaska in 2010 (Table 6.2), using U.S. cancer mortality rates and the U.S. standard population from 2000 (Table 6.3), was 163.1 per 100,000 person-years, not greatly different from the directly standardized rate of 176.9 (Table 6.4). The indirectly standardized rate of cancer mortality for Florida in 2010 was 165.4, close to the directly standardized rate of 165.6. For both of these calculations, 199.6 (to many decimals) was used as the crude cancer mortality rate for the United States in 2000 (see footnote to Table 6.3). Indirectly standardized rates can be obtained from Stata's **istdize** command, which has limitations mentioned earlier for the **dstdize** command.

6.9 THE STANDARDIZED MORTALITY RATIO (SMR)

While indirectly standardized rates are not often presented, the ratio of the indirectly standardized rate for population A to the crude rate of a standard population S is often used and has a special name, the standardized mortality or morbidity ratio (SMR). This ratio is commonly multiplied by 100, but that convention will be ignored here. These ratios are often used in occupational epidemiology (Checkoway, Pearce, and Crawford-Brown 1989 p125) to identify groups of workers who may have mortality rates higher than those of persons of similar age and sex in the general population. Previously we defined C_{Aexp} (Expression 6.4) as the event count expected in population A based on the total person-time of population A, stratum rates from population A, and *person-time weights from the standard population*. If we define Exp_A as the expected count in population A based on total person-time of population A, stratum rates from population S, and *person-time weights from population A*, the SMR has a simple Expression:

SMR comparing population A with standard population S

$=$ indirectly standardized rate of population A/crude rate of population S

$= rate_A \times (sum[rate_{Si} \times T_{Si}]/T_S) \times (T_A/sum[rate_{Si} \times T_{Ai}])/(sum[rate_{Si} \times T_{Si}]/T_S)$ (Ex.6.12)

$= rate_A \times T_A/(sum[rate_{Si} \times T_{Ai}])$

$= C_A/Exp_A$

The final expression in 6.12 is the observed count in population A divided by the expected count if each stratum of population A had the stratum rates of population S. This ratio of two counts is often written as Obs/Exp or O/E. The SMR, like the SRR, can be described as a weighted average of the stratum-specific rate ratios, with weights equal to the expected counts in each stratum of population A if the stratum rates are those of the standard population:

indirectly standardized rate for population A/crude rate for population S

$= SMR_A$

$= C_A/Exp_A$

$= sum[rate_{Ai} \times T_{Ai}]/sum[rate_{Si} \times T_{Ai}]$ (Ex.6.13)

$= sum[(rate_{Ai}/rate_{Si}) \times rate_{Si} \times T_{Ai}]/sum[rate_{Si} \times T_{Ai}]$

$= sum[(rate_{Ai}/rate_{Si}) \times Exp_{Ai}]/sum[Exp_{Ai}]$

One could use a mortality difference equal to the indirectly standardized rate A minus the crude rate for population S. This is not usually done because (1) rate ratios are typically more homogeneous than rate differences across levels of age and sex and (2) even if a summary on a difference scale might be preferred, the SMR is often used out of habit or in deference to tradition.

The SMR for Alaska in 2010, compared with the U.S. 2000 standard population, was 0.817. The Florida SMR was 0.829 and the Alaska/Florida ratio of SMRs was 0.99, which is similar to the ratio of 1.07 for the ratio of rates directly standardized to the U.S. 2000 standard (Table 6.4). The ratio of Alaska to Florida SMRs is equal to the ratio of the indirectly standardized rates for those states: 163.1/165.4 = 0.99. SMRs can be calculated with Stata's **istdize** command.

6.10 ADVANTAGES OF SMRS COMPARED WITH SRRS (RATIOS OF DIRECTLY STANDARDIZED RATES)

In the 19th and early 20th century, SMRs were often used because of computational ease (Yule 1934), compared with calculation of the SRR. This justification seems irrelevant today because computers can be used. Another reason for the use of SMRs is that they only require the observed total count from population A, the stratum rates from the standard population, and the stratum-specific person-time for population A. If the ages are unknown for those who died in population A, the SMR can still be calculated (Breslow and Day 1987 p65) to estimate a ratio of rates that usually removes much of the confounding related to age. But often knowledge about those who had events in population A will be available, making this justification moot.

Another justification for the use of SMRs, instead of SRRs, is related to statistical precision. When events are uncommon in population A, which will often be the case if this population is small, stratum-specific rates from population A will be imprecise. Event rates in strata from the standard population, which is usually large, will be more precise, giving the SMR more stability compared with the SRR.

In the fictional data of Table 6.5, population A has a crude rate of 72 per 100,000, and a directly standardized rate of 189. The ratio of the directly standardized rate for A compared with S is 189/130 = 1.5. In population A, one person age 85 years or older died. Imagine that on review of these data, we found this person was actually age 84 years and we moved their death to the correct age category. The population A rate in the oldest age stratum would change from a lofty 100,000 to 0 and the directly standardized rate would become 108, changing the SRR to 108/130 = 0.8. But if we use the indirect method, which utilizes only the total count of deaths from population A, the SMR comparing population A with S is 33/35.12 = 0.94. Reclassifying the age category for a single death will have no

TABLE 6.5 Hypothetical age-categorized counts and rates of death in population A and a standard population S. Rates are per 100,000 person-years. Rate ratio = Population A rate/Standard population rate.

| AGE (YRS) | POPULATION A | | | STANDARD POPULATION S | | | |
	COUNT	PERSON-TIME	RATE	COUNT	PERSON-TIME	RATE	RATE RATIO
65–74	20	40,000	50	75	150,000	50	1.0
75–84	12	6,000	200	200	80,000	250	0.8
85+	1	1	100,000	25	200	12,500	8.0
All	33	46,001	72	300	230,200	130	0.5

effect on the observed total count or the expected total count, so the SMR will not change at all. A similar example appears in Breslow and Day (1987 pp63–67).

The confidence interval (CI) for an SMR (an indirectly standardized rate ratio) will usually be narrower than for an SRR (a directly standardized rate ratio), because the calculation of the SE of the SMR involves only the total count of events from population A; fluctuations in the counts from one stratum of population A to another are ignored (Breslow and Day 1987 pp63–67). The SE of the SMR is calculated by assuming homogeneity of effect across different strata of age, sex, or any other variable used for standardization. This means that the SE of the SMR uses a variance-minimizing method, unlike the SE for the SRR. This may be considered to be an advantage of the SMR.

6.11 DISADVANTAGES OF SMRS COMPARED WITH SRRS (RATIOS OF DIRECTLY STANDARDIZED RATES)

Obtaining a narrow CI may not be an advantage of the SMR if an assumption of homogeneity of the rate ratios across standardizing categories seems implausible. The SRR may be preferred because it does not rely on an assumption of homogeneity.

Comparison of SMRs may be biased because each SMR relies upon indirect standardization to a different "standard" population. Imagine that we wish to compare the rates of populations A and B, using standard population S. The ratio of the two standardized rates, or SRRs, for A and B will remove confounding by the standardizing variables, such as age, if the strata are sufficiently fine, as both the standardized rates rely upon the person-time distribution of the same standard population S. But the ratio of two SMRs for A and B may be biased, because SMRs use standardizing weights based upon the person-time distribution of A and B, the populations that are to be compared. Direct standardization typically involves a *single* set of standard person-time weights, whereas indirect standardization uses as many sets of "standard" weights are there are groups to be compared.

In 1934 Yule (1934) published an 82-page article titled "On some points relating to vital statistics, more especially statistics of occupational mortality." Yule referred to direct standardization as the "fixed base" method, meaning that a single distribution of person-time was used for standardization. He called indirect standardization the "changing base method," pointing out that since the standardizing weights change from one comparison to the next, "the method is not fully a method of standardization at all … " Other authors (Silcock 1959, Kilpatrick 1963, Breslow and Day 1987 pp72–73, Greenland 1987a, Greenland, Rothman, and Lash 2008b p69) have also noted that since indirect standardizing weights come from each population to be standardized, any comparison of SMRs is *not* standardized using the same weights and a comparison of two or more SMRs may still be biased due to different distributions of the standardizing variable.

Imagine population A1 is a cohort of workers exposed to a chemical and they have the age-specific rates shown in Table 6.6. The crude rate of death in population A1 is greater than the crude rate in standard population S1: $3355/422.5 = 7.9$. In cohort A1, the crude rate of 3355 is close to the rate of 3600 among older persons, because 90% of persons in population A1 were old. In population S1, 90% of people were young, and the crude rate of 422.5 is close to the rate of 400 among young people. So age, which is related both to the rate of death and to the exposure of being in cohort A1, is a confounder that biases the ratio of the crude rates. The rate ratio of 7.9 is almost entirely a comparison of the old people in population A1 with the young people of population S1. Within the age categories the rate ratios comparing A1 with S1 range from 1 to 4, so the unbiased rate ratio should be somewhere between 1 and 4.

The directly standardized rate for population A1, using the person-time distribution of population S1, is 500.9, so the SRR comparing A1 with S1 is $500.9/422.5 = 1.19$. This ratio is close to 1, the rate ratio comparing A1 with S1 among young people, because most person-time in population S1 is in the youngest stratum and the standardizing weights come from population S1. The indirectly standardized

TABLE 6.6   Hypothetical age-categorized counts and rates of death in population A1 and standard population S1. Rates are per 100,000 person-years. Rate ratio = Population A1 rate/Standard population S1 rate.

	POPULATION A1			STANDARD POPULATION S1			
AGE	COUNT	PERSON-TIME	RATE	COUNT	PERSON-TIME	RATE	RATE RATIO
Young	40	10,000	400	40,000	10,000,000	400	1.0
Middle	1,200	100,000	1,200	6,000	1,000,000	600	2.0
Old	36,000	1,000,000	3,600	900	100,000	900	4.0
All	37,240	1,110,000	3,355	46,900	11,100,000	422.5	7.9

rate for population A1 is 1632, using the rates from population S1 and the person-time distribution of population A1, so the SMR comparing A1 with S1 is 1632/422.5 = 3.86, close to the ratio of 4 among the older persons in both populations. In Table 6.6, the SRR of 1.19 differs from the SMR of 3.86. This difference arises because of a combination of two factors: (1) the stratum-specific rate ratios vary substantially from 1 to 4, and (2) the distribution of person-time is very different in populations A1 and S1.

Recall (Expressions 6.9 and 6.13) that both the SRR and the SMR can be expressed as weighted averages of the stratum-specific rate ratios. If the stratum-specific rate ratios comparing population A1 with S1 were all the same, say 2.0, then regardless of the weights used, the weighted average would also be 2.0. So the SRR and SMR will be equal if the stratum-specific rate ratios are the same. In actual data the stratum rate ratios will rarely ever be identical; but unless they differ greatly, the SMR will tend to approximate the SRR.

The SRR and the SMR will also be equal if the person-time distributions of populations A1 and S1 are identical. If the person-time distributions in both populations are equal, the term $(T_A/T_S \times \text{sum}[\text{rate}_{Si} \times T_{Si}])$ can be substituted for the term $\text{sum}[\text{rate}_{Si} \times T_{Ai}]$ near the end of the 4th line of Expression 6.11. If that substitution is done, the 4th line can be reduced to rate_A alone. The crude rate for population A1 and the indirectly standardized rate for population A1 will be equal if populations A1 and S1 have the same distribution of person-time. Those rates will also be equal to the directly standardized rate for A1. Standardization is designed to adjust the rate for population A1 to account for person-time differences between A1 and S1. If there are no differences in those distributions, direct and indirect standardization will not change the rate for population A1. Two populations are not likely to have precisely the same person-time distribution, but unless the differences are substantial, the SRR and SMR will be similar.

We can summarize by saying that for the SMR to differ from the SRR, the variable used for standardization must be a confounder of the association between population membership and the outcome. In Table 6.6, this criteria is fulfilled because old people are more likely, compared with young people, to be in population A1 and death rates increase with age. In addition, the standardizing variable must be an effect modifier. This is also true in Table 6.6 because although the rate of death increases with age in both populations, this increase is greater in population A1, so the effect of being in A1 on death, compared with being in S1, increases from a rate ratio of 1.0 among the young to a rate ratio of 4.0 among the old.

Even though Florida in 2010 had an older age distribution compared with the U.S. population (Figure 6.1, Tables 6.2 and 6.3) in 2000, the SRR comparing cancer mortality in those two populations was 0.84 (165.6/196.53), similar to the SMR of 0.84 (165.4/196.53) for the same comparison. (Earlier I reported an SMR of 0.83 for Florida. The small difference between 0.83 and 0.84 depends on whether the standard used is the U.S. 2000 standard population or the actual U.S. population from the 2000 census. See footnote to Table 6.3.) The Florida SRR and SMR estimates were similar because the Florida and U.S. age distributions are not that different and cancer mortality rate ratios comparing Florida with the United States across age strata did not vary greatly. The SRR and SMR will be similar unless population age distributions differ greatly *and* age-specific rate ratios vary substantially, as in Table 6.6. In many practical applications both of these circumstances will not be present and therefore comparisons of SMRs will not be biased. Yule (1934) discussed this in 1934 and noted that the two methods of standardization will commonly produce similar results. Other authors (Silcock 1959, Kilpatrick 1963, Breslow and Day 1987 pp72–73, Greenland, Rothman, and Lash 2008b p69), who have described the potential for bias if SMRs are compared, acknowledge that the SMR will often approximate the SRR and therefore comparisons of SMRs may often be unbiased.

Given this, should we prefer the SRR or the SMR? My view is that the SRR is the better choice, as it can reliably remove much of any confounding bias related to the stratifying variables and the comparison of two or more SRRs is well justified when the same standardizing weights are used. When the data allow calculation of the SMR, but not the SRR, the SMR will usually perform well. But in that situation, investigators might acknowledge that some potential for bias may exist.

6.12 THE TERMINOLOGY OF DIRECT AND INDIRECT STANDARDIZATION

In Yule's review of standardization (Yule 1934), he remarked that the terms direct and indirect were of little use, as they failed to distinguish one method from the other. He preferred to call these the fixed and changing base method. Both methods can be described in terms of the ratios of two counts and both methods involve weighted averages. The key distinguishing feature is that the direct method uses a standard set of weights that remains the same across all comparisons, while the indirect method uses weights that change from one comparison to the next. It is a shame that Yule's preferred terminology was not adopted.

6.13 P-VALUES FOR DIRECTLY STANDARDIZED RATES

To test the null hypotheses that the directly standardized rate for population A is not different from the crude rate of the standard population S (meaning that the SRR equals 1), we can use a stratified version of the score statistic (Peto and Pike 1973, Shore, Pasternack, and Curnen 1976, Greenland and Rothman 2008c p277), which was described in Chapter 4 (Expression 4.3):

Score statistic

$$= \text{sum}\left[|C_{Ai} - C_{Aexpi}|/\sqrt{C_{Aexpi}}\right]$$

$$= \text{sum}\left[|C_{Ai} - (T_A \times \text{rate}_{Ai} \times T_{Si}/T_S)|/\sqrt{(T_A \times \text{rate}_{Ai} \times T_{Si}/T_S)}\right]$$

(Ex.6.14)

Recall from Chapter 4 that if we assume a count arose from a Poisson process, then the variance of the count is equal to the count itself. The expected count in each stratum is an estimate of the variance for that stratum and these expected counts are used in Expression 6.14.

The mortality rate for population A2 (Table 6.7) is 371.4. Directly standardizing this rate to the age-categorized person-time of population S2 produces a rate of 516.7. The crude rate ratio is 1.59, the SRR 2.21. The score statistic from Expression 6.14 is 3.997 and the upper-tail P-value, from the normal distribution, for a score statistic this large or larger is .000032. The two-sided P-value is twice this amount, .000064. If no bias is present and the counts in Table 6.7 arose from a Poisson process, then the observed rate ratio of 2.21 is unlikely if the true rate in population A2 were in fact equal to that in population S2.

TABLE 6.7 Hypothetical age-categorized counts and rates of death in population A2 and standard population S2. Rates are per 100,000 person-years. Rate ratio = Population A2 rate/Standard population S2 rate.

AGE	POPULATION A2			STANDARD POPULATION S2			RATE RATIO
	COUNT	PERSON-TIME	RATE	COUNT	PERSON-TIME	RATE	
Young	5	2,000	250	1,000	1,000,000	100	2.5
Middle	3	1,000	300	2,000	1,000,000	200	1.5
Old	5	500	1000	4,000	1,000,000	400	2.5
All	13	3,500	371.4	7,000	3,000,000	233.3	1.59

Expression 6.14 assumes that person-time is measured without error. There is some systematic error in census estimates of person-time; for example, there is evidence that homeless persons are undercounted in the U.S. census. But the random error in person-time estimates in census data and many data sets will be small enough, compared with the random error of the count numerators, that we can usually ignore this source of error and treat person-time as if it were not subject to sampling error. Expression 6.14 also assumes that that only the expected counts contribute to the variance. This is justified because under the null hypothesis of no difference, the observed and expected counts should be equal.

6.14 CONFIDENCE INTERVALS FOR DIRECTLY STANDARDIZED RATES

The variance for a directly standardized rate is the weighted average of the stratum specific variances, with weights equal to the square of the person-time proportions in each stratum of the standard population (Keyfitz 1966, Breslow and Day 1987 p59, Armitage, Berry, and Matthews 2002 p662, Murphy, Xu, and Kochanek 2013 p49). Recall that C/T^2, or $rate^2/C$, is the variance of a rate from formula 4 in Table 4.4. Expression 6.15 estimates the variance for the rate of events in population A, standardized to population S:

Variance of a directly standardized rate

$$= sum\left[(T_{Si}/T_S)^2 \times C_{Ai}/T_{Ai}^2\right]$$

$$= sum\left[(T_{Si}/T_S)^2 \times rate_{Ai}^2/C_{Ai}\right]$$

(Ex.6.15)

The standard deviation (SD, equal to the SE here) for the standardized rate is the square root of this variance and this can be used to construct a CI. The standardized rate for population A2 (Table 6.7) is 516.7 per 100,000 person-years with SD 164.1 and 95% CI 194.9, 838.4.

Another method treats the rates as if they were binomial proportions (risks), with the count of events divided by the population estimate, as if that number of persons had actually been followed over time. This is a reasonable approximation for most population mortality rates because the count of events is much smaller than the size of the population (Keyfitz 1966, Cochrane 1977 p108, Kahn and Sempos 1989 pp92–93, Armitage, Berry, and Matthews 2002 p662). Using the same notation as in Expression 6.15, but defining C/T as a risk, not a rate, the formula is modified to use the variance for a binomial proportion in each stratum of age:

Variance of a directly standardized rate

$$= \text{sum}\left[(T_{Si}/T_S)^2 \times C_{Ai}/T_{Ai} \times (1 - C_{Ai}/T_{Ai})/T_{Ai}\right] \qquad \text{(Ex.6.16)}$$
$$= \text{sum}\left[(T_{Si}/T_S)^2 \times \text{risk}_{Ai} \times (1 - \text{risk}_{Ai})/T_{Ai}\right]$$

Using Expression 6.16, the SD for the directly standardized rate of 516.7 is 163.4 with 95% CI 196.4, 837.0. These results from Expressions 6.15 and 6.16 are close to each other.

6.15 P-VALUES AND CIS FOR SRRS (RATIOS OF DIRECTLY STANDARDIZED RATES)

The ratio of the directly standardized rate in population A2 to the crude rate in population S2 is an SRR: 516.7/233.3 = 2.21 (Table 6.7). If population S2 is large compared with A2, random (sampling) errors in the rates for S2 will be tiny compared with the errors for population A2, so the SD of the SRR uses Expression 6.17 for the errors in the rates of population A2 only (Yates 1934, Breslow and Day 1987 p64). The term in the numerator of Expression 6.17 is the square root of the variance from Expression 6.15 and the quantity in the denominator is simply the crude rate for the standard population:

SE of the SRR

$$= \left(\text{sum}\left[(T_{Si}/T_S)^2 \times C_{Ai}/T_{Ai}^2\right]\right)^{.5}/\text{sum}[(T_{Si}/T_S) \times (C_{Si}/T_{Si})] \qquad \text{(Ex.6.17)}$$
$$= \left(\text{sum}\left[(T_{Si}/T_S)^2 \times C_{Ai}/T_{Ai}^2\right]\right)^{.5}/(C_S/T_S)$$

As explained in Chapter 4, it is best to estimate the CI for a rate ratio on the ln scale (see Expression 4.8), because ratios are more symmetrical on that scale. This can be done using Expression 6.18 (Breslow and Day 1987 p64), which is similar to Expression 4.8 in Chapter 4. Expression 6.18 combines Expressions 6.8 and 6.17. Both Expressions 6.18 and 4.8 use the delta method; the SE of the ln of the estimated quantity is equal to the SE of the estimate divided by the estimate.

SE of the ln of the SRR

$$= \text{SE of the SRR}/\text{SRR}$$
$$= \left(\left(\text{sum}\left[(T_{Si}/T_S)^2 \times C_{Ai}/T_{Ai}^2\right]\right)^{.5}/(C_S/T_S)\right)/(\text{sum}[C_{Ai}/T_{Ai} \times T_{Si}]/C_S) \qquad \text{(Ex.6.18)}$$
$$= \left(\text{sum}\left[(T_{Si}/T_S)^2 \times C_{Ai}/T_{Ai}^2\right]\right)^{.5}/((\text{sum}[C_{Ai}/T_{Ai} \times T_{Si}])/T_S)$$
$$= \left(\text{sum}\left[(T_{Si}/T_S)^2 \times C_{Ai}/T_{Ai}^2\right]\right)^{.5}/\text{sum}[C_{Ai}/T_{Ai} \times T_{Si}/T_S]$$

Using Expression 6.17, the SE for the SRR of 2.21 for population A2 (Table 6.7) is 0.70, the ln of the SRR is 0.79, and using Expression 6.18 the SE of the ln of the SRR is 0.32. The ratio of the ln SRR and SE of the ln SRR can be used to compute a Wald statistic of 2.50 and an upper tail P-value of .006 for the hypothesis that the SRR is equal to 1. The two-sided P-value is .012. The 95% CIs for SRR are computed on the ln scale and then exponentiated: 1.19, 4.13.

The ratio of two standardized rates, both standardized to the same population, is equal to the ratio of the SRRs for those rates. The SE of the ln of the ratio of two standardized rates or the two SRRs for those rates (Breslow and Day 1987 p64), one for population A, one for population B, both standardized to the same population S, is the square root of the sum of the variances for the ln of each SRR:

SE of the ln of (SRR_A/SRR_B)

$$= (sum[(T_{Si}/T_S)^2 \times C_{Ai}/T_{Ai}^2]/(sum[C_{Ai}/T_{Ai} \times T_{Si}/T_S])^2 \qquad \text{(Ex.6.19)}$$
$$+ sum[(T_{Si}/T_S)^2 \times C_{Bi}/T_{Bi}^2]/(sum[C_{Bi}/T_{Bi} \times T_{Si}/T_S])^2)^{.5}$$

6.16 LARGE SAMPLE P-VALUES AND CIS FOR SMRS

The observed count of deaths in population A2 was 13 and the expected count based upon the total person-time in A2, the rates in S, and the person-time weights from A2 is 6.0, so the SMR is 13/6 = 2.17 (Table 6.7). Although age is a confounder of the association between being in A2, compared with being in S, and the outcome of death, this association does not change much from one age group to the next; the age-stratified rate ratios range from 1.5 to 2.5, pretty close to the weighted average of the SRR, 2.21. Since the association is not modified much by age, the SMR comparing population A2 with the standard population is 2.17, close to the SRR of 2.21.

The SE of the SMR is (Breslow and Day 1987 p67):

SE of the SMR

$$= C_A^{.5}/Exp_A \qquad \text{(Ex.6.20)}$$

Using Expression 6.20, the SE of the SMR for population A2 (Table 6.7) is 0.60. But, as with the SRR, it is best to do this on the ln scale (Breslow and Day 1987 p67):

SE of the ln SMR

$$= \text{SE of the SMR/SMR}$$
$$= (C_A^{.5}/Exp_A)/(C_A/Exp_A) \qquad \text{(Ex.6.21)}$$
$$= 1/C_A^{.5}$$

The ln of the SMR is 0.77 and using Expression 6.21 the SE of the ln of the SMR is 0.28. Computing the 95% boundaries on the ln scale and exponentiating, the 95% CI for the SMR is 1.29, 3.81. The ratio of the ln SMR and SE of the ln SMR produces a Wald statistic of 2.79 and an upper tail P-value of .0027 for the hypothesis that the SRR is equal to 1. The two-sided P-value is .0053. The SE and P-value for the SMR are both smaller, and the CI narrower, compared with the same statistics for the SRR, because of the homogeneity assumption used by the SMR calculations.

6.17 SMALL SAMPLE P-VALUES AND CIS FOR SMRS

The formulae above will work fairly well when the observed event count is sufficiently large. When the observed count is small a P-value may be calculated by comparing the value of χ in Expression 6.22 with the normal distribution (Rothman and Boice 1979, Breslow and Day 1987 p69). The quantity C_A^* is equal to C_A, the observed count, if C_A is greater than the expected count (Exp_A) and otherwise C_A^* is equal to $C_A + 1$.

$$\chi = (9 \times C_A{}^*)^{.5} \times \left[1 - 1/(9 \times C_A{}^*) - (Exp_A/C_A{}^*)^{1/3}\right]$$

(Ex.6.22)

For the SMR of 2.17 from Table 6.7, $C_A{}^*$ is 13 and Exp_A is 6, so χ is 2.365, the upper-tail P-value is .0090, and the two-sided P-value is .0180, 3-fold larger than the two-sided P-value of .0053 from the Wald statistic.

While computer programs can compute exact CIs for an SMR, good approximations can be found using Expression 6.23 (Rothman and Boice 1979, Breslow and Day 1987 p69). In Expression 6.23 the approximate upper and lower limits are estimated for the count of the outcomes and those counts are divided by the expected count. The quantity $z_{\alpha/2}$ indicates the $100 \times (1 - \alpha)$ percentile of the unit normal distribution; for alpha equal to .10 this quantity is about 1.64 and for alpha equal to .05 it is approximately 1.96.

Lower confidence limit for the SMR

$$= C_A \times \left[1 - 1/(9 \times C_A) - \left(z_{\alpha/2}/\left(3 \times C_A{}^{.5}\right)\right)\right]^3/Exp_A$$

(Ex.6.23)

Upper confidence limit for the SMR

$$= (C_A + 1) \times \left[1 - 1/(9 \times (C_A + 1)) + \left(z_{\alpha/2}/\left(3 \times (C_A + 1)^{.5}\right)\right)\right]^3/Exp_A$$

For the SMR of 2.17 the 95% CI from Expression 6.23 is 1.153, 3.705. These are close to the exact limits of 1.154, 3.705.

6.18 STANDARDIZED RATES SHOULD NOT BE USED AS REGRESSION OUTCOMES

Age-standardized rates are sometimes used as the outcomes of linear regression models in the mistaken belief that doing this will remove age as a potential confounding variable. But adjustment of the outcomes alone, without accounting for how the other regression variables are related to age, will generally produce biased estimates (Rosenbaum and Rubin 1984).

6.19 STANDARDIZATION IS NOT ALWAYS THE BEST CHOICE

Standardization creates summary rates that can be used for comparisons that are relatively free of bias related to population differences in the distribution of the standardizing variables. But standardized rates are not the actual rates for a population; they are approximations of what the rate might have been if the population had a different distribution of the standardizing factors or had the stratum-specific rates of another population. In many situations the actual rate, not the standardized rate, will be desired.

A single summary estimate such as the SRR or SMR may not be the most useful way of comparing two populations. If the rate ratios vary substantially across levels of the standardizing variables, the stratum-specific estimates may be more informative than a summary estimate (Breslow and Day 1987 pp61,75, Greenland and Rothman 2008c pp264–265). This may be true for any method that summarizes associations in the presence of important variation across strata.

Stratified Analysis

Inverse-Variance and Mantel-Haenszel Methods

7

Standardized adjustment, discussed in Chapter 6, creates a weighted-average of stratum-specific rate ratios or differences using weights equal to the person-time distribution of a real or hypothetical population. In this chapter I discuss inverse-variance, Mantel-Haenszel, and maximum-likelihood methods which also create weighted averages of rate ratios or differences. These methods pool stratum-specific ratio or difference estimates using weights that reflect the precision of each stratum estimate. A stratum with lots of data will usually have a more precise estimate and that stratum will get more weight in the analysis compared with strata that contain little information. These methods assume that the individual rate ratios or differences in each stratum all estimate the same true quantity. This is called the assumption of homogeneity or uniformity of effect (Greenland and Rothman 2008c pp270–272). These methods treat any differences in the stratum-specific estimated associations as if they were due to random variation from one stratum to the next.

Inverse-variance, Mantel-Haenszel, and maximum likelihood methods have the advantage, compared with standardization, of being *efficient*. They produce the most precise estimate possible from the data (Rothman 2012 pp189–191). However, if the assumption of homogeneity is not true, the pooled estimates may be biased. Imagine, for example, that we wished to summarize a set of rate ratios that varied across strata because of differences in the true effect of the exposure from one stratum to the next. If we create a summary estimate based upon the precision of each stratum estimate, this would not be likely to estimate the average effect across all the strata. The precision of each stratum estimate is related to the event count in each stratum, but there is no reason to think that in the absence of homogeneity that the precision-related weights would result in a summary estimate that was a true average for the entire population. One option is to use precision-weighted methods to identify sources of heterogeneity and report different estimated associations according to characteristics of the strata that account for this heterogeneity.

7.1 INVERSE-VARIANCE METHODS

Inverse-variance weighting has also been called direct pooling, precision weighting, the Woolf method, weighted least squares (Greenland and Rothman 2008c p271) and information weighting (Greenland 2008a p334). The weights are the inverse of the variance ($1/(\text{standard error})^2 = 1/SE^2$) of each rate difference or ratio (Kleinbaum, Kupper, and Morgenstern 1982 pp341–342,359–361). The variances are equal to the square of the SE (SE^2) of the mean for row 5 (rate differences) or row 10 (rate ratios) in the last column of Table 4.4.

Inverse-variance methods are often used to summarize results from several studies in a meta-analysis, because all that is required from each study is the estimated association and a measure of precision, such as the SE or confidence interval (CI) for each estimate. Mantel-Haenszel methods require the study (or stratum) specific counts and person-time data, which are not always available.

Inverse-variance, Mantel-Haenszel, and maximum likelihood methods all rely on asymptotic normality assumptions; the estimates and their variances are valid when the counts in the data are infinitely large. When overall counts are small, these methods will be biased. Additionally, inverse-variance and maximum-likelihood methods require that within each stratum to be summarized or within the cross-classification of the regression variables (for a maximum-likelihood regression model), the counts should not be too small (Pike, Hill, and Smith 1980, Breslow 1981, Greenland and Robins 1985, Robinson and Jewell 1991, Peduzzi et al. 1996, Greenland, Schwartzbaum, and Finkle 2000, Vittingh-off and McCulloch 2007). As a rule-of-thumb, outcome counts of 10 or more are desirable within each stratum. Having strata with counts of 0 or 1, often called "sparse" data, will likely result in bias when inverse-variance and maximum likelihood methods are used. In contrast, Mantel-Haenszel methods perform well when the data are sparse, even when some rate numerator counts are zero, provided the overall counts are sufficiently large.

7.2 INVERSE-VARIANCE ANALYSIS OF RATE RATIOS

Imagine we have data from 2 randomized trials of Drug A versus a placebo (Table 7.1). To average rate ratios we use the log scale. The letters E and NE can be used as subscripts to indicate exposed and not exposed elements of the data; the letters indicate the two exposure levels that are being compared. The last column of row 10 in Table 4.4 shows us that the variance of the ln rate ratio for the US study is $(1/C_E + 1/C_{NE})$. The inverse of this variance can be expressed as $1/(1/C_E + 1/C_{NE})$ or $(1/C_E + 1/C_{NE})^{-1}$ or $(C_E \times C_{NE})/(C_E + C_{NE}) = 1/(1/20 + 1/60) = 15$. For the French study the inverse variance is $1/(1/12 + 1/30) = 8.571$. If we abbreviate the rate ratios as rrUS and rrFr and the variance for the ln of each rate ratio as varlnrrUS and varlnrrFr, the inverse-variance weighted estimate of the pooled rate ratio for both studies is equal to exponential([(ln(rrUS) x 1/varlnrrUS) + ln(rrFr) x 1/varlnrrFr]/(1/varlnrrUS +1/varlnrrFr)) = exponential([(ln(.5) x 15.0 + ln(.4) x 8.571)]/(15.0 +8.571)) = 0.461.

The variance of the ln of the pooled rate ratio is the inverse of the sum of the inverse-variances of the individual ln rate ratios (Expression 7.1).

Variance of the ln of a pooled rate ratio for k rate ratios

$$= 1/(1/\text{variance}\ln(rr1) + 1/\text{variance}\ln(rr2) + \ldots + 1/\text{variance}\ln(rrk)) \tag{Ex.7.1}$$

$$= 1/\left(1/\text{selnrr1}^2 + 1/\text{selnrr2}^2 + \ldots + 1/\text{selnrrk}^2\right)$$

Using Expression 7.1 and the data in Table 7.1, the lower 95% confidence limit for the pooled rate ratio of 0.461 is:

TABLE 7.1 Counts and rates (per 1 person-time unit) of disease outcome events in two hypothetical randomized controlled trials that compared Drug A with placebo. 95% confidence intervals are shown for the estimates from each study.

STUDY	TREATMENT	COUNT	PERSON-TIME UNITS	RATE	RATE RATIO[a] (95% CI)	RATE DIFFERENCE[b] (95% CI)
US	Drug A	20	20	1	0.5	−1
US	Placebo	60	30	2	(0.30, 0.83)	(−1.67, −0.33)
French	Drug A	12	10	1.2	0.4	−1.8
French	Placebo	30	10	3	(0.20, 0.78)	(−3.07, −0.53)

[a] Rate ratio = Drug A rate/Placebo rate
[b] Rate difference = Drug A rate − Placebo rate

$$\text{exponential}\left(\left[\left(\ln(\text{rrUS}) \times 1/\text{selnrrUS}^2\right) + \left(\ln(\text{rrFr}) \times 1/\text{selnrrUS}^2\right)\right]/\left(1/\text{selnrrUS}^2+1/\text{selnrrFr}^2\right)\right.$$
$$-\left(z \text{ for } 1-\text{alpha}/2\right) \times \left(1/\left(1/\text{selnrrUS}^2 + 1/\text{selnrrFr}^2\right)\right)^{0.5}\right])$$
$$= \text{ exponential}\left(\left[(\ln(.5) \times 15.0) + (\ln(.4) \times 8.571)\right]/(15.0+8.571)\right.$$
$$-\left[(1.96) \times (1/(15.0+8.571))^{0.5}\right])$$
$$= 0.308.$$

Changing the minus sign to a plus sign in this Expression provides the upper confidence limit of 0.690. We can avoid all this busy work by using Stata's **ir** command with the pool option:

```
. ir count rx ptime, pool by(study) istandard
              study |    IRR        [95% Conf. Interval]       Weight
- - - - - - - +- - - - - - - - - - - - - - - - - - - - - - - - - - - - - -
                 US |     .5    .2854585   .8414213            20   (exact)
             French |     .4    .1865091   .8045291            10   (exact)
- - - - - - - +- - - - - - - - - - - - - - - - - - - - - - - - - - - - - -
              Crude | .4740741    .3063497   .7168435               (exact)
   Pooled (direct) | .4610309    .3078979   .6903244
  I. Standardized | .4571429    .3047361   .6857723
- - - - - - - - - - - - - - - - - - - - - - - - - - - - - - - - - - - - - -
Test of homogeneity (direct) chi2(1) =     0.27 Pr>chi2 = 0.6023
```

The "crude" rate ratio reported by the **ir** command is just the ratio of two rates collapsed across study. For those exposed to Drug A, the rate was $(20 + 12)/(20 + 10)$, for those not exposed the rate was $(60 + 30)/(30 + 10)$, and the ratio of these two rates is 0.474. The pooled or inverse variance rate ratio of 0.461 is so close to the crude ratio that they are essentially the same in this example. But they are not identical. The pooled rate ratio is the rate ratio "adjusted" for study, using the inverse-variance method. If we use Poisson regression (see Chapter 9) to estimate the crude rate ratio, omitting study from the model, we get the crude rate ratio of 0.474 reported above. Poisson regression uses person-time weights, not inverse-variance weights. If we adjust for study in Poisson regression, the result is 0.4598; close to the pooled estimate, but not exactly the same.

Assume we know the rates and CIs for the trials in Table 7.1, but the counts and person-time data are unknown to us. This situation might arise in a meta-analysis; the study authors may report the final estimates and CIs, but not the count and person-time information. Or the estimates may be adjusted for other variables, in which case the adjusted rate ratio estimates and their CIs will be what we want for a meta-analysis. The SE for the ln of the rate ratio for the US study can be obtained on the ln scale using the 95% CI and setting z equal to about 1.96, which is the z-score when alpha is equal to .05: SE ln rate ratio (US) = |upper limit – lower limit|/(2 x z for 1-alpha/2) = | ln(0.8294) – ln(0.3014) |/(2 x 1.96) = 0.258. The inverse of the variance for the ln of the rate ratio for the US study is $1/SE^2 = 15.0$. This inverse variance can be estimated in one step as $1/[(\ln(0.8294) - \ln(.3014))/(2 \times 1.96)]^2$. The inverse of the variance of the ln of the rate ratio for the French study can be obtained in the same way and the two ln rate ratios can be pooled as shown previously, along with the variance for the pooled rate ratio. Once the ln of the rate ratios and their SEs are calculated, the final pooling can be done by Stata's **metan** command, a command for meta-analysis, to obtain the same results that were reported by the **ir** command:

```
. metan lnrr se2, fixedi eform nograph
      Study       |  ES    [95% Conf. Interval]    % Weight
- - - - - - - - - - - +- - - - - - - - - - - - - - - - - - - - - - - - - - -
1                 | 0.500    0.301    0.829          63.63
2                 | 0.400    0.205    0.781          36.37
```

```
- - - - - - - - - - - - - - +- - - - - - - - - - - - - - - - - - - - - - - - - - - - - - - -
I-V pooled ES      | 0.461    0.308   0.690     100.00
- - - - - - - - - - - - - - +- - - - - - - - - - - - - - - - - - - - - - - - - - - - - - - -
  Heterogeneity chi-squared =  0.27 (d.f. = 1) p = 0.602
  I-squared (variation in ES attributable to heterogeneity) =  0.0%

  Test of ES=1 : z=  3.76 p = 0.000
```

We can formally test the assumption of homogeneity upon which the pooled estimate relies. The test statistic is a chi-squared statistic that can be compared with a chi-squared distribution with degrees of freedom equal to the number of strata (rate ratio estimates) minus 1; the P-value is the proportion of the chi-square distribution in its upper tail for values larger than the test statistic. We compute the deviations of each stratum estimate from the pooled estimate, divide each deviation by the SE of the stratum estimate, square these quantities, and sum them. A Wald statistic divides an estimate by its SE. The statistic for a test of homogeneity (sometimes called a heterogeneity statistic) is a type of Wald statistic, as it divides each difference between the pooled and stratum estimate by the SE of the stratum estimate and then squares that quantity. In the meta-analysis literature this statistic is often designated by the letter Q (Hedges and Olkin 1985 p123, Sutton et al. 2000 pp38–39, Deeks, Altman, and Bradburn 2001 p293).

Test statistic of the hypothesis of homogeneity of stratum estimates

$$= Q$$
$$= X^2$$
$$= \text{sum}\left[(\text{estimate}_i - \text{pooled estimate})^2 / (\text{SE of estimate}_i)^2\right]$$
$$= \text{sum}\left[(\text{estimate}_i - \text{pooled estimate})^2 / (\text{variance of estimate}_i)\right] \qquad \text{(Ex.7.2)}$$
$$= \text{sum}\left[((\text{estimate}_i - \text{pooled estimate}) / (\text{SE of estimate}_i))^2\right]$$
$$= \text{sum}[\text{estimate}_i^2 / (\text{SE of estimate}_i)^2$$
$$\quad - \text{sum}[((\text{estimate}_i / (\text{SE of estimate}_i)^2)^2] / \text{sum}\left[1 / (\text{SE of estimate}_i)^2]\right]$$

Following Expression 7.2, the test statistic for homogeneity of rate ratios is done on the ln scale:

Test statistic of the hypothesis of homogeneity of rate ratios

$$= X^2 \qquad \text{(Ex.7.3)}$$
$$= \text{sum}\left[(\text{lnrr}_i - \text{pooled lnrr})^2 / \text{selnrr}_i^2\right]$$

For the two rate ratios in Table 7.1 the homogeneity statistic is 0.272 and the P-value (proportion of area in the upper tail of the chi-squared distribution for values greater than 0.272, for 1 degree of freedom) is .60; these were reported earlier by both the **ir** and **metan** commands. This indicates little evidence of any difference in the true rate ratios for the U.S. and French study populations. The rate ratio estimates from the two studies are plausible if the true rate ratio is 0.461 in both populations. A large P-value does not eliminate the possibility that the estimates from the U.S. and French studies are truly different, it only tells us that the available evidence does not strongly reject the view that they are estimates of the same true rate ratio.

Tests of homogeneity have low power in most situations. Studies are often planned to have 80 or 90% power to find a statistically significant deviation of a given size between the estimated association and the null value using all the data. When we stratify the data for a homogeneity test, power is reduced, often greatly, because stratification increases the total variance and within each stratum the smaller sample size reduces the precision of each estimate (Brookes et al. 2004, Greenland and Rothman 2008c p270).

7.3 INVERSE-VARIANCE ANALYSIS OF RATE DIFFERENCES

To get the pooled rate difference for Table 7.1 we do not use the log scale. If the count and person-time information are known, then we can estimate the variance of each rate difference using formula 5 of Table 4.4. The variance of the rate difference (variance rd) for the US study is $C_{EUS}/T_{EUS}^2 + C_{NEUS}/T_{NEUS}^2 = rate_{EUS}/T_{EUS} + rate_{NEUS}/T_{NEUS} = 1/20 + 2/60 = 0.1167$. The inverse-variance weighted summary rate difference is $[(rate_{EUS} - rate_{NEUS}) \times 1/variance\ rd(US)] + [(rate_{EFR} - rate_{NEFR}) \times 1/variance\ rd(FR)]/[1/variance\ rd(US) + 1/variance\ rd(FR)] = [(1-2) \times 1/0.1167 + (1.2-3) \times 1/.042]/[1/0.1167 + 1/.042] = -1.17$.

The variance of the pooled rate difference is the inverse of the sum of the inverse-variances of the individual rate differences (Expression 7.4)

Variance of the pooled rate difference for k rate differences

$$= 1/(1/variancerd1 + 1/variancerd2 + \ldots + 1/variancerdk)$$ (Ex.7.4)

$$= 1/(1/serd1^2 + 1/serd2^2 + \ldots + 1/serdk^2)$$

Using Expression 7.4, the lower 95% confidence limit for the pooled rate difference is

$$\left[(rdUS \times 1/serdUS^2) + (rdFR \times 1/serdFR^2)\right]/(1/serdUS^2 + 1/serdFR^2)$$
$$- \left[(z\ for\ 1 - alpha/2) \times (1/(1/serd1^2 + 1/serd2^2))^{0.5}\right]$$
$$= \left[(-1 \times (1/0.341^2) - 1.8 \times (1/0.648^2))/(1/0.342^2 + 1/0.648^2)\right]$$
$$- \left[1.96/(1/(1/0.341^2 + 1/0.648^2))^{.5}\right]$$
$$= -1.77$$

Changing the last minus sign to a plus provides the upper confidence limit of –0.58. The **ir** command can do the heavy lifting:

```
. ir count rx ptime, by(study) ird pool istandard
            study |      IRD    [95% Conf. Interval]   Weight
------------------+-----------------------------------------------
                1 |       -1    -1.669455   -.3305449     20
                2 |     -1.8    -3.070202   -.5297982     10
------------------+-----------------------------------------------
            Crude | -1.183333   -1.777191   -.5894754
   Pooled (direct) | -1.173913   -1.766148   -.5816784
   I. Standardized | -1.266667   -1.881853   -.6514798
------------------------------------------------------------------
Test of homogeneity (direct) chi2(1) =    1.19 Pr>chi2 = 0.2748
```

If we only know the rate differences and their 95% CIs, we can calculate the SE for the rate difference for the U.S. study using the 95% CI for the rate difference and setting z equal to 1.96: (upper limit – lower limit)/(2 x z for 1-alpha/2) = (–0.331 – (–1.669))/(2 x 1.96) = 0.341. We can compute the SE for the French study rate difference in a similar manner and use these SE values to calculate the pooled rate difference as previously described.

To test the hypothesis of homogeneity of the rate differences we use a version of Expression 7.2 for rate differences:

Test statistic for the hypothesis of homogeneity of rate differences

$$= X^2$$

$$= \text{sum}\left[(rd_i - \text{pooledrd})^2 / serd_i^2\right]$$

(Ex.7.5)

The homogeneity statistic is 1.19, there is 1 degree of freedom, and the P-value is .27, just as reported by the **ir** command. The **metan** command can provide the same results.

7.4 CHOOSING BETWEEN RATE RATIOS AND DIFFERENCES

Homogeneity statistics can be used to help us decide whether to pool estimates on a rate ratio or a rate difference scale. In meta-analyses, summaries on the ratio scale are usually a better fit to the data (Deeks 2002). But considerations other than fit to the data may help drive the choice.

For Table 7.1, the homogeneity statistic for the pooled rate ratio was 0.272 compared with 1.19 for the pooled rate difference. This indicates the pooled rate ratio is a better fit to the data, although the differences in the homogeneity tests in this example are small and not terribly persuasive. Examining the rate ratios and differences themselves leads to the same choice. The U.S./French rate ratios is 0.5/0.4 = 1.25 whereas the ratio of the rate differences, −1/−1.8 = 0.56, is further from the null. An argument can be made that the ratio and difference estimates are pretty similar and the homogeneity statistics failed to reject homogeneity on either scale; therefore pooling is reasonable on both scales and the choice could depend on factors aside from the test statistics. The choice between ratio and difference summaries for Table 7.1 is not clear-cut. In real data the contrast will sometimes be more extreme.

7.5 MANTEL-HAENSZEL METHODS

In 1951 a paper by Jerome Cornfield (1951) showed how a risk ratio could be estimated from case-control data; the odds ratio comparing the exposure history of cases (persons with a disease outcome) and controls (persons without the outcome) will closely estimate the risk ratio for the disease among those exposed compared with those not, provided that the outcome is sufficiently rare in the population from which the cases and controls were selected. This was discussed in Chapter 3 (Table 3.3). Cornfield's insight encouraged the use of the case-control study design, but his paper did not present suitable methods for adjusting the crude odds ratio for potential confounding factors. In 1959 Nathan Mantel and William Haenszel (1959) showed how adjustment could be done and their methods are still in use. Their method dealt with confounding by creating odds ratios within levels of confounding factors and summarizing those odds ratios using special weights. Subsequently, their methods were extended to risk ratios (Nurminen 1981, Tarone 1981, Kleinbaum, Kupper, and Morgenstern 1982 p345, Greenland and Robins 1985, Newman 2001 pp148–149, Greenland and Rothman 2008c pp274–275, Cummings 2009a), risk differences (Greenland and Robins 1985, Newman 2001 pp155–156, Cummings 2011), odds ratios from matched case-control studies (Kleinbaum, Kupper, and Morgenstern

1982 p344), risk ratios from matched cohort studies (Cummings and McKnight 2004, Cummings 2011), rate ratios (Rothman and Boice 1979 pp12–13, Kleinbaum, Kupper, and Morgenstern 1982 p345,361, Breslow 1984, Greenland and Robins 1985, Breslow and Day 1987 pp109–114, Greenland and Rothman 2008c pp273–274) and rate differences (Kleinbaum, Kupper, and Morgenstern 1982 p361, Greenland and Robins 1985, Greenland and Rothman 2008c pp273–274).

As long as the overall counts are large, Mantel-Haenszel methods produce unbiased estimates even when there are many sparse strata; this is an advantage compared with inverse-variance and maximum likelihood estimation (Greenland and Robins 1985, Greenland and Rothman 2008c). For rate ratios, Mantel-Haenszel and maximum likelihood methods produce similar CIs, but for rate differences the Mantel-Haenszel CIs can be much wider (Greenland and Robins 1985, Greenland and Rothman 2008c). Therefore it is best to summarize rate differences using maximum likelihood, unless small stratum counts require the use of Mantel-Haenszel estimators.

7.6 MANTEL-HAENSZEL ANALYSIS OF RATE RATIOS

The letters E and NE will be used as subscripts to indicate exposed and not exposed segments of the data. The Mantel-Haenszel pooled rate ratio (Rothman and Boice 1979 pp12–13, Nurminen 1981, Kleinbaum, Kupper, and Morgenstern 1982 p361, Breslow 1984, Breslow and Day 1987 p109, Newman 2001, Greenland and Rothman 2008c pp273–274) is

$\text{Mantel} - \text{Haenszel rate ratio}$

$$
\begin{aligned}
&= \text{sum}[C_{Ei} \times T_{NEi}/(T_{Ei} + T_{NEi})]/\text{sum}[C_{NEi} \times T_{Ei}/(T_{Ei} + T_{NEi})] \\
&= \text{sum}[C_{Ei}/T_{Ei} \times T_{Ei} \times T_{NEi}/(T_{Ei} + T_{NEi})] \\
&\quad /\text{sum}[C_{NEi}/T_{NEi} \times T_{NEi} \times T_{Ei}/(T_{Ei} + T_{NEi})] \\
&= \text{sum}[\text{rate}_{Ei} \times T_{Ei} \times T_{NEi}/(T_{Ei} + T_{NEi})]/\text{sum}[\text{rate}_{NEi} \times T_{NEi} \times T_{Ei}/(T_{Ei} + T_{NEi})] \\
&= \text{sum}[\text{rate}_{Ei} \times T_{Ei} \times T_{NEi}/(T_{Ei} + T_{NEi})]/\text{sum}[C_{NEi} \times T_{Ei}/(T_{Ei} + T_{NEi})] \\
&= \text{sum}[(\text{rate}_{Ei}/\text{rate}_{NEi}) \times C_{NEi} \times T_{Ei}/(T_{Ei} + T_{NEi})]/\text{sum}[C_{NEi} \times T_{Ei}/(T_{Ei} + T_{NEi})]
\end{aligned}
$$

(Ex.7.6)

The last line of Expression 7.6 shows that the Mantel-Haenszel pooled rate ratio is a weighted average of the stratum rate ratios, with weights equal to the stratum count of events among unexposed persons multiplied by the stratum person-time of the exposed, divided by the total stratum person-time of those exposed and not exposed: $C_{NEi} \times T_{Ei}/(T_{Ei} + T_{NEi})$. The Mantel-Haenszel method does *not* pool rate ratios on the logarithmic scale, unlike the other methods that we have discussed. The Mantel-Haenszel weight for the U.S. study is 24, for French study it is 15, so the Mantel-Haenszel rate ratio is $[(.5 \times 24) + (.4 \times 15)]/(24 + 15) = 0.46154$, similar to the pooled inverse-variance rate ratio of 0.46103; the two methods provide essentially the same result for the data in Table 7.1.

In the textbook by Breslow and Day (Breslow and Day 1987 p109 eq3.16) the formula for the Mantel-Haenszel rate ratio has incorrect subscripts that invert the numerator and denominator. Breslow gives the formula with the correct subscripts in an earlier publication (Breslow 1984).

A formula for the variance of the ln of the Mantel-Haenszel rate ratio was described by Tarone in 1981 (Tarone 1981). Breslow proposed a different formula in 1984 (Breslow 1984) and that formula is given in the Breslow and Day textbook (Breslow and Day 1987 p109). The variance for the ln of the Mantel-Haenszel rate ratio in Expression 7.7 was proposed by Greenland and Robins in 1985 (Greenland and Robins 1985, Rothman 1986a p213, Greenland and Rothman 2008c p273). The variance from Expression 7.7 performs well when the overall counts are large, even if stratum counts are small.

Variance of the ln of the Mantel − Haenszel rate ratio

$$= \text{sum}\left[(C_{Ei} + C_{NEi}) \times T_{Ei} \times T_{NEi}/(T_{Ei} + T_{NEi})^2\right] \quad \text{(Ex.7.7)}$$
$$/[\text{sum}[C_{Ei} \times T_{NEi}/(T_{Ei} + T_{NEi})] \times [\text{sum}[C_{NEi} \times T_{Ei}/(T_{Ei} + T_{NEi})]$$

For the Mantel-Haenszel rate ratio of 0.4615, the ln of the variance is 0.04231 and the 95% CI, with the endpoints calculated on the ln scale and then exponentiated, is 0.3084, 0.6907.

The Mantel-Haenszel statistic for a test of homogeneity of rate ratios, derived from Expression 7.3, is 0.272, similar to the value using the inverse-variance method. The **ir** command can produce all of these results:

```
. ir count rx ptime, pool by(study)
        study |      IRR    [95% Conf. Interval]   M-H Weight
--------------+----------------------------------------------
          US  |       .5    .2854585   .8414213       24 (exact)
      French  |       .4    .1865091   .8045291       15 (exact)
--------------+----------------------------------------------
       Crude  |  .4740741   .3063497   .7168435          (exact)
Pooled (direct)| .4610309   .3078979   .6903244
 M-H combined | .4615385    .308408    .6907011
--------------------------------------------------------------
Test of homogeneity (direct) chi2(1) =    0.27  Pr>chi2 = 0.6023
Test of homogeneity (M-H)    chi2(1) =    0.27  Pr>chi2 = 0.6022
```

7.7 MANTEL-HAENSZEL ANALYSIS OF RATE DIFFERENCES

The Mantel-Haenszel rate difference (Greenland and Robins 1985, Greenland and Rothman 2008c p273) is shown in Expression 7.8.

Mantel − Haenszel rate difference

$$= \text{sum}[(C_{Ei} \times T_{NEi} - C_{NEi} \times T_{Ei})/(T_{Ei} + T_{NEi})]/\text{sum}[T_{Ei} \times T_{NEi}/(T_{Ei} + T_{NEi})]$$
$$= \text{sum}[(\text{rate}_{Ei} \times T_{Ei} \times T_{NEi} - \text{rate}_{NEi} \times T_{Ei} \times T_{NEi})/(T_{Ei} + T_{NEi})] \quad \text{(Ex.7.8)}$$
$$/\text{sum}[T_{Ei} \times T_{NEi}/(T_{Ei} + T_{NEi})]$$
$$= \text{sum}[(\text{rate}_{Ei} - \text{rate}_{NEi}) \times T_{Ei} \times T_{NEi}/(T_{Ei} + T_{NEi})]/\text{sum}[T_{Ei} \times T_{NEi}/(T_{Ei} + T_{NEi})]$$

The last line of Expression 7.8 describes the Mantel-Haenszel rate difference as a weighted average of the stratum rate differences, with weights equal to the stratum person-time of the exposed multiplied by the stratum person-time of the unexposed, divided by the stratum total person-time of those exposed and those not exposed: $T_{Ei} \times T_{NEi}/(T_{Ei} + T_{NEi})$. The Mantel-Haenszel weight is 12 for the U.S. study and 5 for the French study, so the Mantel-Haenszel rate difference is [(1–2) x 12 + (1.2–3) x 5)]/(12 + 5) = −1.2353, a little different from the inverse-variance estimate of −1.1739.

Variance of the Mantel – Haenszel rate difference

$$= \text{sum}\left[\left(C_{Ei} \times T_{NEi}{}^2 + C_{NEi} \times T_{Ei}{}^2\right)/\left(T_{Ei} + T_{NEi}\right)^2\right]$$
$$/\left(\text{sum}[T_{Ei} \times T_{NEi}/(T_{Ei} + T_{NEi})]\right)^2 \qquad \text{(Ex.7.9)}$$
$$= \text{sum}\left[\left(\left(\text{rate}_{Ei}/T_{Ei}\right) + \left(\text{rate}_{NEi}/T_{NEi}\right)\right) \times \left(T_{Ei} \times T_{NEi}/(T_{Ei} + T_{NEi})\right)\right)^2\right]$$
$$/\left(\text{sum}[T_{Ei} \times T_{NEi}/(T_{Ei} + T_{NEi})]\right)^2$$

The variance of the Mantel-Haenszel rate difference is 0.09446, slightly larger than the variance of 0.09130 for the rate difference from the inverse-variance method. The **ir** command can produce the Mantel-Haenszel summary estimate if we create the required weights:

```
. gen double mhwgt = 20*30/(20+30) if study==1
(2 missing values generated)
. replace mhwgt    = 10*10/(10+10) if study==2
(2 real changes made)
. ir count rx ptime, pool by(study) ird standard(mhwgt)
```

study	IRD	[95% Conf. Interval]		Weight
1	-.001	-.0016695	-.0003305	12
2	-.0018	-.0030702	-.0005298	5
Crude	-.0011833	-.0017772	-.0005895	
Pooled (direct)	-.0011739	-.0017661	-.0005817	
Standardized	-.0012353	-.0018377	-.0006329	

Test of homogeneity (direct) chi2(1) =   1.19 Pr>chi2 = 0.2748

The chi-squared statistic for a test of homogeneity described in Expressions 7.2, 7.3, and 7.5 is a Wald-type statistic and the pooled estimate used in those Expressions should be a maximum likelihood estimate. Mantel-Haenszel pooled estimates are not maximum likelihood estimates, however the test statistic will usually work well for Mantel-Haenszel rate ratios. But it is not usually valid for Mantel-Haenszel rate differences (Greenland and Rothman 2008c p279).

7.8 P-VALUES FOR STRATIFIED RATE RATIOS OR DIFFERENCES

The Mantel-Haenszel statistic for testing the overall hypothesis of no association using person-time data is a version of the score statistic in Expressions 4.3 and 6.14. The null hypothesis is that the rates of those exposed and not exposed do not differ; this may be considered a test that the summary rate ratio is 1 or the summary rate difference is 0. As with the version of this test for standardized rates (Expression 6.14), within each stratum we find the difference between the observed and expected count of outcomes among the exposed, divide this difference by the SE for this count, and sum these values in a statistic that can be compared with the upper tail of the normal distribution (Shore, Pasternack, and Curnen 1976, Greenland and Rothman 2008c p277). This statistic is valid even in sparse data, if the total counts are sufficiently large. Let C_{Ei} be the observed count among the exposed and C_{expEi} the expected count among the exposed. C_{expEi} is our best estimate of the count we would observe under the null hypothesis that the rates of the exposed and unexposed are the same, and the variance of C_{expEi} is our best estimate of the variance of C_{Ei}.

Scorestatistic

$= \text{sum}[|C_{Ei} - C_{expEi}|/\sqrt{\text{sum}[\text{variance of } C_{expEi}]}$

$= \text{sum}[|C_{Ei} - [(C_{Ei} + C_{NEi}) \times T_{Ei}/(T_{Ei} + T_{NEi})]|/\sqrt{\text{sum}[(C_{Ei} + C_{NEi}) \times T_{Ei} \times T_{NEi}/T_{Ei}^2]}$

$$(\text{Ex.7.10})$$

For the data in Table 7.1 the score statistic is −3.853 and the upper-tail area under the normal distribution curve for a value of 3.853 or greater is .000058; the two-sided P value is twice this, .00012.

7.9 ANALYSIS OF SPARSE DATA

Data are described as sparse if the outcome counts in the strata to be summarized are small, even when the overall outcome counts in the data are large. Mantel-Haenszel methods have the advantage, compared with other methods, of producing valid estimates in sparse data and for the rate ratio, the Mantel-Haenszel variance estimate is as small as with other methods (Greenland and Robins 1985, Walker 1985). When the stratum numerators are both 0 for those exposed and not exposed, that stratum contributes no information to either the Mantel-Haenszel or the inverse-variance estimates. When the numerator for those exposed is 0, the Mantel-Haenszel rate ratio is 0 (see Expression 7.6) and this ratio is included in the weighted average. When the rate numerator for those not exposed is 0 no estimate of the rate ratio is possible and the Mantel-Haenszel weight for that stratum is 0.

When a 0 is present for either the exposed or not exposed rate numerator, the inverse-variance method cannot estimate a weight for the rate ratio (see Table 4.4, line 10), because 1/0 is not defined for the variance of a rate ratio. In order to use data in strata with 0s, an ad hoc modification of the inverse-variance method is to add 0.5 to the rate numerator of both rates; strata with rates of zero for both exposed and unexposed are ignored.

I simulated data with the following characteristics; there were 50 strata and in each stratum the rate denominator was 0.125 time units for those exposed and 2 time units for those not exposed. The rate count numerator, generated randomly from the Poisson distribution, was 1 for the exposed and 4 for those not exposed, so the true rate ratio was (1/0.125)/(4/2) = 4. In this example stratification was not necessary for the analysis, as there was no variation in the rate ratio across the strata, but this simple situation is easy to simulate and the results easy to interpret. Ten thousand sets of data were simulated. The crude and Mantel-Haenszel rate ratios were estimated without any change to the counts in each simulated set of data. But for the pooled rate ratio based on inverse-variance methods, strata with 0s for both rate numerators were omitted and strata with a 0 for one rate numerator were modified by adding 0.5 to both numerator counts. Averaged on the log scale the simulated crude and Mantel-Haenszel rate ratios were both 3.97, nearly the same as the true rate ratio of 4, whereas the inverse-variance rate ratio was biased upward to 5.24. Using similar methods, Greenland and Robins (Greenland and Robins 1985) showed that inverse-variance rate ratios and rate differences can be notably biased in sparse data.

The ad hoc addition of a constant, typically 0.5, to cell counts of zero has been used for years, but this approach can produce biased estimates (Greenland 2010). A more modern approach is to use quasi-Bayes (also called pseudo-Bayes) smoothing of counts or penalized methods of estimation (Cox 2009, Greenland 2010, Cole et al. 2014).

7.10 MAXIMUM-LIKELIHOOD STRATIFIED METHODS

Maximum-likelihood estimators for stratified rate data have been available for decades but are rarely employed. They have complicated formulae and require iterative solutions. If maximum likelihood is to be used, most investigators turn to Poisson regression and related regression methods for rates. For those who desire the formulae for maximum likelihood estimators suitable for rates, these can be found in several publications (Rothman and Boice 1979 pp11–13, Rothman 1986a, Sahai and Khurshid 1996).

7.11 STRATIFIED METHODS VERSUS REGRESSION

Regression methods have many advantages compared with stratified analysis. In regression we can use continuous explanatory variables in a flexible manner, smooth across many levels of a variable, study and account for lack of homogeneity in effect estimates through the use of interaction terms, and include more variables than is typically possible in a stratified analysis. For these reasons, and others, regression is commonly preferred over stratified methods.

But stratified methods are sometimes preferred. When counts and rates are not available, inverse-variance methods allow the analyst to average or otherwise manipulate rate ratios or differences as long as an estimate of variance is available; this is particularly useful for meta-analysis. Mantel-Haenszel methods are unbiased in sparse data, whereas regression methods for rates will typically require more than 5 or 10 counts per regression variable. Mantel-Haenszel methods can be useful in the early stages of an analysis, even if the final analysis will utilize regression, because stratified methods are more transparent, compared with regression, making it easier for the analyst to study relationships between variables.

Collapsibility and Confounding

8

Chapter 5 discussed criticisms of incidence rates but ignored the fact that rate ratios and differences are usually not collapsible. This is arguably the most serious limitation of incidence rates. I postponed this topic until after stratified analysis methods were introduced, as these are used in this discussion. Many ideas in this chapter are nicely reviewed in two papers by Greenland (Greenland 1987b, 1996).

8.1 WHAT IS COLLAPSIBILITY?

Consider a study in which the exposed and unexposed groups are alike, aside from exposure, in their distribution of risk factors for the outcome. In statistical jargon, the two cohorts are exchangeable. Whichever group is exposed, the estimate of association will be the same (aside from sampling variation). The estimated association is an unbiased estimate of the causal effect of exposure on the outcome. The outcomes of the unexposed group represent, on average, what would have been seen in the exposed group in the absence of exposure. Using different lingo, the outcomes of the unexposed subjects represent the counterfactual outcomes of the exposed; outcomes that are counter to (contrary to) the observed outcomes of the exposed. Conversely, the outcomes of the exposed represent what would have happened to the unexposed, had they been exposed. All these phrases describe a study that is free of confounding bias.

In this unbiased study, if the association between exposure and outcome is estimated using a *risk ratio* or a *risk difference*, the following Statements will be true:

Statement 1. The estimate can be interpreted as the ratio or difference causal effect on average risk of the exposed due to exposure.

Statement 2. Adjusting for (conditioning or stratifying on) any characteristic of the study subjects will not change the size of the estimated association.

    a. In its most restricted form, collapsibility means that if the study subjects are divided into subgroups and the estimated association is the same in each subgroup, then if the data are collapsed across subgroups into a single population, the association in that single population will equal the associations in the subgroups. So if the risk ratio is 2.6 in each of four subgroups, the risk ratio will be 2.6 in the collapsed population.

    b. In a more expansive formulation, collapsibility means that if study subjects are divided into subgroups, the appropriately weighted summary of the subgroup (standardized, conditional) estimates of association will equal the overall (crude, unadjusted, marginal) estimate of association for all subjects. Investigators sometimes assess confounding by comparing the crude (collapsed, unadjusted, marginal) association and the adjusted (standardized, conditional) association. This method is useful in studies where the compared populations are not exchangeable and will work well for risk ratios and risk differences.

However, these Statements will not usually be true in an unbiased study if the association between exposure and outcome is based upon ratios of odds, rates, or hazards, or differences in rates. And for these outcome measures, a comparison of crude and adjusted estimates may mislead us regarding the presence of confounding. This chapter will discuss why this is so.

The examples in this chapter involve nonrecurrent outcomes with censoring of person-time after the outcome occurs, because the Statements will usually not be true for these outcomes. I will try to distinguish between confounding factors and other factors which are associated with outcome risk but are not confounders in the data. Confounding variables are associated with both the treatment or exposure of interest and with the outcome of interest. The presence of a confounding factor means the compared groups are not exchangeable. Variables that influence outcome risk, but are distributed identically in the compared groups, do not prevent exchangeability or produce confounding.

I created data that is devoid of chance (nonsystematic) variation, so that the examples clearly illustrate the discussed ideas. Adjusted and crude associations are therefore exactly equal when they should be. In real data, nonsystematic variation (sometimes called chance or sampling variation) will almost always create some difference between crude and adjusted associations, even though the compared groups should be exchangeable, as in a well-done randomized trial.

8.2 THE BRITISH X-TRIAL: INTRODUCING VARIATION IN RISK

The hypothetical TEXCO study, described in Chapter 3 (Table 3.1, Figures 3.1–3.4), compared persons who, aside from exposure to X, were identical in their risk for death, just like the uranium atoms discussed in Chapter 2. Now imagine British researchers have published a randomized trial of treatment X compared with placebo. This X-Trial is flawless; there are no dropouts or missing data and compliance with taking X or placebo was perfect. The subjects in each arm of a randomized trial do not have the same risk for death, aside from the treatment, as if they were uranium atoms. Instead, they should be alike, on average, in their *distribution* of factors that affect the risk for the outcome. In the British X-Trial, the *only* factor that is related to the risk of death and which varies in the study population, is whether or not a person had a normal or a bad genotype. In this fictional study, and others described in this chapter, the only potential confounding variable is genotype. Otherwise, the compared subjects have the same age, sex, health habits, and so on. The perfectly randomized trial had 10,000 subjects treated with X and 10,000 on placebo and in each arm exactly half of the subjects had the bad genotype and the other half had the normal genotype (Table 8.1). Confounding bias should be eliminated by this perfect balance; the two arms are said to be comparable or exchangeable.

In the British X-Trial, the rate of death among those on placebo was .02 per person-year in persons with a normal genotype and 5 times greater, .10, among those with the bad genotype. For both genotypes, treatment with X was catastrophic, because X increased the mortality rate fivefold. Within each of the 4 groups formed by genotype and exposure to X, the risk of death did not vary, so death occurred at a constant rate in each group. This is equivalent to saying that deaths arose from a Poisson process within each group. Therefore, I used Expression 2.7 for exponential decay to calculate the survival times for the persons in each group. If the trial subjects are followed for 5 years (Table 8.1), the rate in the treated arm is 0.227 deaths per person-year, the rate in the placebo arm is 0.0056, and the rate ratio is 4.0.

The rate ratio was 5.0 in subgroups restricted to normal or bad genotype (Table 8.1), but when the data were *collapsed* over genotype, the rate ratio became 4.0. The ratio of 4.0 is not biased by confounding, because the trial arms were identical in their distributions of genotype. The rate ratio of 4.0 is a correct estimate of the causal ratio effect of exposure to X on the rate outcomes of the exposed persons in the trial. Nevertheless, 4.0 is *not* the ratio causal effect on *average* rate of exposure for the exposed, which is 5.0 in this example. Thus Statement 1 in the list shown earlier is not true for the rate ratio in this unbiased study. Statement 2a in the list is also not true for the rate ratio, because the

TABLE 8.1 The British X-Trial, a randomized trial of treatment X and death. Subjects were followed until death occurred or the end of follow-up at 5 years. Rates are shown with deaths in the numerator and time (person-years, rounded to nearest integer) in the denominator. Rates and rate differences are per 1 person-year. Risk ratios and differences are for 5 years. Adjusted (conditional or standardized) associations are adjusted for genotype. Crude (marginal or collapsed) associations ignore genotype.

TREATMENT	NORMAL GENOTYPE	BAD GENOTYPE	ALL	
X	Number = 5000	Number = 5000	Number = 10,000	
	Rate = 1967/19,675 = .10	Rate = 4590/9178 = .50	Rate = 6557/28,853 = .227	
Placebo	Number = 5000	Number = 5000	Number = 10,000	
	Rate = 475/23,793 = .02	Rate = 1967/19,675 = .10	Rate = 2442/43,468 = .056	
Association			Adjusted	Crude
Rate ratio	5.0	5.0	5.0	4.0
Rate difference	0.08	0.40	0.18[a]	0.17
Risk ratio	4.1	2.3	2.7	2.7
Risk difference	.30	.52	.41	.41
Odds ratio	6.2	17.3	10.2	5.9
Hazard ratio	5.0	5.0	5.0	3.9

[a] Adjusted rate difference standardized to person-time of the exposed. If unexposed person-time is used as the standard, adjusted rate difference is 0.22. A regression model for rate differences produced an estimate of 0.20.

stratum rate ratios were both 5.0, yet the collapsed rate ratio was 4.0. The rate ratio also failed to meet the collapsibility definition of Statement 2b, because the rate ratio adjusted for genotype, 5.0, differed from the crude (unadjusted) rate ratio of 4.0. All these results are consequences of the noncollapsibility of rate ratios.

The difference between the rate ratios of 4.0 and 5.0 has nothing to do with confounding. The difference between crude and adjusted rate ratios appeared when risk was allowed to vary within the exposed and unexposed groups. It arose because, unlike the TEXCO study in Chapter 3, we relaxed the assumption that all study subjects would behave as if they were identical uranium atoms.

8.3 RATE RATIOS AND DIFFERENCES ARE NONCOLLAPSIBLE BECAUSE EXPOSURE INFLUENCES PERSON-TIME

At the start of the British X-Trial, the two trial arms were perfectly exchangeable (Table 8.1), with a 50:50 distribution of persons with normal and bad genes. As time passed, death was more common for those with bad genes and for those receiving X, and most especially for the hapless persons with bad genes and exposure to X (Table 8.1). Not only did treatment X and having a bad genotype increase the counts of the rate numerators, but these factors also influenced the person-time in the rate denominators. Those exposed to X and bad genotype died sooner, so they accumulated less person-time under observation.

A crude rate is a person-time weighted average of stratum-specific rates (Expression 6.1). For those given treatment X, the crude rate is the person-time weighted average of the genotype-specific rates: $[(0.10 \times 19,675) + (0.50 \times 9178)]/(19,675 + 9178) = 0.227$ (Table 8.1). For those on placebo, the crude rate of $0.056 = [(0.02 \times 23{,}793) + (0.10 \times 19{,}675)]/(23{,}793 + 19{,}675)$. A standardized rate ratio (Expression 6.6) uses the same weights for the two populations that are compared. Because the person-time weights for the X-treated cohort (19,675 for normal-gene subjects and 9178 for bad-gene individuals) *differ* from those for the placebo cohort (23,793 for normal-gene folks and 19,675 for bad-gene people), the ratio of the two crude (collapsed or marginal) rates (4.0) does not equal the standardized (adjusted or conditional) rate ratio (5.0).

Another way to explain the noncollapsibility of rate ratios (or differences) is to note that because exposure affects person-time, person-time is an outcome. Using person-time as part of the outcome statistic amounts to adjusting for an outcome variable, which results in bias (Greenland 1996).

The standardized rate difference varies in Table 8.1 depending upon the standard used; this deserves a short comment. The data were created to have identical rate ratios for both genotypes: 5.0. Because the rates under no exposure varied by genotype, this means the rate differences were not identical for both genotypes. Consequently, the choice of standard (the exposed, unexposed, or some other standard), influences the size of the standardized rate differences, but not the size of the standardized rate ratios.

The crucial point is that the crude rate ratio does not equal the stratum-standardized rate ratio, even though the compared populations are exchangeable. This is not due to confounding, but because treatment with X changed not only the numerator of the rate ratios but also their denominators. As the rate numerator grows, it cannibalizes its own denominator. This feature of rates is unimportant when outcome risk is uniform within the exposed and unexposed groups, as it was in the TEXCO example of Chapter 3. But when outcome risk varies, by genotype in this example, the rates are no longer collapsible across risk levels when exchangeable groups are compared.

8.4 WHICH ESTIMATE OF THE RATE RATIO SHOULD WE PREFER?

The X-Trial produced two rate ratios; the crude (marginal or collapsed) rate ratio of 4.0 and the standardized (conditional or adjusted) rate ratio of 5.0. Which is best?

The rate ratio of 4.0 is an unbiased comparison of the rates of the exposed and unexposed groups. The mortality rate really was four times larger for those taking X compared with placebo. The rate ratio of 4.0 accurately describes the causal effect of exposure on the exposed population in the X-Trial. In this example, the rate ratio of 4.0 applies to a population with equal numbers of subjects with the two genotypes. But the rate ratio of 4.0 lacks any interpretation as an *average* causal effect. It not an estimate of the *average* change in rates among the exposed due to exposure or the change in the *average* rate ratio due to exposure (Greenland 1987b, 1996).

As best we can tell, the average causal effect was a rate ratio of 5.0. The data were created so that the rates of the exposed subjects within each genotype were always 5 times greater compared with those taking placebo. So in this perfect trial, adjusting for genotype produced a rate ratio that equals the unbiased average causal effect of exposure on mortality. Why not use the rate ratio of 5.0 as the causal estimate from the trial?

The problem with the rate ratio of 5.0 is that it rests on the assumption that we have fully accounted for (conditioned on or adjusted for) *all* factors that influence the risk for death. This assumption is true in this simple example. Aside from genotype and exposure to X, the subjects in the trial were like the uniform uranium atoms of Chapter 2. But actual humans vary in their age, sex, genetic make-up, diet, alcohol-use, driving behaviors, smoking habits, and an infinity of other factors that affect mortality. We could revise this example to include additional factors related to death, creating additional subgroups, each with its own rate. If we did this, the adjusted (standardized) rate ratio would move further away from 1.0 compared with the crude rate ratio. The adjusted rate ratio would, consequently, differ more from the effect of exposure on the total cohort, but would never equal the average causal effect of exposure on mortality, because we could never account for all variation in mortality risk. In real data the adjusted rate ratio would be in a limbo between the observed effect of exposure on the exposed and the average causal effect.

The inequality between crude and adjusted rate ratios arose because if rates vary with exposure to X and across genetic subgroups, then person-time will accumulate differently across subgroups. Consequently, the standardized rate ratios cannot equal the crude rate ratios. Although this discussion focused on rate ratios, all that has been said applies as well to rate differences. So which estimate is preferred? The ratio of 4.0 is an unbiased description of what happened in the trial, but it is a biased estimate of the average causal effect of X on rates. The adjusted ratio of 5.0 is the causal effect on the average rate, but in data for real humans the adjusted estimate would surely be biased because we could not account for all sources of risk variation.

8.5 BEHAVIOR OF RISK RATIOS AND DIFFERENCES

The risk ratio and risk difference do not suffer from the problems just described for the rate ratios and differences. In the X-trial the crude and adjusted risk ratios of 2.7 at 5 years of follow-up (Table 8.1) are unbiased estimates of the average change in risk among the exposed due to exposure. Because the two study populations were exchangeable at the start of the study, the crude and adjusted risk ratios (and differences) were always the same at each point in time (Table 8.2). Even though the risk for the outcome may vary between trial subjects, so long as the distribution of risk is the same in each trial arm, the risk ratio and risk difference will, on average, fulfill Statements 1, 2a, and 2b, made early in this chapter.

TABLE 8.2 The British X-Trial, a randomized trial of treatment X and death. Subjects were followed until death occurred or the end of follow-up. The frequency of death in the X-treated group is compared with that in the placebo group. Adjusted (conditional or standardized) associations are adjusted for genotype (normal or bad). Crude (marginal or collapsed) associations ignore genotype. Rate differences are per 1 person-year. Adjusted rate differences are standardized to the distribution of the exposed subjects. Risk differences are for total follow-up time at each point in time. Further details in Table 8.1 and text.

ASSOCIATION		FOLLOW-UP TIME (YEARS)					
		0.25	0.5	1	3	5	10
Rate ratio	Crude	4.9	4.9	4.7	4.3	4.0	3.7
	Adjusted	5.0	5.0	5.0	5.0	5.0	5.0
Rate difference	Crude	0.24	0.23	0.22	0.19	0.17	0.14
	Adjusted	0.24	0.23	0.22	0.20	0.18	0.16
Risk ratio	Crude	4.8	4.6	4.3	3.3	2.7	2.0
	Adjusted	4.8	4.6	4.3	3.3	2.7	2.0
Risk difference	Crude	.06	.11	.19	.36	.41	.41
	Adjusted	.06	.11	.19	.36	.41	.41
Odds ratio	Crude	5.1	5.2	5.3	5.7	5.9	6.3
	Adjusted	5.2	5.5	5.9	8.1	10.1	12.4
Hazard ratio	Crude	4.9	4.9	4.7	4.3	3.9	3.4
	Adjusted	5.0	5.0	5.0	5.0	5.0	5.0

8.6 HAZARD RATIOS AND ODDS RATIOS

In the British X-Trial, the crude and adjusted hazard ratios, from a Cox proportional hazards regression model, differed (Tables 8.1 and 8.2). This gulf becomes noteworthy after a year. Robins and Morgenstern pointed out in 1987 (Robins and Morgenstern 1987 p882) that if two groups were initially exchangeable, the crude and adjusted hazard ratios for a causal risk factor would diverge over time as events became common. Others have pointed out that crude and adjusted hazard ratios may not agree, even when the groups compared are exchangeable (Ford, Norrie, and Ahmadi 1995, Schmoor and Schumacher 1997).

In the X-Trial, the crude hazard ratio is similar to the crude rate ratio until four or more years have passed (Table 8.2). The hazard ratio estimates the instantaneous rate across all times. As time passes, the highest risk group, exposed persons with a bad genotype, dwindles. By 4 years 86% of this group is dead. At 4 years and beyond, the crude hazard ratio moves toward 1 faster than the rate ratio, because the hazard ratio gives more weight to the comparison of the exposed and unexposed later in follow-up. In the later years of the study the overall rate of death is lower among the exposed because so many of the exposed people with bad genes are already dead.

The crude (collapsed) and adjusted (standardized) odds ratios also differ in Tables 8.1 and 8.2. Noncollapsibility of the odds ratio was recognized by the 1980s (Miettinen and Cook 1981, Greenland 1987b, Robins and Morgenstern 1987). Numerical examples that demonstrate the collapsibility of risk ratios and noncollapsibility of odds ratios, can be found elsewhere (Cummings 2009b). Several authors have shed light on the properties of the odds ratio (Greenland 1991, Hauck et al. 1991, Hauck, Anderson, and Marcus 1998, Greenland, Robins, and Pearl 1999, Newman 2001 pp33–67).

8.7 COMPARING RISKS WITH OTHER OUTCOME MEASURES

Risks, rates, hazards, and odds are all ratios. A causal exposure will influence the size of the numerator and the denominator for each of these measures. For risks, the exposure does not change the denominator. The risk denominator is the number of subjects at the start of the study and does not change with the passage of time. But for rates, hazards, and odds, a causal exposure that increases the outcome frequency will decrease the size of the denominator. It is this demolition of the denominator that produces noncollapsibility when rates, hazards, or odds are compared, either as ratios or differences. The exposure effect on the denominator will vary if study subjects vary in their risk for the outcome. This variation will not cancel out when two exposure groups are compared, resulting in noncollapsibility.

When outcomes are sufficiently rare (say < 10 or 20% of the noteworthy groups have the outcome), then the rate denominator will shrink only a little: see Expressions 2.11 and 2.12. The same is true for hazards and odds. Thus rate, hazard, and odds ratios will approximate risk ratios when outcomes are not common and the crude and adjusted rate, hazard, and odds ratios or rate differences will be similar when exchangeable groups are compared. This is shown in Table 8.2, where crude and adjusted associations are all similar at 0.25 and 0.5 years of follow-up.

The X-Trial data illustrates why it will usually be true that the odds ratio > rate ratio > risk ratio > 1, as discussed in Chapter 3. We can use follow-up through 1 year (Table 8.2) for this explanation. At time 0 the denominators of the exposed and unexposed risks are set at 10,000 and these remain unchanged at 1 year. By 1 year the count of dead was 2443 in the treated arm and 575 in the placebo arm. Because the denominators of the risks were the same, the risk ratio is 2443/575 = 4.3. For the rate ratio, the maximum possible person-time at 1 year is equal to 10,000 person-years for both trial arms. With each death the person-time shrinks by some amount between 0 and 1 year of person-time. Since the deaths come sooner in the exposed arm, the shrinkage is greater for that group. Assuming deaths followed an exponential decay pattern, at 1 year the person-time for the exposed was 8693 years, less than the 9709 years for the unexposed. Consequently, the rate ratio $(2443/8693)/(575/9709) = 4.7$ is larger than the risk ratio of 4.3. The odds of death at 1 year for the treated is equal to (risk of treated at 1 year)/(1 − risk of treated at 1 year). If we multiply the top and bottom of this ratio by 10,000, the odds ratio is equal to the (count of the dead)/(count of the survivors) $= 2443/(10,000-2443)$. So while the rate ratio loses a quantity *between 0 and 1* for each death from its greatest possible denominator of 10,000, the odds ratio *loses 1* from that denominator with each death. Consequently, the odds ratio, $(2443/7557)/(575/9425) = 5.3$ is further from 1.0 than the rate ratio (4.7).

8.8 THE ITALIAN X-TRIAL: 3-LEVELS OF RISK UNDER NO EXPOSURE

With the publication of the British X-Trial, leaders of the on-going Italian X-Trial were alarmed to learn of the harm produced by X. They stopped their study and analyzed the data. In their initial report, the Italians classified genotypes into two categories, normal and bad. They reported that after 5 years, the crude rate ratio was 3.8, and the adjusted rate ratio (adjusted for normal versus bad genes) was 4.2 (Table 8.3). But a year later clever geneticists in Rome found that persons with the bad genetic allele could be subtyped into those with a lousy gene (mortality rate 0.05 per person-year when not exposed to X) and those with an awful gene (rate 0.25). When this was done, the rate ratio adjusted for all three genotypes was 5.0. This example demonstrates what I claimed earlier; more variation in risk will cause the crude and adjusted rate ratios to differ more and the adjusted ratio will be further from 1. The adjusted rate ratio will fall short of being an unbiased estimate of the causal effect on average rate, because risks under no exposure will always vary more than we can expect to measure. This is why the risk ratio or difference may be preferred as a measure of association when outcomes are common. When comparing exchangeable populations, the crude and adjusted risk ratios and risk differences will be the same and they can be interpreted as an average effect on risk, despite measured or unmeasured variations in the risks of individuals.

8.9 THE AMERICAN X-COHORT STUDY: 3-LEVELS OF RISK IN A COHORT STUDY

Soon after the Italian trial results appeared, U.S. epidemiologists announced results from the American X-Cohort study. In their data, 7000 people had an exceptional genotype with the lowest mortality (rate under no exposure 0.01 per person-year), 10,000 had a normal genotype with a mortality rate of 0.02, and 7075 had an awful allele (rate 0.4). At 5 years of follow-up, the data (Table 8.4) showed something that puzzled the epidemiologists. The rate ratios comparing those exposed to X with those not exposed were 5.0 in the genetic subgroups and the crude rate ratio was also 5.0. Why did the collapsed and standardized rate ratios agree, given the variation in outcome rates by genotype?

Statements 1, 2a, and 2b all involved an assumption of exchangeability; the two groups being compared should have similar distributions of risk factors for the outcome, as they would (on average) in a randomized trial. But the exposed and unexposed groups in the American X-Cohort study differed

TABLE 8.3   The Italian X-Trial: randomized trial of treatment X and death. Subjects were followed until death occurred or the end of follow-up at 5 years. Rates are shown with deaths in the numerator and time (person-years, rounded to nearest integer) in denominator. Rates and rate differences are per 1 person-year. Risk ratios and differences are for 5 years. Crude (marginal or collapsed) associations ignore genotype. Partly adjusted associations are adjusted for bad genotype (including lousy and awful genotypes in one category) versus normal genotype. Adjusted (conditional or standardized) associations are adjusted for all three genotype categories. Adjusted rate and risk differences are standardized to the distribution of the exposed.

TREATMENT	NORMAL GENOTYPE	LOUSY GENOTYPE	AWFUL GENOTYPE	ALL		
X	Number = 5000 Rate = 1967/ 19,675 = .10	Number = 3750 Rate = 2676/ 10,703 = .25	Number = 1250 Rate = 1248/ 996 = 1.25	Number = 10,000 Rate = 5891/31,374 = .188		
Placebo	Number = 5000 Rate = 475/ 23,793 = .02	Number = 3750 Rate = 829/ 16,592 = .05	Number = 1250 Rate = 892/ 3568 = 0.25	Number = 10,000 Rate = 2196/43,953 = .050		
Association				Crude	Partly adjusted	Adjusted
Rate ratio	5.0	5.0	5.0	3.8	4.2	5.0
Rate difference	0.08	0.20	1.0	0.14	0.14[a]	0.15[b]
Risk ratio	4.1	3.2	1.4	2.7	2.7	2.7
Risk difference	.30	.49	.28	.37	.37	.37
Odds ratio	6.2	8.8	250	5.1	6.6	8.0
Hazard ratio	5.0	5.0	5.0	3.6	4.1	5.0

[a] Partly adjusted for bad genotype (lousy plus awful genotype in one category, versus normal genotype). Rate difference standardized to person-time of the exposed. If unexposed person-time is used as the standard, the partly adjusted rate difference is 0.16. A regression model for rate differences produced an estimate of 0.15.

[b] Adjusted rate difference standardized to person-time of the exposed. If unexposed person-time is used as the standard, adjusted rate difference is 0.20. A regression model for rate differences produced an estimate of 0.16.

at the start of follow-up. Persons exposed to X were less likely to have the exceptional gene compared with those unexposed (17 versus 41%), about equally likely to have the normal gene (42 versus 41%), and more likely to have the awful gene (42 versus 17%) (Table 8.4). So there was confounding by genotype at the start of follow-up: persons exposed to X had a more lethal genetic make-up compared with the unexposed. This imbalance was obvious throughout the study, as crude and adjusted estimates of all associations differed at most points in time (Table 8.5). But for the rate ratio (and difference) the estimated associations were collapsible at 5 years. The hazard ratios were collapsible at about 3 years and the odds ratios were collapsible at about 10 years. Only the risk ratios and differences remained noncollapsible over 10 years. This pattern is different from that in Table 8.2, where, except for the risk ratio and difference, the crude and adjusted estimates diverged as follow-up time increased.

To make the rate ratios collapsible in Table 8.4, I created a Stata file with 5000 records for each of the 6 covariate patterns produced by X-exposure (yes, no) and genotype (exceptional, normal, awful). The six rates in Table 8.4 were assigned to each record according to the six covariate patterns. The expected survival time of each subject was calculated using Expression 2.7 for exponential decay times. These steps produced rate ratios of 5.0 within each stratum of genotype. To induce confounding by genotype, the number exposed to X with an exceptional genotype was reduced to 2000 and the number

TABLE 8.4 The American X-Cohort Study of exposure to X and death. Subjects were followed until death occurred or the end of follow-up at 5 years. Rates are shown with deaths in the numerator and time (person-years, rounded to nearest integer) in the denominator. Rates and rate differences are per 1 person-year. Risk ratios and differences are for 5 years. Adjusted (conditional or standardized) associations are adjusted for genotype. Crude (marginal or collapsed) associations ignore genotype.

EXPOSURE TO X	EXCEPTIONAL GENOTYPE	NORMAL GENOTYPE	AWFUL GENOTYPE	ALL	
Exposed	Number = 2000 Rate = 442/8850 = .05	Number = 5000 Rate = 1967/ 19,675 = .10	Number = 4995 Rate = 4995/ 2495 = 2.0	Number = 11,995 Rate = 7404/31,020 = .239	
Unexposed	Number = 5000 Rate = 243/ 24,388 = .01	Number = 5000 Rate = 475/ 23,793 = .02	Number = 2080 Rate = 1799/ 4496 = 0.4	Number = 12,080 Rate = 2517/52,676 = .048	
Association				Adjusted	Crude
Rate ratio	5.0	5.0	5.0	5.0	5.0
Rate difference	0.04	0.08	1.6	0.19[a]	0.19
Risk ratio	4.5	4.1	1.2	1.8	3.0
Risk difference	.17	.30	.14	.22[b]	.41
Odds ratio	5.6	6.2	[c]	7.0	6.1
Hazard ratio	5.0	5.0	5.0	5.0	4.4

[a] Adjusted rate difference standardized to person-time of the exposed. If unexposed person-time is used as the standard, adjusted rate difference is 0.19. A regression model for rate differences produced an estimate of 0.20.

[b] Adjusted risk difference standardized to person-time of the exposed. If unexposed person-time is used as the standard, adjusted risk difference is .21.

[c] No one survived in the group that was exposed to X and had an awful gene, so the odds ratio could not be calculated. The median unbiased estimate from exact logistic regression was an odds ratio of 1 with a 95% confidence interval from 0 to infinity.

unexposed to X with an awful genotype was also changed to 2000. Then small, iterative changes in the counts for those with awful genes were made until the rate ratios produced by Stata's **ir** command became collapsible at 5 years. Collapsibility could be generated at any point in time for any estimate of association, by introducing the necessary imbalance at the start of follow-up.

When a confounding variable has only two levels, collapsibility cannot be induced by the iterative conjuring described above. But if three of more levels are allowed, collapsibility becomes possible. Whittemore used categorical tables to show this in a 1978 publication (Whittemore 1978). Recent examples appear in a textbook (Weiss and Koepsell 2014 pp226,266). The collapsibility of the rate ratios in Table 8.4 looks superficially like the collapsibility of the risk ratios in Table 8.3. But there are differences between Table 8.3, which compares exchangeable populations, and the comparison of cohorts in Table 8.4. The risk ratios are collapsible across any two levels of genotype in Table 8.3. But in Table 8.4, the rate ratios are not collapsible across all combinations of two genotypes. The adjusted rate ratios for exposure to X are 5.0 within each genotype level in Table 8.4. For genotypes exceptional and normal the crude (collapsed) rate ratio was also 5.0. But when genotypes exceptional and awful are combined, the crude rate ratio was 6.8, and for genotypes normal and awful the crude ratio was 3.9. The collapsed ratio that was elevated (6.8) effectively counter-balanced the lesser ratio of 3.9, so that collapsing across all 3 genotypes produced a crude rate ratio of 5.0. Another difference between exchangeable and confounded comparisons is that the collapsibility of the risk ratios persisted over time in Table 8.2, but collapsibility of the rate ratios in Table 8.5 was fleeting.

In Tables 8.1, 8.2, and 8.3, the crude rate ratios all had interpretations as unbiased estimates of the ratio change in rates due to exposure to X. These interpretations were possible because the populations were exchangeable. In Tables 8.4 and 8.5, the crude rate ratios are confounded because the compared populations are not exchangeable; unlike the rate ratios of Tables 8.1, 8.2, and 8.3, these ratios do not estimate the unbiased effect of exposure on the rates (Robins and Morgenstern 1987 p882, Greenland 1996). In the American X-Cohort study, collapsibility of the stratum rate ratios does not correspond to lack of confounding of the crude rate ratio.

A similar example was described by Greenland (1996 p500). Imagine an open, steady-state population in which the age distributions of smokers and nonsmokers are the same. If rate ratios for death associated with smoking are constant across age strata, then crude and age-standardized rate ratios will be the same (collapsible) and it will appear that there is no age-related confounding. This impression will be wrong, because smokers should have a *younger* age-distribution than nonsmokers in the population, due to the lethal effect of cigarettes on mortality. Among all people who smoke starting before age 20 years, fewer of them will reach age 60 due to their smoking, compared with the experience of nonsmokers.

In Tables 8.4 and 8.5, the adjusted rate ratios are unbiased estimates of average causal effect on the rates, because we have stipulated that genotype is the only possible confounder and, in addition, genotype is the only source of variation in risk when not exposed. But real people would not have a uniform risk of death within strata formed by genotype and X-exposure. By 0.25 years, 10% of the entire study population was dead. That proportion will often be small enough that the rate ratio will approximate the average causal effect on risks (see Expressions 2.11 and 2.12). But at 0.25 years in the American X-Cohort, 39% of the exposed persons with the awful genotype were dead. This large proportion in an important subgroup resulted in an adjusted rate ratio of 5.0 which differed notably from the adjusted risk ratio of 4.2 (Table 8.5). At 0.1 years of follow-up (not shown in Table 8.5), 4%

TABLE 8.5 The American X-Cohort study of exposure to X and death. Subjects were followed until death occurred or the end of follow-up. The frequency of death in the X-treated group is compared with that in the placebo group. Adjusted (conditional or standardized) associations are adjusted for genotype (exceptional, normal, awful). Crude (marginal or collapsed) associations ignore genotype. Rate differences are per 1 person-year. Adjusted rate and risk differences are standardized to the distribution of the exposed subjects. Risk differences are for total follow-up time at each point in time. Further details in Table 8.4 and text.

ASSOCIATION		FOLLOW-UP TIME (YEARS)					
		0.25	0.5	1	3	5	10
Rate ratio	Crude	9.9	9.0	7.7	5.4	5.0	5.1
	Adjusted	5.0	5.0	5.0	5.0	5.0	5.0
Rate difference	Crude	0.70	0.61	0.48	0.25	0.19	0.14
	Adjusted	0.62	0.55	0.44	0.25	0.19	0.14
Risk ratio	Crude	9.0	7.7	5.9	3.5	3.0	2.6
	Adjusted	4.2	3.6	2.9	1.9	1.8	1.8
Risk difference	Crude	.16	.25	.34	.39	.41	.46
	Adjusted	.13	.21	.26	.23	.21	.25
Odds ratio	Crude	10.8	10.4	9.3	6.5	6.1	7.4
	Adjusted	6.0	7.1	9.3	8.5	7.0	7.3
Hazard ratio	Crude	9.9	8.9	7.4	4.9	4.4	4.3
	Adjusted	5.0	5.0	5.0	5.0	5.0	5.0

of all study subjects were dead, 18% of exposed persons with awful genes were dead, and the adjusted rate ratio of 5.0 was pretty closer to the adjusted risk ratio of 4.7. So the adjusted rate ratio of 5.0 is close to the average causal rate ratio at 0.1 years of follow-up.

8.10 THE SWEDISH X-COHORT STUDY: A COLLAPSIBLE RISK RATIO IN CONFOUNDED DATA

Now consider the Swedish X-Cohort study (Tables 8.6, 8.7, 8.8). Those exposed to X were more likely to have the exceptional and awful genes and less likely to have normal genes, compared with those unexposed. Although the distribution of genes differed between the compared groups, the *average gene-related* risk of death, ignoring the effect of treatment with X, at 5 years was *the same*, .057, in the compared groups. Exposure to X increased the risk fivefold, so the ratio of average risks was .283/.057 = 5.0. At 5 years of follow-up the collapsibility of the risks means that the crude risk ratio of 5.0 is the unbiased estimate of the ratio change in risks due to X-exposure and the standardized risk ratio of 5.0 can be interpreted as the causal effect of X on the average risk of the exposed. I will justify these claims here.

TABLE 8.6 The Swedish X-Cohort Study of exposure to X and death. Subjects were followed until death or the end of follow-up at 5 years. Rates are shown with deaths in the numerator and time (person-years, rounded to nearest integer) in denominator. Rates and rate differences are per 1 person-year, rounded to three digits. Risk ratios and differences are for 5 years. Adjusted (conditional or standardized) associations are adjusted for genotype. Crude (marginal or collapsed) associations ignore genotype.

EXPOSURE TO X	EXCEPTIONAL GENOTYPE	NORMAL GENOTYPE	AWFUL GENOTYPE	ALL	
Exposed	Number = 72,000 Rate = 8888/ 337,293 = .026	Number = 20,000 Rate = 7226/80,592 = .090	Number = 16,000 Rate = 14,502/ 30,617 = .474	Number = 108,000 Rate = 30,616/ 448,503 = .068	
Unexposed	Number = 62,000 Rate = 1530/ 306,160 = .005	Number = 55,000 Rate = 3974/ 264,943 = .015	Number = 9064 Rate = 1643/41,078 = .040	Number = 126,064 Rate = 7147/612,180 = .012	
Association				Adjusted	Crude
Rate ratio	5.3	6.0	11.8	7.4	5.8
Rate difference	.02	.07	.43	0.059[a]	0.057
Risk ratio	5.0	5.0	5.0	5.0	5.0
Risk difference	.099	.289	.725	.227[b]	.227
Odds ratio	5.6	7.3	43.7	8.8	6.6
Hazard ratio	5.3	6.0	11.8	7.3	5.8

[a] Adjusted rate difference standardized to person-time of the exposed. If unexposed person-time is used as the standard, adjusted rate difference is 0.072. A regression model for rate differences produced an estimate of 0.065.

[b] Adjusted risk difference standardized to person-time of the exposed. If unexposed person-time is used as the standard, adjusted risk difference is the same, .227.

TABLE 8.7   The Swedish X-Cohort study of exposure to X and death. Subjects were followed until death or the end of follow-up. The frequency of death in the X-treated group is compared with the deaths in the placebo group. Adjusted (conditional or standardized) associations are adjusted for genotype (exceptional, normal, awful). Crude (marginal or collapsed) associations ignore genotype. Rate differences are per 1 person-year. Adjusted rate and risk differences are standardized to the distribution of the exposed subjects. Risk differences are for total follow-up time at each point in time. Further details in Table 8.6 and text.

ASSOCIATION		FOLLOW-UP TIME (YEARS)					
		0.25	0.5	1	3	5	10
Rate	Crude	8.6	8.3	7.9	6.6	5.8	4.8
ratio	Adjusted	8.0	7.9	7.9	7.6	7.4	7.0
Rate difference	Crude	.09	.09	.08	.07	.06	.04
	Adjusted	.09	.09	.08	.07	.06	.05
Risk	Crude	8.5	8.2	7.6	6.0	5.0	3.8
ratio	Adjusted	7.7	7.5	7.1	5.8	5.0	4.0
Risk difference	Crude	.02	.04	.08	.17	.23	.30
	Adjusted	.02	.04	.08	.17	.23	.30
Odds ratio	Crude	8.7	8.5	8.2	7.3	6.6	5.7
	Adjusted	8.1	8.2	8.4	8.7	8.8	8.9
Hazard ratio	Crude	8.6	8.3	7.9	6.6	5.8	4.7
	Adjusted	7.5	7.4	7.4	7.3	7.3	7.1

Let me pull back the curtain on the legerdemain that produced the Swedish cohort data. To make the stratified risk ratio equal to 5.0 at 5 years for those with normal genotype, a rate of .015 was selected for the unexposed. The 5 year risk from Expression 2.9 was $1 - \exp(.015 \times 5 \text{ years}) = .072$. This risk was multiplied by 5 and Expression 2.10 was used to compute the rate for those exposed to X: $[-\ln(1-[5 \times (1-\exp(-.015 \times 5 \text{ years}))])]/5 \text{ years}] = .090$. These rates were then used to calculate survival times for the exposed and unexposed subjects with normal genotype, using Expression 2.7 for exponential decay. A lower rate when not exposed (.005) was picked for those with an exceptional genotype, a higher rate (.040) for those with awful genotype, and Expressions 2.9 and 2.10 were used in the same way to calculate the rates of those exposed to X with these genotypes. These calculations produced risk ratios of 5.0 at 5 years within each genotype category. Then the counts of subjects at the start of follow-up were manipulated until the crude risk ratio was also equal to 5.0 at 5 years. There was never any attempt to make the average risk related to genotype alone equal in the exposed and unexposed groups; but that result (Table 8.8) was an inevitable consequence of collapsibility at 5 years.

Contrast the 5-year *risk* ratios from the Swedish study with the 5-year *rate* ratios from the American X-Cohort study. The rate ratios in the American study were collapsible at 5 years (Tables 8.4, 8.5), but the average rates under no exposure were not equal in the two groups (Table 8.8). Average rate among the exposed was 0.883 and 0.883/5 = 0.18, which is not equal to the average rate of 0.081 among the unexposed. Average rate and person-time-weighted average rate are not the same. In the American cohort study, those exposed to X were less likely to have the exceptional genotype, about equally likely to have the normal gene, and more likely to have the awful gene compared with the unexposed (Table 8.8). So the exposed in that study should have worse outcomes at 5 years compared with the unexposed, even in the absence of exposure. But in the Swedish study, while the distributions of genotype differed between the exposed and unexposed, the *average* risk when not exposed to X was the same at 5 years in both groups. The Swedish groups were exchangeable in terms of their risk outcomes at 5 years.

If the Swedish groups were exchangeable regarding 5-year risks, then it should be true that if those unexposed (keeping the counts of subjects unchanged) were assigned the rates of the exposed group,

TABLE 8.8 Comparison of rates at 5 years from the American X-Cohort study with risks at 5 years from the Swedish X-Cohort study. Rates are per person-year, risks are risks at 5 years. Weighted-average rates were weighted by person-time. Weighted-average risks were weighted by the number persons at the start of the study. Average rates and risks can both be thought of as weighted by the number of persons at the start of the study.

| | AMERICAN X-COHORT | | | | SWEDISH X-COHORT | | | |
| | EXPOSED TO X | | UNEXPOSED | | EXPOSED TO X | | UNEXPOSED | |
GENOTYPE	N (%)	RATE	N (%)	RATE	N (%)	RISK	N (%)	RISK
Great	2000 (17)	0.05	5000 (41)	0.01	72,000 (67)	.123	62,000 (49)	.025
Normal	5000 (42)	0.10	5000 (41)	0.02	20,000 (19)	.361	55,000 (44)	.072
Awful	4995 (42)	2.00	2080 (17)	0.40	16,000 (15)	.906	9064 (7)	.181
Weighted average		0.239		0.048		.283		.057
Average		0.883		0.081		.283		.057

and vice versa, the 5-year crude risk ratio should still be 5.0. This was indeed true. In fact, when rates and exposure status were switched, the crude rate ratios at all times (Table 8.7) were unchanged. But swapping the rates of those exposed and unexposed in the American study changed the 5-year rate ratio from 5.0 to 1.1. In that cohort, the two groups were not exchangeable regarding 5-year rate outcomes.

Although the crude risk ratio at 5 years in the Swedish study is a correct estimate of the ratio change in risk due to exposure, the crude ratio estimates at other times lack this interpretation; they are biased by the initial imbalance for genotype. Collapsibility of the risk ratio indicates absence of confounding by genotype only at 5 years of follow-up.

The adjusted rate ratio of 5.0 at 5 years in the American X-cohort is an unbiased estimate of the causal ratio effect of exposure on the average rate, given that aside from genotype there are no other confounders and no other source of variation in risks under no exposure. The limitation of this estimate is that it requires homogeneity of risk (and therefore rates) within the 6 subgroups formed by genotype and exposure to X. This homogeneity is unrealistic in studies of humans.

The adjusted risk ratio at 5 years in the Swedish study is also an unbiased estimate of the causal ratio effect on average risk, assuming the only confounder is genotype. This interpretation does not require homogeneity of risks. Within the six strata formed by genotype and X-exposure, the risks of individuals can vary, so long as they average to the six risks in Table 8.8. If risks between exposed and unexposed subjects vary so that the ratio of the average risks changes from the value of 5.0 in Table 8.8, then the characteristic that produced this variation will be an additional confounder. A confounder in addition to genotype could be a source of bias for any of the associations from the American and Swedish cohort studies. Variation in risk without confounding is a source of bias only for associations based upon rates, hazards, and odds, not for those using risks. To put this another way, variables that cause risks to vary are unimportant for associations based upon risks, unless they are actually confounders. When we use outcomes that devour their denominators (rates, hazards, odds), a variable that produces variation in outcome risk will bias estimates of association, even when it is not a confounder.

8.11 A SUMMARY OF FINDINGS

We have waded deep into the weeds with these examples. It is time to look at the big picture. The examples all show that associations based upon risks will be unbiased under weaker assumptions compared with associations that rely upon outcome measures that cannibalize their denominators: rates, hazards, and odds.

1. Randomized trials. In the British and Italian randomized trials, the crude risk ratios and differences were unbiased estimates of the effect of exposure on the exposed. The adjusted risk ratios and differences were unbiased estimates of the average causal effect. The crude and adjusted associations were equal to each other. Once events were common, crude and adjusted associations based on rates, hazards, and odds were not equal. Adjusted associations based on rates, hazards, and odds were unbiased in our simple examples, but the lack of bias rests upon an assumption of homogeneity of risk that is unrealistic in most trials.
2. Cohort studies. In the American and Swedish cohort studies with populations that were not exchangeable, the adjusted risk ratios and differences were unbiased estimates of average causal effect. This was not true for the other associations.
3. Collapsibility. Collapsibility of the risk ratio or difference on levels of a possible confounder, indicates that the crude (marginal or collapsed) estimates were not biased by confounding. Collapsibility does not correspond to absence of confounding when rates, hazards, or odds are used. The rate ratio, rate difference, odds ratio, and hazard ratio were all collapsible at some point in time in the American X-Cohort study (Table 8.5), but the crude association estimates were all biased.

8.12 A DIFFERENT VIEW OF COLLAPSIBILITY

In the absence of confounding, crude and adjusted associations based upon rates, hazards, and odds will differ even when the compared populations are exchangeable. I have argued that this arises from the mathematical properties of outcome measures that reduce their denominators are numerator events become more common.

Other authors have ascribed noncollapsibility of the hazard ratio (Hernán, Hernández-Diaz, and Robins 2004, Hernán 2010) and the rate ratio (Sjölander, Dahlqwist, and Zetterqvist 2016) to selection bias. In addition, Sjölander and colleagues assert that the mechanisms that induce noncollapsibility for the odds ratio and the rate difference are different, while I contend they are the same. Readers may find these alternative viewpoints interesting. Despite our different views regarding the reasons for noncollapsibility, I regard these papers as useful for pointing out an important problem with rates and suggesting solutions.

8.13 PRACTICAL IMPLICATIONS: AVOID COMMON OUTCOMES

When outcome risk is sufficiently small, say .1 in time interval T, the rate per T-person-units will closely approximate the risk (Expressions 2.11 and 2.12). Over short intervals nearly everyone survives to time T, so the final rate denominator is nearly equal to the original population size multiplied by T. In this situation, rates approximate risks, and rate differences and ratios will approximate risk differences or ratios. Consequently, noncollapsibility will not be an important problem. The outcome must be rare not only in the entire population, but in any noteworthy subgroup used for stratification or adjustment in the analysis. In studies of mortality in open populations, most causes of death are sufficiently rare that studies of mortality may not be afflicted by the problems discussed in this chapter.

In the British X-Trial, the risk and rate ratios agree closely at 0.25 and 0.5 years (Table 8.2); by 6 months 8% of all study subjects and 22% of exposed persons with a bad genotype were dead. The 6-month rate difference of 0.23 deaths per person-year may not seem similar to the risk difference of .11. But the risk difference is for 6 months. If we divide the rate difference by 2 we get a rate difference of 0.115 deaths per 6-months, similar to the risk difference.

If we limit the analysis to a short enough time interval, the noncollapsibility of rate ratios will usually not be important. Unfortunately, this generalization may not always be true. Greenland (1996) points out that competing risks (other factors that eliminate subjects from follow-up) could diminish rate denominators differently in different strata. If this happens, differential changes in stratum-specific rate denominators can result in problems related to noncollapsibility.

8.14 PRACTICAL IMPLICATIONS: USE RISKS OR SURVIVAL FUNCTIONS

If common events are to be studied, it may be best to use risks, not rates, to measure the outcomes. This will often be easy when everyone is followed for the same length of time. But when follow-up time varies, this becomes more complicated. Instead of using rates or hazards, we can compare survival curves or survival times (Robins and Morgenstern 1987, Hernán 2010). This will be discussed in Chapter 25 about hazard ratios. As discussed in Chapter 2, risks can have their own limitations.

8.15 PRACTICAL IMPLICATIONS: CASE-CONTROL STUDIES

Case-control studies compare those with the outcome (cases) with controls (noncases). In these studies, the ratio of cases to controls is usually large, giving the impression that outcomes are common. But if the outcome is rare in the population from which the cases arose, then odds ratios from the analysis will approximate risk ratios for the original population. Since risk ratios are collapsible, the problem of noncollapsibility is usually not a concern.

8.16 PRACTICAL IMPLICATIONS: UNIFORM RISK

In the fictional studies of this chapter, the adjusted rate ratios or differences would probably be biased because risk varies in human populations; people are not uniform atoms of uranium. But an assumption of uniform risk might be reasonable in some studies. Imagine machine parts tested to failure. If the parts are very similar in their quality, and we wished to compare the failure rate of a new version with an old version, it might be reasonable to use rate comparisons and assume that the risk of failure is homogenous for the new and old versions.

8.17 PRACTICAL IMPLICATIONS: USE ALL EVENTS

So far we have discussed collapsibility for nonrecurrent outcomes, with censoring of person-time after the event occurs. If rates are used to study recurrent outcomes and subjects are all followed for the same length of time, the resulting rate ratios or differences will be collapsible (Greenland 1996). In this situation, person-time is not affected by the exposure, so the mechanism that produces noncollapsibility is removed. If everyone is followed for the same length of time, rate ratios will be ratios of outcome counts and rate differences can be expressed as count differences per unit of time equal to the follow-up interval.

Even for recurrent events, noncollapsibility could arise if person-time varies notably for reasons related to the exposure. These reasons could include an exposure that forces some people to leave the study or a competing risk that does the same. Some reasons for variation in follow-up would not be important. For example, if the study must recruit and enroll people over some length of time, but end on a preplanned date, the resulting variation in person-time may have no relation to the exposure and therefore not be a source of noncollapsibility.

Poisson Regression for Rate Ratios

9

In previous chapters I showed that rates can be analyzed by treating the numerator counts and denominator person-time separately. If events are produced by a Poisson process, the counts will fit a Poisson distribution. One important feature of a Poisson process is independence, the idea that the occurrence of one event does not influence the occurrence of other events. A second feature is that the process is stationary; within a given time interval or categories formed by the cross-classification of variables, the risk (and consequently the rate) of an event is constant. If these assumptions are approximately true, we can rely upon the Poisson variance formulae shown in Table 4.4. The person-time denominator does not contribute to the variance of a rate but is used as a weight to summarize or otherwise manipulate rates. The method assumes that if the person-time denominator of population B is double that of population A and if the two populations are otherwise alike, the numerator event count for population B should be twice that of population A. If the event count in population B falls short of or exceeds this expected amount, we can use Poisson regression to try to find factors, other than person-time, that explain the observed difference in the rates of the two populations. Using person-time to explain differences in event counts is usually of little interest; we wish to remove the expected influence of person-time from the analysis and find other factors that may explain observed differences.

Radioactive decay (Chapter 4) fits a Poisson process so well that perhaps it really is a Poisson process. For event counts such as deaths in a population, new patents in a year, or new dropouts from high school, the true process is probably not Poisson, but the approximation may often be close enough to justify Poisson methods. While the overall process that produced the counts not may be Poisson, we may be able to slice up person-time and introduce other variables so that within short time intervals and suitable categories the data do fit a Poisson distribution. As with any statistical method that assumes the data come from a particular distribution, there will often be some discrepancy between the distributional assumptions and reality. In later chapters I will show how some assumptions about the Poisson distribution can be relaxed in regression. But those modifications or extensions build upon the Poisson regression model, which is the topic of this chapter.

9.1 THE POISSON REGRESSION MODEL FOR RATE RATIOS

A multiplicative model such as Expression 9.1 is well suited to estimate ratios of rates: C indicates a count, T represents person-time, the coefficients to be estimated are indicated by the letter B, with subscripts ranging from 0 to k, and the x terms are for explanatory or predictor variables:

$$\text{rate} = C/T = B_0 \times B_1^{X1} \times B_2^{X2} \times \ldots \times B_k^{Xk} \qquad \text{(Ex.9.1)}$$

In Expression 9.1, each 1 unit increment in the value of any explanatory variable, such as x_1, will increase the size of the predicted rate; the predicted rate will be multiplied by the coefficient for that variable. Imagine that B_1 is equal to 3. If the value of x_1 is 0, then $B_1^0 = 1$, and the size of B_1 contributes nothing to the predicted rate. If x_1 is 1, the predicted rate become $B_1^1 = 3$ times larger. If x_1 is 2, the predicted rate is $B_1^2 = 3^2 = 3 \times 3 = 9$ times larger compared with the rate when $x_1 = 0$ and 3 times larger than when $x_1 = 1$. In this model, the ratio change in the rate for any 1 unit increment in the value of any predictor is equal to the size of the coefficient for that variable. The term B_0 is a constant that represents the rate when all the x terms are equal to zero.

Take the logarithm of both sides of Expression 9.1 to get Expression 9.2

$$\ln(C/T) = \ln(B_0) + \ln(B_1)x_1 + \ln(B_2)x_2 + \ldots + \ln(B_k)x_k \qquad \text{(Ex.9.2)}$$

Designate the logarithm of each coefficient B as b, so that $\ln(B) = b$, and rewrite 9.2:

$$\ln(C/T) = b_0 + b_1x_1 + b_2x_2 + \ldots + b_kx_k \qquad \text{(Ex.9.3)}$$

Expression 9.3 is a linear model, meaning that the terms on the right side of the Expression are just summed to predict the outcome, the ln of the rate. The combination of terms on the right side of the Expression is called the linear predictor. Expression 9.3 looks somewhat like expressions for the ordinary least squares linear regression model, except that the outcome is the logarithm of the rate, not the rate. Expression 9.3 is sometimes called a log-linear model, because the estimation is done on the scale of the ln of the rate. (The term log-linear model can also be applied to logistic regression, other regression methods, and methods for the analysis of contingency tables. Because this term has several meanings, I will avoid it.) Because the ln scale is used, the predicted rate will never be less than a rate of 0, a desirable feature because negative event counts and rates are not possible.

Expression 9.3 makes the ln of the rate the outcome, but it has the disadvantage of combining the counts and person-time into a single rate term, rather than keeping them separated for the analysis as was done by the methods described in Chapters 6 and 7. The logarithm of the ratio of two quantities is equal to the log of the numerator minus the log of the denominator, so $\ln(C/T) = \ln(C) - \ln(T)$. Therefore, rewrite Expression 9.3 as Expression 9.4:

$$\ln(C) - \ln(T) = b_0 + b_1x_1 + b_2x_2 + \ldots + b_kx_k \qquad \text{(Ex.9.4)}$$

Move the $\ln(T)$ to the right side of the Expression to make it part of the linear predictor in Expression 9.5:

$$\ln(C) = b_0 + b_1x_1 + b_2x_2 + \ldots + b_kx_k + \ln(T) \qquad \text{(Ex.9.5)}$$

Expression 9.5 is one way to represent the Poisson regression model. The linear predictor on the right side of Expression 9.5 includes person-time, but there is no coefficient to be estimated for this term: no b symbol appears in front of $\ln(T)$. When a term is included in a regression model without a coefficient, it is called an offset, because it moves (offsets), the predicted outcome by a fixed amount. An offset is a model variable with a coefficient constrained to equal 1. If the person-time is doubled in Expression 9.5, the outcome count will also double, which is what we usually desire for estimating rate ratios. Person-time affects the count of outcomes on a multiplicative scale; if person-time doubles or triples, the number of outcomes doubles or triples.

How does Expression 9.5 estimate a rate ratio? Imagine there are 2 observations, one for an exposed (subscript e) person and another for an unexposed (subscript u) person; this exposure variable takes the place of x_1 in Expression 9.5 and exposure is coded as 1, lack of exposure as 0. The two subjects are both alike regarding all the other x variables, 2 through k. The Expressions for the exposed and unexposed persons are:

$$\ln(C_e) = b_0 + b_1(1) + b_2x_2 + \ldots + b_kx_k + \ln(T_e)$$
$$\ln(C_u) = b_0 + b_1(0) + b_2x_2 + \ldots + b_kx_k + \ln(T_u)$$

(Ex.9.6)

To calculate the difference in the estimated logarithms of the rates due to the exposure variable, subtract the second expression from the first and take advantage of the fact that when x is equal to 1, b_1 x 1 = b_1, and when x is equal to 0, then b_1 x 0 = 0. Since the two subjects are alike except for the exposure variable, all the other model terms are removed by the subtraction:

$$\ln(C_e) - \ln(C_u)$$
$$= b_0 + b_1 \times 1 + b_2x_2 + \ldots + b_kx_k + \ln(T_e) - [b_0 + b_1(0) + b_2x_2 + \ldots + b_kx_k + \ln(T_u)]$$
$$= b_1 \times 1 - b_1 \times 0 + \ln(T_e) - \ln(T_u)$$
$$= b_1 + \ln(T_e) - \ln(T_u)$$

(Ex.9.7)

Move the person-time offsets on the right side of the last line of Expression 9.7 to the left side of Expression 9.8 to show that the estimated coefficient b_1 is equal to the ln of the rate ratio:

$$\ln(C_e) - \ln(C_u) - \ln(T_e) + \ln(T_u)$$
$$= [\ln(C_e) - \ln(T_e)] - [\ln(C_u) - \ln(T_u)]$$
$$= \ln(C_e/T_e) - \ln(C_u/T_u)$$
$$= \ln[(C_e/T_e)/(C_u/T_u)]$$
$$= \ln(rate_e/rate_u) = b_1$$

(Ex.9.8)

Expression 9.8 shows that the estimated coefficients are ln rate ratios. For a variable coded as 1/0, the coefficient is the ln of the rate ratio comparing those exposed with those unexposed. For a continuous variable, the coefficient is the ln of the estimated ratio change in rate for each 1-unit increment in the variable; for example, the ln of the ratio change for a 1-year increment in age or for each $1000 increase in family income.

If we exponentiate the last line of 9.8, the rate ratio comparing a person exposed to $x_1 = 1$ with an otherwise similar person not exposed is given by the exponential of b_1:

$$\exp(\ln(rate_e/rate_u)) = rate_e/rate_u = \exp(b_1)$$

(Ex.9.9)

Exponentiated coefficients from the regression model in Expression 9.5 are estimated rate ratios. Statistical software that estimates this model can be instructed to show a table of output for the coefficients, the ln of the rate ratios, or the exponentiated coefficients, the rate ratios. If the explanatory variable falls into well-known and immutable categories, then the interpretation of the rate ratios will be obvious. For example, if authors explain that a variable indicates female sex, the reader can assume that the rate ratio is the estimated ratio change in the rate expected for a female compared with an otherwise similar male. If the explanatory variable is labeled sex or gender, interpretation will not be clear because everyone has a sex and without knowing how female or male sex was coded, the meaning of the coefficient for sex is unclear. It is good practice to label all variables, categorical or continuous, in such a way that interpretation is obvious. For continuous variables, the size of the coefficient will vary depending on the units used. If a continuous variable is age, the size of the exponentiated coefficient for a 1-unit increment in age will be 365 times larger if age is expressed in years rather than days.

The term b_0 is often called the intercept in a regression model with a linear predictor. For the model in Expression 9.5, the intercept is the ln of the rate when all exposures are set to 0. The exponential of b_0 is the rate when all other explanatory variables are equal to 0. More precisely, $\exp(b_0)$ is a rate ratio; the ratio of the rate when all the x_i terms are equal to zero compared with a rate of 1 outcome event per 1 unit of person-time. I will soon illustrate the difference between these two interpretations of $\exp(b_0)$ in an example. On a difference scale the null rate against which other rates are compared is a rate of 0. But on a ratio scale the null rate is 1. Comparing rates on a ratio scale to a null rate of 0 would be intractable, as these comparisons would produce ratios that are undefined.

Expression 9.5 can give the impression that the logarithms of the counts are the outcome in Poisson regression. But zero counts are often found in data and the ln of zero is undefined. Poisson regression handles counts of 0 with ease, because the actual outcomes are the counts, not their logs. If we were to actually estimate the lns of counts or rates, and then average those somehow, we will usually get something different from what is estimated by Poisson regression, because the mean of a ln and the ln of a mean are not the same thing (Lindsey and Jones 1998). Poisson regression estimates the mean count (and also the mean rate), not the mean ln(count); the mean count is not usually equal to the exponential of the mean ln(count). To appreciate that the counts are the outcomes in Poisson regression, we can exponentiate both sides of Expression 9.5 and get Expression 9.10, which shows that the counts are the outcome and the expected count is multiplicatively related to person-time:

$$
\begin{aligned}
C &= \exp[b_0 + b_1x_1 + b_2x_2 + \ldots + b_kx_k + \ln(T)] \\
&= e^{[b0 + b1xi + b2x2 + \ldots + bkxk + \ln(T)]} \\
&= T \times e^{[b0 + b1x1 + b2x2 + \ldots + bkxk]} \qquad\qquad \text{(Ex.9.10)}\\
&= T \times \exp[b_0 + b_1x_1 + b_2x_2 + \ldots + b_kx_k] \\
&= T \times \exp[b_0] \times \exp[b_1x_1] \times \exp[b_2x_2] \times \ldots \times \exp[b_kx_k]
\end{aligned}
$$

So far I have described a multiplicative model that allows us to estimate ratios of rates. This model will not predict negative rates. Expression 9.10 becomes a *Poisson* model if the calculations for the variance, standard errors (SE), confidence intervals (CI), and P-values rely upon the characteristics of the Poisson distribution and use the formulae in Table 4.4. If the counts arise from a Poisson process, as described in Chapter 4, then the variance of the mean count will be equal to the mean count and the estimates of statistical precision from a Poisson regression model will be valid.

9.2 A SHORT COMPARISON WITH ORDINARY LINEAR REGRESSION

The usual Poisson regression model carries out estimation on the ln scale. It assumes that a multiplicative relationship is the best initial approach for estimating the relationship between explanatory variables and rates. In the jargon of generalized linear models, the "link" between the rates and the predictor variables is a log link. The possibility that some relationships are additive and not multiplicative, and therefore not linear on the ln scale, can be relaxed with interaction terms. The variance estimates are based on the assumption that if the data were generated by a Poisson process, the variance is described by the formulae in Table 4.4. In particular, a mean count and its variance will be the same if outcomes arise independently from a constant random process. Because the variance is not separately estimated from the data, as it is in linear regression, the Poisson regression model can estimate a rate and its variance from a single observation, using methods described in Chapter 4. There is no assumption of homoskedasticity; on the contrary, it is assumed that the variance will be greater for larger mean counts.

Linear regression does not use the log scale. It assumes that an additive relationship is the first approach for estimating associations. The link function between the outcome and a linear set of predictors is the identity link, so the model estimates an adjusted mean difference in counts or rates. The model can allow some relationships to be multiplicative, rather than additive, by using interaction terms. The variance is separately estimated from the data, so more than one record is needed to produce an estimate. The errors are assumed to follow a normal distribution. Homoskedasticity is assumed; the variance should be the same at each level of the explanatory variables.

9.3 A POISSON MODEL WITHOUT VARIABLES

To see what a Poisson model estimates and relate the output to formulae in Chapter 4, start with hypothetical data (Table 9.1) for patient falls in three nursing homes that had equal amounts of inpatient-time over 1 year of observation. These are fall rates per nursing-home-year.

Since the nursing-home-time units were equal to 1 for all three observations, I could ignore nursing-home-time and simply carry out an analysis of counts. But I will do an analysis of rates using formulae 4 and 9 from Table 4.4 and as well as Expression 4.8 which tells us that the SE of the ln of the rate is equal to the SE of the rate divided by the rate. Formula 4 in Table 4.4 shows that if the rate is 3 per 1 nursing-home-year, the variance of the rate is $(C/T)T = (9/3)/3 = 1$, and the SE of the rate = $(\sqrt{(C/T^2)})$ or rate/$\sqrt{C}$. Therefore:

rate = total count/total nursing-home-time = C/T = $(5+3+1)/(1+1+1) = 9/3 = 3$
SE of rate = $((C/T)/T)^{.5} = (3/3)^{.5} = 1$
Wald statistic for rate difference = z_{diff} = rate/(SE rate) = 3/1 = 3
P-value (2-sided) for z_{diff} = .0027

Formula 9 from Table 4.4, as well as Expression 4.8, can be used to redo these calculations on the ln scale, which is what Poisson regression does for rate ratios:

ln(rate) = ln(3) = 1.099
SE ln(rate) = $1/\sqrt{C} = 1/\sqrt{9} = 1/3 = 0.333$
SE ln(rate) = SE(rate)/rate = 1/3 = 0.333
Wald statistic for rate ratio = z_{ratio} = ln(rate)/SE ln(rate) = 1.099/0.333 = 3.30
P-value (2-sided) for z_{ratio} = .00098

Here is Poisson regression output on the ln scale from Stata software using data from all three nursing homes. The number of falls is indicated by the variable count and nhtime represents the nursing-home-time. The nhtime variable, the denominator of each rate, is entered as an offset option, called **exposure** or **exp**, with its coefficient constrained to equal 1:

TABLE 9.1 Hypothetical counts, nursing-home-year time units, and rates (per 1 nursing-home-year) of patient falls in three nursing homes that were observed for 1 year. The amount of inpatient time at each nursing home is not known, but it was the same in each institution.

NURSING HOME	FALLS	NURSING HOME YEAR TIME UNITS	RATE
Senior Village	5	1	5
Leisure Life	3	1	3
Golden Years	1	1	1

```
. poisson count, exp(nhtime) nolog pformat(%5.4f)
(output omitted)
```

```
-----------------------------------------------------------------
     count |   Coef.    Std. Err.    z     P>|z|   [95% Conf. Interval]
---------+-------------------------------------------------------
     _cons |  1.098612  .3333333   3.30   0.0010    .445291   1.751934
ln(nhtime) |        1   (exposure)
-----------------------------------------------------------------
```

The regression estimates for the ln of the rate, the SE, Z-statistic and P value are identical to what was calculated on the ln scale using formulae from Table 4.4. By adding the **irr** (meaning incidence rate ratio) option after the comma to the regression command, we can exponentiate the ln of the rate and get:

```
. poisson count, exp(nhtime) nolog pformat(%5.4f) irr
(output omitted)
```

```
-----------------------------------------------------------------
     count |   IRR   Std. Err.    z     P>|z|   [95% Conf. Interval]
---------+-------------------------------------------------------
     _cons |    3        1      3.30   0.0010    1.560944   5.765741
ln(nhtime) |    1   (exposure)
-----------------------------------------------------------------
```

This output estimates the rate as 3 per nursing-home-year and the SE of the rate as 1, just what we obtained using Formula 4 from Table 4.4. But the Z-statistic and P-value are from estimation on the ln (ratio) scale; they are for a test comparing the observed rate ratio of 3/1 = 3 with the null hypothesis that the true rate ratio is 1/1 = 1. Although the constant term in the regression model is the mean rate with all other variables set to 0, it is also the *ratio* of the mean rate to a hypothetical or baseline rate of 1 per 1 time-unit; 3/1 = 3. The regression output suggests this comparison, by reporting that the coefficient for the ln of nursing-home-time is 1 in the table of ln rate ratio coefficients. Recall from Expression 9.5 that that the coefficient for nursing-home-time is constrained to be 1 and is not estimated, and so it has no SE or other statistics. When the **irr** option is added to the **poisson** command, the regression coefficients are exponentiated and reported as rate ratios. But the coefficient of 1 for the ln of nursing-home-time is not exponentiated; that would produce a value of exponential(1) = 2.72. Instead, Stata's output reports a rate ratio of 1 for the ln of nursing-home-time. It might be clearer if Stata could rename the variable nursing-home-time instead of *ln* nursing-home-time, in keeping with Expression 9.10. Using Expression 9.10, the count of falls predicted by the model is total nursing home time x the rate per nursing-home year = 3 × exponential(1.099) = 3 × 3 = 9.

The P-values estimated here are based on methods for large counts. Since the counts are small, these methods are not terribly accurate here, but small counts make the calculations simple and generate P-values large enough to be useful for this example. On the rate difference scale we are comparing the observed total count of 9 with an expected null value of 0 and the Wald-statistic P-value is .003. On the ratio scale we are comparing a count of 9 with an expected null value of 3; the observed rate was 3 per 1 unit of time and the null rate of 1 per time unit means that we expect a fall count of 3 from the 3 nursing homes. Even though the difference between 9 and 0 is larger than between 9 and 3, the P-value from the difference method is larger, .003, than the P-value from the ratio (ln scale) method (.001). This arises because difference methods for counts and rates are statistically less efficient compared with ratio methods.

We can change the time units to see if this affects the results. The original time units were for 1 nursing-home-year with the understanding that all the nursing homes experienced the same amount of inpatient time in a year. It is now revealed that the cumulated inpatient time at each institution over a year was 100 patient-years and we decide to estimate the rate per 1 patient-year. The rates now range from .05 per inpatient-year at Senior Village to .01 at Golden Years. Redoing the calculations:

rate = total count/total person-time = C/T = 9/300 = 0.03
SE of rate = $((C/T)/T)^{.5}$ = $(.03/300)^{.5}$ = 0.01
Wald statistic for rate difference = z_{diff} = rate/(SE rate) = .03/.01 = 3
P-value (2-sided) for z_{diff} = .0027

By changing the time units, the size of the rate and its SE changed, but the Z-statistic and P-value did not change. Z-statistics and P-values are for tests of a specific hypothesis. The Z-statistic is a Wald test for the difference between the observed rate and a rate of zero. This was discussed in some detail in Section 4.6 called "Large sample P-values for counts, rates, and their differences using the Wald statistic" in Chapter 4. There I showed the size of this Wald statistic, rate/SE(rate), is equal to the Wald statistic for the total count in the rate numerator, count/SE(count), and these ratios are the same regardless of the person-time units used for the rate. Despite changing the rate denominator units, the P-value on the difference scale is still for a test that compares the observed count of 9 with a null or expected count of 0.

Now look at the calculations on the ln scale and the Poisson regression output using ptime, as an offset, to indicate 100 patient-years for each nursing home:

ln(rate) = ln(.03) = − 3.51
SE ln(rate) = $1/\sqrt{C}$ = $1/\sqrt{9}$ = 1/3 = 0.333
SE ln(rate) = SE(rate)/rate = .01/.03 = 0.333
Wald statistic for rate ratio = z_{ratio} = ln(rate)/SE ln(rate) = − 3.51/.333 = − 10.52
P-value (2-sided) for z_{ratio} = .000000000

```
. poisson count, exp(ptime) nolog pformat(%5.4f)

Poisson regression                          Number of obs    =          3
                                            LR chi2(0)       =       0.00
                                            Prob > chi2      =          .
Log likelihood = -5.6917406                 Pseudo R2        =     0.0000
---------------------------------------------------------------------------
     count |    Coef.    Std. Err.     z     P>|z|    [95% Conf. Interval]
-----------+---------------------------------------------------------------
     _cons | -3.506558   .3333333   -10.52   0.0000   -4.159879   -2.853237
 ln(ptime) |         1   (exposure)
---------------------------------------------------------------------------


. poisson count, exp(ptime) nolog pformat(%5.4f) irr

Poisson regression                          Number of obs    =          3
                                            LR chi2(0)       =       0.00
                                            Prob > chi2      =          .
Log likelihood = -5.6917406                 Pseudo R2        =     0.0000
---------------------------------------------------------------------------
     count  | Inc. Rate  Std. Err.    z     P>|z|    [95% Conf. Interval]
-----------+---------------------------------------------------------------
     _cons  |      .03        .01   -10.52   0.0000    .0156094    .0576574
 ln(ptime) |        1   (exposure)
---------------------------------------------------------------------------
```

In this output, Poisson regression made use of the formulae from Chapter 4. But changing the rate denominator changed the Wald Z-statistic and the P-value for the estimated ln(rate), because changing the rate denominator changed the size of the null or expected rate. The null rate ratio is 1, so when we used time units equal to 1 nursing-home year, the null rate was 1 fall per 1 nursing-home year. There is not a great contrast between a rate of 3 per each nursing-home time unit (which resulted in the count of 9 falls in Table 9.1) and a rate of 1 per nursing-home time unit (which would produce a count of 3), so the P-value for a null hypothesis that the true rate ratio is 1 was .00098; this is small, but not miniscule. But after changing the rate denominator units to 1 patient-year, we were comparing an observed rate of .03 per 1 patient-year on the ratio scale with an expected rate of 1 per 1 patient-year. In the table of exponentiated regression coefficients, the rate ratio of .03 is compared on a ratio scale with the reported rate ratio of 1 for person-time; the software labels this ln(ptime) meaning the ln of person-time, which is not precisely correct. Expression 9.10 shows that that the rate ratio of 1 is for person-time, not ln person-time.

In order to observe a rate of 1 fall per 1 patient-year over the 300 patient-years, the fall count would have to be a whopping 300! So changing the rate denominator produced a comparison between an observed count of 9 and an expected count under the null hypothesis of 300. The large gap between 9 and 300 increased the Z-statistic to 10.5 and the resulting P-value is so tiny that the software could not distinguish it from zero.

Some books state that the constant term in Poisson regression estimates the baseline rate, the event rate when all other model terms are set to zero. This is true. But the Z-statistics, SEs, P-values and CIs are all for a rate ratio, not for the difference between the observed rate (or event count) with a rate (or event count) of zero. As shown in Chapter 4, changing person-time units does not change the P-values or CIs for a rate when the comparison is on a difference scale with a rate of 0. But Poisson regression, works on a ratio (ln rate) scale, so the baseline rate estimate is a comparison with a rate equal to 1 event per 1 unit of person-time. Changing the person-time units in Poisson regression changes the ratio comparison that is made, and therefore the Z-statistics, P-values, and CIs all change for the constant term.

9.4 A POISSON REGRESSION MODEL WITH ONE EXPLANATORY VARIABLE

Although a change in the rate denominator units will change the size of the Z-statistics and P-values for the constant (intercept) term in Poisson regression, this change will not influence the

TABLE 9.2 Counts, person-time (units of 100,000 person-years), and rates (per 100,000 person-years) of homicide in six fictional counties. Three counties were exposed to a new policing program designed to prevent homicides, while the others were not. The revised counts, person-years, and rates are explained in the text.

EXPOSED TO NEW POLICING PROGRAM	COUNTY	HOMICIDES	PERSON-YEARS (100,000)	RATE	REVISED HOMICIDES	REVISED PERSON-YEARS	REVISED RATE
No	Atlantic	10	2	5	26	1	26
No	Columbus	20	3	6.67	4	4	1
No	Richmond	20	5	4	20	5	4
Yes	Henry	10	5	2	10	5	2
Yes	Adams	20	7	2.86	20	7	2.86
Yes	Essex	10	4	2.5	10	4	2.5

size of the rate ratios, ln rate ratios, variance, SE, Z-statistics, or P-values for explanatory variables in the model. All those statistics remain the same, regardless of the denominator time units used. To show this I will use data for homicide mortality rates in six fictional counties (Table 9.2). Three of the counties had a new policing program intended to reduce homicides and the other three did not. In the counties exposed to the new police program, the overall homicide rate was $(10 + 20 + 10)/(5 + 7 + 4) = 40/16 = 2.5$ per 100,000 person-years. The combined rate in the three not exposed counties was $(10 + 20 + 20)/(2 + 3 + 5) = 50/10 = 5$. The rate ratio comparing exposed counties with those not exposed was $2.5/5 = 0.5$. First examine the output for a model without variables, the constant term only model which I will call Model 0. The variable ptime indicates time in units of 1 person-year; ptime was equal to 200,000 for Atlantic county:

Model 0, constant term only, exponentiated output

. poisson count, exp(ptime) irr nolog

```
Poisson regression                      Number of obs    =             6
                                        LR chi2(0)       =          0.00
                                        Prob > chi2      =             .
Log likelihood = -20.597904             Pseudo R2        =        0.0000
--------------------------------------------------------------------------
      count |    IRR   Std. Err.    z     P>|z|    [95% Conf. Interval]
-----------+--------------------------------------------------------------
      _cons | .0000346  3.65e-06  -97.44  0.000    .0000282    .0000426
   ln(ptime)|       1  (exposure)
--------------------------------------------------------------------------
```

Now use Poisson regression to estimate the rate ratio associated with exposure to the new policing program, using person-time units of 1 person-year:

Model 1, exponentiated output

```
. poisson count exposed, pformat(%5.4f) exp(ptime) irr
Iteration 0:   log likelihood = -15.228563
Iteration 1:   log likelihood = -15.228561
Iteration 2:   log likelihood = -15.228561

Poisson regression                      Number of obs    =             6
                                        LR chi2(1)       =         10.74
                                        Prob > chi2      =        0.0010
Log likelihood = -15.228561             Pseudo R2        =        0.2607
--------------------------------------------------------------------------
      count |    IRR   Std. Err.    z     P>|z|    [95% Conf. Interval]
-----------+--------------------------------------------------------------
    exposed |     .5   .106066   -3.27   0.0011   .3299156    .7577695
      _cons | .00005   7.07e-06  -70.03   0.0000   .0000379    .000066
   ln(ptime)|       1  (exposure)
--------------------------------------------------------------------------
```

The reported constant term is the mean rate of .00005 per 1 person-year that was observed in Atlantic, Columbus, and Richmond counties, the counties not exposed to the new policing program. The estimated rate ratio for homicide was 0.5 comparing county populations exposed to the new policing procedure with those not exposed. If the exposed and unexposed county populations were otherwise similar regarding factors that influence homicide rates, a rate ratio of 0.5 would be an impressive effect of the new program. Here, I show the output for the same model with the coefficients, the ln rate ratios:

```
Model 1, output showing ln rate ratios


- - - - - - - - - - - - - - - - - - - - - - - - - - - - - - - - - - - - - - - - -
      count |     Coef.   Std. Err.    z     P>|z|  [95% Conf. Interval]
- - - - - - - + - - - - - - - - - - - - - - - - - - - - - - - - - - - - - - - - - -
    exposed | -.6931472    .212132   -3.27 0.001  -1.108918   -.277376
      _cons | -9.903488   .1414214  -70.03 0.000  -10.18067   -9.626307
  ln(ptime) |         1 (exposure)
- - - - - - - - - - - - - - - - - - - - - - - - - - - - - - - - - - - - - - - - -
```

The SE of the ln(rate ratio) can be calculated from formula 10 in Table 4.4. Using notation for the event counts of exposed and unexposed subjects, the SE ln(rate ratio) = square root$(1/C_e + 1/C_u)$ = square root$(1/40 + 1/50)$ = .212, which is just what is reported in the regression table. The Z-statistic for the exposed variable is the ratio of the ln(rate ratio)/SE ln(rate ratio) = –.69315/.212132 = –3.27. As described in Chapter 4, the SE(rate ratio) = rate ratio x SE ln(rate ratio) = 0.5 x .212132 = 0.106066, which is what the regression table reported when rate ratios were shown earlier.

What happens if we change the units for person-time from 1 person-year to units of 100,000 person-years? Model 2 uses ptime1 to indicate person-time in units of 100,000 person-years:

```
Model 2, exponentiated output

. poisson count exposed, pformat(%5.4f) exp(ptime1) nolog irr

Poisson regression                        Number of obs     =          6
                                          LR chi2(1)        =      10.74
                                          Prob > chi2       =     0.0010
Log likelihood = -15.228561               Pseudo R2         =     0.2607
- - - - - - - - - - - - - - - - - - - - - - - - - - - - - - - - - - - - - - - - -
      count |    IRR  Std. Err.    z     P>|z|   [95% Conf. Interval]
- - - - - - - + - - - - - - - - - - - - - - - - - - - - - - - - - - - - - - - - - -
    exposed |     .5   .106066   -3.27  0.0011   .3299156   .7577695
      _cons |      5  .7071068   11.38  0.0000   3.789587   6.597024
 ln(ptime1) |      1 (exposure)
- - - - - - - - - - - - - - - - - - - - - - - - - - - - - - - - - - - - - - - - -
```

In Model 2, the constant is now equal to 5, meaning a rate of 5 homicides per 100,000 person-years or, more precisely, a rate ratio that compares the rate of 5 with a rate of 1 homicide per 100,000 person-years. The SE is larger, the Z-statistic smaller, and the P-value larger for the constant term compared with the model that used person-time units of 1 person-year. But for the rate ratio of 0.5 associated with being exposed, the SE, Z-statistic and P-value are all unchanged; their size was not affected by the choice of person-time units. The reason for this is that for all variables in the model, the reference or baseline rate is the rate of the constant term. The constant term is the rate among those not exposed and the rate ratio for the exposed term is the ratio of the rate among those exposed with those not exposed. Since the exposed term is a ratio of two rates that *use the same person-time units*, the choice of person-time units will not change the SE or Z-statistics for the exposed term or for any other term that might be in the model. Another way to think of this is that for the constant term, changing the person-time units changes the size of the count expected from the null rate; thus, the constant term rate ratio is .00005 in Model 1 and 5 in Model 2. But for any additional variables entered into the regression model, changing the person-time units does not change the size of the rate ratio; in both Model 1 and Model 2, the rate ratio for the exposed term is 0.5.

Comparing the exposed and unexposed counties of Table 9.2 in Poisson regression, the rate ratio and its SE is determined by the total counts and person-time in the two groups being compared; the variation of rates within the two compared groups does not affect those statistics. To illustrate this, I revised the counts and person-year quantities in Atlantic and Columbus counties. These counties had a combined total of 30 homicides; I put 26 in Atlantic County and left 4 in Columbus. The total person-time was 500,000 person-years; I assigned 100,000 person-years to Atlantic and the rest to Columbus. The revised homicide rate in Atlantic county became a colossal 26 and the rate in Columbus is now only 1. Recall that a Poisson process generates counts from constant rates. In the three exposed counties the rates are in a fairly narrow range, from 2 to 2.86. In the unexposed counties the rates prior to revision were also fairly similar, from 4 to 6.67, but after revision they ranged from 1 to 26. The revised rates in the unexposed counties suggest that the process generating these rates is not constant and therefore not Poisson. When Poisson regression is applied to the revised data, the output is below:

Model 3 for revised counts and person-years

```
. poisson newcount exposed, pformat(%5.4f) exp(newptime1) nolog irr

Poisson regression                      Number of obs    =          6
                                        LR chi2(1)       =      10.74
                                        Prob > chi2      =     0.0010
Log likelihood = -45.586827             Pseudo R2        =     0.1054
-----------------------------------------------------------------------
    newcount |    IRR  Std. Err.     z    P>|z|   [95% Conf. Interval]
-------------+---------------------------------------------------------
     exposed |     .5  .106066   -3.27   0.0011   .3299156   .7577695
       _cons |      5  .7071068   11.38   0.0000   3.789587   6.597024
ln(newpti~1) |      1  (exposure)
-----------------------------------------------------------------------
```

In Model 3 the rate ratios and their SE values are unchanged from Model 2; they are based upon the total counts and person-time within each exposure group and the variation between counties contributes nothing. In one sense this is a strength of Poisson regression. Even if the data do not come from a Poisson process, the model can correctly estimate the associations of interest. In this case, the rate ratio of 0.5 associated with exposure is correct. Poisson regression is robust in the sense that it can correctly estimate rate ratios even if the data are *not* generated by a Poisson process (Gourieroux, Monfort, and Tognon 1984b, Lloyd 1999 pp85–86, Cook and Lawless 2007 pp82–84, Wooldridge 2008 pp597–598, 2010 pp727–728, Cameron and Trivedi 2013a pp72–73). We could also characterize these results as a weakness of Poisson regression, because the SE is computed based on the Poisson distribution, but here the data in the unexposed counties do not fit this distribution. It can be argued that the SE should account for the variations in rates in the three unexposed counties. Fortunately, it turns out that we can do this, as discussed in Chapter 13. For now I point out that the regression output did not totally ignore the revisions in the rates; compared with Models 1 and 2, the log likelihood and pseudo R-squared statistics both changed. Those changes alone would not alert us to the variations in the unexposed rates, but they indicate that the statistical software recognizes that the data have changed and other statistics can be used to detect that the data are no longer a reasonable fit to the Poisson distribution. I will describe those tests in Chapter 12.

The six county records can be collapsed into just two records; one record for exposed counties has a count of 40 and person-time total of 16, the other has a count of 50 and person-time of 10. A Poisson regression model for these two records has this output:

```
Model 4 for two records

. poisson count exposed, pformat(%5.4f) exp(ptime1) nolog irr

Poisson regression                      Number of obs    =          2
                                        LR chi2(1)       =      10.74
                                        Prob > chi2      =     0.0010
Log likelihood = -5.6420782             Pseudo R2        =     0.4876
------------------------------------------------------------------------
     count |    IRR   Std. Err.      z      P>|z|     [95% Conf. Interval]
---------+--------------------------------------------------------------
   exposed |     .5   .106066     -3.27    0.0011     .3299156   .7577695
     _cons |      5   .7071068    11.38    0.0000     3.789587   6.597024
 ln(ptime1)|      1   (exposure)
------------------------------------------------------------------------
```

As expected, the rate ratio for the exposed term and the SE are unchanged from the previous models, because the previous models all used the counts and person-time totals for the two exposure categories. But the log likelihood and pseudo R-squared statistics are different.

9.5 THE ITERATION LOG

When the "nolog" option is omitted, Stata shows the iteration log. By default, Stata fits the Poisson model using maximum likelihood and the Newton-Raphson fitting algorithm. This iterative process seeks values for the model coefficients that maximize the likelihood, also called the joint probability, of the observed data. It is the log likelihood that is actually maximized, which amounts to the same thing. The fitting process starts with an initial set of values for the coefficients and refines those values in steps. The process stops after a step shows little further change. In the case of our simple model with only six records, the algorithm's initial guess at the regression coefficients produced a log likelihood of −15.228563. At the first iteration the log likelihood changed only in the 6th decimal place; the 3 changed to 1, making the log likelihood slightly larger. In the second iteration the change was so small that the algorithm came to a halt; we could force more steps, but the settings in Stata result in fitted estimates precise enough for most purposes. For most analytic work the iteration log is of little interest and it can be suppressed using the "nolog" option. It would be convenient if Stata omitted the log by default and had an option to show this when it is desired.

9.6 THE HEADER INFORMATION ABOVE THE TABLE OF ESTIMATES

Stata reports the number of observations; 6 for Models 0 through 3, and 2 for Model 4. Then Stata reports a variety of statistics that provide some information about model fit; the final ln likelihood, the likelihood ratio chi-squared statistic, and a P-value for that statistic. To understand these statistics, consider the goals of a statistical model. We can think of data as a spreadsheet with a row for each observation and columns for the variables, much like Table 9.2. If our brains were sufficiently powerful, we could read all the rows and columns and perceive relationships between the outcome variable and all the other variables in each column. This task is usually beyond us and models are a way of summarizing data in an attempt to enhance our understanding. A model with no variables, the null model, estimates the mean outcome, such as a mean rate, but tells us nothing about how other variables are related to the outcomes. A fully saturated model would have a model variable (parameter) for each observation; for example, a unique name identifying each record. Entering all those numbers into a regression model would result in a perfect fit with the observed outcomes but fail to describe how the other column variables were related to the outcomes.

What we want is something in between, a model with some parameters, but not too many, so that we get a useful description of how exposures are related to outcomes. This Goldilocks model is not too small, not too big. The most useful Goldilocks model is usually one that correctly describes the way in which exposures are *causally* related to the outcomes. This model would estimate outcomes; any disagreement between predicted and actual outcomes would be attributed to randomness in the causal mechanism. The difference between the predictions and what actually happened is a measure of the discrepancy between the model and the data. This discrepancy is proportional to twice the difference between the maximum ln likelihood of the fully saturated model and the Goldilocks model that we have fit; this quantity is called the deviance (Bishop, Fienberg, and Holland 1975 pp125–130, McCullagh and Nelder 1989 pp33–34). For linear regression, the deviance is equal to the residual sum of squares.

Two models, such as the empty Model 0 and the single variable Model 1, can be compared using the difference in their deviance statistics. The ln likelihood for the empty model with no variables was –20.5979; see output for Model 0. The ln likelihood for Model 1, with one variable, was –15.2286. The difference between these two log likelihoods, multiplied by –2, is $-2 \times (-20.5979 + 15.2286) =$ 10.74. This quantity is equal to the *difference* in the *deviances* of the two models and is called the *likelihood ratio statistic*. A comparison of two models using their deviances is called the likelihood *ratio* test because it is based upon the ln of the *ratio* of 2 likelihoods: $-2 \times$ (ln likelihood of Model 0 – ln likelihood of Model 1) = $-2 \times$ ln(likelihood of Model 0/likelihood of Model 1). The likelihood ratio statistic can be treated as an approximate chi-squared statistic to test the difference in any two models; this is why Stata gives this value next to the abbreviation "LRchi2" meaning likelihood ratio chi-squared statistic. For Model 1, the statistic is 10.74; this tests Model 1 against a model with coefficients equal to 0 for all variables aside from the constant term (Model 0).

The likelihood ratio P-value is .0010 for a test of the hypothesis that the observed rate ratio of 0.5 comes from a population where the true rate ratio is 1. This P-value is close to the Wald statistic P-value of .0011 for the exposed term in Model 1. In this example, with only 1 variable in the model, the Wald statistic and the difference in deviances are tests of the same null hypothesis, a test that the rate ratio for the exposed term is 1; or a test that the ln rate ratio is equal to 0. The likelihood ratio test is preferred over the Wald test, but in most situations the choice will make little difference. If we had more variables in the model, the likelihood ratio test statistic that Stata calls LRchi2 would be for a test that *all* the variable coefficients were jointly equal to 0.

The output headers for Models 1 and 2 report a pseudo R-squared statistic of 0.26. There are several pseudo R-squared statistics. The one Stata reports for Poisson regression is computed as 1 – (likelihood of the fitted model/likelihood of the empty model). This is a comparison of Models 1 or 2 with Model 0. This has been called the likelihood ratio index and was suggested by McFadden (Hardin and Hilbe 2012 p61). It can be thought of as an attempt to quantify the amount of variation in the outcomes that is "explained" by the variables in the model.

The choice of person-time units in Models 1 and 2 did not change the log likelihood statistic, the likelihood ratio chi-squared statistic, the P-value for the likelihood ratio test, or the pseudo R-squared statistic. But when the counts and person-time were rearranged in Model 3 the pseudo

R-squared statistic became smaller because there was more variation in the rates. Although the rate ratio for the exposed variable was 0.5 in all models, this association "explained" less of the observed variation in rates in Model 3 (R-squared = .11). Conversely in Model 4, there was less variation because the regional rates were collapsed into just 2 rates; in that model the pseudo R-squared value was greater, .49. An R-squared statistic is not a useful measure of the strength of an association, because its size depends not only upon how much the exposure influences the outcome but also upon the amount of variation in the data (Greenland et al. 1986a, 1991).

9.7 USING A GENERALIZED LINEAR MODEL TO ESTIMATE RATE RATIOS

The generalized linear model approach was described by Nelder and Wedderburn in 1972 (Nelder and Wedderburn 1972) and is described in several textbooks (McCullagh and Nelder 1989, Lindsey 1997, Hoffmann 2004, Hardin and Hilbe 2012). Instead of treating linear regression, logistic regression, Poisson regression, and other regressions in isolation, the generalized linear model approach considers these regression methods as similar because all relate an outcome variable to a linear predictor. These regression methods differ in two fundamental ways: (1) the relationship between outcome and the linear predictor is specified differently between different models, and (2) they differ regarding the anticipated distribution of the error terms. The relationship between a continuous outcome and the linear predictor for the linear regression model is specified to be equal. This is called the identity link and the error terms are expected to fit a normal distribution. For Poisson regression the link between outcome and linear predictor is the logarithmic function (see Expressions 9.5 and 9.10) and the errors are expected to follow a Poisson distribution.

Stata's **glm** command can be used to fit a generalized linear model. Applying this to the data in Table 9.2 we can obtain the results for Model 1 earlier:

```
. glm count exposed, link(log) family(poisson) pformat(%5.4f) exp(ptime)
eform

Iteration 0:   log likelihood = -15.263651
Iteration 1:   log likelihood = -15.228572
Iteration 2:   log likelihood = -15.228561
Iteration 3:   log likelihood = -15.228561

Generalized linear models                No. of obs        =          6
Optimization    : ML                     Residual df       =          4
                                         Scale parameter   =          1
Deviance        = 3.459925524            (1/df) Deviance   =  .8649814
Pearson         = 3.523809524            (1/df) Pearson    =  .8809524

Variance function: V(u) = u              [Poisson]
Link function     : g(u) = ln(u)         [Log]

                                         AIC               =   5.742854
Log likelihood   = -15.22856066          BIC               =  -3.707112
```

```
                |            OIM
        count |    IRR    Std. Err.     z     P>|z|    [95% Conf. Interval]
   ---------+----------------------------------------------------------
      exposed |     .5    .106066    -3.27   0.0011   .3299156   .7577695
        _cons |  .00005   7.07e-06   -70.03  0.0000   .0000379   .000066
    ln(ptime) |     1    (exposure)
```

The ln likelihood, rate ratios, SEs, Z-statistics and CIs are identical to those shown earlier for Model 1 using Poisson regression. The glm header reports that optimization was done using ML (maximum likelihood), which is Stata's default for fitting generalized linear models. Compared with the **poisson** command, the **glm** iteration took four steps instead of three and had a different starting value for the ln likelihood. This is because Stata's **poisson** command is specifically designed for Poisson regression and picked a better starting value. Both commands converged to the same values.

The software reported a deviance statistic of 3.46. As explained earlier, this quantity is equal to twice the difference between the ln likelihoods of the saturated model and the fitted model. In order to clarify the meaning of the deviance, the output here is for the fully saturated model with an indicator variable for each county record:

```
. glm count i.county, link(log) fam(p) exp(ptime) eform nolog

Generalized linear models                No. of obs       =          6
Optimization    : ML                     Residual df      =          0
                                         Scale parameter =          1
Deviance     = 3.84814e-14               (1/df) Deviance  =          .
Pearson      = 3.74579e-14               (1/df) Pearson   =          .

Variance function: V(u) = u              [Poisson]
Link function     : g(u) = ln(u)         [Log]

                                         AIC              =   6.499533
Log likelihood  = -13.4985979            BIC              =   3.85e-14
-------------------------------------------------------------------------
                |            OIM
        count |    IRR    Std. Err.     z     P>|z|    [95% Conf. Interval]
   ---------+----------------------------------------------------------
       county |
     Columbus |  1.333333  .5163978   0.74   0.458   .6241224   2.848444
     Richmond |     .8     .3098387  -0.58   0.565   .3744735   1.709066
        Henry |     .4     .1788854  -2.05   0.040   .1664911   .9610122
        Adams |  .5714286  .2213133  -1.44   0.148    .267481   1.220762
        Essex |     .5     .2236068  -1.55   0.121   .2081139   1.201265
              |
        _cons |  .00005    .0000158  -31.32  0.000   .0000269   .0000929
    ln(ptime) |     1    (exposure)
-------------------------------------------------------------------------
```

The output here is for the empty model with no variables:

```
. glm count, link(log) family(p) exp(ptime) eform nolog

Generalized linear models                    No. of obs      =        6
Optimization    : ML                         Residual df     =        5
                                             Scale parameter =        1
Deviance      =  14.1986115                  (1/df) Deviance =  2.839722
Pearson       =  15.58201058                 (1/df) Pearson  =  3.116402

Variance function: V(u) = u                  [Poisson]
Link function     : g(u) = ln(u)             [Log]

                                             AIC             =  7.199301
Log likelihood   = -20.59790365              BIC             =  5.239814
-------------------------------------------------------------------------
             |               OIM
      count  |    IRR     Std. Err.     z    P>|z|    [95% Conf. Interval]
-------------+-----------------------------------------------------------
       _cons | .0000346   3.65e-06   -97.44  0.000   .0000282    .0000426
  ln(ptime)  |        1   (exposure)
-------------------------------------------------------------------------
```

The log likelihood and deviance statistics for all 3 models are shown in Table 9.3. For the saturated model the software reported a deviance of 3.84814×10^{-14}. The deviance of the saturated model is 0 by definition, and the tiny estimated deviance differs from zero only because the Newton-Raphson algorithm stops at a finite, but trivial, distance from perfect fit. The likelihood ratio chi-squared statistic of 10.74 was reported by Stata's **poisson** command for Models 1, 2, and 3, which had a single variable for the policing program. This value equals the null model deviance of 14.20 minus the deviance, 3.46, of the model with the policing program variable only.

The header after fitting the generalized linear model reports that the variance is equal to the mean count using the notation $V(\upsilon) = \upsilon$, where the Greek letter mu is used to indicate the mean count. The link function is reported as the ln of the mean count, $\ln(\upsilon)$. This is expected given the options used for the **glm** command. The number of observations and model degrees of freedom are given. Other statistics include a Pearson chi-squared statistic, scale parameter, the deviance and Pearson statistics divided by the degrees of freedom, and two penalized measures of model fit, the Akaike Information Criteria (AIC) and Bayesian Information Criteria (BIC). I will discuss those statistics in Chapter 12.

TABLE 9.3   Three Poisson regression models were applied to the data in Table 9.2: (1) the null model with no variables, (2) a model with a single variable for the new policing program, and (3) a fully saturated model with an indicator (dummy) variable for each of the six counties.

		MODEL	
STATISTIC	NULL	POLICING VARIABLE ONLY	SATURATED
Ln likelihood	−20.60	−15.23	−13.50
Deviance = 2 x (model ln likelihood – ln likelihood of saturated model)	14.20	3.46	0
Likelihood ratio chi-squared statistic = deviance of null model – model deviance	0	10.74	14.20

The generalized linear model can also be fit using an algorithm for iterated, reweighted least squares. This will provide risk ratio results identical to the maximum likelihood method for this example. Any difference from maximum likelihood estimates can usually be removed by making sure that both algorithms use the same criteria for convergence. There is no particular advantage to using iterated, reweighted least squares to fit a Poisson regression model.

Since Stata's **poisson** command is specifically optimized to fit a Poisson rate *ratio* model, the **poisson** command is usually preferred over the **glm** command. The **poisson** command is designed to seek optimal starting values for rate ratios and it has special options designed for this model. But it is worth learning the generalized linear model method. Using the **glm** command makes it easy to examine different modeling choices, including changes in the link function and choice of expected distribution. Stata's **glm** command has some options that are not available with the **poisson** command. For example, the **glm** command can make use of frequency rates, sampling rates (inverse of the sampling probability), and analytic weights (inversely proportional to the variance). Analytic weights are not available for the **poisson** command.

9.8 A REGRESSION EXAMPLE: STUDYING RATES OVER TIME

Analysts often wish to know whether rates changed over time. This question is frequently answered by comparing the rate in one year with a rate several years in the past. Rates vary from year to year, so the result of this comparison may depend partly on the choice of the two years that are compared. This method ignores the rate information available from years between the first and last. Regression can make use of all the yearly rates during an interval to study any change and doing this will give less weight to the choice of the first and last year.

In about 1997, the U.S. Secretary of Health and Human Services issued a statement saying that hip fracture rates were increasing among the elderly, persons 65 years old and older. Mary Lemier at the Washington State Department of Health wondered if this was true in Washington and she and I created a file of data that contained the number of hospital admissions in the state for hip fractures of seniors 65 years and older by calendar year, patient sex, and patient age. Age was categorized using single year of age categories (the integer part of age) from 65 to 89, a category coded as 92 for those 90 to 94 years, a category coded as 97 for those 95–99, and a category coded as 103 for those 100 and older. Nearly all persons with hip fractures are hospitalized for treatment, so hospital admissions rates for hip fracture are nearly equivalent to hip fracture rates. The hip fracture rates increased over the interval from 1989 to 1995, although in 1990 and 1994 the rate was less than in the previous year (Table 9.4 and Figure 9.1).

TABLE 9.4   Counts, person-years, and rates of hospital admissions for hip fractures in Washington State, 1989–1995, for persons age 65 years or older.

YEAR	COUNT OF ADMISSIONS	PERSON-YEARS	RATE PER 1000 PERSON-YEARS
1989	3813	557,335	6.84
1990	3827	572,279	6.69
1991	4053	585,390	6.92
1992	4223	596,490	7.08
1993	4318	606,255	7.12
1994	4266	614,450	6.94
1995	4409	622,821	7.07

We can use Poisson regression to estimate the ratio change in rates from 1989 to 1995, just using the rates for the first and last year of the data:

```
. poisson count i.year if year==1989 | year==1995, exp(pop) irr nolog
```

```
Poisson regression                          Number of obs   =          112
                                            LR chi2(1)      =         2.38
                                            Prob > chi2     =       0.1225
Log likelihood = -4663.4389                 Pseudo R2       =       0.0003
------------------------------------------------------------------------------
     count |     IRR    Std. Err.     z    P>|z|    [95% Conf. Interval]
-----------+------------------------------------------------------------------
      year |
      1995 | 1.034728  .0228829    1.54   0.123   .9908368   1.080564
           |
     _cons | .0068415  .0001108 -307.81   0.000   .0066277   .0070621
   ln(pop) |        1  (exposure)
------------------------------------------------------------------------------
```

The rate ratio of 1.035 is the rate in 1995 (7.07) divided by the rate in 1989 (6.84). We could have obtained the same result by just dividing the two rates or using stratified methods.

To estimate the change in rates over time with Poisson regression and data from all 7 years, we could enter year as a continuous variable with values of 1989, 1990, ... , 1995. The output table (not shown) reports the ratio change in rate associated with a one-year increment in time: rate ratio 1.00726. To quantify the change over the 6-year interval, we calculate $1.00726^6 = 1.044$. A more convenient approach is to create a variable (let me call it newyr, meaning new year variable), equal to (year−1989)/ 6. This variable has values 0, .1667, .3333, .5, .6667, .8333, 1 for the 7 years. Since newyr has a value of 0 for 1989 and 1 for 1995, we can enter newyr as a linear term and Poisson regression estimates the associated ratio change in rates for the entire 6-year interval, along with a CI:

```
. poisson count newyr, exp(pop) irr nolog
```

```
Poisson regression                          Number of obs   =          392
                                            LR chi2(1)      =         6.02
                                            Prob > chi2     =       0.0142
Log likelihood = -16653.596                 Pseudo R2       =       0.0002
------------------------------------------------------------------------------
     count |     IRR    Std. Err.     z    P>|z|    [95% Conf. Interval]
-----------+------------------------------------------------------------------
     newyr | 1.044363  .0184799    2.45   0.014   1.008764   1.081218
     _cons | .0068039   .000074 -458.91   0.000   .0066605   .0069505
   ln(pop) |        1  (exposure)
------------------------------------------------------------------------------
```

The output above reports the ratio change in rate was 1.044 (95% CI 1.009, 1.081) over the interval from 1989 to 1995 (Figure 9.1). This rate ratio is an estimate of the change over time but uses all the yearly data instead of just comparing 1995 with 1989. A 4.4% ratio increase is not large, but it does appear that the fracture rate increased. Why?

The increase in rates over time may be related to age, which is strongly related to fracture rates. Hip fractures are about twice as common among women compared with men (Figure 9.2). The ratio change in rates from age 65 to 85 years is linear with age for both men and women. I used Poisson regression to estimate the linear change in rates (on the log scale) from age 65 to 85 and the fitted lines

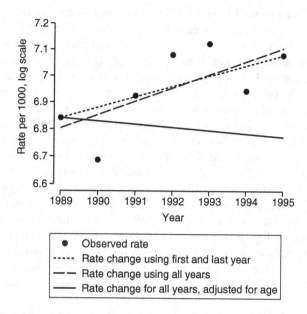

FIGURE 9.1 Rates per 1000 person-years of hospital admissions for hip fracture in Washington State, 1989–1995, for persons age 65 years or older. The solid line is an estimate of what would have happened to fracture rates if the underlying rate was that in 1989 and the population age-distribution did not change over time.

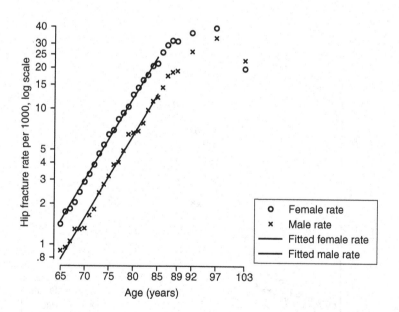

FIGURE 9.2 Rates per 1000 person-years of hospital admissions for a hip fracture in Washington State, 1989–1995, for persons age 65 years or older. The observed rates are shown using O for females and X for males. The solid lines are from Poisson regression models restricted to persons 65 to 85 years, one model for females, another for males. The slope of the lines are nearly the same for both sexes, a ratio change in rate of 4.01 per decade increment in age for females and 4.04 per decade for males. The vertical axis is on the log scale.

are shown with the observed rates in Figure 9.2; the agreement is impressive. The log scale was used for the vertical axis because this makes it easy to visualize relationships for ratios; for each decade increase in age (whether from 65 to 75 or from 72 to 82) the fracture rate increased 4-fold and the vertical distance between rates in the plot is the same for any 10-year change in age up to 85 years. To emphasize this point, Figure 9.3 shows the rates plotted without the log scale, showing exponential curves for men and women. For ages 65 to 85, a rate ratio model fits the data more closely than a rate difference model, as the rate ratio changes are almost constant as age increases (Figure 9.2), whereas the rate difference from one year of age to next increases steadily with older age (Figure 9.3).

Figure 9.2 shows a linear relationship between rates on a log scale as age increases, until the oldest ages where the curves appear to droop. Breslow and Day graphed similar curves for ovarian cancer and age (Breslow and Day 1975, 1987 p129). A linear relationship, sometimes with a drooping tail among the elderly, was shown for gastric cancer rates from four countries in a 1967 paper by Doll and Cook (1967), although they plotted rates on the log scale against age on the log scale; their graph is reproduced in the book by Breslow and Day (1987 p56). Frome and Checkoway graphed the log of the rate of skin cancer against log age (Frome and Checkoway 1985) and reported a straight line for this relationship. For the hip fracture rates, a plot of rates on the log scale against age on the log scale (not shown) looks very similar to Figure 9.2 and model fit statistics suggest that it makes little difference whether we use age or ln age. In these examples rates for biological events fit a log-linear scale remarkably well.

After age 85 the rate change was no longer linear on the log scale. The increase slowed and then rates declined at the oldest ages (Figures 9.2 and 9.3). We can speculate about the reasons for this drop. People older than 90 are often bed-bound or use a wheel-chair, which may reduce their risk of a fall and fracture. Some persons already bed-bound may not be admitted to a hospital when they fracture their hip. Those at highest risk of fracture may be dying of other ailments before they can experience a fracture.

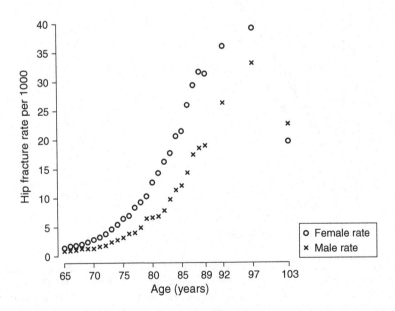

FIGURE 9.3 Rates per 1000 person-years of hospital admissions for a hip fracture in Washington State, 1989–1995, for persons age 65 years or older. The observed rates are shown using O for females and X for males. The rates are the same as those shown in Figure 9.2, but the vertical axis is not on the log scale in this graph.

Because age is powerfully related to fracture rates, a change in the average age of senior citizens over time could increase fracture rates over time. In fact, the mean age of Washington residents age 65 and older increased by 0.5 years, from 74.1 to 74.6 years, over the period 1989–1995. The mean age of those with a hip fracture increased even more, from 81.6 to 82.3. So the oldest citizens were getting even older over time. Was this change enough to increase the fracture rates? To find out, I reestimated the linear change in rates with a model that adjusts for age using indicator (dummy) variables for each age category:

```
. poisson count newyr i.age, exp(pop) irr nolog

Poisson regression                          Number of obs   =         392
                                            LR chi2(28)     =    28669.88
                                            Prob > chi2     =      0.0000
Log likelihood = -2321.6656                 Pseudo R2       =      0.8606
```

count	IRR	Std. Err.	z	P>|z|	[95% Conf. Interval]	
newyr	.9898163	.0175051	-0.58	0.563	.9560947	1.024727
age						
66	1.171202	.0914407	2.02	0.043	1.005021	1.364862
67	1.258296	.0966791	2.99	0.003	1.082386	1.462795
68	1.44882	.1082535	4.96	0.000	1.251452	1.677316
69	1.628578	.1193025	6.66	0.000	1.41076	1.880026
70	1.850501	.1331368	8.55	0.000	1.607121	2.130739
71	2.174609	.1531434	11.03	0.000	1.894247	2.496466
72	2.512113	.1741876	13.28	0.000	2.192894	2.877801
73	3.126447	.2114901	16.85	0.000	2.738237	3.569694
74	3.635865	.242915	19.32	0.000	3.189615	4.144548
75	4.301452	.2836827	22.12	0.000	3.77988	4.894995
76	4.797316	.3145526	23.91	0.000	4.218775	5.455195
77	5.567984	.3616466	26.44	0.000	4.902432	6.323892
78	6.383956	.4117464	28.74	0.000	5.625872	7.24419
79	7.476203	.478082	31.46	0.000	6.595522	8.474479
80	8.789191	.5579758	34.24	0.000	7.76088	9.953753
81	9.768222	.6197425	35.92	0.000	8.626035	11.06165
82	11.21303	.7092644	38.21	0.000	9.905617	12.69301
83	12.70055	.8022714	40.24	0.000	11.22157	14.37446
84	14.88892	.9375081	42.89	0.000	13.1603	16.8446
85	15.76739	.9979777	43.57	0.000	13.92785	17.8499
86	18.9222	1.197259	46.47	0.000	16.71529	21.4205
87	21.78679	1.386162	48.43	0.000	19.23253	24.68028
88	23.76824	1.525194	49.37	0.000	20.95926	26.95368
89	23.85589	1.542449	49.06	0.000	21.01645	27.07894
92	28.81557	1.718385	56.36	0.000	25.63698	32.38827
97	32.48382	2.078273	54.40	0.000	28.65552	36.82357
103	17.27928	1.934828	25.45	0.000	13.87437	21.51979
_cons	.0011767	.0000682	-116.44	0.000	.0010504	.0013182
ln(pop)	1	(exposure)				

It is worth studying the rate ratios reported for the age categories. The rate ratio for age 75, compared with the omitted category of 65, was 4.3, close to the linear change of 4.0 in fracture rate for both men and women. The rate ratio for age 85 was 15.8, close to the change of 4 x 4 = 16 for a two-decade change based upon the linear model for a ratio change in rate with age (Figure 9.2).

After age adjustment, the ratio change in rates over the 6-year interval was 0.99 (Figure 9.1). Essentially there was no change in fracture rates over time if we compare seniors within the same age categories. We can fit more complicated models, by adding a variable for male sex or by adding interaction terms between sex and age to the main effects of those variables; although adding these terms improved model fit, the association of interest between the passage of time and the rates was still 0.99 in these models and the CI was little affected. It is not surprising that adjusting for sex does not influence the estimate of change with time. Although male sex is related to fracture rates (Figures 9.2 and 9.3), sex has almost no relationship to year; the proportion of the senior population that was female did not change appreciably over time. Therefore sex was not a confounder of the association between time and fracture rates.

9.9 AN ALTERNATIVE PARAMETERIZATION FOR POISSON MODELS: A REGRESSION TRICK

Instead of using the count as the outcome, we can use the rate itself as the outcome and use weights to provide the software information needed to correctly estimate the SEs for the Poisson model. There is no reason to use this method to estimate rate ratios and I do not recommend it for that purpose. But in Chapter 10 I will show that this method can be used to estimate adjusted rate differences. Since it also works for rate ratios, I will introduce it here. This method was known before 1987, when Breslow and Day (1987) published their book about the analysis of cohort studies. The method is briefly mentioned on pages 137 and 142–143 of their book in a description of how the Poisson model could be implemented in GLIM (Generalized Linear Interactive Modelling) software, a computer program released in 1974, but no longer distributed.

In Chapter 6 I discussed the rates of cancer in Alaska (884/710,231 = 124.5 per 100,000 person-years) and Florida (41,467/18,801,310 = 220.6) in 2010 (Table 6.2); the crude rate ratio comparing Florida with Alaska is 124.5/220.6 = 1.77. We can estimate this ratio and its CI using Poisson regression, with the variable florida coded as 1 for Florida and 0 for Alaska:

```
. poisson count florida, exp(pop1) irr nolog
```

```
Poisson regression                     Number of obs    =          2
                                       LR chi2(1)       =     342.52
                                       Prob > chi2      =     0.0000
Log likelihood = -10.546528            Pseudo R2        =     0.9420
------------------------------------------------------------------
    count |    IRR     Std. Err.    z     P>|z|   [95% Conf. Interval]

--------+---------------------------------------------------------
  florida | 1.771992   .0602305   16.83   0.000   1.657789   1.894063
    _cons | .0012447   .0000419  -198.87  0.000   .0011653   .0013295
ln(pop1) |        1  (exposure)
------------------------------------------------------------------
```

Now fit this model using the rate as the outcome and omitting the person-time offset. The outcome rate1 in the model indicates the rate per 1 person-year for each state:

```
. poisson rate1 florida, irr nolog
note: you are responsible for interpretation of noncount dep. Variable

Poisson regression                          Number of obs  =           2
                                            LR chi2(1)     =        0.00
                                            Prob > chi2    =      0.9869
Log likelihood = -.02328019                 Pseudo R2      =      0.0058
--------------------------------------------------------------------------
     rate1 |     IRR     Std. Err.      z    P>|z|    [95% Conf. Interval]
-----------+--------------------------------------------------------------
   florida | 1.771992    62.82039     0.02   0.987    1.18e-30    2.66e+30
     _cons | .0012447    .0352798    -0.24   0.813    9.29e-28    1.67e+21
--------------------------------------------------------------------------
```

In this output, Stata warns us that the rates are not counts. This is a useful warning because we can use Poisson regression to estimate ratios of variables that are not counts, but the SE depends on the count information. The model correctly estimated the rate ratio as being 1.77, but the SE for the rate ratio is now an astronomical 62.8, more than 1000-fold greater compared with the previous estimate of 0.06.

To understand why the SE is now 62.8, use formula 10 in Table 4.4, which tells us that the SE of the ln(rate ratio) for the ratio of two rates is the square root of $(1/C1 + 1/C2)$, where C1 and C2 are the counts for the two rate numerators. In the model above we used the rates per 1 person-year for Alaska (0.00124) and Florida (0.00221), so the software merrily computed that the SE for ln of the rate ratio must be the square root$(1/.00124 + 1/.00221) = 35.45$. The SE of the rate ratio is equal to the rate ratio x SE ln(rate ratio) = 1.77 x 35.45 = 62.8. This ridiculous estimate arose because we provided the rates instead of the counts to the software.

We need to offer additional information so that the software can produce the correct SE. One way to do this is to use frequency weights to tell the software that the counts came from 710,231 persons in Alaska and 18,801,310 persons in Florida. Below is the output from a model in which I set frequency weights (fweight) equal to the total person-years from each state and the variable pop1 contains those population (person-year) estimates:

```
. poisson rate1 florida [fweight=pop1], irr nolog
note: you are responsible for interpretation of noncount dep. variable

Poisson regression                          Number of obs  =    19511541
                                            LR chi2(1)     =      342.52
                                            Prob > chi2    =      0.0000
Log likelihood = -277539.04                 Pseudo R2      =      0.0006
--------------------------------------------------------------------------
     rate1 |     IRR     Std. Err.      z    P>|z|    [95% Conf. Interval]
-----------+--------------------------------------------------------------
   florida | 1.77194     .0602278     16.83  0.000    1.657742    1.894005
     _cons | .0012447    .0000419   -198.88  0.000    .0011653    .0013295
--------------------------------------------------------------------------
```

The output above reports that there were 19.5 million observations and the log likelihood has changed compared with the usual Poisson model. But the rate ratio estimate, SE, and CIs are now correct. To compute the SE, the software still thought that each rate per 1 person-year was a count, but it now had information that these supposed small counts (.00124 and .00221) could be multiplied by the person-time estimate from each state. So the new SE of the ln (rate ratio) was equal to the square root of $(1/(.00124 \times 710{,}231) + 1/(.00221 \times 18{,}801{,}310))$ = square root of $(1/884 + 1/41{,}467)$ = 0.034. Therefore, the SE of the rate ratio is $1.77 \times 0.034 = 0.06$, which is correct.

If we divide the rates by 100,000 (creating a variable called rate100k) and divide person-time by the same amount (creating the variable pop100k), we should be able to estimate the same rate ratio. I showed earlier that this could be done using an offset. But the person-time estimates, expressed in units of 100,000 years, will now be fractions and Stata does not allow frequency rates that are not integers. Stata does allow something that it calls **iweights**, or importance weights. These **iweights** can do what we want. Here is a model in which the rates were expressed per 100,000 person-years and person-time was expressed using units of 100,000 person-years:

```
. poisson rate100k florida [iweight=pop100k], irr nolog
note: you are responsible for interpretation of noncount dep. variable


Poisson regression                         Number of obs   =           2
                                           LR chi2(1)      =      342.52
                                           Prob > chi2     =      0.0000
Log likelihood = -703.77842                Pseudo R2       =      0.1957
-----------------------------------------------------------------------
rate100k |     IRR    Std. Err.      z    P>|z|    [95% Conf. Interval]
---------+-------------------------------------------------------------
 florida | 1.771992  .0602305    16.83   0.000    1.657789   1.894063
   _cons | 124.4665  4.186263   143.43   0.000    116.5262   132.948
-----------------------------------------------------------------------
```

By using importance weights, we get the correct number of observations in the header (2) and the correct rate ratio and SE. Compared with a model that uses the count as the outcome and an offset, the weighted method reports a different ln likelihood. But when using ln likelihoods and deviances, we usually care about comparisons between models and not the absolute values of these statistics. So as long as we estimate models in the same way, either using count outcomes and offsets or rate outcomes and weights, we can make valid comparisons.

This weighted method may also be used with the **glm** command and in Chapter 10 we will want the added flexibility of that command to estimate rate differences. Here I show how the **glm** command can use the weighted method:

```
. glm rate100k florida [iw=pop100k], link(log) fam(p) eform nolog
note: rate100k has noninteger values


Generalized linear models                  No. of obs       =          2
Optimization    : ML                       Residual df      =          0
                                           Scale parameter  =          1
Deviance      = 8.18149e-12                (1/df) Deviance  =          .
Pearson       = 3.49028e-12                (1/df) Pearson   =          .

Variance function: V(u) = u                [Poisson]
Link function    : g(u) = ln(u)            [Log]
                                           AIC              =   705.7784
Log likelihood  = -703.7784172             BIC              =   8.18e-12
```

```
             |              OIM
 rate100k |    IRR    Std. Err.    z     P>|z|    [95% Conf. Interval]
---------+----------------------------------------------------------------
  florida |  1.771993   .0602305   16.83   0.000    1.657789    1.894063
    _cons |  124.4665   4.186263  143.43   0.000    116.5262    132.9479
---------------------------------------------------------------------------
```

This weighted method can do more than just compare two rates. Here we see output from a model that uses this method to compare Florida with Alaska but adjusts for the age distribution of the states using indicator variables for the age categories in Table 6.2. The model below uses the rate per person-year (rate1) and the stratum-specific population counts by state and age:

```
. glm rate1 florida i.agecat [iw=pop1], link(log) fam(p) eform nolog
note: rate1 has noninteger values
```

```
Generalized linear models               No. of obs        =        22
Optimization    : ML                    Residual df       =        10
                                        Scale parameter =         1
Deviance       = 48.62187545            (1/df) Deviance =   4.862188
Pearson        = 52.66630784            (1/df) Pearson  =   5.266631

Variance function: V(u) = u             [Poisson]
Link function     : g(u) = ln(u)        [Log]

                                        AIC             =   21302.46
Log likelihood  = -234315.0775          BIC             =   17.71145
```

```
           |              OIM
   rate1 |    IRR    Std. Err.     z     P>|z|    [95% Conf. Interval]
--------+-----------------------------------------------------------------
  florida |  1.020597   .0347775   0.60   0.550    .9546604    1.091087
          |
  agecat |
     1-4 |  1.934418   1.184584   1.08   0.281    .5825028    6.423956
    5-14 |   .949187   .5747612  -0.09   0.931    .2896835    3.110139
   15-24 |  2.654386   1.557032   1.66   0.096    .8407351    8.380484
   25-34 |  6.269495   3.646084   3.16   0.002    2.005434    19.60003
   35-44 |  22.23173   12.86058   5.36   0.000    7.154374     69.0836
   45-54 |  86.82703   50.15182   7.73   0.000    27.98954    269.3482
   55-64 |  227.6192   131.4422   9.40   0.000    73.39553    705.9081
   65-74 |  454.9078   262.6774  10.60   0.000    146.6946    1410.694
   75-84 |  789.7431   456.0162  11.55   0.000    254.6725    2449.005
     85+ |  1220.461   704.7792  12.31   0.000    393.5324     3785.01
          |
   _cons |  .0000134   7.75e-06  -19.40   0.000    4.31e-06    .0000416
---------------------------------------------------------------------------
```

Age was a confounder of the comparison of Florida with Alaska because cancer rates are much higher at older ages (Table 6.2) and Florida had an older population (Figure 6.1). However, within the age categories, most of which cover a 10-year range, there was little difference between the two states, so the

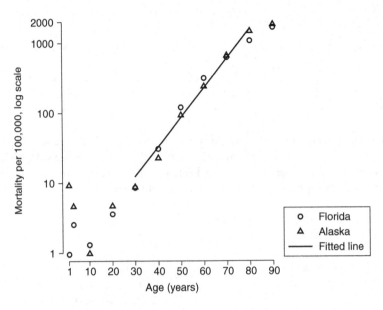

FIGURE 9.4   Cancer mortality rates per 100,000 person-years for Florida and Alaska in 2010, according to age. The solid line is from a Poisson regression model for persons 30 to 80 years in Alaska. The slope of the line is for a ratio change in rate of 2.6 for each decade increase in age. Vertical axis on the log scale.

regression model shown earlier, which compared persons of about the same age, estimated an age-adjusted rate ratio of 1.02. The relationship between age and cancer mortality is approximately linear on the log scale in both states at the older ages where most cancer deaths occur (Figure 9.4). If we create a variable for age with values equal to the approximate middle of each age category of Table 6.2 (1, 3, 10, 20, ... , 90) and enter that variable as a linear term in the model below, we get a rate ratio estimate of 1.00 (95% CI 0.94, 1.07), similar to the previous estimate of 1.02 (95% CI 0.95, 1.09).

```
. glm rate1 florida age [iw=pop1], l(log) f(p) eform nolog
note: rate1 has noninteger values
```

```
Generalized linear models              No. of obs       =         22
Optimization    : ML                   Residual df      =         19
                                       Scale parameter  =          1
Deviance     = 2660.199033             (1/df) Deviance  = 140.0105
Pearson      = 2369.919626             (1/df) Pearson   = 124.7326

Variance function: V(u) = u            [Poisson]
Link function     : g(u) = ln(u)       [Log]

                                       AIC              = 21420.35
Log likelihood  = -235620.8661         BIC              = 2601.469
------------------------------------------------------------------
             |              OIM
     rate1 |    IRR    Std. Err.     z    P>|z|    [95% Conf. Interval]
--------+---------------------------------------------------------
   florida |  1.004916  .0342429   0.14  0.886    .939993   1.074323
```

```
    age |  1.075624    .000329   238.35   0.000    1.07498   1.076269
  _cons |  .0000308   1.20e-06  -266.61   0.000    .0000286   .0000333
```

The fit is superior for the model with indicator variables, but for most purposes the single linear term for age does just as well at removing confounding.

9.10 FURTHER COMMENTS ABOUT PERSON-TIME

At the start of this chapter I wrote that we often assume that rates increase linearly on the ln (ratio) scale as person-time increases and I said that use of person-time to explain differences in event counts is usually uninteresting. What I wrote deserves some qualification. Rates may not increase multiplicatively as person-time increases. There might be data in which doubling person-time quadruples the event count. I did not mean to imply that knowing the relationship between person-time and event counts is never useful. But if the event count quadruples when person-time doubles, we will usually be interested in *why* this happens, and this means we will want to study factors aside from person-time. Furthermore, I do not mean to imply that we can only use person-time as an offset. There might be special situations in which we wish to use person-time both as an offset and also as a variable in the model for rates. But for most analyses of rates, the assumption that the rate changes multiplicatively in relation to person-time will serve us well.

9.11 A SHORT SUMMARY

Poisson rate ratio regression can be used to estimate changes in rates over time and to adjust for age and other variables. This method can be used to describe how rates vary with age or any other factor. Because regression can smooth relationships into lines or curves (as I will show in Chapter 15), it has flexibility beyond the capacity of stratified methods (Frome and Checkoway 1985, Breslow and Day 1987 pp120–153). Poisson regression can correctly estimate rate ratios even if the counts are not from a Poisson process and even when the assumption that mean and variance are equal is violated; the SEs can be adjusted using robust variance methods that will be discussed later. Poisson regression is a flexible method for rates because it gracefully allows the analyst to separate the count numerator from the rate denominator.

Poisson Regression for Rate Differences

10

The choice between rate ratios and rate differences was discussed in Chapter 3. Formulae for rate differences were introduced in Chapter 4. Chapters 6 and 7 presented stratified methods for rate differences. While Poisson regression for rate ratios is explained in some textbooks and used for many studies, Poisson regression for rate differences is not often described and rarely used. Breslow and Day mentioned this method in their 1987 textbook (Breslow and Day 1987 pp137,142–143), but the discussion is so brief that a reader could miss it. Hilbe discussed a model for differences in counts (Hilbe 2011 pp152–155). Some articles refer to a rate difference model (Aranda-Ordaz 1983, Maldonado and Greenland 1994, 1996), but provide little detail. One reason that adjusted rate differences are not often used may be that analysts are unaware that regression models for rate differences even exist.

10.1 A REGRESSION MODEL FOR RATE DIFFERENCES

To estimate adjusted rate differences we can start with a model similar to Expression 9.3 where C indicates a count, T represents person-time, the coefficients to be estimated are indicated by the letter b, with subscripts ranging from 0 to k, and the x terms are for explanatory or predictor variables:

$$\text{rate} = C/T = b_0 + b_1x_1 + b_2x_2 + \ldots + b_kx_k \tag{Ex.10.1}$$

Unlike Expression 9.3, nothing in Expression 10.1 is on the log scale; 10.1 an additive linear model, just like the expression for ordinary least squares linear regression. The mean rate will be equal to the constant b_0 term when all the x variables are equal to zero. Each additional model term adds or subtracts a quantity from the estimated constant rate term. The expression can be rewritten as:

$$C = T \times (b_0 + b_1x_1 + b_2x_2 + \ldots + b_kx_k) \tag{Ex.10.2}$$

Expression 10.2 shows that although the coefficients are added (rather than multiplied as in Expression 9.1 or multiplied after exponentiation as in Expression 9.10), the event count is multiplicatively related to person-time. In Expression 10.2 a doubling of person-time will double the count of the outcomes, just as in Expressions 9.5 and 9.10.

The model in Expression 10.2 would estimate the difference in counts. We want to use something like Expression 10.1 to estimate the difference in rates. We need to modify 10.1 so that we can separately use the information about the counts and the rates, rather than combining them in a single outcome variable. This is needed so that we can account for differences in person-time from one record to the next. It would also be nice if the regression model could estimate standard errors using formulae in Chapter 4 that are suitable for counts from a Poisson process.

10.2 FLORIDA AND ALASKA CANCER MORTALITY: REGRESSION MODELS THAT FAIL

The rates of cancer in Alaska (884/710,231 = 124.5 per 100,000 person-years) and Florida (41,467/18,801,310 = 220.6) in 2010 (Table 6.2) were used in Chapters 6 and 9. The Florida rate was greater by 96.1 per 100,000 person-years. The SE of the Florida minus Alaska rate difference can be calculated using formula 5 from Table 4.4. Using units of 100,000 person-years, the SE of the rate difference = square root((Florida rate/Florida person-time) + (Alaska rate/Alaska person-time)) = square root((220.6/188.801310) + (124.5/7.10231)) = 4.32. So we want a regression model that can estimate the mean difference of 96.1, SE of 4.32, and a Wald (z) statistic of 96.1/4.32 = 22.2.

Generalized linear modeling software allows us to select both a model link function and the type of error distribution we anticipate. For rate ratio models, discussed in Chapter 9, we used generalized linear models with a log link (to estimate ratios) and a Poisson error family. To estimate a rate difference we can use an identity (equality) link to tell the software that the rate should be identical to (equal) a linear combination of terms as in Expression 10.1. We can select the Poisson error family once again. The outcome variable is called "rate100k" to indicate the rate per 100,000 person-years and the only explanatory variable in the model is called florida, coded as 1 for Florida and zero for Alaska. We can apply this model to the 22 age-specific records in Table 6.2:

```
. glm rate100k florida, link(identity) family(poisson) nolog
note: rate100k has noninteger values
```

```
Generalized linear models              No. of obs        =        22
Optimization    : ML                   Residual df       =        20
                                       Scale parameter =         1
Deviance        =   16980.64667        (1/df) Deviance = 849.0323
Pearson         =   19697.10686        (1/df) Pearson  = 984.8553

Variance function: V(u) = u            [Poisson]
Link function    : g(u) = u            [Identity]

                                       AIC          =   777.5924
Log likelihood  = -8551.516921         BIC          =   16918.83
```

```
-----------------------------------------------------------------
             |          OIM
   rate100k |   Coef.  Std. Err.      z    P>|z|   [95% Conf. Interval]
---------- +-----------------------------------------------------
    florida | -44.36075  8.22037   -5.40  0.000   -60.47238  -28.24912
      _cons |  393.8401  5.983614  65.82  0.000    382.1124   405.5677
-----------------------------------------------------------------
```

This output incorrectly estimates that the Florida rate was less than the Alaska rate by 44 deaths per 100,000 person-years; this incorrect difference is even in the wrong direction. This regression model summed the age-specific rates for Alaska (9.2 + 4.6 + ... + 4711) and divided that sum by 11 (for the 11 age groups); a weighted-average with weights equal to 1. This "average" rate was 393.84 for Alaska and 349.48 for Florida, and the Florida – Alaska difference was – 44.36. This flawed method produced an estimated difference which treated the Alaska rate for infants, with 1 death within a 1-year age category, as being equal in importance to the 233 deaths in the 10-year category from 65 to 74 years.

This model used the **family(poisson)** option, so the software treated the outcomes, the mean rates of 393.84 and 349.48, as if they were counts. Because we provided no information about person-time, the software assumed that the person-time denominators for each of the 11 "counts" from each State were equal to 1. Using formula 5 in Table 4.4, the software calculated the SE of the rate difference = square root((349.48/11) + (393.84/11)) = 8.22. This SE is erroneous because the assumptions used to calculate it were not true.

To fix the problems with this model, perhaps we can use an offset? Since we are not working on the log scale, we will try an offset equal to the person-time for each record (in units of 100,000 person-years), not the ln of the person-time. Stata will let us do this using the **offset** option instead of the **exposure** option:

```
. glm rate100k florida, offset(pop100k) link(identity) family(poisson) nolog
note: rate100k has noninteger values
(output omitted)
```

```
-------------------------------------------------------------------------
             |                OIM
    rate100k |    Coef.    Std. Err.    z     P>|z|    [95% Conf. Interval]
-------------+-----------------------------------------------------------
     florida | -54.80712   8.219627   -6.67   0.000   -70.91729   -38.69694
       _cons | 393.6362    5.983613   65.79   0.000   381.9085    405.3638
     pop100k |        1    (offset)
-------------------------------------------------------------------------
```

The attempt to use an offset was foolish. Person-time is part of the rate denominator. Trying to subtract this from each age-state-specific rate produced an estimate even more biased than the previous model.

10.3 FLORIDA AND ALASKA CANCER MORTALITY: REGRESSION MODELS THAT SUCCEED

In order to correctly estimate the Florida minus Alaska rate difference per 100,000 person-years of 96.1, SE of 4.32, and a Wald (z) statistic of 96.1/4.32 = 22.2, we need to somehow use Expression 10.1, which has the rate as the outcome, but convey to the software the separate count and person-time information in Expression 10.2. One way to do this is to multiply both sides of Expression 10.1 by person-time. For each record in Table 6.2, multiply the rate by person-time for that record in units of 100,000 person-years; this will convert the rates to counts of deaths. Also multiply the florida variable, coded 1/0, by the person-time for each record. To complete this process, multiply the constant (intercept) term by person-time. Do this by creating a variable, called pop100k, equal to each record's person-time in units of 100,000 years. This new pop100k variable is entered as an explanatory variable into the model and the software is told to not estimate a constant term for the model. This means the new pop100k variable will be used to estimate a new "constant" (intercept) coefficient multiplied by person-time. The old model based on Expression 10.1 looked like this:

$$rate = b_0 + b_1 \times florida \tag{Ex.10.3}$$

The new model, after the multiplication by person-time, looks like this:

$$
\begin{aligned}
\text{rate} \times \text{T} &= b_0 \times \text{T} + b_1 \times \text{florida} \times \text{T} \\
&= \text{T} \times (b_0 + b_1 \times \text{florida})
\end{aligned}
\qquad\text{(Ex.10.4)}
$$

Here are the commands that generate the new variables multiplied by the person-time in each record and the regression output from the new model. This model correctly estimates the rate difference, SE and Wald Z-statistic:

```
. gen double newrate = rate100k*pop100k
. gen double newflorida = florida*pop100k
. gen double newintercept = pop100k
. glm newrate newflorida newintercept, link(identity) family(poisson) nolog
noconstant
note: newrate has noninteger values
```

```
Generalized linear models              No. of obs      =         22
Optimization    : ML                   Residual df     =         20
                                       Scale parameter =          1
Deviance     = 86914.08247             (1/df) Deviance =   4345.704
Pearson      = 117936.153              (1/df) Pearson  =   5896.808

Variance function: V(u) = u            [Poisson]
Link function     : g(u) = u           [Identity]

                                       AIC             =    3957.27
Log likelihood  = -43527.97066         BIC             =   86852.26
```

```
-----------------------------------------------------------------------------
              |                 OIM
      newrate |    Coef.   Std. Err.     z    P>|z|   [95% Conf. Interval]
--------------+--------------------------------------------------------------
   newflorida |  96.08723   4.324104   22.22  0.000   87.61215   104.5623
 newintercept |  124.4665   4.186263   29.73  0.000   116.2616   132.6715
-----------------------------------------------------------------------------
```

It can be cumbersome to create the new variables as described earlier and coding mistakes are possible. A simpler approach is to use frequency weights that expand the data so that the number of records corresponds to the number of people in the population. The mid-year population estimate is an estimate of person-time, but it is also a good estimate of the number of people in the population in this example. Stata requires that frequency weights must be integers, so for this model the outcome, rate1, is the rate per person-year and the frequency weights will be set equal to the amount of person-time in units of 1 person-year:

```
. glm rate1 florida [fweight=pop1], link(identity) family(poisson) nolog
note: rate1 has noninteger values
```

```
Generalized linear models              No. of obs      =  1.95e+07
Optimization    : ML                   Residual df     =  1.95e+07
                                       Scale parameter =         1
Deviance     = 86914.08247             (1/df) Deviance =  .0044545
Pearson      = 117936.1535             (1/df) Pearson  =  .0060444
```

```
Variance function: V(u) = u                    [Poisson]
Link function     : g(u) = u                   [Identity]


                                        AIC            = .0284703
Log likelihood  = -277747.8078          BIC            = -3.27e+08


- - - - - - - - - - - - - - - - - - - - - - - - - - - - - - - - - - - - - -
             |                OIM
      rate1 |   Coef.    Std. Err.     z     P>|z|     [95% Conf. Interval]
- - - - - - +- - - - - - - - - - - - - - - - - - - - - - - - - - - - - - - -
    florida |  .0009609   .0000432   22.22   0.000     .0008761    .0010456
      _cons |  .0012447   .0000419   29.73   0.000     .0011626    .0013267
- - - - - - - - - - - - - - - - - - - - - - - - - - - - - - - - - - - - - -
```

In this output, the mean difference of .000961 per 1 person-year is correct; it represents a difference of 96.1 per 100,000 person-years, which is what we expected. The SE is correct; multiplying .0000432 by 100,000 produces 4.32. The Wald (z) statistic is the ratio of the mean difference to its SE: .009609/.0000432 = 22.22, which is also correct. Some of the header information is a bit bizarre because Stata now thinks that we are analyzing data from over 19.5 million records instead of 22 records. The estimate of the deviance per degree of freedom is now miniscule, whereas it was quite large using the previous method. It may seem a bit counter-intuitive that expanding the data to represent more than 19.5 million records did not shrink the SE. Recall that Poisson methods do not necessarily gain precision by having more observations. A single record with 100 deaths from 100,000 person-years provides the same information about precision as the combination of 100 records with 1 death each from 1 person-year and 99,900 records with 0 deaths in each from 1 person-year.

In their book about cohort study data, Breslow and Day recommended (Breslow and Day 1987 pp137,142–143) the use of weights to estimate adjusted rate differences with a Poisson model. They used GLIM software and I suspect the weights they used were treated as frequency rates by the software. There are disadvantages to frequency rates. Much of the regression header information will be distorted by this method. Stata will not allow noninteger values for these weights. Worst of all, if we use a robust variance estimator, discussed in Chapter 13, this estimator will create a SE that is too small when frequency rates are used. The method I showed earlier, in which the variables are multiplied by person-time, will work with a robust variance estimator. Frequency weights should be avoided for estimating rate differences or ratios, unless those weights really do represent the number of records.

As shown in Chapter 9, importance weights can be used. These weights are used to tell Stata how much weight to give each observation relative to the others, but Stata will still know the correct number of records used in regression. Stata can use these weights correctly with a robust variance estimator. Here is the output using importance weights (equal to person-years in units of 100,000), showing correct results for the rate difference and SE. The deviance is now large relative to the degrees of freedom: 4345 compared with .0045 when frequency weights were used:

```
. glm rate100k florida [iweight=pop100k], link(identity) family(poisson)
  nolog
note: rate100k has noninteger values

Generalized linear models          No. of obs     =          22
Optimization    : ML               Residual df    =          20
                                   Scale parameter =           1
```

```
Deviance          = 86914.08247        (1/df) Deviance =     4345.704
Pearson           = 117936.1535        (1/df) Pearson  =     5896.808


Variance function: V(u) = u            [Poisson]
Link function     : g(u) = u           [Identity]


                                       AIC            =     3998.489
Log likelihood  = -43981.38211         BIC            =     86852.26
- - - - - - - - - - - - - - - - - - - - - - - - - - - - - - - - - - - - - -
              |                OIM
    rate100k |   Coef.    Std. Err.     z     P>|z|    [95% Conf. Interval]
- - - - - - - - - - - - - - - - - - - - - - - - - - - - - - - - - - - - - -
     florida | 96.08724   4.324104   22.22   0.000    87.61215    104.5623
       _cons | 124.4665   4.186263   29.73   0.000    116.2616    132.6715
- - - - - - - - - - - - - - - - - - - - - - - - - - - - - - - - - - - - - -
```

Importance weights can also be used to estimate adjusted rate differences. After age-category adjustment, the Florida rate was lower than the Alaska rate by a small amount: 0.28 deaths per 100,000 person-years.

```
. glm rate100k florida i.agecat [iweight=pop100k], /* */ link(identity)
   family(poisson)    nolog
note: rate100k has noninteger values

Generalized linear models              No. of obs      =         22
Optimization    : ML                   Residual df     =         10
                                       Scale parameter =          1
Deviance       =  48.8646079           (1/df) Deviance =   4.886461
Pearson        =  51.15611979          (1/df) Pearson  =   5.115612
Variance function: V(u) = u            [Poisson]
Link function     : g(u) = u           [Identity]


                                       AIC            =     50.97938
Log likelihood  = -548.7731753         BIC            =     17.95418


- - - - - - - - - - - - - - - - - - - - - - - - - - - - - - - - - - - - - -
              |                OIM
    rate100k |   Coef.    Std. Err.     z     P>|z|    [95% Conf. Interval]
- - - - - - - - - - - - - - - - - - - - - - - - - - - - - - - - - - - - - -
     florida | -.2821114   .8519406  -0.33   0.741   -1.951884    1.387662
              |
      agecat |
         1-4 | 1.337526    .9656305   1.39   0.166    -.5550752    3.230127
        5-14 | .0049714    .843433    0.01   0.995   -1.648127     1.65807
       15-24 | 2.329053    .8884146   2.62   0.009     .5877923    4.070313
       25-34 | 7.271435   1.003745    7.24   0.000     5.30413     9.23874
       35-44 | 29.09348   1.362983   21.35   0.000    26.42208    31.76488
       45-54 | 117.3741   2.193843   53.50   0.000    113.0742    121.6739
       55-64 | 309.8183   3.672971   84.35   0.000    302.6194    317.0172
       65-74 | 620.672    5.994053  103.55   0.000    608.9238    632.4201
       75-84 | 1078.614   9.88607   109.10   0.000    1059.238    1097.991
```

```
   85+ |  1667.673  19.51857  85.44  0.000   1629.417  1705.929
       |
  _cons |  1.566504  1.011875   1.55  0.122  -.4167335  3.549742
------------------------------------------------------------------
```

10.4 A GENERALIZED LINEAR MODEL WITH A POWER LINK

Both the additive (difference) and multiplicative (ratio) models for rates can be fit using the power link (Breslow and Day 1987 pp137,142–143). The rate outcome is related (linked) to the linear predictor by using the function rate^{power}, where power is some quantity from 0 to 1. If power is set to 1 by using **link(power 1)** as the link function, the link is equivalent to **link(identity)** and the additive (rate difference) model is fit. If the power is set to 0, this corresponds to the log link and the multiplicative (rate ratio) model is used. The command for the rate difference model with importance weights looks like this:

```
glm rate100k florida [iweight=pop100k], link(power 1) family(poisson) nolog
```

The power link can be used to estimate models that are between a purely additive or multiplicative model; Breslow and Day present a detailed example (Breslow and Day 1987 pp143–146). Imagine data that does not adequately fit an additive or multiplicative model. You could estimate the model several times using the power link with power values ranging from 0 to 1 and select the model with the lowest deviance value. If the best model had a power link value between 0 and 1, it would be difficult to interpret the regression coefficients (Royston and Lambert 2011 p119); they would not be rate differences or ln rate ratios. But you could use the best model to estimate predicted rates for each record in your data or another sample. One option would be to estimate predicted rates under the assumption, for a binary exposure, first that everyone in the sample was exposed and then that everyone was not exposed, but otherwise their covariates did not change. You could then use the predicted rates to estimate either a rate ratio or difference. This is called marginal standardization and we will discuss this approach in Chapter 21.

10.5 A CAUTION

This chapter shows how adjusted rate differences can be estimated using Poisson regression. In practice, difficulties can arise with convergence of these regression models. For example, to adjust the difference in the Florida and Alaska cancer mortality rates for age I showed that this could be done using 10 indicator (dummy) variables for the 11 age categories. The adjusted rate difference, comparing Florida with Alaska, was –.28 deaths per 100,000 person-years, a result that agrees fairly well with estimates discussed in earlier chapters. But the software struggled through 404 iteration steps to achieve convergence. When I tried to fit the same model using age as a linear term, the software failed to converge, despite using options to overcome the difficulty. It is perhaps not surprising that a linear age term could not be estimated, because the age category differences vary a great deal and the use of the Poisson error distribution tries to constrain predicted counts to be 0 or more. This convergence problem will get some attention in Chapters 11 and 21.

Poisson regression is well suited for estimating ratios. It is so good at this that many authors (Gourieroux, Monfort, and Tognon 1984b, Lloyd 1999 pp85–86, Cook and Lawless 2007 pp82–84, Wooldridge 2008 pp597–598, 2010 pp727–728) have noted its advantages over other methods, even when the outcomes are not counts, but binary or continuous variables. But Poisson rate difference regression is not necessarily optimal and it may sometimes amount to pounding a square peg into a round hole. If adjusted rate differences are desired, methods such as standardization or stratified methods may be preferred. Another option is to fit a Poisson rate ratio regression model, which may have a superior fit to the data compared with a Poisson rate difference model, then estimate the predicted rates and rearrange these into an adjusted rate difference using marginal methods. Marginal methods will be discussed in Chapter 21.

Although it is rare to see regression-adjusted rate differences in research papers, they can be estimated using Poisson regression methods.

Linear Regression

11

There was an era when ordinary least squares linear regression was used to analyze rates because it was the only regression method available. This changed by the 1980's. Breslow and Day (1987) did not even mention linear regression in their 1987 book about cohort studies; Poisson and Cox proportional hazards regression received all their attention. However, some studies still use linear regression to analyze rates and in this chapter reviews that approach.

11.1 LIMITATIONS OF ORDINARY LEAST SQUARES LINEAR REGRESSION

Ordinary least squares linear regression treats each outcome value as having the same statistical precision. The method assigns no precision to any outcome value in isolation, but estimates precision using a variance formula (Expression 4.2) that compares each observed value with the mean value. This can work well if the outcome is systolic blood pressure, or the weight of laboratory mice, and we have no reason to think that the precision of these measurements varies with their size. To use statistical jargon, ordinary least squares linear regression assumes that the variance of each rate is the same, a property called homoskedasticity.

Imagine that during a year 4 outcome events occurred in a rural town with a mid-year population of 1000: rate 4 per 1000 person-years. During the same year there were 7000 outcome events in a city with a mid-year population of 1 million: rate 7 per 1000 person-years. Surely the rate based on 7000 events is more precise than the rate based on just four events; the formulae in Table 4.4 all assume this is true. Rates are heteroskedastic; rates based on larger counts are more precise. This variation in the precision of rates is built into Poisson regression. In order to apply linear regression to rates, we will somehow need to overcome the assumption that rates are equally precise.

The ordinary least squares linear regression model looks like Expression 11.1, which includes the error term that is often shown for this model:

$$C/T = \text{rate} = b_0 + b_1 x_1 + b_2 x_2 + \ldots + b_k x_k + \text{error} \qquad \text{(Ex.11.1)}$$

As shown in Chapter 10 (Expressions 10.1 and 10.2), we can multiply both sides of Expression 11.1 by person-time to get Expression 11.2:

$$C = T \times (b_0 + b_1 x_1 + b_2 x_2 + \ldots + b_k x_k + \text{error}) \qquad \text{(Ex.11.2)}$$

Expression 11.2 assumes that person-time is an explanatory variable that is free of random error, or at least sufficiently precise that any random error is small compared with other sources of error. The error term represents random error in the outcome counts, not person-time. However, the size of the random error is not constant in this model; it is proportional to person-time, an important feature that will reappear later in this chapter.

The presence of heteroskedasticity can bias the standard errors (SE) in ordinary linear regression, but this alone will not bias the estimated coefficients. However, there is an additional problem. Ordinary linear regression can produce biased estimates when applied to rates, because the method ignores the fact that rates are made up of two quantities, a numerator and a denominator. If a cohort is made up of males with 100 events from 10,000 person-years (rate 1 per 100 person-years) and females with two 2 events from 100 person-years (rate 2 per 100 person-years), ordinary linear regression will produce a rate for the entire cohort by simply averaging the two rates: $(1+2)/2 = 1.5$ per 100 person-years. But the actual rate in the cohort was $(100+2)/(10,000 + 100) = 102/10,100 = 1.01$ per 100 person-years; a person-time weighted average is desired (Expression 6.1).

Ordinary least squares linear regression, applied to rates, suffers from two disadvantages: (1) it fails to account for the greater precision of rates with more outcome events; (2) it fails to average rates by using person-time information. The first problem produces bias in the SEs. The second can bias the estimated coefficients. This chapter will discuss these problems and show that solutions are sometimes available.

11.2 FLORIDA AND ALASKA CANCER MORTALITY RATES

Consider the Florida and Alaska cancer mortality data (Table 6.2) discussed in Chapters 6, 9, and 10. Cancer mortality in Florida was 220.6 (41,467/18,801,310) per 100,000 person-years, greater than in Alaska (884/710,231 = 124.5) by 96.1. Recall (Expression 6.1) that the crude (overall) rate for Florida is equal to a weighted average of the stratum-specific rates (for example, strata based on age) with weights proportional to the person-time for each stratum.

If we use linear regression to estimate the Florida minus Alaska rate difference, using the 11 age-specific rates for each state in the regression model, the Florida rate will be estimated by summing the age-specific rates $(1.0 + 2.5 + ... + 1667.3)$ and dividing by 11. This "average" rate is 349.48, larger than the actual rate of 220.6, because the averaging method assigns equal weight to each age-specific rate; the large rates among those 75 and older were given more weight, relative to person-time weighting, than the smaller rates from the millions of person-years lived by residents younger than 55 years. For Alaska, the use of equal weights for each stratum of age has an even more profound influence, producing an "average" rate of 393.84 compared with the actual rate of 124.5. This occurs because in Alaska there were few elderly residents and linear regression gave equal weight to the rate of 1825.5 from 4711 person-years among those 85 and older and the rate of 4.7 from 106,560 person-years among persons 15 to 24 years. The output below from ordinary least squares linear regression shows these results. The outcome variable rate100k is the age-specific rate per 100,000 person-years and the variable florida is coded 1 for Florida and 0 for Alaska. The model intercept term with a rate of 393.84 is the "average" rate for Alaska, and –44.4 is the estimated Florida minus Alaska rate, far from the actual difference of +96.1.

```
. regress rate100k florida
(header output omitted)
```

```
------------------------------------------------------------------------
 rate100k |   Coef.    Std. Err.     t     P>|t|    [95% Conf. Interval]
----------+-------------------------------------------------------------
  florida | -44.36075   258.7587   -0.17   0.866   -584.122    495.4005
    _cons |  393.8401    182.97     2.15   0.044    12.17125   775.5089
------------------------------------------------------------------------
```

The linear regression estimate of – 44.4 is not useful for several reasons. First, equal weight was given to age categories which are unequal in age range. In effect, the method gives the rate for infants (a 1 year range of age) 10 times more weight compared with the rate from those 55–64 years (a 10 year range), just because the Compressed Mortality data has age categories for those groups. If different age categories were available, a different estimate would be produced. Second, the person-time within each age-category varies. Linear regression gives equal weight to all the age-stratified rates, regardless of the person-time denominator. Third, a rate based upon 1 death from 10,828 person-years for infants in Alaska is a less precise estimate of cancer mortality than a rate of 1074.7 based upon 11,795 deaths from over 1 million person-years among persons 75–84 in Florida. But linear regression treats these rates as if they were equally precise.

The problems described earlier also afflicted the first Poisson regression model for rate differences (which ignored person-time) that was used in Chapter 10 in the section about incorrect regression models. That erroneous Poisson model produced the same intercept estimate and rate difference as the earlier linear regression model. The problems discussed here derive not from the choice of a Gaussian or Poisson error family but from using rates as outcomes without also using information about person-time in the regression model.

11.3 WEIGHTED LEAST SQUARES LINEAR REGRESSION

The limitations of the Poisson and linear regression models described above can be addressed by supplying information about person-time to the statistical software. In Chapter 10 I showed that Poisson regression can estimate the rate difference if we multiply the outcome rates and explanatory variables by person-time, include person-time as an intercept in the model, and suppress the estimation of an additional intercept term (Expression 10.4). We can do the same thing using ordinary least squares linear regression, but instead of multiplying all the rates and variables by person-time, we multiply by the square-root of person-time. This is called weighted least squares linear regression and is described in many textbooks about linear regression (Neter, Wasserman, and Kutner 1990 pp418–420, Draper and Smith 1998 pp223–239, Kleinbaum et al. 1998 pp250–251, Cook and Weisberg 1999 pp204–206). A particularly lucid account can be found in the textbook by Wooldridge (2008 pp276–282).

Weighted least squares linear regression is commonly used to remove heteroskedasticity from an ordinary least squares linear regression model. Homoskedasticity means that the variance for the unobservable errors in linear regression (Expression 11.1) is the same, conditional on the explanatory variables, for all values of the explanatory variables. If systolic blood pressure is the outcome and age is an explanatory variable, homoskedasticity means that the *variance* of the errors, the unobserved difference between the measured blood pressure and the "true" mean blood pressure in the population, is the same for all levels of age; one variance fits all. If this assumption is not true, then heteroskedasticity is present; this will not bias the estimated mean differences (regression coefficients) relating age to blood pressure, but the SEs of the coefficients will be biased. If the variance of the errors is proportional to age, then the true variance can be expressed as a single estimated variance multiplied by age: variance x age. The standard deviation (SD) of the errors can be expressed as $\sqrt{(\text{variance} \times \text{age})}$ or SD x $\sqrt{(\text{age})}$. To remove heteroskedasticity when the variance of the errors is proportional to age, we can *divide* both sides of the regression equation, including the intercept, by $\sqrt{(\text{age})}$ (Wooldridge 2008 pp276–282). So if the outcome is systolic blood pressure, indicated by SBP, and the explanatory variable is age, Expression 11.1 can be replaced by Expression 11.3 in order to remove heteroskedasticity that is proportional to age:

$$SBP/\sqrt{(\text{age})} = b_0/\sqrt{(\text{age})} + b_1 x_1/\sqrt{(\text{age})} + \text{error}/\sqrt{(\text{age})} \qquad (\text{Ex.11.3})$$

Now we turn this idea on its head. To estimate rate differences the problem is the flip side of the heteroskedasticity problem. The ordinary least squares linear regression model assumes that homoskedasticity is true and each observation is an equally precise measure of the underlying rate for each explanatory variables. This assumes that the variance of the error terms for a rate *does not change* with the amount of person-time. But for rates we *expect* heteroskedasticity to be present; the variance of the errors for a count, and therefore the rate based upon that count, increases proportionally (multiplicatively) with person-time as shown by Expression 11.2. Therefore the SD of the errors is proportional to $\sqrt{T}$. To introduce this *expected* heteroskedasticity into Expression 11.1, we *multiply* each side of Expression 11.1 by $\sqrt{T}$, to get Expression 11.4:

$$\text{rate} \times \sqrt{(T)} = b_0 \times \sqrt{(T)} + b_1 x_1 \times \sqrt{(T)} + \ldots + \text{error} \times \sqrt{(T)} \qquad \text{(Ex.11.4)}$$

Because rate $\times \sqrt{T} = C/T \times \sqrt{T} = C/\sqrt{T}$, we can fit the same model and get the same coefficients using either rate $\times \sqrt{T}$ or $C/\sqrt{T}$ as the outcome.

Using weighted least squares linear regression for the analysis of rates is described well in an econometrics textbook by Wooldridge (Wooldridge 2008 pp281–282). The same method is nicely described in an article by Xu et al. (2010), accompanied by results from simulations. Versions of this method have been known for decades; for example, a 1984 article (Rosenbaum and Rubin 1984 p439) about linear regression for the analysis of rates recommended person-time weights in some situations. We can apply this procedure to the Florida and Alaska data, using terms previously defined and person-time in units of 100,000 person-years, indicated by pop100k:

```
. gen double newrate100k = rate100k*pop100k^.5
. gen double newflorida  = florida*pop100k^.5
. gen double newintercept = pop100k^.5
. regress newrate100k newflorida newintercept, noconstant
```

Source	SS	df	MS		
Model	9255732.05	2	4627866.02	Number of obs = 22	
Residual	25564236.8	20	1278211.84	F(2, 20) = 3.62	
				Prob > F = 0.0455	
				R-squared = 0.2658	
Total	34819968.9	22	1582725.86	Adj R-squared = 0.1924	
				Root MSE = 1130.6	

newrate100k	Coef.	Std. Err.	t	P>|t|	[95% Conf. Interval]
newflorida	96.08723	432.1687	0.22	0.826	-805.4009 997.5754
newintercept	124.4665	424.2302	0.29	0.772	-760.4622 1009.395

This output shows the correct rate difference of 96.1 and the correct rate for Alaska as the intercept term. We can fit the same model using a generalized linear model with an identity link and Gaussian (normal) error distribution. If we do this, as shown here, the coefficients and their SEs are identical. Ordinary linear regression treats the coefficient/SE ratio as a t-statistic and computes P-values using the t-distribution and degrees of freedom. Generalized linear models use the same ratios to produce Wald Z-statistics which are compared with the normal distribution to compute P-values. Therefore, the **regress** command and the **glm** command for the same model report slightly different P-values and confidence intervals (CI). The gigantic SEs from both models are biased, not merely because the error terms are not normally distributed, but because I deliberately created a model that violated the assumption of homoskedasticity. I multiplied the model estimated error variance by person-time, which increased the size of the estimated SEs for the coefficients. Fortunately, we can fix the SEs by using a robust variance estimator (not shown here) that is resistant to heteroskedasticity; if we do this in the earlier model or the model here, the SE for the newflorida term will decrease from 432 to 108.

```
. glm newrate100k newflorida newintercept, link(identity) f(gaussian)
  nolog nocons

Generalized linear models                No. of obs     =       22
Optimization     : ML                    Residual df    =       20
                                         Scale parameter = 1278212
Deviance       = 25564236.83             (1/df) Deviance = 1278212
Pearson        = 25564236.83             (1/df) Pearson  = 1278212

Variance function: V(u) = 1              [Gaussian]
Link function    : g(u) = u              [Identity]

                                         AIC            = 16.98536
Log likelihood   = -184.838935           BIC            = 2.56e+07

-----------------------------------------------------------------------
             |              OIM
newrate100k  |   Coef.   Std. Err.    z    P>|z|   [95% Conf. Interval]
-------------+---------------------------------------------------------
  newflorida |  96.08723  432.1687   0.22  0.824  -750.9479   943.1224
newintercept | 124.4665   424.2302   0.29  0.769  -707.0094   955.9425
-----------------------------------------------------------------------
```

In this discussion, weighted least squares linear regression was introduced as a way of removing heteroskedasticity. Then I changed horses in mid-stream; instead of using weighted least squares to remove heteroskedasticity, I used it to introduce heteroskedasticity and explained that the SEs could be corrected by a robust variance estimator. Weighted least squares for rate outcomes is not needed to remove heteroskedasticity; its virtue is that it allows person-time weighted averaging of rates.

11.4 IMPORTANCE WEIGHTS FOR WEIGHTED LEAST SQUARES LINEAR REGRESSION

Instead of multiplying all the regression variables by $\sqrt{T}$, we can use importance weights (**iweights**) and the **glm** command to fit the same model more easily, just as we did in Chapter 10 to estimate rate differences with Poisson regression. The importance weights are equal to person-time (T), not $\sqrt{T}$:

```
. glm rate100k florida [iweight=pop100k], link(identity) family(gaussian)
  nolog

Generalized linear models                No. of obs     =       22
Optimization    : ML                     Residual df    =       20
                                         Scale parameter = 1278212
Deviance       = 25564236.83             (1/df) Deviance = 1278212
Pearson        = 25564236.83             (1/df) Pearson  = 1278212
```

```
Variance function: V(u) = 1              [Gaussian]
Link function   : g(u)  = u              [Identity]

                                         AIC        = 141.3415
Log likelihood  = -1552.757049           BIC        = 2.56e+07

-----------------------------------------------------------------------
             |              OIM
   rate100k  |  Coef.    Std. Err.     z    P>|z|   [95% Conf. Interval]
-------------+---------------------------------------------------------
     florida |  96.08723  432.1687   0.22   0.824   -750.9479   943.1224
       _cons |  124.4665  424.2302   0.29   0.769   -707.0094   955.9425
-----------------------------------------------------------------------
```

The coefficients and SEs in the model here are identical to what we obtained when we carried out regression using the variables with the "new" prefix. The deviance statistics are also the same, but the log likelihood, AIC, and BIC values are not identical. So when comparing models, it is important that the method used be consistent; if **iweights** are used for one model, use them for the other as well.

In Stata, **iweights** do not do the same thing in all commands, so results are not always what you might expect. We can rescale the **iweights** in the model above and get the same coefficient estimates and SEs; for example, you could use person-time in units of 1 person-year. However, the header statistics will change. For the Poisson rate difference model with **iweights**, described in Chapter 10, rescaling the weights changes the SEs. This happens because the Poisson method uses counts and person-time to estimate the SEs; if the outcome rate uses person-time units that differ from the person-time units of the importance weights, the formula for the SE will not get the right result. This variation in the behavior of **iweights** means that they should be used with some care.

If you use Stata's **regress** command, for ordinary least squares linear regression, to fit the model above with the same importance weights in units of 100,000 years of person-time, the software will report that there are 195 observations. The sum of the weights is 195.12 and Stata uses the integer part of that as the number of records and treats the importance weights as if they were frequency weights. This is not what we want for estimating rate differences, because the size of the SEs will change depending upon how we express person-time. To estimate a linear regression model using importance weights, use the **glm** command with an identity link and Gaussian (Normal) distribution.

11.5 COMPARISON OF POISSON, WEIGHTED LEAST SQUARES, AND ORDINARY LEAST SQUARES REGRESSION

Linear regression and Poisson regression are doing different things when they estimate rate differences. A weighted least squares linear regression model estimates a variance *from the data* by comparing each observation with the others. Conditional on the levels of the explanatory variables, the variance is multiplied by the person-time weights and these revised variances are used to average the observations. Poisson regression for rate differences uses the importance weights to effectively convert the outcomes to counts. The Poisson model separates out both components of each rate, the numerator and denominator, and makes use of these for estimating the rate differences. Based on the assumptions of event independence and stationary rates for a Poisson process described in Chapter 4, the variance of each rate is calculated using the formulae in Table 4.4.

If we compare the estimated difference in the Florida and Alaska cancer mortality rates from the weighted least squares models with those from weighted Poisson regression, shown in Chapter 10, they are the same for the first seven digits; they differ in the 8th digit, which was not shown in the output. If a robust estimator is used, both methods produce the same SE for the first 8 digits; remarkable similarity considering the differences between these methods. So these regression methods can produce similar results. But a regression model with only one explanatory variable and 22 records is not a stiff test. Which method is best?

Counts and rates are often not normally distributed. But when linear regression is applied to non-normal data, the Central Limit Theorem tells us that the estimated SEs will be nearly correct if we have a large number of records (Wooldridge 2008 pp172–176). How large? Perhaps only 30 records for one explanatory variable (Lumley et al. 2002), and more records for more variables. Using a robust variance estimator also requires that the number of observations not be too small. So even when rates are not normally distributed, weighted least squares linear regression can provide approximately correct P-values and CIs if there are enough records. Some evidence for this can be found in the simulations by Xu et al. (2010). In addition, linear regression is adept at estimating adjusted differences. As mentioned near the end of Chapter 10, the Poisson regression model for age-adjusted differences converged only after hundreds of iterations when we used age-categories and would not converge at all for a continuous age term. In contrast, linear regression converged quickly for both models. So with a sufficient number of observations, linear regression may perform as well as Poisson regression and linear regression may converge to produce results when Poisson regression will not.

One reason that Poisson regression for rate differences may have convergence problems is that the Poisson model will not allow negative rates. Table 11.1 shows the observed cancer mortality rates and fitted rates for age categories using the Alaska and Florida data of Table 6.2. The fitted rates for Florida from a Poisson rate difference model with importance weights and a similarly weighted least squares linear regression model are identical when rounded to the nearest integer. These predicted rates are close to the observed Florida rates because both regression models give more weight to the more precise rates from Florida. For Alaska both sets of predicted rates are similar, but they differ more from the observed Alaska rates which are relatively less precise and therefore less influential in both regression models. The linear regression model predicted negative rates, which are impossible, for infants and persons age 5–14 years old in Alaska. The Poisson model does not allow negative rates. This is a relative advantage for Poisson regression because it may reduce bias in estimates, but precluding negative rates may make convergence difficult.

Poisson regression for rate differences does not estimate the variance by comparing one observation to another. The variance for each rate is estimated using the count numerator and the person-time denominator and the formula in row 5 of Table 4.4. These SEs will be correct if it is reasonable to assume a Poisson process and if the numerator counts are large enough. This means that with Poisson regression we can obtain correct SEs even if we compare only two rates, provided that the rates themselves are sufficiently precise. Later, in a section about variance weighted least squares regression, we will show examples in which Poisson regression has arguably superior performance compared with weighted least squares.

To illustrate the performance of ordinary least squares, weighted least squares, and Poisson regression, hypothetical data were created regarding job injury rates among 1000 workers (Table 11.2). Among 200 workers (records 1 and 2) who did not receive safety training and were inexperienced, the injury rate was 2 events per worker-year. Workers who were experienced (records 3 and 4) had a lower rate of 1.3 events per worker-year: a rate difference of –0.7 compared with records 1 and 2. When a worker was inexperienced and given safety training, their injury rate decreased by 0.3 events per year compared with the inexperienced and untrained workers in records 1 and 2; see record 5. Records 6 and 7 are also for inexperienced workers who received training; for some the rate was 0.8 and for others it was 2.0. The worker-time weighted average of these rates was $(0.8 \times 1 \times 100) + (2.0 \times 3 \times 100)/[(1 + 3) \times 100] = 6.8/4 = 1.7$, the same rate as in record 5. As far as Poisson regression is concerned, the rate for all inexperienced workers who received the safety training (records 5, 6, and 7) is

TABLE 11.1   Age-categorized counts and rates of deaths due to cancer in Alaska and Florida, 2010. Observed rates are shown as well as rates predicted by a Poisson model for rate differences and a weighted least squares linear regression model. Rates are per 100,000 person-years. Additional information in Table 6.2.

AGE (YRS)	ALASKA					FLORIDA				
	COUNT	PERSON-YEARS (1000S)	OBSERVED RATE	POISSON MODEL RATE	LINEAR MODEL RATE	COUNT	PERSON-YEARS (1000S)	OBSERVED RATE	POISSON MODEL RATE	LINEAR MODEL RATE
<1	1	11	9	2	-1	2	209	1	1	1
1-4	2	43	5	3	0	22	865	3	3	3
5-14	1	102	1	2	-1	29	2,211	1	1	1
15-24	5	107	5	4	1	88	2,457	4	4	4
25-34	9	103	9	9	6	196	2,290	9	9	9
35-44	21	93	23	31	28	746	2,431	31	30	30
45-54	103	111	93	119	116	3,282	2,741	120	119	119
55-64	205	86	239	311	309	7,335	2,338	314	311	311
65-74	233	35	659	622	619	10,734	1,728	621	622	622
75-84	218	15	1465	1080	1077	11,795	1,098	1075	1080	1080
85+	86	5	1826	1669	1666	7,238	434	1667	1669	1669

TABLE 11.2 Hypothetical job injury rates per worker-year, according to whether or not workers were exposed to a safety training program and their level of work experience. Data for 1000 workers.

RECORD NUMBER	SAFETY PROGRAM	EXPERIENCED	RATE PER 1 WORKER-YEAR	WORKER-YEARS	EXPECTED MEAN COUNT	NUMBER OF WORKERS
1	No	No	2.0	1	2.0	100
2	No	No	2.0	2	4.0	100
3	No	Yes	1.3	2	2.6	100
4	No	Yes	1.3	3	3.9	200
5	Yes	No	1.7	1	1.7	100
6	Yes	No	0.8	1	0.8	100
7	Yes	No	2.0	3	6.0	100
8	Yes	Yes	1.0	4	4.0	40
9	Yes	Yes	0.4	2	0.8	80
10	Yes	Yes	1.2	6	7.2	80

a stationary 1.7. Ordinary least squares linear regression treats the rates of 1.7, 0.8, and 2.0 as if they average to 1.5. For the experienced and trained workers in records 8, 9, and 10, the population-weighted average rate was 1, but the average in ordinary least squares linear regression average is (1 × 40) + (.4 × 80) + (1.2 × 80)/(40 + 80 + 80) = 0.84.

I expanded Table 11.2 data into records for 1000 workers, using the number of workers in the last column. When the person-time weighted Poisson rate difference model of Chapter 10 is used, adjusting for worker experience, the result was a correct rate difference of –0.3 injuries per worker-year for a worker exposed to safety training compared with another worker of similar experience. Weighted least squares linear regression produced the same result. But ordinary least squares linear regression estimated a rate difference of –0.48, because the method incorrectly estimated lower average rates for workers who received safety training.

I created simulated sets of data for 1000 workers with the covariates and person-time for each record as described in Table 11.2. The outcome count for each worker was sampled randomly from a Poisson distribution with a mean count equal to the expected mean count in the table. The sampled counts were divided by worker-time to create the rates used by the regression models. Both Poisson and weighted least squares linear regression performed well (Table 11.3); the mean estimated association was unbiased. The 95% CIs from Poisson regression included the true safety program effect estimate of –0.3 in 94.8% of the simulations, close to the ideal of 95%. This is not surprising, as these data were generated by a Poisson process. The robust variance estimator was not quite as accurate in this example, with coverage equal to 95.9%. In an analysis of actual data, the robust variance estimator might be the better choice, unless we can be confident that the Poisson assumptions are true. Coverage from weighted least squares was 96.3%, indicating that the SE from this method was a little larger than desired. Adding the robust variance estimator helped shrink the SE toward its true value, improving coverage to 95.8%.

These simulations were repeated using only 100 workers, based upon counts equal to one-tenth the counts in the last column of Table 11.2. Findings were similar to those when 1000 workers were used (Table 11.3). Poisson regression and weighted least squares linear regression did not always agree. The estimated association between safety education and injury rates differed by as much as 0.24 in the simulations, a meaningful amount in this example. Overall, the Poisson regression model did a little better; in 54% of the simulations the estimated rate difference from that method was closer to the true rate difference of –0.3 compared with the result from weighted least squares. This advantage for the Poisson method is shown graphically in Figure 11.1, where the

TABLE 11.3   Estimates of the association between safety education and injury rate per worker-year, adjusted for worker experience. Simulations based on the covariate patterns and worker-year distribution in Table 11.2. True effect of safety education was a rate reduction of –0.3 injuries per worker year. Coverage refers to the percent of 95% model confidence intervals that included the true effect of –0.3; ideally this should be 95%. Coverage not shown for ordinary least squares because the estimated association was so biased. A robust variance estimator was used to produce the robust confidence intervals. Two sets of simulations were carried out; 50,000 simulations for 1000 workers; 100,000 simulations for 100 workers based upon one-tenth the number of workers in last column of Table 11.2.

REGRESSION METHOD	NUMBER OF WORKERS	TRUE EFFECT OF SAFETY EDUCATION	MEAN RATE DIFFERENCE FROM SIMULATIONS	COVERAGE OF 95% CONFIDENCE INTERVALS (%)	COVERAGE OF 95% ROBUST CONFIDENCE INTERVALS (%)
50,000 simulations					
Poisson	1000	-0.3	-0.30020	94.8	95.9
Weighted least squares	1000	-0.3	-0.30016	96.3	95.8
Ordinary least squares	1000	-0.3	-0.48027	omitted	omitted
100,000 simulations					
Poisson	100	-0.3	-0.30007	95.0	95.4
Weighted least squares	100	-0.3	-0.30012	96.2	95.5
Ordinary least squares	100	-0.3	-0.48000	omitted	omitted

distribution of results from weighted least squares has a lower peak and wider tails compared with results from Poisson regression. But the advantage for Poisson regression was slight in this example. Based upon these results, one might conclude that Poisson regression should be the preferred method. But if that method fails to converge, results from weighted least squares regression should be reasonably close.

In real data the divergence between rate differences based upon the Poisson versus the Gaussian family, using person-time weights, may be notable. One may then have to decide whether to rely upon one error family or another. If it is reasonable to assume that the counts arose from something approximating a Poisson process, the Poisson method may be best. Even if a Poisson process seems doubtful, this will not necessarily mean that an estimate from weighted least squares regression is more accurate.

For both sets of simulations, ordinary least squares linear regression produced biased estimates (Table 11.3). Is this evaluation fair? After all, data were deliberately created so that the rates within some covariate patterns (records 6 and 7, also 9 and 10) were allowed to vary in a manner that was related to worker-time. The variation that we created in the rates within some of the 4 covariate strata of Table 11.2 was constrained so that the worker-time stratified rates would have averages that made it easy to show what the expected mean associations should be from the simulations. In real data variations in rates will not fit this convenient pedagogical pattern. But the example helps show that ordinary least squares linear regression can be biased unless we can *assume that variation in rates is not related to person-time*; this assumption will usually be untrue to some extent. If we have information regarding both the outcome counts and person-time that make up the rates to be analyzed,

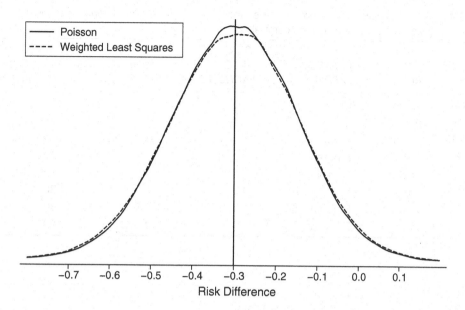

FIGURE 11.1   Distribution of rate difference estimates from Poisson regression (solid line) for rate differences and weighted least squares linear regression (dashed line). Both methods used weights equal to the person-time for each worker record. Results from 100,000 simulations of data for 100 workers with the covariate distributions described in Table 11.2. The distributions of the rate difference estimates were smoothed using a kernel density method.

then we can avoid any assumption about how rates may vary with person-time, by using a regression method weighted by person-time.

11.6 EXPOSURE TO A CARCINOGEN: ORDINARY LINEAR REGRESSION IGNORES THE PRECISION OF EACH RATE

At the risk of beating a dead horse, consider data from two fictional factories where some workers were exposed to a carcinogenic chemical (Table 11.4). Among those not exposed to the chemical the rate of cancer was 10 per 1000 worker-years for young workers and 30 per 1000 person-years for old workers. Regardless of age, the association of chemical exposure with cancer was a rate difference of 10 per 1000 worker-years at MegaChem where there were 70,000 worker-years of observation and 1750 cases of cancer. The same association was 20 per 1000 at MiniPaint with had only 7000 worker-years and 210 cancer diagnoses. Under the assumption of homogeneity, discussed in Chapter 6, the chemical-related differences in cancer rates, 10 and 20 per 1000, are assumed to be estimates of the same true rate difference. Given that the estimated rate difference of 10 from MegaChem is based on a larger number of cancer cases, we expect that the true rate difference should be closer to 10 than 20. Using Poisson regression with importance weights, described in Chapter 10, we can estimate the overall association between chemical exposure and cancer using ratek, the rate per 1000, as the outcome and using pyrsk, worker time in 1000 year units:

TABLE 11.4 Counts of new cancers, worker-time, and cancer rates in two fictional factories, according to worker age and exposure to a carcinogenic chemical.

FACTORY	AGE	CHEMICAL EXPOSURE	COUNTS OF NEW CANCER DIAGNOSES	WORKER-YEARS (1000 YEARS)	RATE PER 1000 WORKER-YEARS
MegaChem	Young	Unexposed	300	30	10
MegaChem	Old	Unexposed	150	5	30
MegaChem	Young	Exposed	100	5	20
MegaChem	Old	Exposed	1200	30	40
MiniPaint	Young	Unexposed	30	3	10
MiniPaint	Old	Unexposed	15	0.5	30
MiniPaint	Young	Exposed	15	0.5	30
MiniPaint	Old	Exposed	150	3	50

```
. glm ratek chemical [iweight=pyrsk], /*
     */ link(id) family(poisson) nolog
(header output omitted)
```

```
------------------------------------------------------------------
             |               OIM
      ratek  |    Coef.    Std. Err.      z     P>|z|   [95% Conf. Interval]
-------------+----------------------------------------------------
    chemical |  25.19481   1.149919    21.91   0.000   22.94101   27.44861
       _cons |  12.85714   .5778856    22.25   0.000   11.72451   13.98978
------------------------------------------------------------------
```

In the output above, the association between chemical exposure and cancer is a rate difference of 25.2 per 1000 worker-years. This crude estimate cannot be right because the average association must fall between the factory-specific stratum estimates, 10 at MegaChem and 20 at MiniPaint. The estimate of 25.2 is biased because chemical exposure was more common among old workers and old workers had higher cancer rates, 30 per 1000 worker years, aside from exposure to the carcinogen. We can remove age-related confounding by adjustment in the model below where old = 1 for older workers and old = 0 for younger workers:

```
. glm ratek chemical old [iweight=pyrsk], link(identity) family(poisson)
nolog
```

```
------------------------------------------------------------------
             |               OIM
      ratek  |    Coef.    Std. Err.      z     P>|z|   [95% Conf. Interval]
-------------+----------------------------------------------------
    chemical | 10.90909   1.595144     6.84   0.000    7.782666   14.03552
         old |       20   1.639466    12.20   0.000   16.78671   23.21329
       _cons |       10   .5427033    18.43   0.000    8.936321   11.06368
------------------------------------------------------------------
```

In this regression table, the estimated association between chemical exposure and cancer was a rate difference of 10.9 per 1000 worker-years. This estimate falls between the two factory-specific estimates of 10 and 20 and it is much closer to the estimate of 10 from MegaChem, where the rate difference was more precise because MegaChem had 8 times as many cancer cases as MiniPaint.

Ordinary least squares linear regression treats the rate differences of 10 and 20 as if they were equally precise and averages them to get a difference of 15. The rate based upon 1750 cancer cases was given the same weight as the rate based upon 210 cases, when information about person-time is ignored:

```
. regress ratek chemical, noheader
```

```
------------------------------------------------------------------------------
     ratek |     Coef.    Std. Err.     t     P>|t|     [95% Conf. Interval]
-----------+------------------------------------------------------------------
  chemical |       15     8.660254    1.73    0.134     -6.190878    36.19088
     _cons |       20     6.123724    3.27    0.017      5.015786    34.98421
------------------------------------------------------------------------------
```

If we adjust for age, the estimated association for chemical exposure is still 15 in ordinary linear regression, as shown below. Confounding by age seems to have disappeared because we divided the outcome counts by the person-time that produced the counts. We paid a price for doing this, because the model gives equal weight to two rate differences, 10 and 20, that are not equally precise.

```
. regress ratek chemical old, noheader
```

```
------------------------------------------------------------------------------
     ratek |     Coef.    Std. Err.     t     P>|t|     [95% Conf. Interval]
-----------+------------------------------------------------------------------
  chemical |       15     3.162278    4.74    0.005      6.871106    23.12889
       old |       20     3.162278    6.32    0.001     11.87111     28.12889
     _cons |       10     2.738613    3.65    0.015      2.960172    17.03983
------------------------------------------------------------------------------
```

The key point here is that ordinary least squares linear regression ignores the precision of each rate; weighted Poisson regression and weighted least squares linear regression can remedy this problem.

11.7 DIFFERENCES IN HOMICIDE RATES: SIMPLE AVERAGES VERSUS POPULATION-WEIGHTED AVERAGES

In 2010, the homicide rate was higher in the 8 Southern States compared with the 6 New England States (Table 11.5). The person-time-weighted rate (which weighted Poisson and weighted least squares regression can both estimate) in the South was 6.31 per 100,000 person-years, compared with 2.93 in New England; a difference of 3.38. The unweighted average rate (which ordinary least squares linear regression estimates) for the South was 6.69 and 2.37 for New England: a South–New England difference of 4.32. The person-time-weighted average rate for the South (6.31) was less than the unweighted average (6.69) for the South because weighted averaging gave more weight to the large

TABLE 11.5 Counts of homicide death, person-time, and rates for the six New England states and eight Southern States in 2010. States are ordered by their rates.

REGION	STATE	HOMICIDE DEATHS	PERSON-YEARS (MILLION)	RATE PER 100,000 PERSON-YEARS	PERSON-TIME WEIGHTED AVERAGE RATE[a]	AVERAGE RATE[b]
New England	Vermont	8	0.63	1.28		
New England	New Hampshire	18	1.32	1.37		
New England	Maine	26	1.33	1.96	2.93	2.37
New England	Rhode Island	27	1.05	2.57		
New England	Massachusetts	203	6.55	3.10		
New England	Connecticut	141	3.57	3.95		
South	Kentucky	199	4.34	4.59		
South	North Carolina	533	9.54	5.59		
South	Florida	1093	18.80	5.81		
South	Tennessee	406	6.35	6.40	6.31	6.69
South	Georgia	633	9.69	6.53		
South	South Carolina	320	4.63	6.92		
South	Alabama	390	4.78	8.16		
South	Mississippi	282	2.97	9.50		

[a] The person-time weighted average rate is sum(rate$_i$ x person-time$_i$)/sum(person-time$_i$) = sum(count$_i$)/sum(person-time$_i$)

[b] The average rate is sum(rate$_i$)/(number of states)

population of Florida (rate 5.81) and less weight to the smaller population of Mississippi (rate 9.50). The weighted-average New England rate (2.93) was higher than the unweighted rate (2.37) because the weighted-average gave more weight to two New England states with large populations and higher rates: Massachusetts (rate 3.10) and Connecticut (rate 3.95).

Weighted Poisson and weighted least squares linear regression both estimate that during 2010 the South experienced a greater homicide rate compared with New England. The Poisson method estimates a SE that is justified by Poisson assumptions (Table 4.4):

```
. glm rate100k south [iweight=pop100k], /*
     */ link(identity) family(poisson) nolog

note: rate100k has noninteger values
(output omitted)

-------------------------------------------------------------------------
             |               OIM
   rate100k  |    Coef.   Std. Err.      z    P>|z|   [95% Conf. Interval]
-------------+-----------------------------------------------------------
      south  |  3.384417  .1749505   19.34   0.000    3.04152    3.727313
      _cons  |  2.928376  .1423825   20.57   0.000    2.649312   3.207441
-------------------------------------------------------------------------
```

```
. glm rate100k south [iweight=pop100k], link(identity) family(gaussian)
nolog
(output omitted)
```

```
-----------------------------------------------------------------
            |               OIM
  rate100k  |    Coef.   Std. Err.      z    P>|z|    [95% Conf. Interval]
------------+----------------------------------------------------
    south   | 3.384417   .7626285    4.44   0.000    1.889692    4.879141
    _cons   | 2.928376   .6858342    4.27   0.000    1.584166    4.272587
-----------------------------------------------------------------
```

We know that homicide rates vary by sex, age, and other factors. We can think of 3.38 as the difference in the homicide rates for a person randomly sampled from the South compared with the rate for a randomly sampled person from New England. The sampling probability for an individual is equal to the inverse of the *regional* person-time; a Massachusetts resident has the same chance of being sampled as a Vermont resident. We interpret 3.38 as the difference in rates for the entire population of each region.

Ordinary least squares linear regression estimates that the average homicide rate in the Southern states was greater than that in the New England states by 4.32 per 100,000:

```
. regress rate south, noheader
```

```
-----------------------------------------------------------------
  rate100k  |    Coef.   Std. Err.      t    P>|t|    [95% Conf. Interval]
------------+----------------------------------------------------
    south   | 4.318825   .7322976    5.90   0.000    2.723286    5.914365
    _cons   | 2.368941    .553565    4.28   0.001    1.162826    3.575055
-----------------------------------------------------------------
```

We can interpret 4.32 as the difference in homicides rates experienced by a person sampled from the Southern states, compared with the New England states, with the probability of sampling proportional to the inverse of each *state's* person-time. So a Mississippi resident is more likely to be sampled (or equivalently, contributes more to the regional rate estimate) than a Florida resident by an amount equal to 18.80/2.97 = 6.3. We can think of 4.32 as the difference between an average (or randomly selected) *state* in the South and an average state in New England, with each state given equal weight.

Both estimates, 3.38 and 4.32, may be useful. If we wish to compare regional homicide rates, we will usually select 3.38 as the desired statistic. But estimating what happened in the average state, with a difference of 4.32, may be suitable for studies of state-level policies or for other purposes. Unfortunately, ordinary least squares linear regression estimates this average difference by treating all rates as if they were equally precise. Treating state rates as equally precise is analogous to a meta-analysis of randomized-trials which gives equal weight to each study, regardless of the precision of each study's estimate of the association between treatment and the outcome. A more defensible approach is to estimate the average rate for a state using a method that also accounts for the precision of each rate. One fixed-effects precision-weighted method is variance weighted least squares regression, which will be discussed later in this chapter. Random effect methods, another choice, will be discussed in later chapters.

11.8 THE PLACE OF ORDINARY LEAST SQUARES LINEAR REGRESSION FOR THE ANALYSIS OF INCIDENCE RATES

When information is available for both the counts and person-time that make up a set of rates, there is little reason to use ordinary least squares linear regression. If adjusted rate differences are desired, person-time-weighted Poisson regression or weighted least squares linear regression are preferred for their abilities to correctly average rates and to account for the precision of different rates. Poisson regression and its variations are available for rate ratios. If one desires to estimate an association for the average unit of analysis, such as a county or a state, better methods than ordinary least squares, such as variance weighted least squares or random-effect models, are available.

Sometimes an analyst may have rate information without knowledge of the numerator counts and person-time denominators. Using weights approximately equal to person-time may still be possible in some instances. If not, an analysis using ordinary least squares linear regression may be preferable to no analysis. In this situation, it might be worth stating that this method may produce biased estimates because it assumes that the size of the rates does not vary systematically with their person-time denominators and it assumes that assigning equal precision to all rates will not produce important bias for either the estimated association or its variance.

11.9 VARIANCE WEIGHTED LEAST SQUARES REGRESSION

In 2010 the homicide rate in the South was 6.31 per 100,000 person-years (3856 deaths/61,082,315 person-years) and in New England it was 2.93 (432/14,444,865). The SD of a rate is $\sqrt{(C/T^2)} = \sqrt{(rate/T)}$ (Table 4.5). So the SD of the rate per 100,000 for the South is $\sqrt{(2.93/144.45)} = 0.1017$ and that for New England is 0.1424. To estimate the difference in these rates, we can use variance weighted least squares which Stata implements with the **vwls** command. Previously calculated SDs can be provided to the software with the **sd** () option. The rate difference of 3.38 and SE of 0.17 are just what we obtained previously using person-time weighted Poisson regression:

```
. vwls rate100k south, sd(sd)
```

```
Variance-weighted least-squares regression      Number of obs   =        2
Goodness-of-fit chi2(0)   =    .                 Model chi2(1)   =  374.23
Prob > chi2               =    .                 Prob > chi2     =  0.0000
```

rate100k	Coef.	Std. Err.	z	P>|z|	[95% Conf. Interval]	
south	3.384417	.1749505	19.34	0.000	3.04152	3.727313
_cons	2.928376	.1423825	20.57	0.000	2.649312	3.207441

Variance-weighted least squares uses previously calculated variance information. The weights used are the inverse of the variance of each rate. This has been called information weighted least squares, inverse-variance weighting, and precision-weighting. The analyst must predigest the data and disgorge the SD results to the software, just as some birds feed their young. The method assumes that the rates within each stratum are independent of those in the other strata, so there is no covariance to be estimated. Although we have only shown a model with a single variable, variance-weighted least squares regression can create adjusted estimates using additional variables, provided that the SDs can be calculated for the rate outcomes of each covariate or each level of a continuous variable used in the regression model.

The variance-weighted output used only two rates, one for the South and the other for New England. Instead we can use the data for the 14 states in Table 11.5, with a separate SD for each state, as shown here:

```
. vwls rate100k south, sd(sd)

Variance-weighted least-squares regression      Number of obs  =      14
Goodness-of-fit chi2(12)    = 145.34            Model chi2(1) = 450.24
Prob > chi2                 = 0.0000            Prob > chi2    = 0.0000
----------------------------------------------------------------------------
   rate100k |    Coef.   Std. Err.      z     P>|z|    [95% Conf. Interval]
----------+-----------------------------------------------------------------
      south | 3.554478  .1675157    21.22    0.000    3.226153    3.882803
      _cons | 2.598401  .1341209    19.37    0.000    2.335529    2.861273
----------------------------------------------------------------------------

. lincom _cons+south

 (1)  south + _cons = 0
----------------------------------------------------------------------------
   rate100k |    Coef.   Std. Err.      z     P>|z|    [95% Conf. Interval]
----------+-----------------------------------------------------------------
        (1) |  .152879  .1003648    61.31    0.000    5.956168    6.349591
----------------------------------------------------------------------------
```

According to the output above, the rate for New England was 2.60 per 100,000 person-years and the rate for the South was 2.60 + 3.55 = 6.15. These do not equal the regional average rates or the person-time weighted average rates (Table 11.5). The precision-weighted method of pooling assumes that each state-specific rate in New England is an estimate of the same true rate, using the homogeneity assumption discussed in Chapter 6. The difference between the rate in Vermont and the rate in Connecticut is attributed to chance variation around a true common rate. The method is variance-minimizing; the variance of the pooled estimate is the smallest possible variance for any weighted average of the state rates. When using Poisson methods, person-time weights are used (Expression 6.1) to average state rates: $\text{sum}(\text{rate}_i \times T_i)/\text{sum}(T_i) = \text{sum}(C_i)/\text{sum}(T_i) = C/T$. If we use variance weighting, the pooled (inverse-variance weighted) average of the New England state rates is calculated using formulae in Expression 11.5:

Pooled average of rates

$$= \text{sum}(\text{rate}_i \times 1/\text{variance}_i)/\text{sum}(1/\text{variance}_i)$$
$$= \text{sum}(\text{rate}_i \times T_i \times T_i/C_i)/\text{sum}(T_i \times T_i/C_i)$$
$$= \text{sum}(C_i/T_i \times T_i \times T_i/C_i)/\text{sum}(T_i \times T_i/Ci)$$
$$= \text{sum}(T_i)/\text{sum}(T_i \times T_i/C_i)$$
$$= T/\text{sum}(T_i/\text{rate}_i)$$
$$= 1/[\text{sum}(T_i/\text{rate}_i)/T]$$
$$= 1/[\text{sum}(1/\text{rate}_i \times T_i)/\text{sum}(T_i)]$$

(Ex11.5)

The first three lines of Expression 11.5 show that the pooled average uses weights equal to the inverse of the variance of each rate. The last line shows this equals the reciprocal of the person-time weighted average of the *inverse* of the rates. This estimation method corresponds to the fixed-effects estimate of association that is often used in meta-analysis, a method that assumes that each study-specific estimate is an attempt to measure the same true association. To show the relationship to inverse-variance meta-analysis, we can use Stata's **metan** command (Bradburn, Deeks, and Altman 2009, Harris et al. 2009) to summarize the state rates and their SDs. The **metan** command estimates pooled average rates and CIs that are the same as those estimated by the **vwls** command, and provides information about the heterogeneity of the rates. The output shows the state-specific rates under the heading "ES", meaning effect size; that generic heading is used because the software can summarize many statistics, such as risk ratios or risk differences. The "I-V pooled ES" estimates show the inverse-variance-weighted pooled rates for New England and the South, with the same CIs that were estimated by the **vwls** command:

```
. metan rate100k sd, nograph by(south) label(namevar=state)

       Study        |    ES    [95% Conf. Interval]  % Weight
-----------------+-----------------------------------------
    New England     |
Vermont             |  1.278   0.393   2.164        3.16
New Hampshire       |  1.367   0.736   1.999        6.22
Maine               |  1.957   1.205   2.710        4.38
Rhode Island        |  2.565   1.598   3.533        2.65
Massachusetts       |  3.100   2.674   3.527       13.64
Connecticut         |  3.945   3.294   4.596        5.85
   Sub-total        |
   I-V pooled ES    |  2.598   2.336   2.861       35.90
-----------------+-----------------------------------------
    South           |
Kentucky            |  4.586   3.949   5.223        6.11
North Carolina      |  5.590   5.115   6.064       11.02
Florida             |  5.813   5.469   6.158       20.88
Tennessee           |  6.398   5.775   7.020        6.41
Georgia             |  6.534   6.025   7.043        9.57
South Carolina      |  6.918   6.160   7.676        4.32
Alabama             |  8.159   7.350   8.969        3.78
Mississippi         |  9.504   8.394  10.613        2.02
   Sub-total        |
   I-V pooled ES    |  6.153   5.956   6.350       64.10
-----------------+-----------------------------------------
Overall             |
   I-V pooled ES    |  4.877   4.719   5.034      100.00
-----------------+-----------------------------------------

Test(s) of heterogeneity:
            Heterogeneity  degrees of
              statistic     freedom       P     I-squared**
New England     47.66          5        0.000     89.5%
South           97.68          7        0.000     92.8%
Overall        595.58         13        0.000     97.8%
Overall Test for heterogeneity between sub-groups:
              450.24          1        0.000
** I-squared: the variation in ES attributable to heterogeneity)
```

```
Considerable heterogeneity observed (up to 92.8%) in one or more sub-
groups,

Test for heterogeneity between sub-groups likely to be invalid
(some output omitted)
---------------------------------------------------------------
```

The **metan** command can estimate a random-effects pooled average of state-specific rates within a larger region, such as New England, using the method of DerSimonian and Laird (1986, Fleiss 1993). Because the state-specific rates have large count numerators, they have a lot of precision and most of their variation cannot be attributed to chance. Consequently the random-effects pooled rates are close to the average rate estimates in Table 11.5 that gave equal weight to each state.

Ordinary least-squares linear regression pools rates by just averaging them, a method that ignores the precision of each rate. Inverse-variance weighting creates a weighted average that uses information about precision. This may be a useful choice for some study questions. If variance-weighted least squares regression is to be used, but person-time-weighted average rates are desired, two preliminary steps are needed: first collapse the data into a single rate for each covariate pattern using person-time weights, then compute the SDs.

Variance-weighted least squares regression is a large-sample method that involves an assumption of approximate normality. Rates are typically not normally distributed, but the normality assumption of variance-weighted least squares will be satisfied if there are many individual observations or if the variance estimates of the rates are sufficiently precise. In the homicide data, the second requirement is met because of the large number of deaths in each state. Just the comparison of the two rates for New England and the South, a model with only two observations, should produce valid SEs because of the large rate numerator counts for each region. These details and others are described by Zhu, Chu, and Greenland (2011).

11.10 CAUTIONS REGARDING INVERSE-VARIANCE WEIGHTS

Stata's **vwls** command has an option for computing SDs for covariate patterns, but this option is a poor choice for estimating rate differences. In the output below all 14 state-level rates were used but no SDs were provided to the software. The software then combined the rates for the six New England states and the eight Southern states by averaging them within each region as if they were equally precise. As a result, the estimates for each region are just what ordinary least squares estimates, but the SEs are different, because they were computed separately within each region, not across all regions. The results are no better than those estimated by ordinary least squares regression.

```
. vwls rate100k south

Variance-weighted least-squares regression        Number of obs   =      14
Goodness-of-fit chi2(0)   =     .               Model chi2(1)   =   39.03
Prob > chi2               =     .               Prob > chi2     = 0.0000

--------------------------------------------------------------------------
rate100k |      Coef.    Std. Err.      z      P>|z|    [95% Conf. Interval]
```

```
- - - - - - - +- - - - - - - - - - - - - - - - - - - - - - - - - - - - - - - - - - - - - - - - - - -
     south |   4.318825    .6912736    6.25    0.000    2.963954    5.673697
      _cons |   2.368941    .4250272    5.57    0.000    1.535903    3.201979
- - - - - - - - - - - - - - - - - - - - - - - - - - - - - - - - - - - - - - - - - - - - - - - - -

. lincom _cons+south

 ( 1)  south + _cons = 0

- - - - - - - - - - - - - - - - - - - - - - - - - - - - - - - - - - - - - - - - - - - - - - - - -
rate100k |      Coef.    Std. Err.      z     P>|z|    [95% Conf. Interval]
- - - - - - - +- - - - - - - - - - - - - - - - - - - - - - - - - - - - - - - - - - - - - - - - - - -
      (1) |   6.687766    .5451706   12.27    0.000    5.619252    7.756281
- - - - - - - - - - - - - - - - - - - - - - - - - - - - - - - - - - - - - - - - - - - - - - - - -
```

Stata can incorporate inverse-variance weights into most regression models by using what the Stata developers call analytic weights or **aweights**. Doing this in an ordinary least squares linear regression with a single explanatory variable will result in estimates that are the same as those from variance weighted least squares, but the SEs will differ. Variance weighted least squares makes no attempt to estimate the variance; it meekly accepts the predigested values. But when **aweights** are used by ordinary least squares linear regression, the software calculates a single shared variance of the errors and multiplies this by weights equal to the variance. This was described by Wallenstein and Bodian in 1987 (Wallenstein and Bodian 1987), with a later correction (Greenland and Engelman 1988, Wallenstein 1988), but their article does not mention rates or variance weighted least squares. A clear discussion was presented by Zhu, Chu, and Greenland (2011) with a worked example for a single variable model to estimate the change in a set of rates over time. That article explains that when inverse-variance weights are used in ordinary least squares linear regression with one variable, the incorrect SEs can be corrected by dividing them by the square root of the mean square error of the residuals, which is also called the root mean square error (RMSE). This will work in some software packages: SAS, for example. In Stata software this correction requires that the SE be divided by the root mean square error multiplied by the square root of the mean of the weights, which are themselves equal to the inverse of the variance for each rate: in other words, SE corrected = SE/(RMSE x mean(weight)) = SE/(RMSE x mean(1/SD of each rate). This cumbersome correction can be avoided by using Stata's **vwls** command.

The difference between use of variance weighted least squares and ordinary least squares with analytic weights is described in Stata's description of the **vwls** command and also in the discussion about weighted estimation. The Stata manuals offer a nice example showing that in a model with two explanatory variables, the regression coefficients differ between variance-weighted least squares and ordinary least squares regression with inverse-variance weights. The moral here; don't expect inverse-variance weighting in ordinary least squares linear regression to provide the same rate difference estimates or SEs as variance weighted least squares.

11.11 WHY USE VARIANCE WEIGHTED LEAST SQUARES?

A need for variance weighted least squares will arise if several rates and variances are calculated from data with a complex sampling design and the analyst wants to use the design-based variance in a regression model; variance weighted least squares can save the day. An example of this situation appeared in an article that examined trends in rates of emergency department visits (Tang et al. 2010). The authors of that study used inverse-variance weights in ordinary least squares linear regression. A better method, using variance-weighted least squares, was subsequently described by Zhu, Chu, and Greenland (2011).

Imagine a situation in which the numerator count is large, for example the number of deaths in traffic crashes in a year, but the denominator, a survey estimate of vehicle miles of travel is much less precise. In this instance nearly all the random error for the estimated rate of deaths per mile can be attributed to the denominator and variance-weighted least squares could be used to analyze such data.

If we desire a fixed-effects rate difference for an association averaged across units with varying person-time contributions, such as states or factories or schools, this could be done using variance weighted least squares.

11.12 A SHORT COMPARISON OF WEIGHTED POISSON REGRESSION, VARIANCE WEIGHTED LEAST SQUARES, AND WEIGHTED LINEAR REGRESSION

From 2000 to 2012 the rate of traffic crash death per billion miles of vehicle travel declined (Figure 11.2) (National Highway Traffic Safety Administration 2013). When analyzing trends over time, we can create a variable called "iyr" (for "indicator year") equal to the year minus the first year divided by the number of

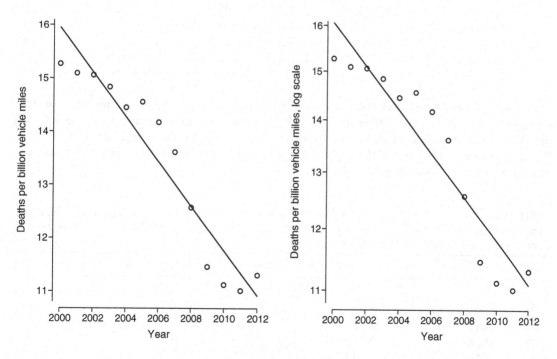

FIGURE 11.2 Traffic crash deaths in the United States per billion vehicle miles of travel, for the years 2000–2012. Both plots show the same observed rates as circles. Plot on the left shows a fitted line from an additive (rate difference) Poisson model. Plot on the right uses the log scale for the vertical axis and shows a fitted line from a multiplicative (rate ratio) Poisson model.

years minus 1: iyr = (year-2000)/(13–1). This variable takes the value 0 for the first year (2000), 1 for the last year (2012), and has intermediate values equally spaced across all other years. When this variable is used in regression of rate differences, the estimated coefficient is the linear rate difference across the entire time interval, using data from all the years. For crash deaths per billion miles, the estimated linear change was plotted from additive (difference) and multiplicative (ratio) Poisson models (Figure 11.2). The fitted lines and the fitted values do not differ much (Table 11.6), but the Akaike Information Criteria statistic suggests the additive model is a better fit to these data. The additive model regression results are shown here, with rateb indicating deaths per billion miles and miles in units of 1 billion:

```
. glm rateb iyr [iweight=miles], /*
        */ link(identity) family(poisson) nolog
note: rateb has noninteger values

Generalized linear models                No. of obs        =          13
Optimization      : ML                   Residual df       =          11
                                         Scale parameter =           1
Deviance          = 732.6958739          (1/df) Deviance = 66.60872
Pearson           = 732.3084012          (1/df) Pearson   = 66.57349

Variance function: V(u) = u              [Poisson]
Link function     : g(u) = u             [Identity]
                                         AIC               =   13066.99
Log likelihood    = -84933.4042          BIC               =   704.4814
-----------------------------------------------------------------------
             |             OIM
   rateb |    Coef.    Std. Err.      z     P>|z|     [95% Conf. Interval]
---------+-------------------------------------------------------------
     iyr |  -5.032411   .0607807   -82.80   0.000    -5.151539   -4.913283
   _cons |  15.94823    .0378389   421.48   0.000    15.87407     16.0224
-----------------------------------------------------------------------
```

The additive Poisson model estimates that over the 12-year interval, the rate of traffic crash death declined by 5.03 deaths per billion miles of vehicle travel. The multiplicative model using a log link (output not shown), estimated a rate ratio of 0.69, meaning that the mortality rate fell by 31%. We can produce results close to the additive Poisson model estimates using variance-weighted least squares regression, as shown here:

TABLE 11.6 Traffic crash death rates per billion vehicle miles of travel. Observed rates and rates fitted using an additive (rate difference) Poisson model and a multiplicative (rate ratio) Poisson model. To save space, rates are shown for only every third year in these data.

YEAR	OBSERVED RATES	RATES FROM ADDITIVE MODEL	RATES FROM MULTIPLICATIVE MODEL
2000	15.27	15.95	16.06
2003	14.84	14.69	14.64
2006	14.17	13.43	13.34
2009	11.46	12.17	12.16
2012	11.30	10.92	11.09

```
. gen double sd = (deaths/miles^2)^.5

. vwls rateb iyr, sd(sd)

Variance-weighted least-squares regression        Number of obs    = 13
Goodness-of-fit chi2(11)   = 733.25                Model chi2(1)   = 7070.74
Prob > chi2                = 0.0000                Prob > chi2     = 0.0000
------------------------------------------------------------------------------
     rateb |      Coef.   Std. Err.       z    P>|z|    [95% Conf. Interval]
-----------+------------------------------------------------------------------
       iyr |  -5.040884   .0599479    -84.09   0.000   -5.158379   -4.923388
     _cons |   15.93328   .0374932    424.96   0.000    15.85979    16.00676
------------------------------------------------------------------------------
```

The result from variance-weighted least squares is slightly different from the Poisson model; a rate decrease of 5.04 instead of 5.03 deaths per billion miles. The small difference between the two methods arises because the Poisson model weights each rate by the miles of travel for that year, whereas the variance-weighted method weights each rate by the inverse of its variance, a quantity equal to $miles^2$/ deaths for each year.

Weighted least squares linear regression (output shown below) with importance weights equal to yearly miles produced a somewhat different estimate, a rate decrease equal to 4.95 deaths per billion miles. Weighted least squares used the importance weights, but also estimated a variance from the data, which slightly altered the estimated rate difference over 12 years. This example shows that weighted Poisson regression and weighted least squares will not necessarily produce the same estimates:

```
. glm rateb iyr [iweight=miles], link(identity) f(gaussian) nolog

Generalized linear models                  No. of obs       =         13
Optimization       : ML                    Residual df      =         11
                                           Scale parameter =  874.6661
Deviance        =  9621.32663              (1/df) Deviance =  874.6661
Pearson         =  9621.32663              (1/df) Pearson  =  874.6661

Variance function: V(u) = 1                [Gaussian]
Link function     : g(u) = u               [Identity]
                                           AIC             =  24755.87
Log likelihood    = -160911.1497           BIC             =  9593.112
------------------------------------------------------------------------------
           |                 OIM
     rateb |      Coef.   Std. Err.       z    P>|z|    [95% Conf. Interval]
-----------+------------------------------------------------------------------
       iyr |  -4.954832    .489899    -10.11   0.000   -5.915016   -3.994647
     _cons |   15.90897   .2905821     54.75   0.000    15.33944    16.4785
------------------------------------------------------------------------------
```

11.13 PROBLEMS WHEN AGE-STANDARDIZED RATES ARE USED AS OUTCOMES

Some studies use a linear regression model with age-standardized rates as the outcome. Levene et al. (2010) used ordinary least squares linear regression to estimate associations between several factors (proportion of the population that smoked, proportion with known hypertension) and the age-standardized rate of coronary heart disease in regions in England.

The use of age-standardized rates as a linear regression outcome was discussed by Rosenbaum and Rubin in 1984 (Rosenbaum and Rubin 1984). They pointed out that if age-standardized rates are used as the outcome, and age is omitted from the list of explanatory values, then the regression model fails to account for the relationships between age and the other explanatory variables. The outcome is adjusted for age using the standardizing method, but the explanatory variables are not age adjusted. This can bias the coefficient estimates.

It is common to see a study in which authors use information about regions or other population groups (counties, states, countries, companies, schools, or other entities) and use a regression method to estimate how regional factors are associated with event rates, such as mortality. The variables used in the regression may be regional characteristics that can be reasonably thought of as being the same for everyone in the region; examples include laws regarding alcohol sales or vehicle licensing, or an index of air pollution. Explanatory variables which are the same for everyone within a region can be thought of as age-standardized; since they have the same value for everyone, a weighted average based on any age distribution will be equal to the original value. So if the explanatory variables are all regional in nature, then using age-standardized rates as the outcome will not be a source of bias.

But it is common for studies of regional rates to also adjust for regional differences in characteristics of individuals, such as age, sex, ethnic group, income, or other factors. Rosenbaum and Rubin (1984) argue that if age-adjusted rates are used as the outcome, then any explanatory variables which are not constant across residents of the same region should also be age-adjusted. Unfortunately, this is rarely done and will often be impossible.

Mortality data for the United States and many other countries is now available in computerized files with deaths and person-time stratified on age, sex, and some categories related to race or ethnicity. In these data, age-adjustment can be done by a regression model, so it is not necessary to use age-standardized rates as an outcome. Analyses of mortality can be done using age-stratified data.

11.14 RATIOS AND SPURIOUS CORRELATION

Chapter 1 describe the problem that may arise when ratios are used as both outcomes and explanatory variables in regression; if both the outcome and the explanatory variable are divided by the same quantity, a relationship ("spurious correlation") may appear between two otherwise unrelated quantities. Rates are ratios; a count of events divided by person-time. It is not uncommon to see ratios used as explanatory variables in analyses of rates from regions or institutions. For example, instead of entering the number of unemployed persons into the regression model, the investigators enter the unemployed proportion, the number of unemployed persons divided by the population size (which is equal to the person-time estimate).

To learn whether this is a problem in the analysis of rates, I carried out a simulation study of regression results (Table 11.7). Counts of deaths by homicide during 2010 in the 50 U.S. states and the

TABLE 11.7 Proportion of P-values < .05 from a simulation study of regression models using U.S. state-level data for counts and rates of homicide in 2010. Data were used from all 50 states and the District of Columbia; each region was represented twice, so there were 102 regions used. Each proportion was based upon 20,000 simulations. Ideally the proportion of P-values < .05 should be .05; proportions of .04, .05, and .06 are in boldface.

MODEL TYPE[a]	COUNT RELATED TO PERSON-TIME[b]	DISTRIBUTION[c]	USUAL VARIANCE[d] EXPLANATORY VARIABLE[e]		ROBUST VARIANCE[d] EXPLANATORY VARIABLE[e]	
			COUNT	RATIO	COUNT	RATIO
Linear	No	Uniform	.02	.07	**.05**	.20
		Normal	.02	.00	**.05**	.00
		Poisson	.03	.00	**.05**	.00
	Yes	Uniform	.00	.02	.00	**.05**
		Normal	.00	.02	.00	**.05**
		Poisson	.00	**.05**	.00	**.06**
Poisson	No	Uniform	.71	.90	**.05**	.14
		Normal	.71	1.00	**.05**	.00
		Poisson	.70	1.00	**.06**	.00
	Yes	Uniform	.43	.71	.00	**.05**
		Normal	.51	.71	.00	**.05**
		Poisson	1.00	.75	.00	**.06**

[a] Two models were used: (1) a generalized linear model for rate differences with an identity link, Gaussian errors, importance weights equal to state population estimates, and the state homicide rates as the outcome, or 2) a Poisson model for rate ratios with the count of deaths in each state as the outcome and person-time as an offset.

[b] The counts used as explanatory variables in the regression models were drawn from six pseudo-random distributions:

1. Uniform distribution ranging from 0 to 1000.
2. Normal distribution with mean 100,000 and SD 10,000.
3. Poisson distribution with mean 100,000.
4. Uniform distribution ranging from 0 to the population estimate for each state.
5. Normal distribution with mean equal to half of each state's population estimate, with SD equal to 1/10th each state's population estimate.
6. Poisson distribution with mean equal to half of each state's population estimate.

Methods 1–3 generated counts that were not related to the person-time estimates and methods 4–6 generated counts that were larger for states with larger populations.

[c] Distribution indicates the distribution from which the counts were drawn using a pseudo-random method.

[d] All models were estimated with the usual variance estimator and again with a robust variance estimator.

[e] The sole explanatory variable in each model was either (1) the untransformed count drawn for each region from a pseudo-random distribution or (2) a *ratio* created by dividing that count by the state population.

District of Columbia were used, along with the person-time (population) estimates for each state in that year. I used each state twice, so there were 102 records in each regression model; this was done because robust variance estimators have better performance in larger samples. It is common to examine state-level data, so these data exemplify the population size variation often encountered in a study of rates. The largest state was California (population 37,253,956) and the smallest was Wyoming

(563,626). The choice of homicide counts as the outcome was arbitrary, but using actual counts added an element of realism to the simulations. The largest count of homicide deaths was 1905 in California and the smallest was 8 in Vermont.

The only explanatory variable used in each regression model was a pseudo-random count drawn, for each of the 102 regions in each simulation, from six distributions:

1. Uniform distribution ranging from 0 to 1000.
2. Normal distribution with mean 100,000, SD 10,000.
3. Poisson distribution with mean 100,000, SD 10,000.
4. Uniform distribution ranging from 0 to the population estimate for each state.
5. Normal distribution with mean equal to half of each state's population estimate and SD equal to 1/10th of each state's population estimate.
6. Poisson distribution with mean equal to half of each state's population estimate.

In this list, the first three methods generated explanatory counts that were not related the state population size. Examples in real data might be pollen counts, the average count of E. Coli bacteria in water, a measure of water hardness, or a count of storks in the state. Counts such as these would not necessarily be proportional to population size. The last three methods in the list generated counts that should be larger, all other things being equal, in a state with more people. The number of unemployed persons or the number with a high school diploma are examples of this kind of population-related count.

Two types of regression model were used: (1) a generalized linear model for rate differences with an identity link, Gaussian error distribution, importance weights equal to the state population estimate, and homicide rates as the outcome, and (2) a Poisson model for rate ratios with the count of homicides as the outcome and person-time as an offset. Each model was estimated both with and without a robust variance estimator. The only explanatory variable in each model was either the randomly selected count or a ratio created by dividing the count by the state population. Because these variables were created without regard to the homicide rates, they should have no systematic association with the rates; on average, 5% of the P-value for these variables should be $< .05$ in the simulations. The only information collected from the simulations were the P-values for the association between the explanatory count (or ratio) and the outcome rate. Each set of P-values was based upon 20,000 simulations (Table 11.7).

Finding that small P-values were too common would indicate the "spurious correlation" problem that concerned Karl Pearson. But for the person-time weighted linear rate difference models with the usual variance, there was no evidence of this problem. For a ratio explanatory variable, the proportion of P-values that were small $(< .05)$ was generally too small, not too large, when the usual variance estimator was used; the proportions were .07, .00, .00, .02, .02, and .05. When Poisson rate ratio regression was used with the usual variance estimator, there were too many small P-values; 43 to 100% of P-values were $< .05$ whether counts or ratios were used. This is not an indication of "spurious correlation," but rather evidence that the usual variance estimator did a terrible job when the variation in outcome rates was greater than expected from a Poisson process.

For both model types, linear difference model and Poisson ratio model, the robust variance estimator showed better performance. More details about this estimator are in Chapter 13. When the robust variance estimator was used for weighted linear rate difference models or Poisson rate ratio models, the correct P-value proportion of .05 was obtained when (1) a count unrelated to population size was used as an explanatory variable or (2) a count related to population size was divided by person-time and the resulting ratio was used as an explanatory variable. These results suggest that some counts should not be divided by person-time and others should be. Fortunately, these results fit with common sense. There seems to be no reason, for example, to create a ratio of the pollen count to population size. But it seems intuitive that we would be more interested in the proportion of the population that is unemployed rather than the count of employed people. The results of Table 11.7 are worth some study.

11.15 LINEAR REGRESSION WITH LN (RATE) AS THE OUTCOME

Poisson regression models for rate ratios use a log link, so the explanatory variables are linear on the log scale and the outcomes are non-negative counts, including counts of 0. Some studies use the log of the rate as the outcome in linear regression to estimate rate ratios, a sort of poor-man's Poisson regression. This approach was understandable before Poisson regression models became widely available in software, but there is now little justification for this strategy.

If there are no events, the outcome rate is 0. But log(0) cannot be estimated. To deal with this difficultly, some investigators omit records with no events, an approach that can introduce bias. Another tactic is to replace zero counts with a small quantity such as .01 or .00001. This may be satisfactory in some situations, but these quantities differ substantially on the log scale and the choice for the small quantity may be a source of bias: $\ln(.01) = -4.6$, $\ln(.00001) = -11.5$. Poisson regression for rate ratios handles counts of zero without difficulty.

Sometimes a linear regression model that uses the log of the rate as the outcome is estimated and then the regression coefficients are transformed back to the original scale by exponentiation to produce a rate ratio. But since the average of a group of ln(rates) is not necessarily equal to the ln of the average rate (Lindsey and Jones 1998), this method may produce biased estimates of the desired ratios.

The event rate in Table 11.8 was greater among those exposed (110 events in 2 million person-years) compared with those not exposed (100 events in 2 million person-years): rate ratio 1.10. If we express the rates among those exposed and not exposed on the ln scale, average them for those exposed and those not, and compare the antilogs of those averages, the rate ratio becomes 0.63 (Table 11.8), implying fewer events among those exposed. Poisson regression for rate ratios will produce an estimate of 1.10, whereas ordinary least squares linear regression and population-weighted linear regression will both produce biased estimates of 0.63 when the ln(rate) is used as the outcome. (Credit for this example goes to Fisher and van Belle (1993 p466).)

We could try to use variance weighted least squares with ln(rate) as the outcome for the data in Table 11.8. Each ln(rate) is weighted by the inverse of the variance, which means the weights are equal to the numerator count of each rate (see Formula 9 in Table 4.4). This produces a rate ratio equal to $\exp([(\ln(1) \times 10 + \ln(10) \times 100)/(10 + 100)] - [(\ln(5) \times 50 + \ln(5) \times 50)/(50 + 50)]) = 1.62$.

If we collapse groups 1 and 2 into a single rate (110 per 2 million person-years) and do the same for groups 3 and 4 (rate 100 per 2 million person-years), then no averaging of the rates will occur in the regression models and all four methods (Poisson regression, ordinary and weighted linear regression, and variance weighted least squares) will produce the same rate ratio of 1.10 when the last three of these methods use the ln(rate) as the outcome. But this simple situation is of little interest, as we can easily compare two rates without resorting to any regression model.

TABLE 11.8 Hypothetical event counts, person-time and rates for four groups: two exposed, two unexposed. Mean rate is the person-time weighted average. Mean ln(rate) is just the average of two ln(rate) values.

EXPOSED	GROUP	COUNT	PERSON-YEARS (10^6)	RATE PER 10^5 PERSON-YEARS	MEAN RATE	RATE RATIO	LN (RATE)	MEAN LN (RATE)	ANTILOG MEAN LN (RATE)	RATE RATIO
Yes	1	10	1	1	5.5		0.00	1.15	3.16	
Yes	2	100	1	10			2.30			
No	3	50	1	5		1.10	1.61			0.63
No	4	50	1	5	5.0		1.61	1.61	5.00	

The chief message here is that if rate ratios are desired, some version of Poisson regression, perhaps Poisson regression with a robust variance, will usually be preferred. When the robust variance estimator is used, this method is sometimes called Poisson pseudo-maximum likelihood or quasi-maximum likelihood estimation. Linear regression with the ln(rate) should not be used. Many authors have made this point in one way or another (Gourieroux, Monfort, and Tognon 1984b, Miller 1984, Lloyd 1999 pp85–86, Cameron and Trivedi 2005 pp668–669,682–683, Santos Silva and Tenreyro 2006, Cook and Lawless 2007 pp82–84, Wooldridge 2008 pp597–598, Cameron and Trivedi 2009 pp560–561, Wooldridge 2010 pp727–728, Nichols 2010, Gould 2011). In many respects linear regression is the Monarch of difference models. But Poisson regression is the Emperor of models for ratios.

Sometimes rates are derived from a complex survey and we wish to use the survey design based estimate of variance. There may be good reasons to think the rates are better summarized as an adjusted rate ratio, rather than a rate difference. In this situation, variance weighted least squares with the ln(rate) as the outcome may be a reasonable choice, despite concerns that averaging ln(rates) may introduce some bias. Zhu et al. (2015 p5811) took this approach in a study of driver licensing laws.

The rate ratio of 0.63 (Table 11.8) from the linear regression approach cannot be justified. But a reasonable argument could be made that the estimate of 1.62 from variance weighted least squares regression should be preferred over the estimate of 1.10 from Poisson regression. Whether or not we should collapse the rates in groups 1 and 2 will depend, in part, on the possible reasons for the apparent variation (heterogeneity) in the rates among these two exposed groups. Heterogeneity will receive more attention in later chapters.

11.16 PREDICTING NEGATIVE RATES

As shown for the data in Table 11.1, a linear regression model for rate differences with Gaussian errors can predict negative rates. This can be an advantage for achieving convergence and the fact that a few predicted rate values may be negative may not be an important source of bias for estimating associations in many applications. But this can be a source of bias in some situations. For this reason, Poisson regression for rate differences may be preferred provided estimates can be obtained.

But if the goal is to predict rates, linear regression may do a poor job, particularly if some rates are based on small counts and negative rates are predicted. If the model is to be used, for example, to estimate what happens when an exposure is set to zero, negative rates may arise and result in biased predictions (Weiss and Koepsell 2014 p364).

11.17 SUMMARY

Here is a short summary of the ideas in this long chapter:

1. Avoid using ordinary least squares linear regression to estimate rate differences, as the estimates may be biased.
2. Instead, use person-time weighted least squares linear regression or person-time weighted Poisson regression for rate differences. The former method may converge when the Poisson regression will not. Otherwise, the Poisson model may be preferable, as it does not allow the prediction of negative rates.
3. Variance weighted least squares linear regression can be used to estimate rate differences. This may be helpful for rates that have variances from the design of a complex survey.

4. Do not confuse variance weighted least squares linear regression with a regression model that incorporates weights proportional to the inverse of the variance.
5. Do not let variance weighted least squares linear regression estimate the SD from the data.
6. Avoid age-standardized rates as a regression outcome. Adjust for age instead.
7. In some situations these suggested rules cannot be followed. Consider whether a possibly biased analysis is better than no analysis at all.

The most important idea in this chapter, underlying most of these suggestions, is that we should prefer regression models that use information both about the rate numerator and about the rate denominator.

Model Fit

12

During 2003–2005 a randomized controlled trial was conducted to assess whether an exercise program would prevent falls (Shumway-Cook et al. 2007). Sedentary persons age 65 years or older were randomly assigned to exercise on three days of each week (n = 226) or a control group (n = 227). Trial participants kept a diary of their falls in each month. The planned year of follow-up was completed for 442 (98%) of the subjects (Table 12.1); rates were based on all available follow-up time, including time from 11 subjects who dropped out prior to 1 year of follow-up. The rate of falls was 297/222.67 person-years = 1.33 in the exercise group, less than the rate of 398/224.53 person-years = 1.77 in the control arm: a rate ratio of 0.75 and a rate difference of –0.44 falls per person-year.

12.1 TABULAR AND GRAPHIC DISPLAYS

Is it reasonable to use confidence intervals (CI) that assume the fall counts are from two Poisson processes, one for the exercise group, another for the control group? If a Poisson process with a mean rate of 1.33 generated counts from 222.67 person-years of time, there would be fewer counts of zero and more counts of 1, 2, and 3 compared with the observed counts in the exercise group (Figure 12.1). The same is true for the control group. Figure 12.1 is a common method for displaying count data. We can also plot the proportion of all falls for each per-subject fall count (Figure 12.2). In the exercise group there were fall counts as large as 13 and 61 falls were observed from 6 subjects with counts of 9 or more (Table 12.1). If the falls were from a Poisson process, on average the proportion of falls among persons with a count of 9 or more would be .000077, compared with the observed proportion of .205 (61/297). (Methods for generating expected counts and proportions were described in Chapter 4.) Among controls one count of 45 was observed and subjects with 9 or more falls accounted for a third of all falls (132/398 = .332) compared with an expected proportion of .0005. It would be reasonable to ask whether the count of 45 is even plausible. In addition to helping the analyst, something like Table 12.1 can be helpful to the reader of a study, because it reveals much more than the rates alone. A table similar to Table 12.1 appeared in the report of the fall trial (Shumway-Cook et al. 2007).

Because the counts vary more (more zero counts, more large counts) than would be expected if they were generated by a single Poisson process within each trial arm, we call these counts overdispersed. The counts violate the assumption that the falls are produced by a constant rate within each group; a constant rate of 1.77 should hardly ever produce counts of 9 or more in a study of this size. The counts violate the assumption of independence; instead of seeing counts that are sprinkled over the subjects by a random Poisson process, we see them bunched, clustered, or correlated within some individuals with large counts. The concepts of independence, constant rate, overdispersion, and clustering are interrelated. The overdispersion shown in the figures might vanish if we were smart enough to better classify study subjects according to their propensity for falling. In this sense over-dispersion is not so much a property of the data as it is a reflection of our ignorance about predicting falls. Lack of independence or extra-Poisson variation do not necessarily

TABLE 12.1 Number of persons according to the number of falls they had during a randomized controlled trial that compared persons assigned to an exercise program with a control group. Follow-up time was 1 year for all persons except for 13 subjects who dropped out early, as described in footnotes.

COUNT OF FALLS DURING FOLLOW-UP	EXERCISE N = 226 NO. (%)	CONTROL N = 227 NO. (%)
0[a]	102 (45)	97 (43)
1[b]	56 (25)	59 (26)
2[c]	37 (16)	29 (13)
3	12 (5)	12 (5)
4	3 (1)	12 (5)
5[d]	5 (2)	5 (2)
6	3 (1)	3 (1)
7	1 (0)	2 (1)
8	1 (0)	1 (0)
9	3 (1)	3 (1)
10	1 (0)	0 (0)
11	1 (0)	0 (0)
13	1 (0)	1 (0)
20	0 (0)	1 (0)
27	0 (0)	1 (0)
45	0 (0)	1 (0)

[a] Four persons in the exercise group had follow-up of .108, .152, .308, .860 years. Two persons in the control group had follow-up of .001, .078 years.
[b] Two persons in the exercise group had follow-up of .759 and .798 years.
[c] One person in the exercise group had follow-up of .683 years. One person in the control group had follow-up of .458 years.
[d] One person in the control group had follow-up of .997 years.

reflect anything intrinsic about falls; rather, these concepts are descriptions of reasons for not relying on Poisson assumptions to estimate quantities such as the SE, P-values, and confidence-intervals.

Other graphical methods can be used to assess whether rates are better described on a multiplicative (ratio or log scale) or an additive (difference or linear scale). One example was in Figure 11.2. Chapter 21 shows how this can be done for a set of predicted rates after fitting a regression model and applying marginal methods.

12.2 GOODNESS OF FIT TESTS: DEVIANCE AND PEARSON STATISTICS

In addition to graphic and tabular examination of the count data we can use goodness of fit tests, starting with the Poisson regression model for a rate ratio:

```
. poisson fallcnt exercise, irr exp(time) nolog
```

```
Poisson regression                              Number of obs  =        453
                                                LR chi2(1)     =      13.90
                                                Prob > chi2    =     0.0002
Log likelihood = -1045.5595                     Pseudo R2      =     0.0066
```

```
-------------------------------------------------------------------------
  fallcnt |       IRR    Std. Err.      z    P>|z|     [95% Conf. Interval]
----------+--------------------------------------------------------------
 exercise |  .7524891    .0576996   -3.71   0.000     .6474877    .8745183
    _cons |  1.772553    .0888501   11.42   0.000     1.606691    1.955537
 ln(time) |         1   (exposure)
-------------------------------------------------------------------------
```

```
. estat gof
```

```
      Deviance goodness-of-fit  =  1434.583
      Prob > chi2(451)          =    0.0000

      Pearson goodness-of-fit   =  2816.012
      Prob > chi2(451)          =    0.0000
```

In this output, the rate ratio that compares the exercise group with the control group is 0.75. Poisson regression will produce the correct estimate of association even when the data are not from a Poisson process. The goodness-of-fit statistics are both large, with miniscule P-values, suggesting that these data did not arise from a Poisson process. This means the SEs are not correct and consequently the P-values and the CIs are not correct. The deviance statistic is equal to twice the maximum possible likelihood of a saturated model with an observation for each trial participant minus twice the likelihood of the fitted model: deviance = 2 x [ln(maximum fitted likelihood) − ln(model likelihood)]. The deviance for a Poisson model can be calculated from Expression 12.1 (Breslow and Day 1987 p137, McCullagh and Nelder 1989 pp33–34, Lindsey 1997 p210) without actually fitting the saturated model:

$$\text{Deviance} = 2 \times \text{sum}[C_i \times \ln(C_i/(\text{fitted count})) - C_i + (\text{fitted count})] \qquad (\text{Ex.12.1})$$

The deviance is well named, as it is a measure of how much the model predicted counts deviate from the observed counts. The fitted counts in Expression 12.1 are the model predicted counts per 1 time unit multiplied by the observed time for each subject; these equal the rates per 1 person-year for the exercise (1.33) and control (1.77) subjects followed for a year. For a control subject followed for 0.5 years, the fitted count is 0.5 x 1.77. When the observed count is 0 for an observation, $0 \times \ln(0/(\text{mean count}))$ is considered to equal 0 and for that observation the expression reduces to 2 x the fitted count. Fitted counts are also called expected or predicted counts. For the trial subjects, the deviance statistic for the Poisson model is 1434, which is treated as a chi-squared statistic with degrees of freedom equal to the number of records (453) minus the number of model terms, including the constant term: degrees of freedom = 453−2 = 451. The deviance is compared with the chi-squared distribution to obtain a P-value. For the falls data the fit is awful because the observed counts are often far from the predicted counts (Figures 12.1 and 12.2); these data are not from a Poisson process. We have used the deviance statistic for a Poisson model; for other models, such as the logistic model, the deviance statistic has a different formula.

The Pearson goodness-of-fit statistic is calculated by comparing the observed and expected counts using Expression 12.2:

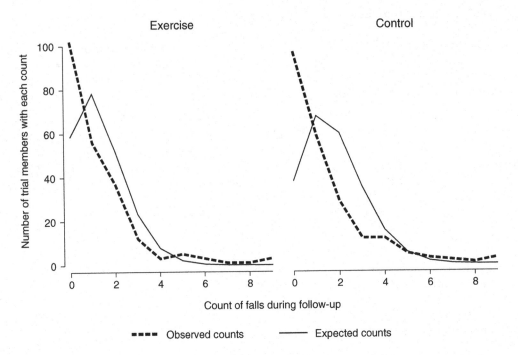

FIGURE 12.1 Observed distribution of fall counts from a randomized controlled trial of an exercise program among elderly adults. Also shown are the expected counts from a Poisson process with a rate of 1.33 per person-year for the exercise group and a rate of 1.77 for the control group. Fall counts as large as 45 were observed, but counts greater than 9 are omitted from the graphs.

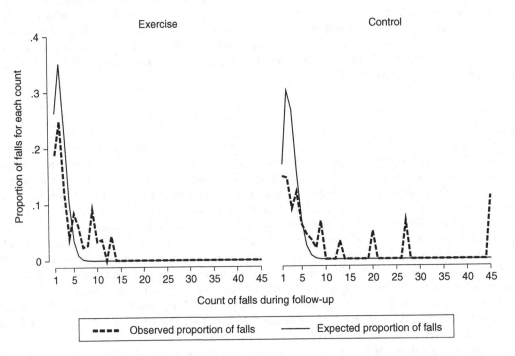

FIGURE 12.2 Observed proportions of fall events; the number of falls for each per-person count of falls divided by the total number of falls. Data from a randomized controlled trial of an exercise program among elderly adults. Also shown are the expected proportions from a Poisson process with a rate of 1.33 per person-year for the exercise group and a rate of 1.77 for the control group.

$$\text{Chi--squared} = \text{sum}\left[(\text{Observed count}_i - \text{Expected count}_i)^2/(\text{Expected count}_i)\right] \qquad \text{(Ex.12.2)}$$
$$= \text{sum}\left[(C_i - \text{Exp}_i)^2/\text{Exp}_i\right]$$

The expected counts in Expression 12.2 are just the same as the fitted (model predicted) counts in Expression 12.1. We called them expected counts here because that terminology is often used for Pearson chi-squared tests and that terminology was used in Chapter 4. The Pearson statistic is 2816, nearly twice the size of the deviance statistic. To obtain a P-value the statistic is compared with a chi-squared distribution for 451 degrees of freedom. Which fit statistic should we prefer? As with the Pearson chi-squared statistic for a 2 x k contingency table, small expected counts make this statistic unreliable. Having expected counts < 5 is often a rule of thumb for not using this statistic. In the falls data, many expected (predicted or fitted) counts were less than 5. If the degrees of freedom is large, as it is here, the Pearson statistic may not perform well (Scribney 1997). Hilbe (2014 pp78–79) argues that the Pearson statistic should be used to assess dispersion, which I will discuss later, not goodness-of-fit.

12.3 A CONDITIONAL MOMENT CHI-SQUARED TEST OF FIT

Andrews (Andrews 1988a, 1988b) described a modification of Pearson's chi-squared test which accounts for the uncertainty of the model estimates. This test has been described in textbooks (Cameron and Trivedi 2005 pp266–267, 2013a pp193–196) and implemented in a Stata command for count models, **chi2gof** (Manjón and Martínez 2014). The command allows the user to categorize the outcome counts into strata and then test the null hypothesis that the frequency distribution of the observed counts matches the frequency distribution of the model predicted counts. It is best to use strata in which the counts are not too small. This command can be used after Stata's **poisson** and **nbreg** (negative binomial regression) commands. When the command is used after the Poisson regression model for the fall count data, and if cell counts of 0, 1, 2, … , 7, and 8 or more are chosen as the strata, the output looks like this:

```
. chi2gof, cells(9) table

Chi-square Goodness-of-Fit Test for Poisson Model:

    Chi-square chi2(8)  =  124.40
    Prob>chi2           =    0.00
```

Cells	Abs. Freq.	Rel. Freq.	Fitted Rel. Freq.	Abs. Dif.
0	199	.4393	.2166	.2227
1	115	.2539	.3262	.0724
2	66	.1457	.2507	.105
3	24	.053	.131	.078
4	15	.0331	.0524	.0192
5	10	.0221	.017	.005
6	6	.0132	.0047	.0085
7	3	.0066	.0011	.0055
8 or more	13	.0331	2.9e-04	.0328

In this output, we see the counts of subjects in the Abs(olute) Freq(uency) column, who had fall counts of 0, 1, … , up to 8 or more. For example, 199 subjects had 0 falls and 115 had 1 fall. The next column shows the relative frequencies; these are observed proportions of subjects in each fall-count stratum. The table then lists the predicted proportions, or fitted relative frequencies, from the Poisson model. The output shows that the Poisson model predicts fewer 0 counts than were observed, and more counts of 1, 2, 3, and 4 falls. This was shown in Figure 12.1, but the **chi2gof** command has the advantage of producing this information with just a few key strokes. Unfortunately, the command only works for ratio models.

12.4 LIMITATIONS OF GOODNESS-OF-FIT STATISTICS

The large deviance and Pearson statistics tell us that given the fitted model, the data do not appear to arise from a Poisson process. This does not mean that the data could not have been generated by several Poisson processes. An analyst might be able to add variables to the model, possibly including interaction terms, and create a model in which the data could be from a Poisson process within each of several covariate patterns. The many zero counts and the few large counts might be explained by a set of variables that allows for different fall propensities. But if the goal is to estimate the association between the exercise program and the fall outcomes, this more complete model is not relevant. Given that goal, the deviance and Pearson statistics are useful because they warn us that the Poisson SE is not valid.

The size of goodness-of-fit statistics will change if we group the data differently in the records used for analysis (Scribney 1997). The Poisson model shown earlier used the fall counts and person-time information (Table 12.1) for each of the 453 persons in the trial. But we could collapse the data according to sex (or any other grouping variable), creating the four records in Table 12.2. If we fit the same Poisson rate ratio model shown earlier, using these four records only, the regression coefficients are identical. The deviance, however, shrinks to 13.00, with a P-value, using three degrees of freedom, of .0015. The Pearson statistic changes to 13.72, close to the deviance value, with a P-value of .0010. The fit is now better, because the rates in Table 12.2 range only modestly from 1.26 to 2.28, compared with the range from 0 to 45 (Figures 12.1 and 12.2) using individual records. If we collapse these data further into a single record for each trial arm, the rate ratio and SE from the regression model will remain the same, but the deviance and Pearson statistics will be equal to zero, with no P-value. Collapsing the data into fewer records removes evidence of the variation in rates that produced the large goodness-of fit-statistics.

Regrouping of data into fewer records can also influence the size of goodness-of-fit statistics in logistic regression (Simonoff 1998, Belloco and Algeri 2013). With Poisson regression, regrouping the data into fewer records may hide variation in the counts and reduce the size of the fit statistics. With

TABLE 12.2   Counts and person-time from a randomized controlled trial that compared persons assigned to an exercise program with a control group. These data are the same as those in Table 12.1, collapsed into four records by trial arm and sex.

TRIAL ARM	SEX	COUNT OF FALLS DURING FOLLOW-UP	PERSON-YEARS	RATE PER PERSON-YEAR
Exercise	Women	216	172.048	1.26
Exercise	Men	81	50.620	1.60
Control	Women	275	170.535	1.61
Control	Men	123	54.000	2.28

logistic regression, grouping records into a few categories can reveal variation in risks that will increase the deviance compared with using individual records; Simonoff (Simonoff 1998) gives an example using data from the sinking of the *Titanic*.

12.5 MEASURES OF DISPERSION

Dividing the deviance and Pearson statistics by the model degrees of freedom can help assess whether data are under or over-dispersed. These ratios should be close to 1 for equidispersed data, greater than 1 if the data are overdispersed, and less than 1 if the data are underdispersed. For the regression model shown earlier, the dispersion statistic based upon the deviance is 1435.5/451 = 3.18 and the dispersion from the Pearson statistic is 6.24. Both of these ratios suggest a lot of overdispersion. Both dispersion statistics will change in size depending upon how the data are grouped, as described previously.

If the data are indeed from a Poisson distribution, then on average the difference between the observed and expected counts squared, divided by the expected counts (Expression 12.2), will be described by the standard normal distribution. The area under that distribution is 1, so when the data are from a Poisson distribution the average value for the Pearson goodness-of-fit statistic will be 1 for each record and the statistic will be equal to 1 multiplied by the number of records. Dividing that sum by the degrees of freedom will be close to 1 unless there are few records or a great many variables in the model relative to the number of records.

Which is better? Hilbe (2014 p43) prefers the Pearson dispersion statistic, arguing that in simulation studies that he has performed, it is close to 1.0, on average, when the data are from a Poisson process, whereas the dispersion measure based upon the deviance is slightly larger, with values ranging from 1.03 to 1.13.

Another way to study dispersion is to compare the expected and observed variance of the counts. If the counts are from a Poisson process, the mean count and its variance are the same (Formula 2 in Table 4.4), so the variance of the mean count for the control group should be 1.77. We can use Expression 4.2 to get the variance for the observed counts, weighting the counts by each subject's follow-up time, and modifying the formula in Expression 4.2 to divide by n–1 instead of n. The result is a variance of 16.71. Since the variance of the observed rates is much greater than the expected Poisson variance, the counts are overdispersed. This method is easy for a model that just compares two rates but would become complicated for a model with several variables.

12.6 ROBUST VARIANCE ESTIMATOR AS A TEST OF FIT

Since the fall events do not appear to arise from a Poisson process, one excellent remedy for this problem is to use a robust variance estimator, which does not assume the counts fit a Poisson distribution. Details about this estimator will be discussed in Chapter 13. Here we just note that the SE for the constant term, which is the rate among the controls, in the Poisson model previously shown, was 0.0889. When the robust variance estimator is applied just to the control data the SE becomes 0.2727. The variance for the control rates using the robust variance estimator for a regression model with rates only from the control group is 16.70, close to the variance of 16.71 reported in the preceding paragraph about a weighted variance from Expression 4.2.

Because the robust estimator can correct the SE when the data are not from a Poisson process, this solution can be used to identify the problem. First fit a Poisson model and then fit the same model using the robust variance. Finding a noteworthy difference between the Poisson and robust SEs, or CIs, acts like a canary in a coal mine, suggesting that a problem exists, even before any examination of the deviance, dispersion statistics, or count distributions.

12.7 COMPARING MODELS USING THE DEVIANCE

Chapter 9 reviewed the use of the likelihood ratio test to compare models. This involves computing the ln of the ratio of two likelihoods, one for a larger or fuller model, the other for a smaller or reduced model with fewer variables. The models to be compared with this test have the same link and distribution family, are applied to the same data, and share a common set of variables, except that the full model has one or more additional variables. The reduced model is described as nested within the full model. The ratio of the two log likelihoods is compared with a chi-squared distribution with degrees of freedom equal to the number of additional variables in the full model. The likelihood ratio statistic is equivalent to the difference in the deviance statistics of the two models (McCullagh and Nelder 1989 pp118–119, Greenland 2008b p426), as described in Expression 12.3:

$$
\begin{aligned}
\text{Likelihood ratio statistic} &= -2 \times \ln(\text{likelihood}_{\text{reduced}}/\text{likelihood}_{\text{full}}) \\
&= -2 \times [\ln(\text{likelihood}_{\text{reduced}}) - \ln(\text{likelihood}_{\text{full}})] \\
&= \text{deviance}_{\text{reduced}} - \text{deviance}_{\text{full}} \\
&= \text{deviance statistic comparing the two models}
\end{aligned}
$$

(Ex.12.3)

The validity of this test depends upon several assumptions (McCullagh and Nelder 1989 pp118–119, Greenland 2008b p426). The number of observations must be large enough to justify the use of maximum likelihood methods. The choice of error family (residual distribution) should be correct. This assumption, as we have shown, was violated when the Poisson rate ratio model was applied to the fall data. The full regression model should be approximately correct in some sense.

The deviance goodness-of-fit statistic described previously is just a likelihood ratio test that compares the fitted (reduced) model with a full model that is saturated, meaning that the full model has so many terms that it reproduces the observed data. The use of deviance tests to compare models is analogous to the use of F-tests to compare linear regression models.

12.8 COMPARING MODELS USING AKAIKE AND BAYESIAN INFORMATION CRITERION

Information criteria can be used to compare models that are applied to the same data, but differ in the variables used, the link function, or the choice of error family. We may wish, for example, to compare a model for rates that is multiplicative (a rate ratio model) with a model for rates that is additive (a rate difference model). We can fit both models using the Poisson error distribution but use the log link for the ratio model and the identity link for the difference model. Or we can fit a rate difference model with an identity link but compare a version with the Poisson error distribution with a model that uses the normal distribution. Two commonly used statistics (Hilbe 2014 pp116–122), the Akaike Information Criterion (AIC) (Lindsey and Jones 1998) and the Bayesian Information Criterion (BIC) (Schwarz 1976), both use the ln(likelihood) to assess model fit. As the number of model terms increases, the ln(likelihood) increases, so reliance on the likelihood alone would always lead us to favor the more complex model with more terms. To compensate for this, both the AIC and the BIC contain penalties for making the model more complex.

The formula for the AIC differs across textbooks and statistical software packages; depending on the formula used, a larger or smaller AIC indicates superior model fit. Stata uses Expression 12.4, with a smaller AIC indicating better fit.

$$\text{Akaike Information Criterion(AIC)} = -2 \times \ln(\text{likelihood}) + 2 \times \text{model degrees of freedom}$$
$$= -2 \times \ln(\text{likelihood}) + 2 \times \text{number of model variables}$$

(Ex.12.4)

The model degrees of freedom is the number of model variables, including the constant (intercept) term. In Expression 12.4, the AIC becomes smaller as the model ln(likelihood) increases, indicating better fit to the data. We expect fit will improve as the number of variables is increased, so the statistic penalizes any improvement by adding a term equal to 2 x the number of model variables. The AIC statistic will shrink if the ln(likelihood) becomes greater by 1 or more for each variable added to a model.

Stata's **glm** command reports a different AIC statistic, Expression 12.5, which is the AIC as defined in Expression 12.4, divided by the number of observations. This is the change in AIC per observation or record and I will call this the AIC per record:

AIC reported by **glm**

$= \text{AIC per record}$

(Ex.12.5)

$= (-2 \times \ln(\text{likelihood}) + 2 \times \text{number of model variables})/\text{number of records}$

Additional modifications of the AIC have been described (Hilbe 2014 pp116–119).

To compare two models using either the AIC or BIC, the likelihood functions of both models should define outcome events in the same way. For example, the Cox proportional hazards model does not define outcome events in the same way as the Poisson regression model, so comparing these models using information criteria would not be valid. If we compare Poisson regression models with other parametric models for count data, this is usually not a concern.

The BIC penalizes the likelihood by the ln of the number of observations multiplied by the number of variables. Expression 12.6 is used by Stata software:

Bayesian Information Criterion(BIC)

$= -2 \times \ln(\text{likelihood}) + \ln(\text{number of observations}) \times \text{model degrees of freedom}$ (Ex.12.6)

$= -2 \times \ln(\text{likelihood}) + \ln(\text{number of observations}) \times \text{number of model variables}$

Stata's **glm** command reports a different version of the BIC based upon the deviance (Hilbe 2014 pp121–122) rather than the likelihood. I will call this the deviance BIC:

BIC reported by **glm**

$= \text{deviance BIC}$

$= \text{deviance} - \ln(\text{number of observations}) \times (\text{number of observations} - \text{number of variables})$

$= \text{deviance} - \ln(\text{number of observations}) \times (\text{model degrees of freedom})$

(Ex.12.7)

A smaller BIC (Expression 12.6 or 12.7) indicates better model fit. The BIC (Expression 12.6) will shrink if, for each additional variable, the ln(likelihood) increases by a quantity greater than 2 multiplied by the natural log of the number of observations in the data. The definition of the number of observations in the data is not always obvious for several reasons. For example, if you have 1000 records but you consider them to be clustered into 100 groups, within which there is no variation, then there are really only 100 independent observations; you have to decide whether to use 1000 or 100 to calculate the BIC. Stata software discusses this topic in the help files for the BIC statistic. In addition, the size of the AIC and BIC will vary depending upon how many records are used to describe the outcome counts and person-time information; regrouping the data can change both the size of the ln(likelihood) and the number of observations.

Should we prefer the AIC or the BIC? If we are comparing models that differ with regard to the link function or the error family, or both, the choice of AIC or BIC makes no practical difference. Both statistics will rely upon the same likelihoods and use the same number of observations, so picking the lower value for either statistic should result in the same choice. This is equivalent to picking the model with the largest likelihood, the largest ln likelihood, or the smallest deviance. If information criteria are used to select among candidate variables for inclusion in a model, the AIC will admit a variable with $P < .16$ for a continuous or binary variable, whereas the BIC will use a P-value cutoff of about .05 for 50 observations and smaller P-values as the sample size increases (Vittinghoff et al. 2012 p398). Which behavior you prefer may vary with your goals.

12.9 EXAMPLE 1: USING STATA'S GENERALIZED LINEAR MODEL COMMAND TO DECIDE BETWEEN A RATE RATIO OR A RATE DIFFERENCE MODEL FOR THE RANDOMIZED CONTROLLED TRIAL OF EXERCISE AND FALLS

Earlier in this chapter Stata's **poisson** command was used to produce a rate ratio for falls of trial subjects (Table 12.1) randomized to an exercise program compared with a control group. If we use the generalized linear model command, **glm**, to fit the same model, additional information about model fit is reported:

```
. glm fallcnt exercise, link(log) family(poisson) exp(time) eform nolog
```

```
Generalized linear models                No. of obs       =        453
Optimization      : ML                   Residual df      =        451
                                         Scale parameter  =          1
Deviance        = 1434.583364            (1/df) Deviance  =   3.180894
Pearson         = 2816.011836            (1/df) Pearson   =   6.243929
Variance function: V(u) = u [Poisson]
Link function    : g(u) = ln(u)          [Log]
                                         AIC              =   4.624987
Log likelihood   = -1045.559496          BIC              = -1323.684
```

```
              |                OIM
    fallcnt   |    IRR     Std. Err.      z     P>|z|    [95% Conf. Interval]
--------------+----------------------------------------------------------------
    exercise  | .7524891   .0576996    -3.71    0.000    .6474877    .8745183
       _cons  | 1.772553   .0888501    11.42    0.000    1.606691    1.955537
    ln(time)  |        1   (exposure)
--------------+----------------------------------------------------------------
```

. estat ic
Akaike's information criterion and Bayesian information criterion

```
------------------------------------------------------------------------------
     Model |     Obs    ll(null)  ll(model)     df        AIC          BIC
-----------+------------------------------------------------------------------
         . |    1022       .      -2089.599      2     4183.198     4193.057
------------------------------------------------------------------------------
```

The **glm** command reports both the deviance and Pearson goodness-of-fit statistics by default; these are identical to the statistics reported by the **estat gof** command after we fit the poisson rate ratio model. To obtain P-values for the null hypothesis of good fit, these statistics can be compared with a chi-squared distribution with 451 degrees of freedom. The **glm** command reports both the deviance and Pearson dispersion statistics. The AIC per record (Expression 12.5) and deviance BIC (Expression 12.7) are shown by default in the header. To obtain the AIC using Expression 12.4 and the BIC using Expression 12.6, we can use the **estat ic** (**estat** for estimation statistics, **ic** for information criteria) command after fitting the model, as shown earlier.

Now fit the rate difference model. Recall from Chapter 10 that we can do this by using the rate as the outcome and introducing person-time as an importance weight:

. glm rate exercise [iweight=time], link(identity) family(poisson) nolog
note: rate has noninteger values

```
Generalized linear models                    No. of obs      =        453
Optimization       : ML                      Residual df     =        451
                                             Scale parameter =          1
Deviance           = 1434.583364             (1/df) Deviance = 3.180894
Pearson            = 2816.01188              (1/df) Pearson  = 6.243929

Variance function : V(u) = u                 [Poisson]
Link function      : g(u) = u                [Identity]

                                             AIC             = 4.620079
Log likelihood     = -1044.447971            BIC             = -1323.684
```

```
------------------------------------------------------------------------------
         |                OIM
    rate |    Coef.    Std. Err.      z     P>|z|    [95% Conf. Interval]
---------+--------------------------------------------------------------------
exercise | -.4387262   .1178327    -3.72    0.000   -.6696741   -.2077783
   _cons |  1.772553   .0888501    19.95    0.000    1.59841     1.946696
------------------------------------------------------------------------------
```

```
. estat ic

Akaike's information criterion and Bayesian information criterion

- - - - - - - - - - - - - - - - - - - - - - - - - - - - - - - - - - - - - - - -
     Model |    Obs   ll(null)   ll(model)    df        AIC          BIC
- - - - - - - + - - - - - - - - - - - - - - - - - - - - - - - - - - - - - - - -
         . |   1022       .     -2040.648     2     4085.296    4095.155
- - - - - - - - - - - - - - - - - - - - - - - - - - - - - - - - - - - - - - - -
```

The header information for the rate ratio and rate difference models are nearly identical. The rate difference model warns us that the rate outcomes are not counts; we can ignore this warning. The deviance and Pearson statistics are identical for the ratio and difference models (Table 12.3), as are the dispersion statistics and deviance BIC that are based upon those measures. The ln likelihoods are slightly different, as are the three information criteria that use the ln likelihood in their formulae. Because both models were fit to the same data, and the deviance and fit statistics are identical, the models really should have the same ln likelihood statistics. The small differences in the ln likelihoods arose because the convergence algorithm did not quite achieve the same maximum likelihood for each model. The ratio model used the canonical link, meaning the log link for the Poisson error family; we can usually expect good convergence for this model. The difference model, which used the identity link, faced a tougher chore and consequently we ended up with a small difference in maximum likelihood. Basically, there are no important differences between the two models. Both show poor fit and overdispersion, neither is clearly superior.

These results were expected. When we compare the crude (unadjusted) rates for two groups, it should not make any substantial difference whether we carry out the comparison by using the ratio or difference of the two rates. In the regression tables, the Z-statistics differ notably for the constant (intercept) term.

TABLE 12.3 Fit statistics for two models used to compare the fall rates of persons in a randomized controlled trial of exercise to prevent falls. Study data in Table 12.1. One model estimated the rate ratio using a log link and the other model estimated the rate difference using an identity link. The difference column shows the rate ratio model statistic minus the rate difference model statistic.

MODEL STATISTIC	RATE RATIO MODEL	RATE DIFFERENCE MODEL	DIFFERENCE
Deviance	1434.58	1434.58	0
Deviance P-value for fit	.0	.0	0
Pearson statistic	2816.01	2816.01	0
Pearson P-value for fit	.0	.0	0
Deviance/degrees of freedom	3.18	3.18	0
Pearson/degrees of freedom	6.24	6.24	0
Ln(likelihood)	−1045.559	−1044.448	−1.11
AIC (Expression 12.4)	2095.12	2092.90	2.22
AIC per record (Expression 12.5)	4.625	4.620	.005
BIC (Expression 12.6)	2103.35	2101.13	2.22
Deviance BIC (Expression 12.7)	−1323.68	−1323.68	0
Poisson SE for exercise term	0.06	0.12	a
Robust SE for exercise term	0.14	0.31	a
Poisson Z-statistic for exercise term	−3.7086	−3.7233	.015
Robust Z-statistic for exercise term	−1.534	−1.436	−098

[a] Differences in model SEs for the rate ratio and rate difference are not relevant. What matters is the difference in the Poisson and robust SEs for the same model.

Recall from Chapter 9 that the Z-statistic of 11.42 from the rate ratio model is for a comparison of the rate of 1.77 with a rate of 1, while the Z-statistic of 19.95 from the rate difference model is for a comparison of the rate of 1.77 with a rate of 0. Because 1.77 is further from 0 than 1, the rate difference model reports a larger Z-statistic for the constant term. For the exercise term, 0.75 in the ratio model and –0.44 in the difference model, which is compared with the rate of 1.77 in both models, the Z-statistics are almost the same, –3.71 and –3.72 (Table 12.3). When only one binary variable is used, fitting a ratio or a difference model for rates is a matter of convenience or preference, not model fit.

The statistics for both models suggest poor fit and overdispersion. To correct this problem, a robust variance estimator can be used by adding the option **vce(robust)**.

```
. glm fallcnt exercise, link(log) family(poisson) exp(time) eform nolog
vce(robust)

Generalized linear models                    No. of obs       =       453
Optimization      : ML                       Residual df      =       451
                                             Scale parameter =         1
Deviance          = 1434.583364              (1/df) Deviance =  3.180894
Pearson           = 2816.011836              (1/df) Pearson  =  6.243929

Variance function: V(u) = u                  [Poisson]
Link function     : g(u) = ln(u)             [Log]

                                             AIC              =  4.624987
Log pseudolikelihood = -1045.559496          BIC              = -1323.684

------------------------------------------------------------------------------
             |               Robust
     fallcnt |       IRR   Std. Err.       z    P>|z|     [95% Conf. Interval]
-------------+----------------------------------------------------------------
    exercise |  .7524891   .1394513    -1.53   0.125     .5233058    1.082044
       _cons |  1.772553   .2724257     3.72   0.000     1.311527    2.395639
    ln(time) |         1  (exposure)
------------------------------------------------------------------------------
```

Using a robust variance changes nothing in the header information, except that the log likelihood is now called a log pseudolikelihood; the deviance, AIC, and other statistics are unchanged. The rate ratio is unchanged. The only thing that changed is the SE and the statistics derived from this: Z, P, and the CI. The 95% CI has now increased from 0.65, 0.87 to 0.52, 1.08. This is the regression table output from the rate difference model using the robust variance:

```
. glm rate exercise [iweight=time], link(identity) family(poisson) nolog
vce(robust)
(output omitted)

------------------------------------------------------------------------------
             |               Robust
        rate |     Coef.   Std. Err.       z    P>|z|     [95% Conf. Interval]
-------------+----------------------------------------------------------------
    exercise | -.4387262   .3054377    -1.44   0.151    -1.037373     .1599206
       _cons |  1.772553   .2724257     6.51   0.000     1.238609    2.306498
------------------------------------------------------------------------------
```

The Z-statistic from the rate difference model is −1.44, not very different from the value of −1.53 for the rate ratio model. The P-values are similar. The robust SEs and CIs for both the ratio or the difference model are much larger than those from the models that assumed a Poisson process (Table 12.3). These changes indicate poor model fit using the Poisson error family. Both the rate ratio and rate difference are unbiased in this example. Poor model fit just means that SEs based upon Poisson assumptions are not reliable, a problem that is remedied by using the robust variance.

12.10 EXAMPLE 2: A RATE RATIO OR A RATE DIFFERENCE MODEL FOR HYPOTHETICAL DATA REGARDING THE ASSOCIATION BETWEEN FALL RATES AND AGE

Consider a slightly more complicated example. I created data for 1022 subjects who ranged in age from 65 to 90 years. The number of subjects decreased as age increased. Stata's **rpoisson** function was used to create pseudo-random counts of fall events from a Poisson distribution with a mean count of 1 at age 65 years. The mean count of this Poisson distribution increased linearly by 0.4 for each 1-year increase in age; mean count = 1 + 0.4 × (age − 65). It was assumed that everyone was followed for 1 year, so the fall rate per person-year for each subject was their randomly generated fall count divided by 1. On average this method will produce data in which the mean rate of falling increases linearly by 0.4 falls per person-year for each 1-year increase in age. A single simulated data set was created. The output below shows results from a rate ratio model applied to these data. This model assumes that the rate increase was linear on a ln scale:

```
. glm fallcnt age, link(log) family(poisson) exp(time) eform nolog
Generalized linear models                    No. of obs      =       1022
Optimization      : ML                       Residual df     =       1020
                                             Scale parameter =          1
Deviance          =  1130.89274              (1/df) Deviance =   1.108718
Pearson           =  1032.103235             (1/df) Pearson  =   1.011866

Variance function : V(u) = u                 [Poisson]
Link function     : g(u) = ln(u)             [Log]

                                             AIC             =   4.093149
Log likelihood    = -2089.598996             BIC             =  -5937.214

- - - - - - - - - - - - - - - - - - - - - - - - - - - - - - - - - - - - - - -
             |                OIM
     fallcnt |      IRR   Std. Err.       z    P>|z|     [95% Conf. Interval]
- - - - - - -+- - - - - - - - - - - - - - - - - - - - - - - - - - - - - - - -
         age |  1.085055   .0025505    34.73   0.000     1.080068    1.090066
       _cons |  .0097724   .0017493   -25.85   0.000     .0068807    .0138795
    ln(time) |        1   (exposure)
- - - - - - - - - - - - - - - - - - - - - - - - - - - - - - - - - - - - - - -
```

TABLE 12.4 Fit statistics for two models used to estimate how the rate of falling was associated with increasing age. Hypothetical data created for 1022 persons assuming a Poisson process with a linear increase in fall rate of 0.4 falls per year for each 1-year increment in age. One model estimated the rate ratio using a log link and the other model estimated the rate difference using an identity link. The difference column shows the rate ratio model statistic minus the rate difference model statistic.

MODEL STATISTIC	RATE RATIO MODEL	RATE DIFFERENCE MODEL	DIFFERENCE
Deviance	1130.89	1032.99	97.90
Deviance P-value for fit	.01	.38	−.37
Pearson statistic	1032.1	952.3	79.8
Pearson P-value for fit	.39	.94	−.55
Deviance/degrees of freedom	1.11	1.01	0.10
Pearson/degrees of freedom	1.01	0.93	0.08
Ln(likelihood)	−2090	−2041	−49
AIC (Expression 12.4)	4183.20	4085.30	97.90
AIC per record (Expression 12.5)	4.1	4.0	0.1
BIC (Expression 12.6)	4193.06	4095.16	97.90
Deviance BIC (Expression 12.7)	−5937.21	−6035.12	97.90
Poisson SE for age term	.00255	.0116	[a]
Robust SE for age term	.00277	.0113	[a]
Poisson Z-statistic for age term	34.73	34.41	0.32
Robust Z-statistic for age term	31.92	35.37	−3.45

[a] Differences in model SEs for the rate ratio and rate difference are not relevant. What matters is the difference in the robust and Poisson SEs for the same model.

There is only one explanatory variable, age in years as a continuous term, in the model above. This model describes the association on a multiplicative scale and estimates that the fall rate increases by a ratio equal to 1.085 for each additional year of age. A chi-squared test of the deviance, 1130.89 on 1020 degrees of freedom, produced a P-value of .009, evidence that the fit is not optimal (Table 12.4). The Pearson statistic, 1032, produced a P-value of .4, suggesting a satisfactory fit. In this instance, the deviance statistic did a better job of recognizing that these data are not linear on the ln (multiplicative) scale. The deviance divided by degrees of freedom is 1.11, consistent with some overdispersion, but the Pearson dispersion statistic of 1.01 suggests no overdispersion. Negative binomial regression will be discussed in Chapter 17, but here I note that when a negative binomial model was fit to these data, the estimated association with age was a rate ratio of 1.086 (95% CI 1.081, 1.091), similar to the estimate from the Poisson ratio model. Negative binomial regression can be used to deal with overdispersed count data, but it is of little help here as overdispersion is not the problem.

Next fit a model that assumes a linear rate difference:

```
. glm rate age [iweight=time], link(identity) family(poisson) nolog

Generalized linear models                    No. of obs       =      1022
Optimization       : ML                      Residual df      =      1020
                                             Scale parameter =         1
Deviance        = 1032.990882               (1/df) Deviance = 1.012736
Pearson         =  952.320978               (1/df) Pearson   =  .933648

Variance function : V(u) = u                 [Poisson]
Link function     : g(u) = u                 [Identity]
```

```
                                          AIC          =  3.997354
Log likelihood    = -2040.648067          BIC          = -6035.116

- - - - - - - - - - - - - - - - - - - - - - - - - - - - - - - - - - - - - - - -
             |                OIM
     rate    |    Coef.   Std. Err.       z     P>|z|      [95% Conf. Interval]
- - - - - - -+- - - - - - - - - - - - - - - - - - - - - - - - - - - - - - - - -
      age    |  .3984845   .0115817    34.41    0.000     .3757848    .4211843
    _cons    | -24.80449   .8110135   -30.58    0.000    -26.39405   -23.21493
- - - - - - - - - - - - - - - - - - - - - - - - - - - - - - - - - - - - - - - -
```

This model estimated that for each 1-year increment in age, the fall rate increased by 0.398, close to the true age effect of 0.400 falls per person-year used to produce the data. The deviance chi-squared P-value of .4 offers no evidence of poor fit (Table 12.4). The dispersion statistics are both close to 1. The ln likelihood is larger with this model and all the information criteria, which are based upon the ln likelihood, favor this rate difference model compared with the rate ratio model. The difference in the deviance, 97.90, is the same as the difference for 3 of the information criteria. This indicates that both models are using the same estimate for the likelihood of the saturated model. This is different from the previous example where the deviance statistics were identical, but the ln likelihoods differed. These hypothetical data were generated on the linear (difference) scale, which made it easier to fit a model using the identity link. In summary, all the statistics favor the rate difference model.

For the rate difference model, the Poisson and robust SEs are similar and the Z-statistics for these models are close (Table 12.4). This suggests that when the identity link is used, the SE based upon

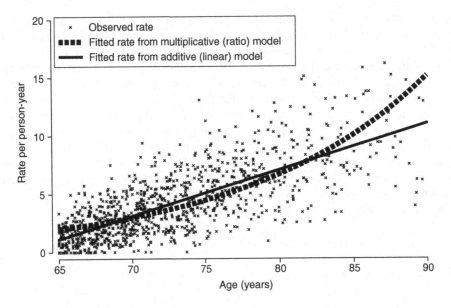

FIGURE 12.3   Hypothetical data for 1022 subjects who were followed for 1 year. Counts of fall events for each hypothetical subject were generated from a pseudo-random Poisson process in which the true rate of falling was 1 per person-year for persons age 65 years and increased by 0.4 for each additional year of age. Each black mark indicates the fall rate for a single subject. The solid line shows the fitted fall rate from a model which correctly assumed the fall rate changed linearly with age. The dashed line is from a multiplicative (ratio) model fit to the same data.

Poisson assumptions is a reasonable choice. These data really were produced by a Poisson process which generated counts that were linearly related to age and the fit statistics confirm this.

We can show the fit of the two models graphically (Figure 12.3). Interpreting a fitted curve can be perilous, as subjective biases and visual mistakes can fool us. While keeping in mind the possibility of subjective bias, graphical displays are often useful. The rates from the multiplicative (ratio) model seem too high at age 65 years compared with the observed rates. From about age 68 to age 84, the rates predicted by both models are not terribly different. But among the few subjects age 85 and older, the curve from the ratio model seems too high.

12.11 A TEST OF THE MODEL LINK

Example 2 compared a rate ratio model with a log link to a rate difference model with an identity link. The models differed only in their link functions. Stata has a command for testing the model link, **linktest**, based upon an idea suggested by Pregibon in 1979 in a doctoral dissertation (Hilbe 2011 p156). Pregibon later published a revised version of this test (Pregibon 1980, Hardin and Hilbe 2012 pp50–51), but Stata's command implements the earlier, better version.

When the relationship between age and fall rates was modeled on a log (multiplicative or ratio) scale, the predicted event count increased linearly with ln age; see Expression 9.5. Although fit statistics suggested this model was less than perfect, the estimated rate ratio was statistically significant (p < .001) and the fit was fairly decent for most values of age. Figure 12.3 showed rates on the vertical axis, but in this example time was always equal to 1, so rates are identical to counts. Now create a variable equal to the model predicted ln of the counts and use this variable to predict the observed ln fall counts in a new model which also has a log link. If the model fit is adequate, this new predictor variable should be closely related to the fall counts; ideally it would predict them perfectly. We can add more flexibility to the new model by adding a term for the square of the predicted ln counts; a quadratic curve will be fit. If the original model between age and falls really was *linear* on a ln scale, the *quadratic* curve should not be needed. Hence the P-value for the square of the fitted ln counts will be large, indicating that this additional term is superfluous.

To carry out all these steps, start with the rate ratio model:

```
. glm fallcnt age, link(log) family(poisson) exp(time) eform nolog
(output omitted)
```

```
- - - - - - - - - - - - - - - - - - - - - - - - - - - - - - - - - - - - - - - -
              |                OIM
      fallcnt |      IRR   Std. Err.       z    P>|z|     [95% Conf. Interval]
- - - - - - - + - - - - - - - - - - - - - - - - - - - - - - - - - - - - - - - -
          age |  1.085055   .0025505    34.73   0.000     1.080068    1.090066
        _cons |  .0097724   .0017493   -25.85   0.000     .0068807    .0138795
     ln(time) |         1  (exposure)
- - - - - - - - - - - - - - - - - - - - - - - - - - - - - - - - - - - - - - - -
```

Next, calculate the predicted ln of the fall counts (called plncnt, meaning predicted ln count) and the square of each predicted ln count (plncnt2) from the ratio model. Stata's **predict** command with the **xb** option will do the heavy lifting; this prediction accounts for the use of time as an offset, although the offset is not important in this example because time was always 1:

```
. predict double plncnt, xb

. gen double plncnt2 = plncnt^2
```

Then use plncnt and plncnt2 in a model with the ln count of falls as the outcome; the model link (log) and family should be those of the original rate ratio model:

```
. glm fallcnt plncnt plncnt2, link(log) family(poisson) nolog
(output omitted)
```

```
- - - - - - - - - - - - - - - - - - - - - - - - - - - - - - - - - - - - - - - -
            |                OIM
    fallcnt |   Coef.    Std. Err.     z     P>|z|      [95% Conf. Interval]
- - - - - - +- - - - - - - - - - - - - - - - - - - - - - - - - - - - - - - - - -
     plncnt |  2.735362   .1906752   14.35   0.000     2.361646    3.109079
    plncnt2 | -.5335145   .0580186   -9.20   0.000    -.6472289   -.4198002
      _cons | -1.270126   .1474427   -8.61   0.000    -1.559108   -.9811433
- - - - - - - - - - - - - - - - - - - - - - - - - - - - - - - - - - - - - - - -
```

If the original rate ratio model perfectly predicted the observed counts, then the model linear prediction, plncnt, would have a coefficient of 1 with a P-value of zero: plncnt has the values of the predicted ln counts and since the ln link was used, the outcome is the observed ln counts. If the linear predictions are perfect, the plncnt2 term would have a coefficient of 0 with a P-value of 1 because the quadratic curve term would be superfluous. But the plncnt2 coefficient was −.5 with a P-value < .001, suggesting that a linear relationship alone failed to describe the relationship between the predicted log counts and observed ln counts. These results signal a problem with the log link in the original rate model, but they do not tell us what link would be better.

Instead of going through these steps, we can use a generalized linear rate ratio model and then use **linktest**, with the results shown here:

```
. glm fallcnt age, link(log) family(poisson) exp(time) eform nolog
(output omitted)
```

```
. linktest, link(log) family(poisson) nolog
```

```
Generalized linear models                No. of obs       =      1,022
Optimization      : ML                   Residual df      =      1,019
                                         Scale parameter =          1
Deviance          = 1041.379085          (1/df) Deviance =   1.021962
Pearson           = 960.0954462          (1/df) Pearson  =   .9421938

Variance function : V(u) = u             [Poisson]
Link function     : g(u) = ln(u)         [Log]

                                         AIC             =   4.007519
Log likelihood    = -2044.842168         BIC             =  -6019.799
```

```
            |                 OIM
   fallcnt  |    Coef.    Std. Err.      z     P>|z|     [95% Conf. Interval]
------------+----------------------------------------------------------------
       _hat |   2.735362   .1906752    14.35   0.000     2.361646    3.109079
     _hatsq |  -.5335145   .0580186    -9.20   0.000    -.6472289   -.4198001
       _cons|  -1.270126   .1474427    -8.61   0.000    -1.559108   -.9811432
------------+----------------------------------------------------------------
```

Stata labels the predicted ln count term "_hat". Observed values of an outcome are often designated by "y" in statistical notation and predicted values indicated by y with a ^ over the y. The ^ symbol is called a caret and when placed over a letter it is called a circumflex diacritical mark. In statistics and mathematics it is called a hat, house, or roof when placed over a letter, because of how it looks. So statisticians sometimes speak of the set of predicted outcome values as y-hat.

Stata's discussion of the **linktest** command, at least through version 15.1, advises that all options used for the original model should be used for the subsequent **linktest** command. But the **exp(time)** option *should not be used*, because the calculation of the linear predictor (plncnt) already accounts for person-time. Using a time offset option with **linktest** will produce biased results. (In this example, the use of **exp(time)** is unimportant, because time is always equal to 1.) If the **poisson** command is used to fit the same rate ratio model, the link and family information is part of the command. So when **linktest** is used after the **poisson** command, the link and family options should be omitted for **linktest**; if these options are used, **linktest** will report an error.

If we fit the model for age and falls using the identity link and then run the **linktest** command, we get this output:

```
. linktest, link(identity) family(poisson) nolog
(output omitted)
```

```
            |                 OIM
      rate  |    Coef.    Std. Err.      z     P>|z|     [95% Conf. Interval]
------------+----------------------------------------------------------------
       _hat |   1.031787   .1042268     9.90   0.000     .8275058    1.236067
     _hatsq |  -.0036633   .0115367    -0.32   0.751    -.0262747    .0189482
       _cons|  -.0497701    .187419    -0.27   0.791    -.4171047    .3175645
------------+----------------------------------------------------------------
```

The _hat (fitted ln count) term is close to 1 and statistically significant, but hat-squared is close to 0 and not statistically significant. This indicates that adding the curved line produced by _hatsq is not statistically superior to a linear fit alone. The null hypothesis for this test was that the identity (linear) link was sufficient. The test provides no evidence against this hypothesis. This does not prove that the identity link model is the correct or true or best model. But we have no evidence that this link choice is not correct.

In the example above with a single variable, over a 1000 observations, and a fairly strong association, all the statistics supported the identity link. In actual data the association of interest may be weaker, the sampling errors greater, many variables may be involved, measurement error may distort relationships, and confounding bias may be present. Using the data alone to decide between an additive (identity or difference) model and a multiplicative (log or ratio) model may be difficult and other considerations may play a role in this choice (Breslow and Day 1987 p124).

Because the link-test relies on statistical significance, it can be misleading when there are many outcome counts; trivial deviations from a perfect log-linear or linear relationship could produce a statistically significant link test. When there are few outcomes, the test may have limited power to detect inadequate links.

12.12 RESIDUALS, INFLUENCE ANALYSIS, AND OTHER MEASURES

The difference between the observed rate for each subject and the model fitted rate is called a residual (Breslow and Day 1987 pp138–139, Lindsey 1997 pp222–226, Hardin and Hilbe 2012 pp51–55, Hilbe 2014 pp108–112). After using the **glm** command, Stata users can invoke the **predict** command to calculate deviance, Pearson, or Anscombe residuals and variations of these. Stata also has a command to calculate Cook's distance (**predict, cooksd**), a measure of each observation's influence on the predicted values (Draper and Smith 1998 pp211–214, Hardin and Hilbe 2012 p49).

A useful measure which requires a little work by the analyst is to calculate delta-beta, an estimate of how much each observation affects the estimate of the main exposure of interest (Greenland 2008b p428). For the data in Table 12.1, the estimated rate ratio was 0.75. We can drop each observation in turn and re-estimate this rate ratio. Delta-beta is the ratio of the rate ratio estimated when each observation is omitted, divided by the rate ratio based upon all observations. The largest delta-beta is 1.12 for the subject with 45 falls. When that subject is omitted, the rate ratio becomes 0.75 × 1.12 = 0.84. Of course, we did not need delta-beta analysis to find this subject; this was obvious from Table 12.1. But for more complex models this approach can identify subjects who have covariate patterns which most influence the estimate of interest. Finding such subjects may alert investigators to recheck that entered data for a few subjects is correct. A delta-beta quantity can be computed for a rate difference as well.

When dealing with rates, it is worth remembering that an observation with a large amount of person-time will have a greater influence on fit than an observation with little person-time, because rates are averaged using person-time weights (Expression 6.1) (Breslow and Day 1987 p139,150).

12.13 ADDING MODEL TERMS TO IMPROVE FIT

It may be possible to improve the fit by adding additional variables or interaction terms (Breslow and Day 1987 pp145–146, Hardin and Hilbe 2012 pp204–209). For example, event rates often vary a great deal with age. This may mean that we should adjust finely for age, perhaps by using more than just a few categories of age or a single linear term for age. And perhaps we should consider interaction terms between age and other model variables. Allowing different rates at different age levels may account for the overdispersion found in the aggregate rates. If a multiplicative model seems to require many interaction terms to produce a better fit, this may be an indication that a linear model should be considered (Breslow and Day 1987 p142). Interaction, also called effect modification, may be present on the multiplicative scale but not on the additive scale, or vice versa.

12.14 A CAUTION

Tests of model fit can help us chose among models and help us identify problems with models. They cannot, however, prove that we have the best model or that the estimated associations are unbiased causal effects (Greenland 2008b p427). For the randomized trial of exercise and falls (Table 12.1), the deviance and dispersion statistics suggested a problem with the model. But the model itself, simply a ratio or difference comparison of two rates, was justified by the randomized trial design. We needed to fix the CIs, but the basic model was correct. In Chapter 9 I presented a study of how hip fracture rates varied with time. After adjustment for age, I mentioned that model fit was improved by adding terms for sex as well as interaction terms for sex and age. But doing this had almost no influence on the size or precision of the estimated association between time and fracture rates, so these extra terms were omitted. Fit statistics know nothing about the study goal, study design, or possible study biases. While fit statistics can alert us to problems we may need to address, our goal is not necessarily the best fitting model, but the model that best answers our study question.

12.15 FURTHER READING

The statistics and tests described in this chapter are used for all models fit with maximum likelihood, not just count models. Further useful advice and references can be found in textbooks by McCullagh and Nelder (1989), Lindsey (1997), Harrell (2001), Long and Freese (2014), and Hardin and Hilbe (2012), among others.

Adjusting Standard Errors and Confidence Intervals

13

If assumptions about a Poisson process are not true, several methods can be used to correct the variances, standard errors (SE), P-values, and confidence intervals (CI) for rate ratios or differences.

13.1 ESTIMATING THE VARIANCE WITHOUT REGRESSION

Imagine that we have a set of rates for a sample of subjects or populations. Designate the number of observations as n, the count for subject i as C_i, the total count as C, the person-time for subject i as T_i, and T as the total person-time. We can estimate the variance of these rates using a time-weighted version of Expression 4.2 with n-1 in the denominator. The weights in this calculation are $n \times T_i/T$:

variance for a sample of rates

$$= \text{sum}\left[(\text{weight}_i) \times (\text{rate}_i - \text{mean rate})^2\right]/(n-1) \qquad \text{(Ex.13.1)}$$
$$= \text{sum}\left[(n \times T_i/T) \times ((C_i/T_i) - C/T)^2\right]/(n-1)$$

The SE of the mean rate is then $\sqrt{(\text{variance}/T)}$. The Poisson variance formulae in Table 4.4 play no role in these calculations. We can use Expression 4.8 to calculate the SE of the ln(rate) = (SE of mean rate)/(mean rate). This allows us to make further calculations on the ln scale.

Using the data from the randomized trial of exercise for the prevention of falls (Table 12.1) (Shumway-Cook et al. 2007), the person-time-weighted rate and its variance can be calculated using Stata's **summarize** command. For this command we must use what Stata calls **aweights**, or analytic weights, to get results that correspond to those from Expression 13.1. For the control group, designated as exercise==0, the commands are:

```
. summarize rate [aweight=time] if exercise==0

    Variable |      Obs      Weight        Mean    Std. Dev.      Min        Max
-------------+----------------------------------------------------------------
        rate |      227   224.534884    1.772553    4.087816        0         45

. scalar rate0 = r(mean)
. di "SE of mean time-weighted rate = " sqrt(r(Var)/r(sum_w))

SE of mean time-weighted rate = .27280316

. * calculate SE of ln(rate0)
. scalar selnrate0 = sqrt(r(Var)/r(sum_w))/rate0
```

The commands above calculate the rate (rate0) and the SE of the ln(rate) (selnrate0). Stata's **summarize** command with **aweight=time** computes the variance (**r(Var)**) using Expression 13.1 for a sample of rates. Dividing the variance by the total person-time, **r(sum_w)**, and taking the square root, produces the SE of the mean rate. The result for the SE of the mean rate is close to the SE produced if we summarize the rates using ordinary least squares linear regression using **iweight=time**: these two SE estimates only differ after 4 digits. Dividing the SE from Expression 13.1 by the rate, **r(mean)**, produces the SE of the ln(rate) (Expression 4.8). The word **scalar** is Stata's lingo for a quantity that is calculated to the greatest precision Stata allows and stored for later use. Repeating these commands for the exercise group produces the scalar quantities rate1 and selnrate1. To obtain the ln of the rate ratio, we just subtract the ln(rate0) of the control group rate from the ln(rate1) of the exercise group rate. The SE for the ln(rate ratio) is calculated by squaring the SEs for each rate, summing these, and taking the square root of the sum. If we want a CI for alpha (the false positive fraction) = .05, we use the expression **invnormal**(1 − alpha/2) = **invnormal**(1 − .05/2) to determine ~1.959964 to great precision. This is used to compute a 95% CI. The Stata commands are:

```
. * calculate the ln(rate ratio)
. scalar lnrr = ln(rate1) - ln(rate0)

. * calculate the SE of the ln(rate ratio)
. scalar selnrr = sqrt(selnrate0^2 + selnrate1^2)

. * calculate the lower and upper CI boundaries
. scalar lower = lnrr - invnormal(1-.05/2)*selnrr

. scalar upper = lnrr + invnormal(1-.05/2)*selnrr

. di "Rate ratio: " %6.3f exp(lnrr) " SE: " %6.3f exp(lnrr)*selnrr /*
>     */ " 95% CI:" %6.3f exp(lower) "," %6.3f exp(upper)
Rate ratio: 0.752 SE: 0.140 95% CI: 0.523, 1.083
```

The rate ratio is 0.75 with 95% CI 0.52, 1.08 (Table 13.1). For the discussion in this chapter I will call this the variance without regression method.

13.2 POISSON REGRESSION

To obtain the SE and related statistics under the assumption that the data are from a Poisson process, we can use the SE formulae in Table 4.4: formula 4 and Expression 4.8, or formula 9. Starting with the control group, Stata commands can do most of the heavy lifting:

```
. * calculate total time for the controls
. egen double tottime0 = sum(time) if exercise==0
(226 missing values generated)

.* calculate the total count of falls for the controls
. egen double totcount0= sum(fallcnt) if exercise==0
(226 missing values generated)
```

TABLE 13.1   Confidence intervals for the rate ratio of 0.75 for fall events, comparing persons randomly assigned to exercise with controls. Data from Table 12.1. Bootstrap and randomization intervals were based on 199,999 replications.

CONFIDENCE INTERVAL METHOD	EXERCISE RATE RATIO
Variance without regression	0.52, 1.08
Poisson regression	0.65, 0.87
Rescaling using Pearson dispersion	0.52, 1.10
Robust variance	0.52, 1.08
Bootstrap normal	0.52. 1.08
Bootstrap percentile	0.52, 1.08
Bootstrap bias corrected	0.52, 1.07
Bootstrap bias corrected & accelerated	0.50, 1.04
Bootstrap-*t*	0.48, 1.07
Randomization to nearly equal groups	0.51, 1.10
Randomization using study site and blocks	0.52, 1.09

```
. * calculate the rate for controls
. scalar rate0 = totcount0/tottime0

. * calculate the SE of the control rate using Poisson assumptions
. scalar serate0 = (totcount0/tottime0^2)^.5

. * calculate the SE of the ln of the control rate using the delta method
. scalar selnrate0 = serate0/rate0 = √(1/totcount0)
```

We can repeat these commands for the exercise group and then proceed with commands similar to those shown in the previous section to get the following:

Rate ratio: 0.75 SE rate ratio: 0.06 95% CI: 0.65, 0.87

Chapter 12 showed the output from Poisson regression; it is numerically identical to the above results. I also showed evidence that the Poisson 95% CI of 0.65, 0.87 is too narrow due to overdispersion.

13.3 RESCALING THE VARIANCE USING THE PEARSON DISPERSION STATISTIC

When Stata's **glm** command uses a Poisson error family, the output header reports "Variance function: V(u) = u." This means the variance of the mean count, V(u), is equal to the mean count, u. For models using the Poisson error family, Stata reports "Scale parameter = 1" in the header information. The scale parameter (SP) is a multiplier of the expected variance. When SP is equal to 1, then V(u) = SP × u = 1 × u = u. By default, Stata uses a SP of 1 for discrete distributions (binomial, Poisson, negative binomial) and an SP equal to the Pearson dispersion statistic for continuous distributions (Gaussian, gamma). To correct the Poisson variance for under or overdispersion, the variance can be multiplied by the Pearson dispersion statistic, sometimes called the Pearson dispersion estimator (Wooldridge 2010 p513). This statistic, described in Chapter 12, is the generalized Pearson chi-squared statistic (Expression 12.2), divided by the model degrees of freedom. For a set of rates to be summarized as a mean rate, the expected counts are just the mean rate, C/T, and using weights defined for Expression 13.1, Expression 12.2 becomes Expression 13.2:

Pearson dispersion statistic

$$= \text{sum}\left[(\text{weight}_i) \times (\text{Observed rate}_i - \text{expected rate})^2 / (\text{expected rate})\right]/(n-1) \qquad \text{(Ex.13.2)}$$

$$= \text{sum}\left[(n \times T_i/T) \times (C_i/T_i - C/T)^2/(C/T)\right]/(n-1)$$

The Poisson variance of the total count is C; divide this by T, the time offset. Multiply C/T, the mean rate, by the dispersion statistic as shown in Expression 13.3:

Poisson variance/T × Pearson dispersion statistic

$$= (C/T) \times \text{sum}\left[(\text{weight}_i) \times (C_i/T_i - C/T)^2/(C/T)\right]/(n-1)$$

$$= \text{sum}\left[(n \times T_i/T) \times (C_i/T_i - C/T)^2\right]/(n-1) \qquad \text{(Ex13.3)}$$

$$= \text{variance from Expression 13.1}$$

So rescaling the variance using the Pearson dispersion statistic (equivalently, rescaling the standard deviation using the square root of the dispersion statistic), is a variance estimator that can account for under or overdispersion. This approach has been described in many books (Agresti 2002 pp150–151, Fleiss et al. 2003 p362, Cook and Lawless 2007 pp82–84, Wooldridge 2008 p598, 2010 pp727–730, Hilbe 2011 pp158–163, Hardin and Hilbe 2012 p232, Cameron and Trivedi 2013a pp37–38, Hilbe 2014 pp92–96).

Poisson regression models can correctly estimate rate ratios without relying upon the assumption that the data arise from a Poisson distribution(Gourieroux et al. 1984b, Lloyd 1999 pp85–86, Cook and Lawless 2007 pp82–84, Wooldridge 2008 pp597–598, 2010 pp727–728, Cameron and Trivedi 2013a pp72–73). This idea was discussed in Chapter 9. When maximum likelihood is used to estimate rate ratios, but the variance is estimated without relying upon assumptions regarding the Poisson distribution, the method is called quasi-likelihood, quasi-maximum likelihood, quasi-maximum likelihood estimation, quasi-Poisson regression, or pseudo-maximum likelihood (Gourieroux et al. 1984b, McCullagh and Nelder 1989). Rescaling is an example of a quasi-maximum likelihood method.

Software makes rescaling easy. Let us fit the Poisson rate ratio model to the exercise and falls data:

```
. glm fallcnt exercise, link(log) family(poisson) exp(time) eform nolog

Generalized linear models                No. of obs      =         453
Optimization       : ML                  Residual df     =         451
                                         Scale parameter =           1
Deviance           = 1434.583364         (1/df) Deviance = 3.180894
Pearson            = 2816.011836         (1/df) Pearson  = 6.243929

Variance function: V(u) = u              [Poisson]
Link function    : g(u) = ln(u)          [Log]

                                         AIC             =    4.624987
Log likelihood     = -1045.559496        BIC             =   -1323.684
------------------------------------------------------------------------
             |          OIM
     fallcnt |      IRR   Std. Err.      z    P>|z|   [95% Conf. Interval]
-------------+----------------------------------------------------------
    exercise | .7524891  .0576996    -3.71   0.000   .6474877  .8745183
       _cons | 1.772553  .0888501    11.42   0.000   1.606691  1.955537
    ln(time) |        1  (exposure)
------------------------------------------------------------------------
```

Below is the regression table output for the ln rate ratios:

```
 --------------------------------------------------------------------
        |              OIM
fallcnt |    Coef.   Std. Err.      z    P>|z|    [95% Conf. Interval]
--------+-----------------------------------------------------------
exercise | -.2843688  .0766783   -3.71   0.000   -.4346556   -.134082
   _cons |  .5724209  .0501255   11.42   0.000    .4741768    .6706651
ln(time) |         1  (exposure)
 --------------------------------------------------------------------
```

This model has poor fit with a large Pearson dispersion statistic of 6.24. The variances (and SEs, P-values, and CIs) are too small because the counts are more spread out than expected from a Poisson process. We can correct the Poisson SEs by multiplying them by the square-root of the scale parameter. Multiplying each Poisson variance by the Pearson dispersion statistic, about 6.24 in this example, will do this. The rescaled SE for the rate ratio for exercise is square-root(variance of ln(rate ratio) × Pearson dispersion) × rate ratio = SE ln(rate ratio) × square-root(Pearson dispersion) × rate ratio = .07667 × square-root(6.2439) × 0.75249 = 0.144. We can avoid these calculations by just adding the **scale(x2)** option to the regression command. Stata uses **x2** to denote the Pearson dispersion statistic, as this is a Pearson chi-squared (χ-squared or χ^2) statistic.

```
. glm fallcnt exercise, link(log) family(poisson) exp(time) eform nolog
scale(x2)
```

```
Generalized linear models                       No. of obs      =        453
Optimization        : ML                        Residual df     =        451
                                                Scale parameter =          1
Deviance            =  1434.583364              (1/df) Deviance  =   3.180894
Pearson             =  2816.011836              (1/df) Pearson   =   6.243929

Variance function: V(u) = u                     [Poisson]
Link function     : g(u) = ln(u)                [Log]

                                                AIC             =   4.624987
Log likelihood      = -1045.559496              BIC             =  -1323.684
 -------------------------------------------------------------------------
         |              OIM
 fallcnt |     IRR    Std. Err.      z    P>|z|    [95% Conf. Interval]
---------+---------------------------------------------------------------
exercise | .7524891   .1441789   -1.48   0.138    .5169014    1.09545
   _cons | 1.772553   .2220172    4.57   0.000   1.386704    2.265764
ln(time) |        1   (exposure)
 -------------------------------------------------------------------------
(Standard errors scaled using square root of Pearson X2-based dispersion.)
```

The header statistics are all the same in the output here, compared with the previous version of this model. Stata does not modify the formula for the variance in the header and reports the scale parameter as 1, even though it is now 6.24. The rate ratios are unchanged, because quasi-maximum likelihood fits the model just like maximum likelihood; only the SEs and statistics related to the SEs change. The note below the regression table reports that the SEs were scaled (or rescaled) using the square root of the Pearson dispersion statistic. The SEs, Z-statistics, P-values, and CIs have been changed because they use the rescaled SE. The 95% CI from this method is 0.52, 1.10, pretty close to the results from the variance without regression method.

Since multiplication of the Poisson variance by the Pearson dispersion statistic recreates the variance from Expression 13.1, why doesn't the rescaling method get *exactly* the same SEs and CIs as the variance without regression method? The results differ a bit because I first applied Expression 13.1 only to the controls to compute the variance. Then I used data only from the exercise group. I treated the exercise and control groups as independent samples and allowed each group to have its own Poisson variance and its *own* Pearson dispersion statistic. In contrast, rescaling allowed the exercise and control groups to have different Poisson SEs, but assumed that both groups had the same amount of overdispersion and multiplied the different Poisson SEs by the same dispersion factor, 6.24.

Which method is better? This is akin to the choice that must be made when a two-sample t-test is conducted. Should we assume each sample has a different variance or should we assume they share a common variance (Armitage et al. 2002 pp106–109)? If we believe that the exercise program might affect the mean fall rate, but not the spread of the rates, then the rescaling method, which assumes a common dispersion, may be a good choice. But if the exercise program may reduce the possibility of large fall rates, so both the mean rate and spread of the rates will be influenced, then the variance without regression method may be preferred.

Information that allows for a perfectly rational choice may not be available. Fortunately, the choice makes little difference in this example (Table 13.1).

Rescaling using the Pearson dispersion statistic has been described as using the NB1 (negative binomial of type 1) variance function. If C indicates a mean count, the Poisson distribution assumes the variance = C. Instead, we could imagine that the variance is equal to $C + alpha \times C^{power}$. If we set power = 1, this new variance can be written as $C + alpha \times C = (1 + alpha) \times C$. Using the Pearson dispersion statistic in place of (1 + alpha) corresponds to a negative binomial model called type 1. Not surprisingly, there is an NB2 variance function = $C + alpha \times C^2$, which can also be used to rescale standard errors (Gourieroux et al. 1984b, 1984a). This is nicely explained by Cameron and Trivedi (2013a pp74–76) and they provide Stata code for the NB2 method on the internet (Cameron and Trivedi 2013b). As a practical matter, few will need to use the NB2 rescaling method and the NB1 method corresponds to the rescaling method already discussed. This is mentioned in case you come across this terminology in the literature. The negative binomial distribution and negative binomial regression gets more attention in Chapter 17.

It is possible to fit a model which rescales SEs for a non-constant dispersion factor, but the rate ratios for this model will be different from, and have a different interpretation, than the rate ratios from a Poisson model (Fleiss et al. 2003 pp362–363). This chapter is about adjusting SEs of rate ratios or differences that can be interpreted as the overall ratio change or difference change related to different levels of an exposure.

13.4 ROBUST VARIANCE

The robust variance estimator goes by many names (Wooldridge 2008 p267, Hardin and Hilbe 2012 pp37–38): the Huber (1967), Eicker (1967), or White (1980, 1982) estimator, some combination of these three names, the heteroskedasticity-robust estimator, the survey estimator, and the sandwich estimator. The last name, a bit of statistical whimsy, refers to the appearance of the three matrices that make up this estimator; the outer two are the same and have been called the bread for a sandwich. When the robust estimator is used for a Poisson regression model, the estimated associations are not affected, but the Poisson variance assumptions are ignored. Therefore this is a quasi-likelihood method. In Stata this estimator can be invoked by adding **vce(robust)** as an option to the regression command. Many textbooks describe this estimator (Wooldridge 2008 pp266–271, 2010 pp297–298,727–728, Hardin and Hilbe 2012 pp37–38).

In a large enough sample, the robust estimator, which is calculated from the residuals (Vittinghoff et al. 2012 p281), converges to Expression 13.1. For the exercise group the rate was 1.334 with SE of 0.138 from Expression 13.1. The robust SE was 0.138. For the control group, the rate was 1.773 with SE 0.273 from Expression 13.1; the robust SE was 0.273. The SE of the rate ratio from the variance without regression method was 0.138. The robust SE was 0.138. The CIs from the two methods are the same for the three digits shown in Table 13.1. Close enough.

Robust SEs may be smaller or larger than Poisson SEs. If there is underdispersion, the robust SEs will be smaller; the Poisson SEs are too big. The reverse is true when overdispersion is present.

Why not always use the robust SEs? You could. This approach is becoming more common in the literature. The robust method may be the most common way of correcting SEs when Poisson methods are used. But when the data really are from a Poisson process, the Poisson SE may be preferred as it will generally provide more statistical power in this situation; the P-values and CIs will be smaller. To use statistical jargon, the Poisson variance is more efficient if it is reasonable to think the data really are produced by a Poisson process (Carroll et al. 1998). A helpful review (Farcomeni and Ventura 2012) and textbook (Heritier et al. 2009) discuss the topic of robust methods.

13.5 GENERALIZED ESTIMATING EQUATIONS

Generalized Estimating Equations (GEE) (Zeger and Liang 1986, Liang and Zeger 1993) are a method for dealing with observations that are clustered; i.e., not statistically independent in some sense. In Chapter 5 we discussed a paper (Windeler and Lange 1995) which appeared in the British Medical Journal in 1995; the authors pointed out that recurrent events for the same person were unlikely to be independent. A year later Glynn and Buring (1996) published a discussion of statistical methods that can account for this lack of independence; GEE was mentioned prominently in their article. Stata implements GEE in models for panel data; for example, the **xtgee** and **xtpoisson, pa** commands can fit GEE or population averaged models to cross-sectional panel data in which the panels might be individuals who are followed over time for events that recur. But these models cannot be applied to the exercise and falls data because each subject only provides a single rate which summarizes all their falls; there is no panel variable.

Instead of providing a GEE command that works for the exercise and falls data, Stata provides a robust variance estimator with the **vce(robust)** option. This sandwich estimator of variance is Stata's version of the GEE approach for data that are not in panels. If you happen to use SAS software, you would use the commands for GEE to get the robust variance estimates. The results from Stata and SAS may not agree exactly, although they will be close. The key point here is that GEE is a method for correcting CIs when observations are not independent, but if you are using Stata for data that does not fit a cross-sectional panel structure, using **vce(robust)** is essentially equivalent to the GEE approach in other software.

13.6 USING THE ROBUST VARIANCE TO STUDY LENGTH OF HOSPITAL STAY

Imagine we want to know how long patients are in the hospital after open heart surgery to replace the aortic value. We also want to know how length of stay is related to age. We obtain data for 50 hypothetical patients, age 50 to 80 years, who had aortic valve replacement at Heart Repair Medical Center. If the date of surgery is designated as Day 1, the earliest discharge was on Day 4. If we ignore Days 1, 2, and 3, and recode Day 4 as 0, Day 5 as 1, and so on, perhaps the association between age and length of stay can be estimated using a Poisson regression ratio model. Using age greater than 50 years in units of 10 years as a continuous variable, labeled age10, the regression output looks like this:

```
. glm days age10, link(log) family(poisson) eform nolog

Generalized linear models                No. of obs      =        50
Optimization     : ML                    Residual df     =        48
                                         Scale parameter =         1
Deviance         =  48.0518395           (1/df) Deviance =   1.00108
Pearson          =  41.18775557          (1/df) Pearson  = .8580782

Variance function: V(u) = u              [Poisson]
Link function    : g(u) = ln(u)          [Log]

                                         AIC             =  3.357041
Log likelihood   = -81.92601696          BIC             = -139.7253

------------------------------------------------------------------------
              |               OIM
        days  |     IRR   Std. Err.      z    P>|z|    [95% Conf. Interval]
--------------+---------------------------------------------------------
       age10  | 1.458608   .1924998    2.86   0.004    1.126163    1.889192
       _cons  | 1.122636   .2771306    0.47   0.639    .6920121    1.821227
------------------------------------------------------------------------
```

At age 50 years the average days in hospital, after Day 4 post-surgery, was 1.12. The number of days in the hospital, after Day 4, increased by a ratio of 1.46 (95% CI 1.13, 1.89) for each 10-year increment in age beyond 50 years. The deviance goodness-of-fit test produced a P-value of .47, the deviance dispersion was 1.00, and the Pearson dispersion was 0.86. So we have no evidence to reject the view that length of stay, after Day 4, may be generated by a Poisson process. In fact, these data did come from a Poisson process, using a random generator of counts from a Poisson distribution with a mean count of 1 day (close to 1.12) at age 50 and a ratio of 1.5 days (close to 1.46) for each 10-year age increment.

Hospital days are measures of time, not indivisible integer counts; this was discussed in Section 2.5, "Numerators that may be mistaken for counts", in Chapter 2. Hospitals usually record the time of admission and discharge to the nearest minute. If we had that information we could analyze length of stay in hours. Let us multiply days by 24 to obtain hours in the hospital and see what happens using the same Poisson model for hours:

```
. glm hours age10, link(log) family(poisson) eform nolog

Generalized linear models                No. of obs      =        50
Optimization     : ML                    Residual df     =        48
                                         Scale parameter =         1
Deviance         = 1153.244158           (1/df) Deviance =  24.02592
Pearson          = 988.5061478           (1/df) Pearson  =  20.59388

Variance function: V(u) = u              [Poisson]
Link function    : g(u) = ln(u)          [Log]

                                         AIC             =  28.17819
Log likelihood   = -702.4546681          BIC             =  965.4671
```

hours	IRR	OIM Std. Err.	z	P>|z|	[95% Conf. Interval]	
age10	1.458608	.0392939	14.01	0.000	1.383592	1.537692
_cons	26.94326	1.357657	65.37	0.000	24.40948	29.74005

Now the dispersion statistics suggest a lot of dispersion and the deviance goodness-of-fit statistic produced a P-value < .0001. A tabular examination shows 6 patients with 0 hours, 14 patients with 24 hours, 12 with 48, 13 with 72, 1 with 96, 2 with 120, and 2 with 144 hours; this distribution is not Poisson. In this example, grouping time into days concealed the non-Poisson distribution of time in hours. The idea that grouping can hide or reveal information was discussed in Section 12.4, "Limitations of goodness-of-fit statistics", in Chapter 12. If we had real data about length of stay in hours, the distribution of time in hours would not be so discrete, but it would not likely be Poisson. Changing time units from days to hours divided the SEs and CIs by $\sqrt{(1/24)}$. The point here is that if counts of time units are treated as if they were indivisible counts, estimates of precision will be influenced by the choice of units: days, minutes, months. A simple remedy for this problem is to use a robust variance. If we do this for the outcome of days, the regression output then shows:

. glm days age10, link(log) family(poisson) eform nolog vce(robust) noheader

days	IRR	Robust Std. Err.	z	P>|z|	[95% Conf. Interval]	
age10	1.458608	.2127068	2.59	0.010	1.095996	1.941191
_cons	1.122636	.283389	0.46	0.647	.6844921	1.841235

Above the SE for age10 is 10% larger compared with the Poisson SE; the Poisson variance is more efficient when the data are from a Poisson process. But if hours are used as the outcome, the robust SE for age10 does not change at all:

hours	IRR	Robust Std. Err.	z	P>|z|	[95% Conf. Interval]	
age10	1.458608	.2127068	2.59	0.010	1.095996	1.941191
_cons	26.94326	6.801337	13.05	0.000	16.42781	44.18964

In the output above, the Z-statistic and P-value did change for the constant term. That is because the constant term in the model using days as the outcome is an estimate of the ratio of length of stay in days for a person age 50 compared with a length of stay of 1 day (24 hours). But in the model that used hours as the outcome the constant term estimated the ratio of length of stay in hours for a 50-year-old compared with 1 hour (1/24th of a day). This larger ratio has a larger Z-statistic.

This example is not about incidence rates. The estimated associations are ratios of intervals of time. I picked this example because Poisson models have been used to examine length of stay as if hospitals days were discrete counts. The example shows that (1) an analysis will produce different results depending on the time units used, (2) time units are not discrete counts, and (3) if we use a robust estimator, we can use the Poisson model to estimate the ratio of quantities that are not counts. While linear regression is the usual initial choice for regression analysis of differences, Poisson regression with a robust variance will often be the best choice for estimating ratios (Gourieroux et al. 1984b, Lloyd 1999 pp85–86, Cook and Lawless 2007 pp82–84, Wooldridge 2008 pp597–598, 2010 pp727–728, Cameron and Trivedi 2013a pp72–73).

13.7 COMPUTER INTENSIVE METHODS

Confidence intervals are often calculated by adding and subtracting, from the estimated association, the SE multiplied by some quantity: 1.64 for a 90% CI, 1.96 for a 95% CI, 2.58 for a 99% CI, and so on. This common method assumes that the estimated association has a normal distribution that is symmetrical around the estimate. This assumption can be justified in infinitely large samples, but we study finite samples. Our goal when estimating a X% CI is to find an interval which will bracket the true association in X% of repeated samples from the study population. The common method using the SE is not always the best estimate of this interval.

Before video games and social media, computers were created to crunch numbers. They excel at this and statisticians have devised clever methods that use computing power to estimate CIs and related statistics. Computer intensive methods for estimating any statistic include the bootstrap, permutation, and randomization. The words resampling or permutation are sometimes used to describe all of these methods. I will describe how several of these methods can be applied to estimate CIs for the rate ratio from the trial of exercise and falls. Information about theory and implementation can be found in several textbooks (Efron and Tibshirani 1993, Mooney and Duval 1993, Lunneborg 2000, Manly 2007). Carpenter and Bithell (2000) have published a short, practical review of bootstrap methods.

13.8 THE BOOTSTRAP IDEA

The investigators who studied exercise and falls (Table 12.1) wanted to estimate a ratio of fall rates. In planning the trial, they assumed that fall counts would follow a Poisson distribution. The study data suggest their assumption was wrong. We do not know the distribution of fall counts in the hypothetical population of all persons who might have entered this study. The idea that underlies the bootstrap is that the best information about the distribution of fall rates is contained in the collected data. By resampling many times from the observed data, the underlying distribution can be estimated. Because the available data are used to estimate the distribution, the method is akin to lifting yourself by your bootstraps.

Although there are several ways in which bootstrap resampling can be done, the most common is to randomly sample *with replacement* from all the observed records. The fall data contain 453 records so each bootstrap sample will have 453 records. After randomly sampling a record, the sampled record is returned to, or replaced in, the data and can be sampled again. Consequently, the first record in the data may appear three times in a single bootstrap sample, the second record may be omitted, and so on. In a bootstrap sample from the fall data, the trial subject who fell 45 times might appear 0, 1, 2, 3, ..., up to 453 times.

Although the resampling is done using a pseudo-random number generator, Stata allows the user to set the starting point, called a seed, in the random sequence. If the original data are in the same sort order at the start of resampling, use of the seed means the bootstrap sampling can be exactly replicated. Stata's pseudorandom number generator is a good one and there is valuable practical advice about the **set seed** command in the manuals.

How many bootstrap samples are needed? Books about the bootstrap discuss this topic and there is a Stata command, **bssize** (Poi 2004), that calculates the number of bootstrap samples using a method published by Andrews and Buchinsky (2000).

Twenty years ago, the advice that only a few hundred or a few thousand replications was adequate was reassuring, because desktop computers were slow. To obtain the bootstrap CIs in Table 13.1, I used 199,999 replications. This was far more than needed, but the price was trivial; a desktop computer completed the chore in 6.4 minutes. Many research studies will require weeks, months, or years of work by several people. If a computer has to run overnight to produce 100,000 replications, that added cost is easy to justify. This ensures that whatever errors remain in the study and analysis, an insufficient number of bootstraps samples is not of concern. In statistical jargon, using many replications reduces "Monte Carlo error." By using many replications, it means that another researcher using the same data will get the same results to several decimals, even if they do not use the same random number seed or the same software. As computing power increases, use of many replications will probably become commonplace (Berry et al. 2014 p367).

Bootstrap methods can construct a distribution for any statistic. In the examples below we will estimate the 95% CI for the rate ratio of 0.75 from the study of exercise and falls. Stata has a **bootstrap** command which makes it easy to produce bootstrap CIs using 4 methods: the normal, percentile, bias corrected, and biased corrected and accelerated CIs.

13.9 THE BOOTSTRAP NORMAL METHOD

The normal method has been called the normal approximation method or the standard method. Resample the fall data 199,999 times and compute the ln rate ratio in each of these samples. Then use Expression 13.1 to calculate the SE of the 199,999 bootstrap ln rate ratios. Finally, add and subtract this bootstrap SE × 1.96 from the ln rate ratio of 0.75 from the analysis of the original data. One advantage of this method is that if the original data sample is small, the bootstrap estimate of the SE may be more accurate than the estimate obtained from the original sample using large sample methods. In addition, this method can be used even if we do not have a formula for the SE of the statistic in the original sample.

This method assumes that the ln rate ratio from resampling has a normal and symmetrical distribution. Since a goal of the bootstrap is to substitute computing power for distributional assumptions, the normal method may amount to shooting oneself in the foot (or boot).

The normal method produced a 95% CI of 0.52 to 1.08. The log scale was used for estimation. When the bootstrapped ln rate ratios are plotted against the inverse normal distribution, the fit is excellent except for mild deviations for a few large values. Stata's command for this plot is **qnorm**; this is called a normal quantile plot. Miller (1997 pp10–15) calls this a probit plot and discusses the value of this approach. When rate ratios were used, instead of ln rate ratios, the 95% CI was 0.47, 1.03, and the normal quantile plot showed poor fit to a normal distribution for both tails of the bootstrapped risk ratios. There are two lessons here; (1) the normal method works well if the bootstrapped distribution is indeed normal, and (2) to estimate the CI for a ratio, use the ln scale.

13.10 THE BOOTSTRAP PERCENTILE METHOD

Sort the 199,999 bootstrapped ln rate ratios from smallest to highest. Then the lower limit for the 95% CI is the .025 x (199,999+1) = the 5000th value and the upper limit is the .975 x (199,999+1) = the

195,000th value. It does not matter if the ln rate ratios or the rate ratios are used; either way the CI results will be the same. This method does not require any assumption of normality, but it assumes that the bootstrap distribution is symmetric around the original rate ratio. Because of the symmetry assumption, this is sometimes called the naïve percentile method. In this example symmetry is close to true and the 95% CI is 0.52, 1.08.

13.11 THE BOOTSTRAP BIAS-CORRECTED PERCENTILE METHOD

This is also called the bias-corrected, BC, or percentile method. Collect the same 199,999 bootstrap ln rate ratios as before. Calculate the "bias," which is the mean ln rate ratio from the 199,999 bootstrap samples minus the ln rate ratio in the original sample. This bias is then used, in a somewhat complicated expression that involves the inverse normal distribution, to move the CI endpoints. The degree of movement can differ for the upper and lower endpoints. Discussion and illustration of this method and the calculations can be found in several places (Mooney and Duval 1993, pp37–40, Carpenter and Bithell 2000, Lunneborg 2000 pp157–162, Manly 2007 p52–56), including the Stata manuals and an online file related to this chapter. You don't need to study these calculations, however, as Stata's **bootstrap** command does the work for you. Unfortunately, this method will often perform poorly; the accelerated method, described next, is usually preferred (Carpenter and Bithell 2000).

13.12 THE BOOTSTRAP BIAS-CORRECTED AND ACCELERATED METHOD

This has been called the accelerated bias-corrected percentile or the adjusted percentile method. It is sometimes abbreviated as BCA or BC_a. This percentile method utilizes the estimated bias, but adds a term, called the acceleration, to not only permit asymmetry, but to allow the shape of the distribution to vary with the size of the estimated statistic, in this case the rate ratio. Recall the person who reported 45 falls; the acceleration is supposed to account for the influence of this extreme value. Details are in several books (Efron and Tibshirani 1993 pp178–188, Davison and Hinkley 1997 pp203–207, Lunneborg 2000 pp157–166, Manly 2007 pp57–60). This method, which Stata implements in its **bootstrap** command, produced 95% CI limits (0.50, 1.04) that are shifted downward toward 0 compared with the other bootstrap methods discussed so far.

13.13 THE BOOTSTRAP-T METHOD

This is also called the Studentized pivotal method. The "t" refers to Student's t-distribution and the formula for a t-statistic. Start with the same bootstrap sample of 199,999 ln rate ratios. In addition, calculate and collect the SE for each ln rate ratio. Calculate a t-statistic for each ln rate ratio: the bootstrap ln rate ratio minus the original sample ln rate ratio, divided by the SE of the bootstrap ln rate ratio. Sort the t-statistics from smallest to largest and find the ln rate ratios that correspond to the 2.5th and 97.5th percentiles of the ordered t-statistics; those ln rate ratios are the limits for the 95% CI.

One problem with this method is that it requires that we have a formula for the SE of the statistic of interest. If we do not, a second order bootstrap can calculate the SE for each of the ln rate ratios in the original sample. If this is done using 25 additional bootstraps, as suggested by Carpenter and Bithell (2000), then the computing chore will be 25 times larger. For rate ratios, of course, SEs are available.

A second problem is that this method may perform poorly if the SEs are correlated with the bootstrap t-statistics. This can be checked with a scatterplot. In the fall data, the SE decreases as the size of the bootstrap ln rate ratio increases; the Pearson correlation coefficient is −.48. A variance-stabilizing transformation is needed so that the size of the SEs is not related to the size of the bootstrap ln rate ratios (Carpenter and Bithell 2000), but it is not clear what form this transformation should take. The 95% CI from the bootstrap-t is 0.48, 1.07, but because of this is not based on a variance-stabilizing method, it may not be accurate.

13.14 WHICH BOOTSTRAP CI IS BEST?

Theory and simulations suggest that the bias-corrected and accelerated method and the bootstrap-t are preferred (Davison and Hinkley 1997 p214, Carpenter and Bithell 2000, Lunneborg 2000 p157). Because we do not have a bootstrap-t CI based upon a variance-stabilizing method, the CI of 0.50, 1.04 from the bias-corrected and accelerated method may be a good choice. But arguments can be made for preferring the randomization methods discussed below.

13.15 PERMUTATION AND RANDOMIZATION

Ronald Fisher (1880–1962) made prodigious contributions to statistical theory and practice. One of these is the permutation test for contingency tables, often called the Fisher exact test. In 1936, Fisher (1936) explained how significance tests were related to permutation tests. To compare the heights of 100 Englishmen with 100 Frenchmen, we can calculate the average difference. Then, Fisher wrote, we can ask "Could these [two] samples have been drawn at random from the same population?" We calculate a probability to answer this question. If this probability (a P-value) is sufficiently small, we conclude that the answer "no" is reasonable, and if it is large, we conclude that "yes" is possible. We are never entirely certain about either answer. Fisher explained that one way to compute this probability is to determine every possible permutation of the 200 height measurements into two equal groups, calculate the mean height difference for each permutation, and compare the observed mean difference with the distribution of the permuted differences. Fisher wrote that no statistician would perform this labor, "but his conclusions have no justification beyond the fact that they agree with those which could have been arrived at by this elementary method." Fisher was saying that methods that rely upon distributional assumptions are shortcuts that bypass onerous calculations that produce the *correct* answers. Several statisticians have expressed views similar to those of Fisher (Edgington 1995 pp10–13). Even Efron and Tibshirani, pioneers of bootstrap methods, argue that when permutation is appropriate, as in the comparison of two groups, this is an excellent method that avoids mathematical assumptions (Efron and Tibshirani 1993 pp202, 218).

The permutation task Fisher described is so large that a desktop computer (in 2018) would be overwhelmed. But something sufficiently close to this can be done. Instead of trying to produce all possible permutations, we could repeatedly randomize the 200 English and French men into two groups of 100 each and compute the mean difference in height between these groups after each randomization.

This is sometimes called re-randomization. If enough randomizations are done, the resulting distribution of the differences should be close to the entire permutation distribution. The generated distribution of mean differences is a random sample, with replacement, of the mean differences from all possible permutations of the data (Piantadosi 1997). If the observed height difference is extreme compared with the randomized distribution of height differences, this is evidence against the null hypothesis that English and French subjects come from populations with the same height distribution.

13.16 RANDOMIZATION TO NEARLY EQUAL GROUPS

The study of exercise and falls (Shumway-Cook et al. 2007) had 226 persons assigned to the exercise program and 227 controls. Assignment was entirely random, so the observed deviation of the rate ratio from 1 is due to a combination of two factors: (1) the causal effect of the exercise intervention and (2) random chance. We cannot know how much each of these factors contributed to the final rate ratio of 0.75, but calculation of a CI helps us understand where this balance may lie.

The observed rate ratio was 0.75. To estimate the 95% CI we can repeatedly re-randomize the 453 study subjects, each with their observed rate information, to two new groups, 226 persons who could hypothetically have received exercise, and 227 who could have been controls. A desktop computer took 68 seconds to create 199,999 rate ratios using simple re-randomization. The lower bound for the 95% CI for the rate ratio is the exponential of the observed ln rate ratio from the original data (ln(0.75) = -.28437) minus the ln rate ratio at the 97.5 centile of the distribution (+0.38223) = 0.51 (Manly 2007 p19). The upper bound is the exponential of the observed ln rate ratio minus the 2.5 centile of the distribution (−0.38281) = 1.10.

The CI based on randomization is easy to obtain from a computer. Its validity relies only on the assumptions that (1) the original assignment of the study subjects to the intervention was random and (2) the fall outcomes of each subject were independent of those of the other subjects. Both these assumptions are easy to defend in this example.

13.17 BETTER RANDOMIZATION USING THE RANDOMIZED BLOCK DESIGN OF THE ORIGINAL STUDY

In the falls study (Shumway-Cook et al. 2007), elderly persons were enrolled at two centers. A separate set of random assignments was generated for each center, using randomized blocks of size 4 or 6. This randomization method would result in a different set of permutations compared with the simpler method already described. I wrote a program that created new block sizes for the subjects at each enrollment center. The program then randomized the study subjects within each block. The program accounted for the fact that the last block at each treatment center was not necessarily completed; for example, a block that should have had six subjects might only have two because trial enrollment was terminated using predetermined criteria. It took a few hours to write this program and it took the computer 1.75 hours to create 199,999 rate ratios. The 95% CI was then calculated as described in the previous section about randomization: 0.52, 1.09. This is the CI that was given in the published report of the study (Shumway-Cook et al. 2007), using the same method and 20,000 rerandomized rate ratios.

The CI based on repeated randomization has nice features. It makes no distributional assumptions or any assumption about the shape of a distribution. Although it is not technically an exact method, because the full permutation distribution was not determined, with 199,999 replications this is effectively an exact method (Piantadosi 1997 p220, Manly 2007 p15). In small samples, an exact method can produce a 95% CI with coverage that may exceed 95% because of the discrete nature of the permuted distribution. But in a study of over 400 subjects, any overcoverage will be trivial because so many permutations are possible that the resulting distribution is nearly continuous. Among the 199,999 generated rate ratios, 147,354 were distinct. The method assumes only that it is reasonable to rerandomize the study subjects. The method is certainly valid if the original assignment to treatment was random; under the null hypothesis of no treatment effect, the observed fall rates for each study subject are unrelated to treatment and we can freely exchange the outcomes of subjects from the exercise group with those in the control group (Piantadosi 1997 pp218–220). One could argue that this method is ideal for the analysis of a randomized trial.

13.18 A SUMMARY

When the data are not from a Poisson process, we have numerous methods for estimating valid P-values and CIs. All the methods in Table 13.1 produced similar results except for ordinary Poisson regression. Among these methods, the randomization method that accounted for the original block design and study sites can be easily justified; that would be my choice for these data. But the approach of using the rate variances without regression or the robust variance estimator, both of which required almost no time and little thought, produced nearly the same 95% CI. Clever statisticians have invented several useful solutions when Poisson assumptions are not true. Our main problem may be selecting from the embarrassment of riches in Table 13.1.

Storks and Babies, Revisited

14

Chapter 1 presented fictional data (Table 1.2) about storks and babies that Jerzy Neyman used in 1952 (Neyman 1952) in a paper about spurious correlation. Different analyses in Chapter 1 suggested that more storks were associated with (1) more babies, (2) fewer babies, or (3) had no relationship with the number of babies. I now return to these data.

14.1 NEYMAN'S APPROACH TO HIS DATA

(Neyman 1952) did not use a regression model to analyze the stork data (Table 1.2). Instead, he pointed out that in the first three counties, which all had female population counts of 10,000, there was no relationship between the stork counts and the baby counts. The counts of babies were 10, 15, and 20, while the stork counts were always 2. The same was true in counties 4, 5, and 6, where the baby counts were again 10, 15, and 20, and the stork counts were all 3. The same pattern is repeated in each group of three consecutive counties. This means that a linear regression analysis with baby counts as the outcome and stork counts as the explanatory variable, will estimate a coefficient of 0 for the stork count variable if we adjust for the number of women. To illustrate this, I divided the population counts by 10,000 to create a variable called women10k, with units equal to 10,000 women and show the linear regression output here:

```
. regress babies storks women10k, noheader
```

babies	Coef.	Std. Err.	t	P>|t|	[95% Conf. Interval]	
storks	-6.34e-15	.6618516	-0.00	1.000	-1.328723	1.328723
women10k	5	.8271569	6.04	0.000	3.339413	6.660587
_cons	10	2.020958	4.95	0.000	5.942757	14.05724

This model shows no association between storks and babies. That is the result Neyman wanted and it fits our belief that storks have nothing to do with babies. The coefficient for storks is essentially 0; it differs from 0 only because a computer stores numbers in binary format and the regression table is in decimal format.

But some aspects of the model are troubling. The intercept (constant) term does not go through 0, so when the female population is 0, there will be 10 babies born. That is not possible. We may be willing to overlook this problem if we think the model fits the data well over the range of births in the data.

The number of women in each county is treated as an explanatory variable in the model. The model estimates that when the female population is 10,000, the birthrate per 10,000 women is 15. The birthrate decreases with increasing population or person-time: 10 for 20,000 women, 8.3 for 30,000 women, 7.5 for 40,000, 7 for 50,000, and 6.7 for 60,000. While birthrates could vary by regional population size, this is not very informative. It seems doubtful that a woman's fertility would change just by moving to a larger or smaller county. We usually want to study other variables, aside from person-time, that might explain *why* this pattern is present.

14.2 USING METHODS FOR INCIDENCE RATES

Neyman used his fictional data to make an important point about the relationships between 3 variables. He picked variables that would add humor to his argument and he was not thinking in terms of incidence rates or woman-time. In addition, he wanted an example in which the "best" analysis yielded a result that fit our expectations; despite stories told to children and cartoons on greeting cards, no one believes that storks bring babies.

A birthrate is an incidence rate and the female population counts can be treated as person-time estimates. This topic has been discussed extensively in earlier chapters. For example, see the first paragraph of Chapter 9 and Section 9.10, titled "Further comments about person-time." When we analyze incidence rates, we customarily treat person-time as an offset or weight and examine other variables, aside from person-time, to explain any variations in rates. We usually use models for incidence rates in which variation in the outcome rate is not a function of person-time; doubling person-time doubles the outcome count but the rate is unchanged.

If we were given the data in Table 12.1 and were told that the population counts were estimates of women-years and the births were observed over a year, how might we approach the analysis? I hope that Chapters 2 through 13 have convinced you that a good choice would be to use a count model and to treat person-time as an offset or weight, not as an explanatory variable. A simple approach would be to compare Poisson ratio and difference models, with the count of storks as the explanatory variable. The Poisson ratio model is shown here:

```
. glm babies storks, link(log) family(poisson) exp(women10k) eform nolog

Generalized linear models              No. of obs      =        54
Optimization     : ML                  Residual df     =        52
                                       Scale parameter =         1
Deviance         = 55.83943189         (1/df) Deviance = 1.073835
Pearson          = 58.4214701          (1/df) Pearson  = 1.12349
Variance function: V(u) = u            [Poisson]
Link function    : g(u) = ln(u)        [Log]

                                       AIC             = 6.198428
Log likelihood  = -165.3575457         BIC             = -151.5877
-------------------------------------------------------------------
             |              OIM
     babies |   IRR    Std. Err.    z    P>|z|   [95% Conf. Interval]
-----------+-------------------------------------------------------
     storks |  .9041434  .0123298  -7.39  0.000   .8802975   .9286352
      _cons |  16.09404  1.579244  28.32  0.000   13.27822   19.50698
ln(women10k)|       1  (exposure)
-------------------------------------------------------------------
```

The ratio model estimates that for each additional stork the birthrate declines by about 10%. The difference model is shown next, using birthrate per 10,000 women-years as the outcome, brate10k:

```
. glm brate10k storks [iweight=women10k], link(identity) family(poisson)
nolog
note: brate10k has noninteger values
```

```
Generalized linear models                    No. of obs      =         54
Optimization     : ML                        Residual df     =         52
                                             Scale parameter =          1
Deviance         = 60.63627592               (1/df) Deviance = 1.166082
Pearson          = 64.72218226               (1/df) Pearson  = 1.244657
Variance function: V(u) = u                  [Poisson]
Link function    : g(u) = u                  [Identity]

                                             AIC             =  14.81128
Log likelihood   = -397.9044779              BIC             = -146.7909
```

```
-----------------------------------------------------------------------------
             |                 OIM
    brate10k |      Coef.    Std. Err.      z    P>|z|     [95% Conf. Interval]
-------------+---------------------------------------------------------------
      storks |  -.7521217    .1110902    -6.77   0.000    -.9698545   -.5343889
       _cons |   13.33689    .8687008    15.35   0.000     11.63426    15.03951
-----------------------------------------------------------------------------
```

The difference model estimates that the birthrate is 13.3 babies per 10,000 women-years when there are no storks, and for each additional stork we subtract 0.75 per 10,000 women-years from this rate.

TABLE 14.1   Fit statistics for two models used to assess the association between *stork counts* and birthrates in the fictional data of Table 1.2. The rate ratio model used a log link and the difference model used an identity link. The difference column shows the rate ratio model statistic minus the rate difference model statistic.

MODEL STATISTIC	RATE RATIO MODEL	RATE DIFFERENCE MODEL	DIFFERENCE
Deviance	55.8	60.6	–4.8
Deviance P-value for fit	.33	.19	.14
Pearson statistic	58.4	64.7	–6.3
Pearson P-value for fit	.25	.11	.14
Deviance/degrees of freedom	1.07	1.17	–.09
Pearson/degrees of freedom	1.12	1.24	–.12
Ln(likelihood)	–165	–398	233
AIC (Expression 12.4)	335	800	–465
BIC (Expression 12.6)	339	804	–465
Poisson SE for stork count term	0.012	0.11	a
Robust SE for stork count term	0.014	0.13	a
Poisson Z-statistic for stork count term	–7.4	–6.8	–0.6
Robust Z-statistic for stork count term	–6.6	–6.0	–0.6

a Differences in model SEs for the rate ratio and rate difference are not relevant. What matters is the difference in the Poisson and robust SEs for the same model.

Which model is better? Deviance and Pearson fit statistics (Table 14.1) do not "reject" either model at the .05 level, but all the statistics suggest that the ratio model is a better choice. There is evidence of overdispersion for both models, but it is minimal for the ratio model. This model might make sense if "storks" were actually counts of family planning centers.

14.3 A MODEL THAT USES THE STORK/WOMEN RATIO

A small simulation study was described near the end of Chapter 11 in Section 11.14, called "Ratios and spurious correlation," with results in Table 11.7. One finding was that when a Poisson model for rate ratios is used and the explanatory counts are related to population size, then it may be best to use an explanatory term that is a ratio (counts/population); an example would be the unemployment proportion. Stork counts may not fall into this category, but nevertheless I created a variable, the storkratio, equal to the county stork count divided by the female population in units of 10,000. The storkratio ranges from 1.3 to 4 and the ratio regression model using this variable is:

```
. glm babies storkratio, link(log) family(poisson) exp(women10k) eform
nolog
```

Generalized linear models			No. of obs	=	54
Optimization	: ML		Residual df	=	52
			Scale parameter =		1
Deviance	= 62.6303318		(1/df) Deviance = 1.204429
Pearson	= 69.53837167		(1/df) Pearson = 1.337276
Variance function: V(u) = u			[Poisson]
Link function	: g(u) = ln(u)		[Log]
			AIC	= 6.324185
Log likelihood = −168.7529956			BIC	= −144.7968

```
-----------------------------------------------------------------------
             |               OIM
      babies |    IRR    Std. Err.     z    P>|z|   [95% Conf. Interval]
-------------+---------------------------------------------------------
   storkratio | 1.381786  .0622636   7.18  0.000   1.264985   1.509372
        _cons | 4.31666   .3861718  16.35  0.000   3.622419   5.143953
  ln(women10k)|       1   (exposure)
-----------------------------------------------------------------------
```

The difference model is shown here:

```
. glm brate10k storkratio [iweight=women10k], link(identity) fam(poisson)
nolog
note: brate10k has noninteger values
```

| Generalized linear models | | | No. of obs | = | 54 |
| Optimization | : ML | | Residual df | = | 52 |

```
                                     Scale parameter =          1
Deviance       = 62.84113486         (1/df) Deviance = 1.208483
Pearson        = 69.30010513         (1/df) Pearson  = 1.332694

Variance function: V(u) = u          [Poisson]
Link function    : g(u) = u          [Identity]


                                     AIC             =  14.85211
Log likelihood  = -399.0069073       BIC             = -144.586


- - - - - - - - - - - - - - - - - - - - - - - - - - - - - - - - - - - - - - - -
             |               OIM
   brate10k  |  Coef.   Std. Err.     z    P>|z|   [95% Conf. Interval]
- - - - - - -+ - - - - - - - - - - - - - - - - - - - - - - - - - - - - - - - - -
 storkratio  | 2.962996  .477819    6.20   0.000    2.026488   3.899504
      _cons  | 2.495531  .8558106   2.92   0.004    .8181728   4.172889
- - - - - - - - - - - - - - - - - - - - - - - - - - - - - - - - - - - - - - - -
```

While an increasing stork count is associated with lower birth rates, an increasing stork ratio is associated with higher birth rates. Some statistics (Table 14.2) suggest that the ratio model is superior. We could go on to models (not shown) that include both the stork count and the stork ratio; these show evidence of underdispersion. But we can stop here. The key point is that the linear regression approach was useful for the point Neyman was trying to make, but this is usually not what we want for an analysis of incidence rates. It is usually preferable to treat person-time so that it influences the rate numerator in a simple multiplicative manner, but is not itself an explanatory variable.

TABLE 14.2 Fit statistics for two models used to assess the association between the *stork ratio* (stork count/ number of women) and birthrates in the fictional data of Table 1.2. The rate ratio model used a log link and the difference model used an identity link. The difference column shows the rate ratio model statistic minus the rate difference model statistic.

MODEL STATISTIC	RATE RATIO MODEL	RATE DIFFERENCE MODEL	DIFFERENCE
Deviance	62.6	62.8	−0.2
Deviance P-value for fit	.15	.14	.004
Pearson statistic	69.5	69.3	0.2
Pearson P-value for fit	.052	.055	−.00
Deviance/degrees of freedom	1.20	1.21	−0.00
Pearson/degrees of freedom	1.34	1.33	0.00
Ln(likelihood)	−169	−399	230
AIC (Expression 12.4)	342	802	−461
BIC (Expression 12.6)	345	806	−461
Poisson SE for stork ratio term	0.06	0.48	[a]
Robust SE for stork ratio term	0.06	0.51	[a]
Poisson Z-statistic for stork ratio term	7.2	6.2	1.0
Robust Z-statistic for stork ratio term	6.9	5.9	1.0

[a] Differences in model SEs for the rate ratio and rate difference are not relevant. What matters is the difference in the Poisson and robust SEs for the same model.

Flexible Treatment of Continuous Variables 15

This chapter discusses quadratic splines and fractional polynomials, two methods for the flexible treatment of continuous explanatory variables in regression. These can be used in any regression model and so this material is not essential for a book about incidence rates. But these techniques are so useful, yet unfamiliar to many, that they are described here. In a regression analysis of incidence rates, these methods are often particularly helpful for dealing with calendar time and age. Other methods for smoothing continuous data, such as generalized additive models (Hastie and Tibshirani 1990) and additional nonparametric approaches (Tarter and Lock 1993, Green and Silverman 1994, Simonoff 1996), are available, but not discussed here.

15.1 THE PROBLEM

We may wish to adjust for systolic blood pressure, age, or family income in regression, to remove any confounding influence of these quantities. Using continuous linear terms may be inadequate if the relationships between these variables and the outcomes are not linear. For example, studies have reported that drinking alcohol is related to cardiovascular mortality by a U- or J-shaped curve; mortality is lowest for those who drink alcohol at a low level, somewhat higher for teetotalers, and considerably higher for heavy drinkers. A single linear term will not capture these relationships and therefore may not remove all of the confounding influence of alcohol drinking from regression estimates.

One flexible approach is to reduce a continuous variable to two or more categories and introduce these categories as indicator (factor or dummy) variables. But this approach makes assumptions that may not be realistic. It assumes that within each category the association with the outcome rate does not vary, but between categories that association is allowed a vary abruptly. A smooth relationship is usually more plausible.

15.2 QUADRATIC SPLINES

Imagine that we wish to adjust for age in a regression model with subjects who range from age 0 to 100 years. To create a single smooth curve, we enter age and age^2. But a more pliant relationship can be created using several quadratic curves which join at their boundaries. The selected boundaries, which are called knots, may reflect prior knowledge regarding age and the model outcome. If we pick knots at 20, 50, and 80 years, we can enter the following terms into a regression model:

age (a linear team without any transformation)

$age2 = age^2$

$age20 = 0$ if age ≤ 20, otherwise $= (age - 20)^2$

$age50 = 0$ if age ≤ 50, otherwise $= (age - 50)^2$

$age80 = 0$ if age ≤ 80, otherwise $= (age - 80)^2$

Using the 5 terms listed above will result in a curved relationship between age and the outcome up to age 20. Then from age 20 to 50 another curve is created, but the start of this curve joins the end of the previous curve. Two more curves, one from 50 to 80 years, another from 80 to 100 years, are allowed. One problem with this approach is that a few observations in the tails of the data, from 0 to 20 years and from 80 to 100 years, may have excessive influence on the curves, resulting in bias. To prevent this, we can constrain both tails (age 0 to 20, 80 to 100) to be linear (Greenland 1995) by using the following variables:

age (a linear team without any transformation)

$age20 = 0$ if age ≤ 20, otherwise $= (age - 20)^2 - (age - 80)^2$

$age50 = 0$ if age ≤ 50, otherwise $= (age - 50)^2 - (age - 80)^2$

The three terms listed here will produce straight lines for the age-outcome association (on the ln scale for ratio models) for those younger than age 20 and older than 80 years. From 20 to 50 and from 50 to 80 two different curves are allowed. This flexible approach requires the same number of regression terms as would the use of four age categories (0–20, 21–50, 51–80, 80–100) as dummy or indicator variables.

Olson, Cummings, and Rivara (2006), used conditional Poisson regression (a method discussed in Chapter 20) to estimate the association between air bag presence and risk (not rate) of death within 30 days of a traffic crash. Among persons in a crash, age has a U-shaped relationship with death; risk is greatest among the elderly, falls to a minimum among teenagers, and rises again among younger children. To remove any confounding influence that age might have on the relationship between exposure to an air bag and death, the authors used quadratic splines. Figure 15.1 shows the risk ratio for death for each year of age compared with age 30 years as the reference category; these risk ratios were adjusted for use of a seat belt or car seat, presence of an air bag, sex, and seat position. A fitted curve is also shown, created by using quadratic splines with knots at ages 5, 10, 15, 20, 40, 60, and 80 years and tails constrained to be linear. We can afford to be extravagant with the number of knots terms because there were 128,208 subjects in the data with 45 to 6323 subjects in each 1-year age interval. The flexible curve in Figure 15.1 provides a close fit to the data, while reducing 98 possible 1-year age categories to just seven regression terms.

Further details about linear and quadratic splines, with helpful advice, can be found in a review by Greenland (1995). Cubic splines can be even more flexible, but in epidemiology and biology the degree of flexibility provided by cubic splines may be more than is reasonable. The goal is to smooth the data in a credible way, not to slavishly follow chance fluctuations in the finite samples that we study. Because cubic splines can be overly flexible, a variation known as restricted cubic splines is sometimes used. These can be created using Stata's **mkspline** command or user written commands **rcsgen** and **splinegen**.

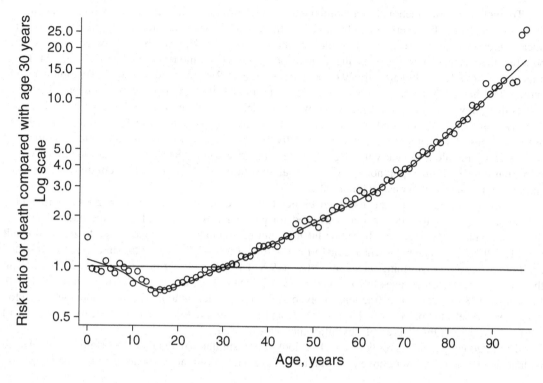

FIGURE 15.1 Quadratic spline example: adjusted risk ratios for death comparing persons at each year of age with persons age 30 years. The fitted line is from quadratic splines with linear tails and knots at 5, 10, 15, 20, 40, 60, and 80 years of age. The circles are the adjusted risks ratios for each year of age. Data for 128,208 persons in 53,249 vehicles that crashed during 1990–2002. Comparisons were made within the same vehicle to control for crash and vehicle characteristics. Risk ratios adjusted for use of a seat belt or car seat, presence of an air bag, passenger sex, and seat position.

15.3 FRACTIONAL POLYNOMIALS

The idea of transforming a variable to improve regression model fit is well known; many books suggest transformations of continuous variables, such as $x^{0.5}$, $\ln(x)$, or x^2. In 1994 Royston and Altman (1994) reviewed this use of transformations and showed how a systematic search among a restricted set of polynomial transformations could produce flexible curves that often fit data closely and avoid spurious performance in the tails of the data. The authors dubbed the method "fractional polynomials" because their approach included the use of polynomial terms that were sometimes fractions rather than integers.

The default set of polynomial terms suggested by Royston and colleagues is –2, –1, –.5, 0, .5, 1, 2, 3. The polynomial 0 is taken to indicate $\ln(x)$, not x^0. The user can select 1, 2, 3, or more of these terms and combine them in the same model; the number selected is called the "dimension" of the fractional polynomial transformation of x. A polynomial choice can be repeated, but each repeated value is multiplied by $\ln(x)$. So if the chosen dimension for a group of fractional polynomial terms is 3 and the best choice for the first polynomial term is x^{-1}, the second term could be $\ln(x) \times x^{-1}$, and the third term could be $\ln(x) \times \ln(x) \times x^{-1}$.

To pick the best fractional polynomial terms, the analyst makes an initial decision about the dimension and then fits every possible model in turn. Models are compared using partial F-tests (for linear regression), or deviance statistics and likelihood ratio tests. This can be a chore as the number of possible models becomes large as the dimension increases: 8 models for 1 dimension, 44 for 2 dimensions, 164 for 3 dimensions, 494 for 4 dimensions, 1286 for 5 dimensions. To minimize this chore, Stata has an **fp** command which automates the model fitting and presents a condensed table of results that allows the analyst to readily see which model is best based on the deviance or on P-values that are approximately adjusted to account for the many comparisons. The **fp** command has many useful options; for example, it can automatically recenter the x variable to aid interpretation and automatically rescale x to deal with negative values or large values. Stata has an additional command, **mfp** (multiple fractional polynomials), which allows fitting of two or more continuous variables simultaneously using fractional polynomials.

Using the traffic crash data discussed earlier (Olson, Cummings, and Rivara 2006), a fractional polynomial model of four dimensions was used for passenger age (Figure 15.2). Age had values of 0 for those younger than their first birthday; $\ln(0)$ cannot be computed and values close to zero can result in undesirably large quantities when transformed by the power -2. The **fp** command therefore rescaled age to (age+1)/10, transforming its values to 0.1 to 9.8. The selected four powers were 1, 2, 3, and 3, so the model used the terms (age+1)/10, $[(age+1)/10]^2$, $[(age+1)/10]^3$, and $[(age+1)/10]^3 \times \ln((age+1)/10)$. Fitting the 1286 models for a fractional polynomial with five terms took about an hour on a desktop computer and selected powers of -1, -1, $-.5$, $-.5$, and 3. These five terms produced a curve (not shown) with a dip at age 1; this degree of flexibility may be excessive.

The fitted curves in Figures 15.1 and 15.2 look pretty similar. The goal of the original study was to include age in the model to remove confounding by age and to estimate associations of air bag exposure

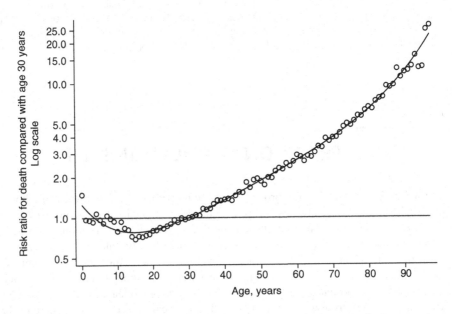

FIGURE 15.2 Fractional polynomial example: adjusted risk ratios for death comparing persons at each year of age with persons age 30 years. The fitted line is from a fractional polynomial model with four dimensions: age was rescaled to (age+1)/10 and the selected powers were 1, 2, 3 and 3. The circles are the adjusted risks ratios for each year of age. Data for 128,208 persons in 53,249 vehicles that crashed during 1990–2002. Comparisons were made within the same vehicle to control for crash and vehicle characteristics. Risk ratios adjusted for use of a seat belt or car seat, presence of an air bag, passenger sex, and seat position.

with death within specific age groups. Both the spline and fractional polynomial approaches show a similar ability to do this for the overall association of air bags with death at all ages. Choosing between these approaches would require more analyses using the additional terms and interactions that were used by Olson, Cummings, and Rivara (2006).

Additional information about fractional polynomials can be found in articles (Royston, Ambler, and Sauerbrei 1999, Sauerbrei and Royston 1999) and a textbook (Royston and Sauerbrei 2008).

15.4 FLEXIBLE ADJUSTMENT FOR TIME

When analyzing rates, there may be interest in studying changes over calendar time or a need to remove potential confounding bias related to calendar time. Several aspects of this topic have been helpfully reviewed by Greenland (1987c) and by Altman and Royston (1988).

Both splines and polynomials can be used to flexibly model calendar time. Rates may be based on information aggregated into fixed intervals; annual mortality rates are an example. If several years of data are available, flexible treatment of calendar year may be appropriate. Calendar time can be expressed in several ways. For example, in a study of homicides in Columbia, Villaveces and colleagues (2000) calculated homicide incidence rates for calendar time units of 6 hours, adjusted for month using 11 indicator variables, adjusted for day of the week using 27 indicators for the 28 intervals of 6 hours, and adjusted for overall trends by modeling calendar day with fractional polynomials. It is also possible to introduce calendar time into a model for longitudinal data and estimate whether the association of interest varied with calendar time by using interaction terms.

Many cohort studies and clinical trials have date of study entry for individuals and date of an outcome. In some studies flexible adjustment may be desired for three measures of time: time since birth (age), time from study entry to study exit, and calendar time, so that compared subjects have the same age, are observed for the same length of time, and are compared at the same moment in calendar time. Time from study entry to exit is equal to follow-up time and for an analysis of rates, this time is typically used as an offset or weight. Alternatively, time to an event can be treated as the outcome and estimates produced by a Cox proportional hazards model, piecewise Poisson model, or Royston-Parmer model (Royston and Parmar 2002). This last group of methods will appear in Chapter 25, and in some examples the assumption of proportional hazards will be relaxed to allow interactions between time and model variables (Royston and Lambert 2011). Fractional polynomials and splines can be used to create flexible time interactions.

15.5 WHICH METHOD IS BEST?

In many instances the choice between quadratic splines and fractional polynomials will make little difference in adjusted estimates. Stata's **fp** command is so fast that it can be used for initial analyses to see how variables are related to each other. Information from these analyses can then be used to create quadratic splines for the final analysis. This is just one of several options.

The two methods described in this chapter are relatively simple to implement and interpret in any statistical software package. Both are easy to use in regression models. The learning curve is short and these tools can help in many analyses.

Variation in Size of an Association

16

Sometimes we want to know if an estimated association varies according to the level of some other characteristic. For example, the association between an exposure and an outcome might vary by the age or sex of the study subjects, by calendar time, or by geographic region. This variation in the size of an association is sometimes called heterogeneity or heterogeneity of effect. It is also called interaction, a name that comes from the use of stratified analysis or regression product (interaction) terms between the exposure and levels of the factor across which the association may vary. Epidemiologists sometimes use the term effect modification, meaning that the size of any exposure effect is modified by some other characteristic. Equivalently, the term subgroup analysis is often used, particularly in relation to randomized controlled trials.

Principled methods for studying heterogeneity of effect and interpreting the results have been described in many articles and books. But the use of inferior methods is so common that problems related to this topic are discussed here, even though they are not strictly necessary in a book about rates.

16.1 AN EXAMPLE: SHOES AND FALLS

In a fictional cohort study of falls and footwear, females who wore sensible shoes had the lowest rate of falling, 0.002 falls per person-week (Table 16.1). Among men with sensible footwear the fall rate was 1.5-fold greater, 0.003. The fall rate was threefold greater, compared those with the lowest rate, among women who wore risky shoes. The highest rate, 0.015, was for men wearing risky shoes. Thirty thousand cohort members were followed for a week. No cohort member fell more than once. The outcome was sufficiently rare that we can assume the falls arose from a Poisson process.

We can use Poisson regression to estimate the association of risky shoe wearing with falls. Create a regression term for risky shoes (riskyshoes, coded 1 for risky, 0 for sensible) and fit Model 1 with riskyshoes as the only term:

```
Model 1
. poisson falls riskyshoes, irr exp(time) nolog
```

```
Poisson regression                          Number of obs  =    30,000
                                            LR chi2(1)     =     54.46
                                            Prob > chi2    =    0.0000
Log likelihood = -1047.9987                 Pseudo R2      =    0.0253
---------------------------------------------------------------------
      falls |    IRR    Std. Err.     z    P>|z|   [95% Conf. Interval]
------------+--------------------------------------------------------
 riskyshoes |   3.375   .6075694    6.76   0.000    2.371592    4.802945
      _cons | .0026667  .0004216  -37.49   0.000    .0019561    .0036354
   ln(time) |       1   (exposure)
---------------------------------------------------------------------
```

Now adjust by adding a term for male sex (male = 1, female = 0) to Model 2:

Model 2
. poisson falls riskyshoes male, irr exp(time) nolog
(output omitted)

```
------------------------------------------------------------------------
      falls |    IRR    Std. Err.    z    P>|z|    [95% Conf. Interval]
------------+-----------------------------------------------------------
 riskyshoes | 4.393228   .8158937   7.97   0.000   3.052824    6.322163
       male | 2.29613    .3655103   5.22   0.000   1.680729    3.136861
      _cons | .0014305   .0002935  -31.93  0.000   .0009569    .0021386
   ln(time) |      1    (exposure)
------------------------------------------------------------------------
```

We can see that there was confounding by sex, as the risky shoe rate ratio changed from 3.4 to 4.4 when adjustment for sex was added in Model 2. Women, who fell less often than men, contributed more person-time to the fall rate of the risky shoe wearers, decreasing the rate of that group. Men contributed more person-time to the fall rate of sensible shoe wearers, increasing the fall rate in that group. Failure to adjust for sex produced a biased rate ratio that confused the lower fall rates of women and the higher fall rates of men with the effect of wearing a risky shoe; this biased the crude (unadjusted) rate ratio downward toward 0.

Assuming there are no additional confounding factors or other sources of bias, is the rate ratio of 4.4 for risky shoe wearing a good estimate for *all* or should we prefer separate estimates for women and men? In other words, does sex modify the association of risky shoe wearing with falls? To answer these questions we create an interaction term between male sex and risky shoes: mxriskyshoes is coded 1 for males with risky shoes and 0 for all others. Then we fit Model 3, which includes the interaction term and the main effect term for male sex, and use Stata's **lincom** command to produce separate estimates for the risky shoe association for men and women:

Model 3
. poisson falls riskyshoes male mxriskyshoes, irr exp(time) nolog
(output omitted)

```
------------------------------------------------------------------------
        falls |    IRR    Std. Err.   z    P>|z|    [95% Conf. Interval]
--------------+---------------------------------------------------------
   riskyshoes |      3    1.024695   3.22   0.001   1.535962    5.859519
         male |    1.5    .5477226   1.11   0.267    .7332911   3.068359
 mxriskyshoes | 1.666667  .6735753   1.26   0.206    .7548136   3.680084
        _cons |   .002    .0006325 -19.65  0.000    .0010761    .0037171
     ln(time) |      1   (exposure)
------------------------------------------------------------------------
```

. lincom riskyshoes + mxriskyshoes, irr
(output omitted)

```
------------------------------------------------------------------------
      falls |    IRR    Std. Err.    z    P>|z|    [95% Conf. Interval]
------------+-----------------------------------------------------------
        (1) |     5    1.080123    7.45   0.000   3.274081     7.63573
------------------------------------------------------------------------
```

TABLE 16.1 Hypothetical data from a cohort study of falls and footwear. Shoes were classified by the researchers as sensible (good support, short heels, and nonslip sole) or risky (flimsy, high heels, slippery soles). All subjects (30,000) used only a single pair of shoes for one week of follow-up. No one fell more than once.

SEX	FOOTWARE	PERSONS	FALLS	RATE PER PERSON-WEEK
Female	Sensible	5,000	10	0.002
Male	Sensible	10,000	30	0.003
Female	Risky	10,000	60	0.006
Male	Risky	5,000	75	0.015

The riskyshoes term in the regression output table for Model 3 is the rate ratio for risky shoe wearing of *women only*, because the relevant information about the men with risky shoes was contained in the interaction term. The model estimated the rate ratio for risky shoe wearing by females as 3.0. For men, the rate ratio for falls when wearing risky shoes, compared with sensible shoes, was the product of the rate ratio for women (3.0) multiplied by the rate ratio for the interaction term: $3.0 \times 1.667 = 5.0$. The **lincom** (for linear comparison) command carries out the computations for us, including statistics that account for the covariance of the riskyshoes and mxriskyshoes terms.

Should we prefer the risky shoe rate ratio of 4.4 for all persons or the separate ratios of 3.0 for women and 5.0 for men? In summarizing the results, it would be fair to say something like this: "In this cohort the rate of falling was greater for those wearing risky shoes compared with otherwise similar persons who used sensible shoes: rate ratio 4.4 (95% confidence interval (CI) 3.1, 6.3)." If this was the first study of this topic and if there was no particular reason to think that the association varied by the sex of the shoe user, we might also add a second sentence: "We found no evidence that the association varied by sex: a test of homogeneity produced P = .21." If there was interest in knowing how the association varied by sex, perhaps because of a theory proposed by shoe engineers, we might revise the second sentence to say:

Although the rate ratio associated with risky shoes was greater for men (5.0) than for women (3.0), the difference in these ratios was not statistically significant: P = .21 from a test of interaction between subject sex and use of risky shoes.

We might even give the CIs for the separate estimates, so that the separate rate ratios can be compared with those from future studies or summarized in a future meta-analysis.

The key point here is that we judge whether the association varies by sex using a formal test of whether the estimated associations for men and women differ significantly from the null hypothesis that they are the same. The P-value for the interaction term, mxriskyshoes, provides this test. Alternatively, we could use a likelihood ratio test comparing models without and with the interaction; that P-value is .22.

16.2 PROBLEM 1: USING SUBGROUP P-VALUES FOR INTERPRETATION

A common problem that arises when subgroups are examined is the incorrect use of the *subgroup* P-values for interpretation. In Model 3, the P-value for the interaction term was .21; this term tests the null hypothesis that the association for risky shoes does not vary by sex. Finding a small P-value would be evidence of heterogeneity by sex. Unfortunately, authors often ignore the interaction P-value and focus instead upon the subgroup P-values, reporting something like this: "Wearing a risky shoe was associated with a threefold increase in the fall rate among women (rate ratio 3.0, 95% CI 1.5, 5.9, p=.001) and an even greater rate increase among men (rate ratio 5.0, 95% CI 3.3, 7.6, p<.001)." This sentence is correct, as far as it goes, but ignores the fact that a formal test of the difference between the rate ratios of 3 and 5 produced a large P-value. Model 3, alone, provides little evidence that the association of risky shoe wearing with falling varies by sex. Many articles (Altman and Matthews 1996, Matthews and Altman 1996a, 1996b, Pocock et al. 2002, Altman and Bland 2003, Brookes et al. 2004) and books (Pocock 1983 pp213–215, Fisher and van Belle 1993 pp619–620, MacMahon and Trichopoulos 1996 pp279–280,284–286, Matthews 2000 pp97–105, Rothman, Greenland, and Lash 2008c pp61–62,72–76,258–259,270,279–280,402–404) have eloquently explained why reliance upon subgroup P-values, or analyses limited to subgroups, as opposed to formal tests of homogeneity of effect, are misleading approaches to judging whether or not variation in association is present. The paper by Brookes et al. (2004) describes the results of simulation studies; formal tests of homogeneity performed well, whereas separate interpretations based upon subgroup P-values were frequently in error.

16.3 PROBLEM 2: FAILURE TO INCLUDE MAIN EFFECT TERMS WHEN INTERACTION TERMS ARE USED

When interaction terms are used in a model the main effects terms should be as rich (meaning complete or thorough), or richer, as the interaction terms in the model. Omitting or abridging main effect terms can produce estimates that confuse main effects with the interaction estimates. Imagine, for example, that an analyst looked at Model 3, shown earlier, and decided that as the P-value for the male sex term was large (.27), this term should be omitted from the model. Results are in Model 4, shown here:

Model 4

```
------------------------------------------------------------------
      falls |     IRR   Std. Err.      z    P>|z|    [95% Conf. Interval]
------------+-----------------------------------------------------
 riskyshoes |    2.25   .4592793    3.97   0.000    1.508106   3.356861
mxriskyshoes |    2.5   .4330127    5.29   0.000    1.780359   3.510528
      _cons | .0026667   .0004216  -37.49   0.000    .0019561   .0036354
   ln(time) |       1   (exposure)
------------------------------------------------------------------
```

. lincom riskyshoes + mxriskyshoes, irr
(output omitted)

```
------------------------------------------------------------------
      falls |    IRR   Std. Err.      z    P>|z|    [95% Conf. Interval]
------------+-----------------------------------------------------
        (1) |  5.625   1.101313   8.82   0.000    3.832363   8.256166
------------------------------------------------------------------
```

Model 4 shows a rate estimate of 0.0027 for the constant or intercept term; this is the person-time weighted average fall rate per person-week for all persons, male and female, who wore sensible shoes. The riskyshoes term with the rate ratio of 2.25 compares women who wore risky shoes (rate 0.006 in

Table 16.1) with men *and* women who wore sensible shoes: 0.006/0.002667 = 2.25. This is smaller than the correct estimate, 3.0, because the effect of risky shoe wearing is now mixed up with the effect of sex. Similarly, the interaction term, mxriskyshoes, has also changed its meaning. In Model 3 this term was a ratio estimate of the amount by which the fall rate ratio for men wearing risky shoes differed from that for women who wore risky shoes; the variable was coded 1 for men who wore risky shoes and otherwise coded zero for each of 3 groups; women in sensible shoes, women in risky shoes, and men in sensible shoes. All 3 of those zero or baseline groups were in Model 3. But in Model 4, only two of these groups are in the model; men and women combined in sensible shoes, and women in risky shoes. Consequently, the effect of male sex on fall rates is mixed up with the effect of risky shoes; the result was a rate ratio of 5.6, biased from the correct estimate of 5.0.

When interaction terms are used, the main effects that make up the interaction term should all be in the model, so that the interaction represents what we expect. This does not guarantee an unbiased estimate, but at least we are estimating what we intended to estimate. This means that if we use three-way interaction terms, then all lesser two-way interactions should be in the model as well as all the main effect terms. An additional corollary is that interaction terms do not need to be as complete as main effect terms. For example, if we wanted to know if any association between wearing risky shoes and falling varied with age, we might use several quadratic spline terms to account for the main effects of age, and then only use two or three age categories to examine interactions between age and shoe type.

16.4 PROBLEM 3: INCORRECTLY CONCLUDING THAT THERE IS NO VARIATION IN ASSOCIATION

Assuming Model 3 contains our best estimates regarding risky shoes and falls, it would be a mistake to say: "The association between risky shoe wearing and falls did not vary by sex." The association *did* vary by sex: it was 3.0 for women, 5.0 for men. A claim that the association did not vary would only be true if the rate ratios were identical for men and women. The finding of a large P-value, .21, from a test of heterogeneity, means that the difference in the two rate ratios might readily arise because we do studies in finite samples. The observed difference in these rate ratios may be entirely or partly due to what we loosely call chance. Given the P-value, we do not have good evidence to support a claim that there *is* variation by sex. But finding a large P-value does not prove that chance explains all, or even part, of the observed difference in the two rate ratios. Large P-values do not prove a null-hypothesis of no difference is true, they only tell us that we do not have strong evidence to reject the null hypothesis (Altman and Bland 1995, Alderson 2004, Hauer 2004, Cummings and Koepsell 2010). No study can ever be large enough to prove that two rate ratios or differences do not differ.

16.5 PROBLEM 4: INTERACTION MAY BE PRESENT ON A RATIO SCALE BUT NOT ON A DIFFERENCE SCALE, AND VICE VERSA

Near the end of Chapter 3, I pointed out that effect modification may exist on the difference scale but not on the ratio scale, and vice versa. If there is an association between exposure and outcome and if the outcome rate when not exposed is different for two groups, then absence of effect modification on the ratio scale implies that there must be effect modification on the difference scale. Similarly, if there is no variation in the association on the difference scale, there must be some variation on the ratio scale if the rates when not exposed differ. This is true for the data in Table 16.1. A rate difference model is shown here:

```
. glm rate riskyshoes male mxriskyshoes [iw=time], link(identity) f(poisson)
nolog
(output omitted)
```

```
                 |              OIM
           rate  |   Coef.   Std. Err.     z    P>|z|    [95% Conf. Interval]
-----------------+----------------------------------------------------------
     riskyshoes  |   .004       .001     4.00   0.000    .00204     .00596
           male  |   .001     .0008367   1.20   0.232   -.0006398   .0026398
   mxriskyshoes  |   .008     .0020736   3.86   0.000    .0039357   .0120643
          _cons  |   .002     .0006325   3.16   0.002    .0007604   .0032396
```

This rate difference model estimates that the fall rate among women with sensible shoes was .002 falls per week. For a woman, wearing risky shoes increased their rate by +.004 falls. The risky shoe rate increase for women, however, was significantly less (P<.001 for the interaction term) than the rate increase induced by risky shoe wearing for men, +.004 + .008 = +.012 additional falls per week. So our previous statement about the homogeneity test for Model 4 should perhaps be revised to say "We found no evidence that the *rate ratio* for the association of risky shoe wearing with falls varied by sex: a test of homogeneity produced p = .21." We might consider whether we prefer a rate difference model for these data.

A more detailed discussion of how variation in associations depends upon the choice of scale may be found in a chapter by Greenland, Lash, and Rothman (2008a).

16.6 PROBLEM 5: FAILURE TO REPORT ALL SUBGROUP ESTIMATES IN AN EVENHANDED MANNER

For problem 5, I will discuss a published study that did not use incidence rates, but which I hope readers will find thought-provoking. In February 1999 an article by Schulman et al. (1999) appeared in the New England Journal of Medicine with the title "The effect of race and sex on physicians' recommendations for cardiac catheterization." The investigators used eight actors who recounted a scripted history of chest pain in a filmed interview. Two actors were white men, two were white women, two were black men, and two were black women. Within each of these pairs by race and sex, one actor portrayed a patient of age 55 and the other played a patient age 70 years. The filmed interviews were shown to physicians at two national meetings in 1996 and 1997. Only one actor, assigned at random, was seen by each physician; the filmed history for each of the eight actors was shown to 90 physicians. The physicians knew that they were participating in a study of clinical decision-making, but they were not told that patient race and sex were of interest. Additional data were provided to the doctors, such as information about smoking history and the results of a cardiac stress test. After being given all the clinical data, each physician was asked whether they would refer the patient for cardiac catheterization. The abstract of the article reported

Logistic-regression analysis indicated that women (odds ratio, 0.60; 95 percent CI, 0.4 to 0.9; P=0.02) and blacks (odds ratio, 0.60; 95 percent CI, 0.4 to 0.9; P=0.02) were less likely to be referred for cardiac catheterization than men and whites, respectively. Analysis of race-sex interactions showed that black women were significantly less likely to be referred for catheterization than white men (odds ratio, 0.4; 95 percent CI, 0.2 to 0.7; P=0.004).

The study received extensive media coverage; an article in the *New York Times* (1999) was representative of many media statements:

A new study of 720 physicians found that with all symptoms being equal, doctors were 60 percent as likely to order cardiac catheterization for women and blacks as for men and whites. For black women, the doctors were 40 percent as likely to order catheterization …

A few months later the *New England Journal* printed a multipage critique (Schwartz, Woloshin, and Welch 1999) of the way in which the study data were reported. The main criticism was that the media had mistaken odds ratios for risk ratios, a problem that might have been avoided if risk ratios had been given in the journal article. The proportion of actor-patients referred for cardiac catheterization was 90.6% for white male actors (Table 16.2), 90.6% for black males, and 90.6% for white females. Only among black females was the referred proportion less, 78.9%. These were the crude proportions, but further adjustment for other variables in the study did little to change the ratios or differences in these proportions. Because the outcome of referral was so common, the odds ratios given by Schulman et al. (1999) were much further from 1 compared with risk ratios for the same outcome. Analyses of age-adjusted risk ratios and risk differences (Table 16.3), without any interaction term, estimated that physicians were 5% less likely to refer blacks or females, compared with white males, far from the 40% less likely reported in the media. While any amount of bias is reprehensible, over 95% of physicians seemed to make referral decisions without regard to race or sex of the patient.

The critics of the article, Schwartz, Woloshin, and Welch (1999), argued that risk ratios for a referral should have been presented in lieu of odds ratios. But when outcomes are common, risk ratios will necessarily be close to 1 (Cummings 2009b). One option would be to use no referral as the study outcome (Table 16.3); when this is done, the odds ratios and risk ratios are not far apart. Another option would be to estimate risk differences. Risk differences, combined with a clear presentation of the crude referral proportions, should make the findings clear, and risk differences have the advantage of being the same, aside from being negative or positive, regardless of whether referral or no referral is used as the outcome. (The topic of symmetry of measures of association was discussed in Section 3.9.)

TABLE 16.2 Data regarding how the race and sex of actor-patients was related to referral for cardiac catheterization by physicians who participated in a study of clinical decision making.

ACTOR NUMBER	RACE	SEX	AGE (YRS)	REFERRED NO. (%)	NOT REFERRED NO. (%)
1	White	Male	55	82 (91.1)	8 (8.9)
2	White	Male	70	81 (90.0)	9 (10.0)
3	Black	Male	55	82 (91.1)	8 (8.9)
4	Black	Male	70	81 (90.0)	9 (10.0)
5	White	Female	55	83 (92.2)	7 (7.8)
6	White	Female	70	80 (88.9)	10 (11.1)
7	Black	Female	55	76 (84.4)	14 (15.6)
8	Black	Female	70	66 (73.3)	24 (26.7)

TABLE 16.3 Estimates of the association between the race and sex of actor-patients and their referral for cardiac catheterization by physicians in a study of clinical decision making. The outcome was referral for catheterization. Model 1 compared all blacks with white males and all females with white males; there was no interaction term between race and sex. Model 2 included an interaction between race and sex, so three groups were compared with white males. Model 3 was identical to Model 1 and Model 4 identical to Model 2, except that for Models 3 and 4 the outcome was *not* being referred for cardiac catheterization. Data used are in Table 16.2. All estimates adjusted for actor-patient age, 55 or 70 years.

ACTOR/PATIENT GROUP	ODDS RATIO	RISK RATIO	RISK DIFFERENCE
Model 1: outcome = referred for cardiac catheterization			
White male	1.0 (reference)	1.0 (reference)	0 (reference)
Black	0.6	0.95	−.05
Female	0.6	0.95	−.05
Model 2: outcome = referred for cardiac catheterization			
White male	1.0 (reference)	1.0 (reference)	0 (reference)
Black male	1.0	1.00	.00
White female	1.0	1.00	.00
Black female	0.4	0.87	−.11
Model 3: outcome = NOT referred for cardiac catheterization			
White male	1.0 (reference)	1.0 (reference)	0.0 (reference)
Black	1.7	1.6	+.05
Female	1.7	1.6	+.05
Model 4: outcome = NOT referred for cardiac catheterization			
White male	1.0 (reference)	1.0 (reference)	0 (reference)
Black male	1.0	1.0	.00
White female	1.0	1.0	.00
Black female	2.6	2.2	+.11

Schulman et al. (1999) reported in the abstract that the odds ratio for referral of black women, compared with white males, was 0.4 (Model 2, Table 16.3). The abstract said nothing about the associations for black males and white females compared with white males; both were odds ratios of 1.0. The subgroup analysis from Model 2 suggests that physicians refer white males, black males, and white females without regard to skin color or sex. But for some reason they don't make similar referral decisions for black women: the proportion referred was 11% smaller compared with the proportions for any of the other 3 groups. Two descriptions of the results were presented by Schulman and colleagues: (1) either there was some reluctance to refer blacks and females, compared with whites and males, as shown by Model 1 (2) or all groups were treated equally except for black females, as suggested by Model 2. The reader of the abstract cannot possibly discern the difference between these descriptions, because most of the subgroups were omitted from the abstract. Most readers of the full paper probably found this confusing; both models appear in Table 5 of the paper, but the model with the interaction term was described in just 1 sentence.

Which model of the results should we prefer? The authors reported (Schulman et al. 1999 p623) that the P-value for the interaction term was .06. They never state which model they think is best, but in their discussion section and in the conclusion of the abstract, they seem to prefer Model 1, as they repeatedly say that both patient race and sex influenced referrals. Given that position, the presentation of the subgroup analysis for black women only in the abstract seems unwise; it seems to be there for its shock value only, as the authors do not adopt Model 2 as their main model. The authors presented only the subgroup comparison that suggested bias and failed to mention the other subgroups that suggested equitable referrals for three of the four patient groups.

Several critics of Shulman's study (Schulman et al. 1999) argued that Model 2 (Table 16.3) should be the correct choice (Schwartz, Woloshin, and Welch 1999 pp280–281, Helft, Worthley, and Chokron 1999, Grima 1999). They reasoned that since the unadjusted referral proportions were the same for white men, black men, and white women, we should accept that the risk ratios were 1.0 for any two of those groups compared with the others. This reasoning seems to use subgroup estimates to make conclusions about interactions. This view overlooks the uncertainty in the subgroup estimates: for example, when black men were compared with white men, the odds ratio was 1.0, but the 95% CI was 0.5, 2.1, suggesting a lot of imprecision in this ratio. (The age-adjusted 95% CI for the risk ratio was 0.5, 1.9.) This violates the approach to heterogeneity that I described earlier, which argues that we consider main effects first and accept interaction terms only when they meet some criteria for statistical significance; a P-value of .06 does not meet the usual criteria of alpha = .05. A choice between Models 1 and 2 is made more difficult because the P-value of .06 is close to .05; how rigid should we be about using P<.05 as the cutoff for accepting Model 2? The choice between Models 1 and 2 can be endlessly debated with these data.

The original study (Schulman et al. 1999), the lengthy criticism by Schwartz, Woloshin, and Welch (1999 pp280–281), and the related letters (Curfman and Kassirer 1999, Davidoff 1999, Helft, Worthley, and Chokron 1999, Grima 1999, Persaud 1999, Schulman, Berlin, and Escarce 1999, Woloshin, Schwartz, and Welch 1999) are worth reading. These papers could be used for a journal club discussion.

The point that I wish to emphasize here is that if the association of interest varies across subgroups, the results from *all* subgroups should be presented in a neutral manner. Presenting or highlighting the estimates that are most dramatically different from the null ignores the fact that any variation (heterogeneity) means that other estimates must have moved closer to the null, compared with the overall association based upon all subgroups.

Related to this idea is the question of whether or not subgroup analysis is useful if the overall association is close to the null. Imagine that there is no association between exposure and outcome; the rate ratio is 1.0. In that case, is it meaningful to examine variation in association? Any variation would mean that the exposure is harmful in some subgroups but beneficial in others. Weiss (2008) discusses this situation and argues that it is uncommon that an exposure that can cause disease in some may prevent the same disease in others. Therefore, when the overall association is close to the null, evidence of variation should be treated with skepticism. There are situations in which this may be true; for example, first generation air bags reduced the risk of death for adults, but probably increased the risk of death for young children (Olson, Cummings, and Rivara 2006). Nevertheless, this situation is unusual.

Negative Binomial Regression

17

The negative binomial distribution has been known for a century. It has been described as an extension or version of (1) the binomial distribution (in contrast to the usual binomial distribution, which has been called the positive binomial) (Yule 1910, Greenwood and Yule 1920, Fisher 1941, Haldane 1941, Cook 2009), (2) the geometric distribution (Yule 1910, Rice 1995 pp38–39, Cook 2009, Forbes et al. 2011), and (3) the Poisson distribution (Greenwood and Yule 1920, Fisher 1941, Bliss and Fisher 1953, Cook 2009). By about 1940, statisticians realized that the negative binomial distribution could be described as a mixture of a Poisson distribution and a Gamma distribution (Haldane 1941, Greenwood 1950, Ross and Preece 1985, McCullagh and Nelder 1989 p199). Negative binomial regression began to appear in statistical software packages in 1992 (Hilbe 2011 p8).

Expression 9.10 showed a multiplicative model for rate ratios that predicts the outcome counts (C) from the estimated regression coefficients (the b terms) and person-time (T) information. The Poisson model treated person-time as an ancillary variable. Time entered into the formula so that any change in person-time had a multiplicative effect on the outcome count, but time was not used in the maximum likelihood estimates. For the next few pages, I will ignore person-time, because it simplifies the discussion, and only discuss the estimation of counts. Person-time could be ignored in real data if, for example, observed counts always arose from the same amount of person-time. When person-time is omitted, Expression 9.10 for the Poisson model becomes Expression 17.1:

$$C = \exp[b_0 + b_1x_1 + b_2x_2 + \ldots + b_kx_k] = e^{[b0 + b1xi + b2x2 + \ldots + bkxk]} \tag{Ex.17.1}$$

If counts are from a Poisson process, the mean predicted count for each covariate pattern will have a variance equal to the mean count; mean count = variance (Table 4.4). But if there is more dispersion in the observed counts than would be expected from a Poisson process, this Poisson variance will be too narrow. To allow for this overdispersion, we could assume that the counts arose in a different way.

Assumption 1: For every observation in the data, the event counts are from a Poisson process; that is, for each person or geographic region or institution, the counts were produced by a process which was constant and the occurrence of each event did not influence the occurrence of the next event.

Assumption 2: From one observation to the next, the rate at which the counts were produced can vary. The Poisson process is constant for each observation, but it varies between observations. Assumption 2 is about variation in event rates that is not accounted for by measured variables, such as sex, age, or calendar time, in the regression model.

Assumption 3: Expression 17.1 can be modified to allow the mean Poisson count to vary between observations. One way is to create an imaginary term that allows for random variation; I will call this term RV for random variable. The exponentiated values of the RV terms (exp(RV) or e^{RV}) are described by a gamma distribution; these exp(RV) terms have a mean of 1, RV terms have a mean of 0 (McCullagh and Nelder 1989 p199, Hilbe 2011 pp188–189, Cameron and Trivedi 2013a p74).

Under these assumptions, the revised expression for predicted counts (omitting any time variable) is shown in Expression 17.2:

$$C = \exp[b_0 + b_1 x_1 + b_2 x_2 + \ldots + b_k x_k + RV]$$

$$= e^{[b0 + b1\ xi + b2\ x2 + \ldots + bk\ xk + RV]}$$

$$= e^{RV} \times e^{[b0 + b1\ x1 + b2\ x2 + \ldots + bk\ xk]}$$ (Ex.17.2)

$$= \exp(RV) \times \exp[b_0 + b_1 x_1 + b_2 x_2 + \ldots + b_k x_k]$$

$$= \exp[(b_0 + RV) + b_1 x_1 + b_2 x_2 + \ldots + b_k x_k]$$

$$= \exp[b_0^* + b_1 x_1 + b_2 x_2 + \ldots + b_k x_k]$$

The last two lines of Expression 17.1 show that this is a random intercept model (Fitzmaurice, Laird, and Ware 2011 p191). The intercept b_0 is the usual model intercept term, the mean count when all other variables equal zero. The RV terms have an average of zero; adding RV to b_0 represents each observation's *deviation* from that intercept. Heterogeneity between observations is introduced by allowing the intercept for the mean count to vary randomly from one observation to the next.

Since the mean of the exp(RV) terms is constrained to equal 1, the mean count predicted by Expression 17.2 will be the same as the mean count predicted by a Poisson model (Expression 17.1). But predicted counts may be greater or smaller depending upon the exp(RV) value for each observation, so the counts will be more spread out (more dispersed) than counts from a Poisson process. Expression 17.2 will produce more small counts and more large counts compared with Expression 17.1. Expression 17.2 will predict fewer counts in the middle of the distribution, near the mean count.

The Gamma distribution is used in Assumption 3 because it is flexible and is mathematically tractable (Cook and Lawless 2007 p36,79); it is used because it works. A regression model created by combining Poisson and gamma distributions corresponds to a negative binomial regression model. In this model the variance of the mean count is a combination of the usual Poisson variance, C, plus the gamma variance of the additional RV terms. There are two common options, among many, for this additional gamma variance. The first is a gamma variance equal to a constant term, delta (estimated by maximum likelihood), which is multiplied by the mean count, C. This is added to the Poisson variance (Hilbe 2014 p135):

$$\text{Variance of } C = \text{Poisson variance} + \text{gamma variance}$$

$$= C + \text{delta} \times C$$ (Ex.17.3)

$$= C \times (1 + \text{delta})$$

This model can be fit in Stata software by specifying the option **dispersion(constant)** when invoking Stata's command, **nbreg**, for negative binomial regression. Stata calls this the constant dispersion model, because the dispersion is 1 + delta for all observations that share the same covariate pattern. Hilbe labels this the linear negative binomial (Hilbe 2014 p127). Cameron and Trivedi (1998, 2013a) dub this the NB1 model because the power applied to the count is 1 in Expression 17.3.

The second common option is to express the gamma variance as alpha x C^2. The alpha term is estimated by maximum likelihood and is not equal to the previously discussed delta term. This model is called the negative binomial *mean* dispersion model in Stata. The dispersion for each observation is 1 + alpha × $\exp[b_0 + b_1 x_1 + \ldots + b_k x_k]$ and this can vary between observations. The variance function for the mean count is now quadratic (McCullagh and Nelder 1989 p199). Hilbe calls this the quadratic negative binomial (Hilbe 2014 p127,135). Cameron and Trivedi call it the NB2 model (Cameron and Trivedi 1998, 2013a); 2 designates the power to which the count is raised in the variance expression. When this model is used, the variance express becomes:

Variance of C = Poisson variance + gamma variance

$$= C + alpha \times C^2 \qquad (Ex.17.4)$$
$$= C \times (1 + alpha \times C)$$

The delta and alpha terms are called dispersion or overdispersion parameters. The larger they are, the more dispersed or spread out the counts become, compared with the Poisson distribution. If delta or alpha is equal to 0, the model reduces to the Poisson model.

When negative binomial regression is used, the quadratic or NB2 version is the usual choice (Hilbe 2014 p130). This is the default choice made by Stata's **nbreg** command; Stata calls this the *mean dispersion model*. This NB2 version is the more flexible choice, allowing the extra-Poisson dispersion to vary across observations. It provides consistent estimates of the regression coefficients for count data even when the data do not fit the negative binomial distribution (Cameron and Trivedi 2013a pp84–85). Regression coefficient estimates from the linear (constant dispersion or NB1) model will be biased unless the data really are negative binomial. More details about the mathematical derivation and properties of these Poisson-gamma mixture models can be found elsewhere (Cook and Lawless 2007 pp36,76–82, Winkelmann 2008 pp20–24, Cook 2009, Lord and Park; Hilbe 2011 pp187–199, Cameron and Trivedi 2013a pp80–84,117–119).

17.1 NEGATIVE BINOMIAL REGRESSION IS A RANDOM EFFECTS OR MIXED MODEL

Negative binomial regression is a mixed model, because it estimates fixed effects, the regression coefficients, and it estimates random effects which follow a gamma distribution. These random effects are also called random heterogeneity or latent variables. Negative binomial regression is a random-intercept mixed model (Diggle et al. 2002 pp186–187, Cameron and Trivedi 2013a pp111–119). The gamma distribution allows the constant or intercept term to vary from one observation to the next. Gardiner, Luo, and Roman (2009) describe negative binomial regression as a random effects model and they distinguish this from a mixed model; the meaning of this distinction is discussed in Chapter 18.

17.2 AN EXAMPLE: ACCIDENTS AMONG WORKERS IN A MUNITIONS FACTORY

In a paper about the negative binomial distribution, Greenwood and Yule (1920) provided data (Table 17.1) regarding the accident frequency of women who manufactured 6-inch artillery shells. The data were from a government report by Greenwood and Woods (1919 Table 2). Observed person-time was the same (5 weeks) for all 647 women and the accident rate was 301/647 = 0.465 accidents per woman over 5 weeks. I entered these data as 6 records for accident counts from 0 to 5 (no woman had more than 5) and used Poisson regression, with frequency weights for the number of women with each count, to estimate the predicted distribution of the events under the assumption that the accidents arose from a uniform Poisson process:

TABLE 17.1 Data regarding the accident counts of 647 women who were followed for 5-weeks at a munition factory that produced 6-inch artillery shells during World War I. Rate was 301/647 = 0.465 accidents per woman over 5 weeks. Data from Greenwood, M., and H. M. Woods. 1919. The Incidence of Industrial Accidents Upon Individuals with Special Reference to Multiple Accidents. Report No. 4. London: Medical Research Committee, Industrial Fatigue Research Board, Her Majesty's Stationary Office.

ACCIDENT COUNT FOR EACH WOMAN	OBSERVED COUNTS OF WOMEN NO. (%)	PREDICTED COUNTS OF WOMEN FROM POISSON DISTRIBUTION NO. (%)	PREDICTED COUNTS OF WOMEN FROM NEGATIVE BINOMIAL DISTRIBUTION NO. (%)
0	447 (69.1)	406 (62.8)	446 (68.9)
1	132 (20.4)	189 (29.2)	135 (20.8)
2	42 (6.5)	44 (6.8)	44 (6.8)
3	21 (3.3)	7 (1.1)	15 (2.3)
4	3 (0.5)	1 (0.1)	5 (0.8)
5	2 (0.3)	0 (0.0)	2 (0.3)

```
. input accidents women

         accidents     women
  1.             0       447
  2.             1       132
  3.             2        42
  4.             3        21
  5.             4         3
  6.             5         2
  7. end

. poisson accidents [fweight=women], irr nolog
```

```
Poisson regression                          Number of obs  =        647
                                            LR chi2(0)     =       0.00
                                            Prob > chi2    =          .
Log likelihood = -617.18432                 Pseudo R2      =     0.0000

------------------------------------------------------------------------
 accidents | Inc. Rate  Std. Err.      z    P>|z|    [95% Conf. Interval]
-----------+------------------------------------------------------------
     _cons | .4652241   .0268151  -13.28   0.000    .4155275     .5208644
------------------------------------------------------------------------
```

```
. estat gof
      Deviance goodness-of-fit =   781.0058
      Prob > chi2(646)         =     0.0002
      Pearson goodness-of-fit  =   960.7575
      Prob > chi2(646)         =     0.0000
```

Use the model to predict the proportion of accidents with each count:
```
. predict pprop, pr(accidents)
```

Use the predicted proportions to get the model predicted counts
. gen pcount = round(pprop*647)

Obtain predicted proportions (probabilities) from a Poisson distribution
function
. gen double pprob2 = poissonp(exp(_b[_cons]),accidents)

All women were followed for 5 weeks, so person-time was omitted from the model; this will have no effect on the estimates. The goodness-of-fit tests provide evidence that the counts are not from a Poisson process. The **predict** command was used to estimate the proportion (pprop) of the accidents in each count category. Equation 4.1 showed how the distribution of event counts could be calculated from a mean count that is assumed to come from a Poisson distribution; the **predict** command after Poisson regression makes this easy. Counts were generated by multiplying the predicted proportions (pprop) by the total count of 647 and rounding to the nearest integer (Table 17.1). I also used the statistical function, **poissonp**, to estimate the predicted proportions for each accident count when the mean count, exp(_b[_cons]), is equal to 0.4652241. Doing this was superfluous, as the values of pprob2 and pprop are the same, but it shows the relationship between what is predicted by Poisson regression and by the statistical function **poissonp**. Compared with the observed counts, the Poisson distribution predicted an insufficient number of women with 0 accidents, a surfeit with 1 accident, and too few with 3, 4, and 5 accidents.

Negative binomial regression was then used in the same way:

. nbreg accidents [fweight=women], irr nolog

```
Negative binomial regression              Number of obs  =        647
                                          LR chi2(0)     =       0.00
Dispersion     = mean                     Prob > chi2    =          .
Log likelihood = -592.2671                Pseudo R2      =     0.0000
```

```
------------------------------------------------------------------------------
  accidents |      IRR   Std. Err.      z    P>|z|     [95% Conf. Interval]
------------+-----------------------------------------------------------------
      _cons |  .4652241  .0332524  -10.71   0.000     .4044098    .5351836
------------+-----------------------------------------------------------------
    /lnalpha|  .1448919  .2152907                    -.2770702     .566854
------------+-----------------------------------------------------------------
      alpha |  1.155915  .2488577                     .7580013    1.762713
------------------------------------------------------------------------------
Likelihood-ratio test of alpha=0:  chibar2(01) = 49.83 Prob>=chibar2 = 0.000
```

. predict nbprop, pr(accidents)

. gen nbcount = round(nbprop*647)

. di e(alpha)
1.1559146

. di 1/e(alpha)
.86511582

. di 1/(1+ exp(_b[_cons]))*e(alpha))

```
.65029681

. gen double nbprob2 = /*
>     */ nbinomialp(1/e(alpha),accidents,1/(1+ e(alpha)*exp(_b[_cons])))
```

The intercept only negative binomial model estimated the same mean count (the rate per 5-weeks of woman-time) of 0.465 that was estimated by Poisson regression. This was expected from Expression 17.2, because the mean of the exp(RV) terms is constrained to equal 1. The standard error (SE) of 0.0333 is larger than the Poisson SE of 0.0268, because the negative binomial variance is larger than the Poisson variance when alpha is larger than zero. The regression table shows the estimated value for alpha, 1.16. The output reports a likelihood ratio test for the hypothesis that alpha is equal to 0; the test result, P <.001, provides evidence against this hypothesis. This test is a handy way of assessing whether overdispersion is present. Some authors suggest using the robust variance estimator when fitting a negative binomial model (Cameron and Trivedi 2013a p85, Hilbe 2014 p125), because of concern that if the data do not fit a negative binomial distribution, the SEs may not be correct. When I did this, the SE shrank a bit from 0.0333 to 0.0327. This small change suggests the negative binomial model accounted well for the extra-Poisson dispersion. The good fit of the predicted counts is apparent from the predicted proportions and counts in Table 17.1, predictions that are close to the observed values.

In the output, I used the statistical function command, **nbinomialp()**, to calculate the probability of each count. The values of nbprob2 from **nbinomialp()** are equal to those in nbprop, the predictions from the negative binomial model. The **nbinomialp** function used the overdispersion parameter, alpha, the count of accidents for each observation, and the inverse of the dispersion for each observation: $1/(1 + alpha \times exp[b_0 + b_1x_1 + ... + b_kx_k]) = 1/(1 + alpha \times C)$.

The negative binomial model output above used the mean dispersion or NB2 method which includes a quadratic term in the variance expression (Expression 17.2). If the constant (NB1) dispersion model is used, all the statistics for the intercept are unchanged (output not shown). With constant dispersion, Stata reports a value for delta (0.538) that is not equal to alpha (1.16), but the likelihood ratio test for the hypothesis that delta=0 has the same chi-squared value of 49.83. For a constant (intercept) only model, the linear and quadratic variance approaches produce equivalent results. The mean dispersion model allows variation in the dispersion for different sets of covariates, but for the constant only model there is only one model term, the intercept, so the mean and constant dispersion models are essentially the same.

A generalized linear model can estimate the same negative binomial model as the mean dispersion model shown earlier:

```
. glm accidents [fweight=women], link(log) family(nb ml) nolog eform
```

```
Generalized linear models                No. of obs      =        647
Optimization      : ML                   Residual df     =        646
                                         Scale parameter =          1
Deviance          = 517.0218672          (1/df) Deviance =   .8003434
Pearson           = 624.7775259          (1/df) Pearson  =   .9671479
Variance function : V(u) = u+(1.1559)u^2 [Neg. Binomial]
Link function     : g(u) = ln(u)         [Log]

                                         AIC             =   1.833901
Log likelihood    = -592.2670972         BIC             =  -3664.114
```

```
- - - - - - - - - - - - - - - - - - - - - - - - - - - - - - - - - - - - - - - -
            |                OIM
  accidents |     IRR   Std. Err.       z    P>|z|    [95% Conf. Interval]
- - - - - - + - - - - - - - - - - - - - - - - - - - - - - - - - - - - - - - - -
      _cons |  .4652241  .0332524  -10.71   0.000    .4044098   .5351836
- - - - - - - - - - - - - - - - - - - - - - - - - - - - - - - - - - - - - - - -
Note: Negative binomial parameter estimated via ML and treated as fixed once
      estimated.
```

The **glm** model used the log link and an option for the negative binomial family, **family(nb ml)**. The **ml** part of that option told the software to produce estimates using maximum likelihood. The alpha quantity is reported inside the variance function in the output: V(u) = u+(1.1559)u^2. This variance function is Stata's notation for Expression 17.4. The alpha value of 1.1559 is the same as that estimated by the **nbreg** command.

There is an option for a negative binomial link with the **glm** command. If we use the negative binomial link, the link function becomes g(u) = ln(u/(u+(1/1.1559))) and the model estimates the exp (_cons) term as 0.350. This link does not estimate the mean count and it *not* the model we want for an analysis of rates (Hilbe 2014 p127).

Greenwood and Woods (1919) argued that extra-Poisson variation in accident counts was evidence that people had different propensities for an accident. Greenwood and others believed that accidents might be reduced if accident prone people could be identified (Burnham 2009). Greenwood and Woods (1919) suggested that those with frequent accidents should be removed from risky jobs. But years later Greenwood (1950) pointed out that mixing several Poisson processes could produce a set of rates that appear to fit a negative binomial distribution. If measurable factors such as age, work experience, or visual acuity could be incorporated into a regression model, the overdispersion in a set of rates might be explained by these variables. Doing this was beyond the methods available to Greenwood before his death in 1949.

17.3 INTRODUCING EQUAL PERSON-TIME IN THE HOMICIDE DATA

Expression 9.10 showed how person-time could be used as an offset in Poisson regression. The offset enabled bookkeeping for time; time contributed in a multiplicative fashion to counts, but time was not involved in the maximum-likelihood estimates or variance functions. In similar fashion, time can be introduced as an offset to a negative binomial model, modifying Expression 17.2 to become Expression 17.4:

$$
\begin{aligned}
C &= \exp[b_0 + b_1 x_1 + b_2 x_2 + \ldots + b_k x_k + \ln(T) + RV] \\
&= e^{[b0 + b1xi + b2x2 + \ldots + bkxk + \ln(T) + RV]} \\
&= T \times e^{RV} \times e^{[b0 + b1x1 + b2x2 + \ldots + bkxk]} \\
&= T \times \exp(RV) \times \exp[b_0 + b_1 x_1 + b_2 x_2 + \ldots + b_k x_k] \\
&= \exp[(b_0 + RV) + b_1 x_1 + b_2 x_2 + \ldots + b_k x_k + \ln(T)] \\
&= \exp[b_0^* + b_1 x_1 + b_2 x_2 + \ldots + b_k x_k + \ln(T)]
\end{aligned}
\qquad \text{(Ex.17.5)}
$$

In Expression 17.5, there is no coefficient for time; it is constrained to equal 1. Time enters the calculations but does not appear to be involved in the maximum likelihood estimation process.

Homicide data from 2010 was presented in Table 11.5. In the six New England states, there were 423 deaths, an average of 423/6 = 70.5 per state. If we use Poisson regression to estimate this average count, the constant only regression model produces the number 70.5 with SE = 3.4. If we fit a negative binomial model, we get the same average of 70.5, with SE = 29.9. In effect, the model assumed that the person-time for each state was equal to 1 and the "rate" was 70.5 deaths per 1 state-year. All this was expected from what has been said so far regarding negative binomial regression.

Now let me introduce person-time. First, I assigned a person-time to each state equal to 1 million person-years. So Vermont, which actually had a population of 0.6 million, and Massachusetts, which had 6.5 million, were given equal amounts of person-time. Using the rates per 100,000 person-years the states actually had, I multiplied those rates by 1 million/100,000 to get new counts that would be expected for those rates. The new counts ranged from 12.8 in Vermont to 39.5 in Connecticut. Then I used Poisson regression with a person-time offset (newpop100k = 1 million/100,000 = 10 for each state) to estimate the person-time averaged rate per 100,000 person-years for all six states:

```
. poisson newcount, exp(newpop100k) irr nolog
note: you are responsible for interpretation of noncount dep. variable

Poisson regression                          Number of obs   =        6
                                            LR chi2(0)      =    -0.00
                                            Prob > chi2     =        .
Log likelihood = -26.152328                 Pseudo R2       =  -0.0000


------------------------------------------------------------------------
    newcount | Inc. Rate  Std. Err.     z    P>|z|   [95% Conf. Interval]
-------------+----------------------------------------------------------
       _cons | 2.368941   .1987017   10.28   0.000    2.00982    2.79223
ln(new~100k) |        1  (exposure)
------------------------------------------------------------------------
```

The person-time weighted-average rate was 2.37 per 100,000 person-years. Following Expression 6.1, this equals the total count of homicide deaths (142.1) divided by the total person-time (6 × 10 units of 100,000 person-years = 60). Now apply negative binomial regression:

```
. nbreg newcount, exp(newpop100k) irr nolog
note: you are responsible for interpretation of non-count dep. variable

Negative binomial regression                Number of obs   =        6
                                            LR chi2(0)      =     0.00
Dispersion     = mean                       Prob > chi2     =        .
Log likelihood = -21.74999                  Pseudo R2       =   0.0000


------------------------------------------------------------------------
    newcount | Inc. Rate  Std. Err.     z    P>|z|   [95% Conf. Interval]
-------------+----------------------------------------------------------
       _cons | 2.368941   .3889615    5.25   0.000   1.717092   3.268247
ln(new~100k) |        1  (exposure)
-------------+----------------------------------------------------------
```

```
/lnalpha |  -2.124092   .7751651                 -3.643388   -.6047965
---------+-------------------------------------------------------------
   alpha |   .1195414   .0926644                  .0261636    .5461856
---------------------------------------------------------------------
```

Note: Estimates are transformed only in the first equation.
LR test of alpha=0: chibar2(01) = 8.80   Prob >= chibar2 = 0.002

Both regression models produced the same intercept rate. The key difference was the change in SE from 0.20 in Poisson regression to 0.39 in the negative binomial model. If the robust variance is used, the SE becomes 0.43 for both models. This is close to the SE from negative binomial regression, so that model did a good job of accounting for heterogeneity. But negative binomial regression had no advantage over the Poisson model with a robust variance.

We can draw a few lessons. First, if person-time does not vary, Poisson regression and negative binomial regression get the same estimates. Second, when rates are heterogenous (they vary), negative binomial may do a good job of accounting for this variation; it did well in this example. Third, heterogeneity of rates, alone, does not cause regression intercept estimates from Poisson and negative binomial models to differ.

17.4 LETTING PERSON-TIME VARY IN THE HOMICIDE DATA

Person-time varied in the six New England states (Table 11.5), from 0.6 million in Vermont to 6.5 million in Massachusetts. Fit a Poisson model, using a variable pop100k to indicate state population in units of 100,000 person-years to estimate the New England rate:

```
. poisson count, exp(pop100k) irr nolog

Poisson regression                          Number of obs   =        6
                                            LR chi2(0)      =     0.00
                                            Prob > chi2     =        .
Log likelihood = -35.644214                 Pseudo R2       =   0.0000
------------------------------------------------------------------------
      count | Inc. Rate  Std. Err.     z   P>|z|   [95% Conf. Interval]
------------+-----------------------------------------------------------
      _cons | 2.928376   .1423825   22.10  0.000   2.662196    3.221171
ln(pop100k) |        1  (exposure)
------------------------------------------------------------------------
```

The Poisson model estimated a mean rate of 2.93 per 100,000 person-years. This is equal to the person-time weighted-average rate, which equals the sum of the deaths in the New England states (423) divided by the total person-time in those states (144.4 person-years). Now fit the negative binomial model:

```
. nbreg count, exp(pop100k) irr nolog

Negative binomial regression                Number of obs   =        6
                                            LR chi2(0)      =     0.00
Dispersion      = mean                      Prob > chi2     =        .
Log likelihood = -25.046322                 Pseudo R2       =   0.0000
```

```
------------------------------------------------------------
     count|  Inc. Rate  Std. Err.     z    P>|z|    [95% Conf. Interval]
---------+--------------------------------------------------
     _cons|  2.457094   .394098    5.60   0.000    1.794303    3.364709
ln(pop100k)|        1  (exposure)
---------+--------------------------------------------------
  /lnalpha| -2.054866  .7099831                   -3.446407   -.6633246
---------+--------------------------------------------------
     alpha|    .12811  .0909559                    .0318599    .5151358
------------------------------------------------------------
```

Note: Estimates are transformed only in the first equation.
LR test of alpha=0: chibar2(01) = 21.20   Prob >= chibar2 = 0.000

Now the rate for the New England rate is 2.46, smaller than the observed rate. It does not matter if we fit the NB1 or NB2 models; results are the same. The predicted counts from the negative binomial model sum to 354.9, smaller than the observed number of deaths, 423. The predicted counts varied from 15.4 to 160.9, a spread that was 28 less than the spread of the Poisson predicted counts. Previously I wrote that negative binomial regression estimates the same mean count but spreads the counts more widely around that mean. That was true in the examples with constant person-time. But in this model, the smaller spread was accompanied by a mean count that was less by 28.

Why did negative binomial regression estimate a mean rate that was (1) different from Poisson regression and (2) different from the observed rate in the data? Look at the $T \times \exp(RV)$ term in Expression 17.5. If time is equal to 1 (or, equivalently, omitted from the model) then the mean rate will equal the mean from Poisson regression, because the $\exp(RV)$ terms average to 1: the equation for the mean count just becomes $\exp(RV) \times \exp(b_0) = 1 \times \exp(b_0)$. If time is not equal to 1, but is constant for all observations, this will just multiply the mean count, increasing or decreasing its size, so that the mean count will have an interpretation as a rate in units corresponding to those used for time. But if time varies from one observation to the next, then although the exponentiated random variable terms sum to 1, multiplying them by the person-time for each observation will result in a sum that is likely to be different from 1. In Poisson regression, person-time played a simple bookkeeping role. In negative binomial regression, person-time is entangled with the random variable used to create overdispersed counts; person-time is embedded in the maximum likelihood estimation.

Think of this as a reweighting of the rates. Imagine we summarized the rates using an inverse-variance method. Negative binomial regression adds an extra quantity to the Poisson variance. This will tend to result in a more equal weighting of the rates. In the New England homicide data, the states with smaller populations (Vermont, New Hampshire) had lower rates, while states with larger populations (Massachusetts, Connecticut) had higher rates. More weight was given to smaller states, less weight to larger states, resulting in a smaller mean rate. The rate of 2.46 from negative binomial regression was intermediate between the observed rate (2.93) and the average rate of 2.37 (Table 11.5) produced by simply weighting each state equally.

The amount of reweighting is related to the size of the counts for each state. Using the homicide counts and person-time from the six New England states (Table 11.5), I multiplied the counts by amounts as small as .18 and as large as 100. For each set of new counts, with the original person-time for each state, negative binomial regression was used to estimate the mean (intercept) rate. These mean rates were rescaled by division with the same quantity used to multiply the counts. When the counts were small, the mean rate was equal to the observed rate (2.93), which equals the person-time weighted-average rate. But as counts became larger, the mean rate decreased until it reached the simple average rate, 2.37 (Figure 17.1). A similar multiplication of person-time, keeping the original counts unchanged and rescaling the estimated mean rates by multiplication instead of division, always resulted in an estimated mean rate of 2.46. So changing the size of person-time did not affect the weighting.

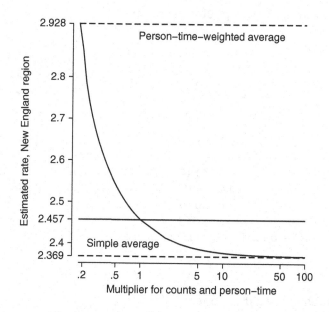

FIGURE 17.1   Rate of homicide per 100,000 person-years in the 6 New England states, 2010, estimated by negative binomial regression. Data from Table 11.5. When the counts for all six states were multiplied by .18, the estimated rate (rescaled by division with .18) was equal to the person-time-weighted average rate, 2.928. This equals the observed rate. When counts were multiplied by 50 or more, (and the means rescaled by division) the estimated rate was 2.369, a simple average of the six rates. Using the original data (a multiplier of 1), the rate was 2.457, indicated by a horizontal line.

Imagine that the data for each state consisted of five records instead of just one. This might occur if we had data for five age categories within each state. I created four new records for each of the New England states. The counts and person-time for each of the five records within each state contained 1/5th of the original counts and 1/5th of the person-time for that state; this made the counts smaller. Poisson regression applied to these 5 × 6 = 30 records estimated the same average rate of 2.93. But negative binomial regression now estimated 2.87, instead of 2.46. To complicate this example, imagine that the data had only 1 record for the 4 smallest states, Vermont, New Hampshire, Maine, and Rhode Island. But the data now has 10 records for Massachusetts and 10 for Connecticut, each with 1/10th the original count and person-time of those states. Applied to these data, the mean rate is still 2.93 with Poisson regression. If the 24 rates now in the data are given equal weight, the simple average is 3.23. Negative binomial regression estimates the mean as 3.06. The key points here are that: (1) expanding or collapsing the data will change the size of the outcome counts in each record. This will not change estimates from Poisson regression, but will change estimates from negative binomial regression. And (2) estimated mean rates from negative binomial regression will fall somewhere between the person-time weighted-average and the simple average.

17.5 ESTIMATING A RATE RATIO FOR THE HOMICIDE DATA

Use Poisson regression to estimate the rate ratio comparing the eight Southern states with the six New England states (Table 11.5):

```
. poisson count south, exp(pop100k) irr nolog

Poisson regression                              Number of obs   =        14
                                                LR chi2(1)      =    275.98
                                                Prob > chi2     =    0.0000
Log likelihood = -120.66222                     Pseudo R2       =    0.5335


----------------------------------------------------------------------------
      count |     IRR     Std. Err.      z    P>|z|    [95% Conf. Interval]
------------+---------------------------------------------------------------
      south |  2.155731   .1104148    15.00   0.000    1.94983     2.383376
      _cons |  2.92837    .1423825    22.10   0.000    2.662196    3.221171
ln(pop100k) |        1   (exposure)
----------------------------------------------------------------------------
Note: _cons estimates baseline incidence rate.

. lincom _cons + south, irr

( 1)  [count]south + [count]_cons = 0
----------------------------------------------------------------------------
      count|     IRR    Std. Err.      z    P>|z|      [95% Conf. Interval]
-----------+----------------------------------------------------------------
       (1)|  6.312793  .1016607   114.42    0.000      6.116653    6.515222
----------------------------------------------------------------------------
```

In the output above, the New England rate was 2.93, in the South it was 6.31, and the ratio was 6.31/2.93. The regional rates are just the observed rates (equal to the person-time weighted-average rates) shown in Table 11.5. Now use negative binomial regression:

```
. nbreg count south, exp(pop100k) irr nolog

Negative binomial regression                    Number of obs   =        14
                                                LR chi2(1)      =     19.08
Dispersion     = mean                           Prob > chi2     =    0.0000
Log likelihood = -73.162314                     Pseudo R2       =    0.1153


----------------------------------------------------------------------------
      count|     IRR   Std.   Err.      z    P>|z|      [95% Conf. Interval]
-----------+----------------------------------------------------------------
      south|  2.652991  .4060419    6.37   0.000      1.965436    3.581069
      _cons|  2.514678  .3072749    7.55   0.000      1.979119    3.195162
ln(pop100k)|        1 (exposure)
-----------+----------------------------------------------------------------
   /lnalpha| -2.735984  .4743686                     -3.66573   -1.806239
-----------+----------------------------------------------------------------
      alpha|  .0648302  .0307534                      .0255855    .1642708
----------------------------------------------------------------------------
Note: Estimates are transformed only in the first equation.
Note: _cons estimates baseline incidence rate.
LR test of alpha=0: chibar2(01) = 95.00          Prob >= chibar2 = 0.000
```

```
. lincom _cons + south, irr

( 1)  [count]south + [count]_cons = 0
-----------------------------------------------------------------
      count|     IRR    Std. Err.    z    P>|z|    [95% Conf. Interval]
---------+-------------------------------------------------------
        (1)|  6.671418  .6133431  20.64  0.000    5.571371   7.988664
-----------------------------------------------------------------
```

In this output, the rate in New England was 2.51, a bit different from 2.46 when the data were limited to the New England states. The difference arose because when all 14 states were included, the exp(RV) terms differ from those used previously.

The intercept (constant term) now represents the rate in New England. It is 2.51, different from the person-time weighted average rate of 2.93 and different from the simple average rate of 2.37 (Table 11.5) The rate for the Southern states is 6.67, nearly equal to the simple average rate of 6.69. This arose because the homicide counts were fairly large for the Southern states, therefore the reweighting treated each state nearly equally. In the South the smaller states with higher rates were given more weight and the larger states with lower rates were given less weight. The reweighting moved the estimated rate higher, compared with the observed rate of 6.31.

This example shows that when person-time varies, negative binomial regression will produce average rates that are closer to simple average rates within strata created by covariates. Poisson regression produces average rates weighted by person-time. Consequently, the rate ratios from negative binomial regression may not agree with those from Poisson regression; they may be larger or smaller depending upon how person-time varies with the rates within each covariate pattern. In these homicide data, the rate ratio comparing the South with New England was 2.16 from Poisson regression and 2.65 from negative binomial regression. The estimated rate ratio from Poisson regression has a clear interpretation; it tells us that the total homicides in the South divided by the total person-time in the South, a quantity that equals the observed rate for the Southern region, was 2.16-fold greater on a ratio scale compared with the same quantity for New England. The estimate from negative binomial regression has a different interpretation; it is a ratio comparison of what the rate was in the average Southern state compared with a rate that is between the rate for the average New England state (2.37) and a rate that is the person-time averaged rate (2.93) for New England.

To summarize, negative binomial regression does two things. First, it adjusts the variance to account for overdispersion. This is desirable but given that other methods for doing this are available (Chapter 13), including the simple option of a robust variance estimator, negative binomial regression may offer little practical advantage. Second, negative binomial regression gives more weight to smaller populations and less to larger populations. This reweighting tends to give more weight to less precise rate estimates, as counts from smaller amounts of person-time will generally be smaller and their rates less precise. The degree of reweighting is less when outcome counts are small, greater when outcome counts are large (Fig. 17.1). The reweighting will change the size of estimated rates and rate ratios and may make it hard to interpret results.

17.6 ANOTHER EXAMPLE USING HYPOTHETICAL DATA FOR FIVE REGIONS

To clarify the findings so far, I created hypothetical data for five geographic regions (Table 17.2). In regions 4 and 5 the population was exposed to some factor that may influence the outcome counts. The

TABLE 17.2   Hypothetical data for three scenarios in five geographic regions. Person-time in units of 100,000 person-years. Rates per 100,000 person-years.

		SCENARIO 1			SCENARIO 2			SCENARIO 3		
REGION	EXPOSED	COUNT	PERSON-TIME	RATE	COUNT	PERSON-TIME	RATE	COUNT	PERSON-TIME	RATE
1	0	20	1	20	20	1	20	20	1	20
2	0	50	1	50	50	1	50	50	1	50
3	0	80	1	80	80	1	80	80	1	80
4	1	150	1	150	150	1.5	100	100	4	25
5	1	150	1	150	150	0.5	300	30	0.1	300

goal is to estimate the rate ratio for outcome events in the two exposed regions (4 and 5) compared with the three regions without exposure (1, 2, and 3). In scenario 1 the person-time weighted average rate was (20 × 1 + 50 × 1 + 80 × 1)/(1 + 1 + 1) = 50 events per 100,000 person-years in the 3 unexposed regions. The rate was 150 in the two exposed regions. The rate ratio, comparing those exposed with those not, was 150/50 = 3 from both Poisson and negative binomial regression; just what we expect, because person-time did not vary between regions.

In scenario 2 (Table 17.2) the person-time quantities changed for regions 4 and 5, producing rates of 100 in region 4 and 300 in region 5. The person-time weighted rate for both regions is still (100 × 1.5 + 300 × 0.5)/(1.5 + 0.5) = 150, so Poisson regression estimates a rate ratio of 3 for the exposure:

```
. poisson count exposed, exp(ptime) irr nolog
(output omitted)
------------------------------------------------------------------
    count |    IRR   Std. Err.      z    P>|z|    [95% Conf. Interval]
----------+-------------------------------------------------------
  exposed |     3        .3     10.99   0.000    2.466046   3.649568
    _cons |    50   4.082483   47.91   0.000   42.60589   58.67733
ln(ptime) |     1   (exposure)
------------------------------------------------------------------
```

But negative binomial regression now estimates a rate ratio of 3.98:

```
. nbreg count exposed, exp(ptime) irr nolog

Negative binomial regression            Number of obs   =          5
                                        LR chi2(1)      =       5.11
Dispersion    = mean                    Prob > chi2     =     0.0237
Log likelihood = -25.468544            Pseudo R2       =     0.0913


------------------------------------------------------------------
    count |    IRR    Std. Err.     z    P>|z|    [95% Conf. Interval]
----------+-------------------------------------------------------
  exposed | 3.975302  1.913081   2.87   0.004    1.547878   10.20948
    _cons |    50    15.40834   12.69   0.000   27.33115   91.47071
ln(ptime) |     1    (exposure)
----------+-------------------------------------------------------
```

```
/lnalpha |  -1.328402   .6432871                -2.589221   -.0675821
---------+----------------------------------------------------------
   alpha |   .2649003    .170407                 .0750785    .934651
---------+----------------------------------------------------------
LR test of alpha=0: chibar2(01) = 104.43            Prob >= chibar2 = 0.000
```

Negative binomial regression estimated that the rate was 50 in the unexposed regions; the person-time was the same for these three regions. But for the exposed regions the negative binomial model assigned nearly equal weight to the region 4 and 5 rates: (100+300)/2 = 200, close to the rate 3.975302 × 50 = 198.8 reported in the regression output.

In scenario 3 (Table 17.2), the observed rate among those not exposed is still 50. But the counts, person-time, and rates all changed in regions 4 and 5. The person-time weighted-average rate among the exposed is now (25 × 4 + 300 × 0.1)/(4 + 0.1) = 31.7. The rate ratio comparing those exposed with those not, from Poisson regression, is 31.7/50 = 0.63:

```
. poisson count exposed, exp(ptime) irr nolog
(output omitted)

-------------------------------------------------------------------
   count |    IRR    Std. Err.      z    P>|z|   [95% Conf. Interval]
---------+---------------------------------------------------------
 exposed | .6341463  .0759891    -3.80   0.000   .5014076   .8020253
   _cons |      50   4.082483    47.91   0.000   42.60589   58.67733
ln(ptime)|       1  (exposure)
-------------------------------------------------------------------
```

Negative binomial regression estimated that the rate among the exposed is 3.1165 × 50 = 155.8, pretty close to the simple average of (25+300)/2 = 162.5. The rate ratio from negative binomial regression was 3.1, quite different from the rate ratio of 0.63 from Poisson regression:

```
Negative binomial regression             Number of obs   =          5
                                          LR chi2(1)      =       2.10
Dispersion      = mean                    Prob > chi2     =     0.1476
Log likelihood = -25.731727               Pseudo R2       =     0.0392

-------------------------------------------------------------------
   count |    IRR    Std. Err.      z    P>|z|   [95% Conf. Interval]
---------+---------------------------------------------------------
 exposed | 3.116502  2.303358    1.54   0.124   .7320784   13.26713
   _cons |       50  22.94137    8.53   0.000   20.34302   122.8923
ln(ptime)|       1  (exposure)
---------+---------------------------------------------------------
/lnalpha |  -.49173   .5936352                 -1.655234   .6717736
---------+---------------------------------------------------------
   alpha | .6115675    .363048                  .1910474   1.957706
-------------------------------------------------------------------
LR test of alpha=0: chibar2(01) = 102.89            Prob >= chibar2 = 0.000
```

The simple data in Table 17.2, helps illustrate how negative binomial regression reweights data, producing results that can differ substantially from those based upon person-time weighting.

17.7 UNOBSERVED HETEROGENEITY

Sometimes authors describe negative binomial regression as a method for dealing with unobserved heterogeneity. The word unobserved refers to variation in counts or rates that is not accounted for, or observed, by variables used in the regression model. The homicide data in Table 11.5 shows variation across states, but variation by sex, age, or other factors, is concealed because there is only a single record for each state. In Chapter 12, I pointed out that assessment of goodness-of-fit depends upon how much variation is revealed, or concealed, by the available data. When Poisson regression is used, collapsing the data into fewer records within covariate patterns will not affect rate ratio estimates, but reduces variability, improves apparent fit, and narrows confidence intervals (CI). With negative binomial regression collapsing the data does not always narrow the CI, because collapsing can change not only the variance but also the estimated rate ratio.

To illustrate how the rate ratio can change depending upon how records are collapsed, I used homicide data for the same states used in Table 11.5, but I created a new data set (not shown) that covered a 15-year period 1999–2013. Records were acquired separately for men and women in 6 age categories (15–19, 20–24, 25–34, 35–44, 45–54, 55–64) within each state: 2 sex groups x 6 age groups x 14 states = 168 records with counts of homicide and person-time. The online data source available to the public (CDC WONDER) suppresses counts smaller than 10 to preserve confidentiality. I replaced 10 suppressed counts, all in smaller states, with a count of 3. There is a lot of variation in the rates of the 168 records: the lowest rate per 100,000 person-years was 0.3 for Rhode Island women age 55–64, the highest was 38.0 for Mississippi men age 20–24. For all women the rate was 3.5, for men it was 13.1. In the 6 age groups, the lowest rate was 3.6 for those age 55–64 and the highest was 15.4 for persons age 20-24 years.

These 168 homicide records were used to estimate the rate ratio for homicide in 8 Southern states compared with six New England states (Table 17.3). All regression models included an indicator for the Southern states (vs. New England) and no other variables. The robust variance option was always used. A Poisson model was fit using the data collapsed to 14 records; one for each state. The next model used data expanded on sex to 28 records. A third model used the data expanded by age group; 14 x 6 = 84 records. The fourth model was expanded on both sex and age, using 168 records. In all Poisson models the rate ratio was the same, 2.72 (Table 17.3). Expansion of the data into more records usually increased the size of the SE, which resulted in a smaller Z-statistic. There was an exception to this behavior; when the data were expanded from 28 records by state and sex, to 168 records by state, sex, and age, the SE shrank from 0.87 to 0.50.

TABLE 17.3   Rate ratios comparing homicide rates in eight Southern states with rates in six New England states. State level mortality data for the years 1999–2013. In the first analysis with each regression method the data are grouped by state only, in the next by state and sex, in the third by state and age, and finally by state, sex, and age. All analyses used a robust variance estimator.

REGRESSION METHOD	DATA GROUPING	NUMBER OF RECORDS	RATE RATIO	SE	Z-STATISTIC
Poisson	State	14	2.72	0.32	8.4
Poisson	State, sex	28	2.72	0.87	3.2
Poisson	State, age	84	2.72	0.45	6.1
Poisson	State, sex, age	168	2.72	0.50	5.4
Negative binomial	State	14	3.34	0.58	6.9
Negative binomial	State, sex	28	3.36	0.89	4.6
Negative binomial	State, age	84	3.18	0.47	7.9
Negative binomial	State, sex, age	168	3.18	0.51	7.3

Negative binomial regression was used to fit the same single-variable model to the four different sets of records (Table 17.3). With negative binomial regression, the rate ratio for Southern versus New England states was always larger than the person-time weighted rate ratio of 2.72 and the size of the rate ratio changed with the number of records. When 84 or 168 records were used, the rate ratio from negative binomial regression (3.18) was closer to the Poisson rate ratio (2.72), because the counts became smaller for each record and negative binomial regression therefore produced estimates closer to those weighted by person-time.

Negative binomial regression is sometimes described as being more conservative, in the sense that it will produce larger P-values and wider CIs, and is therefore less prone to Type I error, compared with Poisson regression. When only 14 state-level records were used, negative binomial regression was indeed more conservative, with a Z-statistic of 6.9 compared with 8.4 from Poisson regression (Table 17.3). But when the data were expanded to 28, 84, and 168 records, Poisson regression was more conservative, as judged by the Z-statistic. With expansion of the data on sex, age, or both, the robust Poisson and negative binomial SEs were similar, but because the rate ratios were larger from negative binomial regression, the corresponding Z-statistics were also larger. An analogy can be made to meta-analysis. Random effects meta-analysis is sometimes described as more conservative compared with fixed effects meta-analysis. But random effects meta-analysis not only adds a random component to the variance, it also reweights the data records more equally compared with the fixed effects summary (Greenland 1994). Consequently, random-effects meta-analysis can sometimes produce a smaller P-value compared with fixed-effects analysis of the same data (Poole and Greenland 1999).

Both Poisson and negative binomial regression can modify the variance when the data are presented in records that reveal heterogeneity. But they can only use information that is shown or "observed" by the data format. In the homicide example, heterogeneity of rates by sex and age were characteristics revealed by using records for both sexes and several age groups. But the data lacked information about variation in homicide rates by income, education, or an infinite number of other characteristics. In a sense, the term "unobserved heterogeneity" is a misnomer. A regression model can only account for heterogeneity that is observed and can be seen in the data records. Since variation is ubiquitous, our ability to account for variations in rates will often face practical limitations.

17.8 OBSERVING HETEROGENEITY IN THE SHOE DATA

Table 16.1 showed data regarding shoe type, sex, and fall rates. I expanded these data into 30,000 records for individuals, all followed for 1 week; 175 had 1 fall and the rest had no falls. The data were analyzed using Poisson regression in Chapter 16. When I tried to study the same 30,000 records with negative binomial regression, maximum likelihood failed to converge. These data can be collapsed into four records as shown in Table 16.1. For example, the first record for women with sensible shoes had a fall count of 10 and person-time of 5000 person-weeks. With this grouping, negative binomial regression will converge and it can recognize the variation in the fall rates across the four records. Using these four records, four models were estimated using both Poisson and negative binomial regression: (1) constant only, (2) constant term plus risky shoes, (3) constant plus male sex, and (4) constant, risky shoes, and male sex (Table 17.4). In the first three models, the estimates differed between Poisson and negative binomial regression, and the SEs were always larger with negative binomial regression. But the estimates and SEs were identical, to many decimal places, for both methods in the fourth model which included a constant term, risky shoes, and male sex. Putting these terms into the model accounted for all the heterogeneity that can be observed in these four records. To put this another way, both Poisson regression and negative binomial regression assume the data in each record are from a Poisson process, absent any information that might reveal whether this is true or not.

TABLE 17.4 Analyses of the data regarding falls and shoes in Table 16.1, comparing Poisson and negative binomial regression results. The data were collapsed into just four records. The usual variance estimators were used for all models.

| REGRESSION METHOD | RATE RATIO (SE) FOR MODEL VARIABLES | | |
	CONSTANT TERM	RISKY SHOES	MALE
Poisson	0.0058 (0.0004)		
Poisson	0.0027 (0.0004)	3.4 (0.6)	
Poisson	0.0047 (0.0006)		1.5 (0.2)
Poisson	0.0014 (0.0003)	4.4 (0.8)	2.3 (0.4)
Negative binomial	0.0065 (0.0024)		
Negative binomial	0.0026 (0.0007)	4.0 (1.6)	
Negative binomial	0.0041 (0.0019)		2.2 (1.4)
Negative binomial	0.0014 (0.0003)	4.4 (0.8)	2.3 (0.4)

17.9 UNDERDISPERSION

If the variability in the rates is less than would be expected from a Poisson process, then the data are underdispersed. This would arise, for example, if the outcome can only occur once, such as death, and the outcome is common. This was discussed in Chapter 4. In the presence of underdispersion, the negative binomial model should estimate alpha as zero and the negative binomial model will become the Poisson model; the result may be P-values and CIs that are too large. One simple way to deal with underdispersion is to use a robust variance estimator.

17.10 A RATE DIFFERENCE NEGATIVE BINOMIAL REGRESSION MODEL

Chapter 10 showed how Poisson regression can estimate a rate difference. We can compare the homicide rates in the eight Southern states with six New England states, using the data with 168 records classified by state, sex, and 6 age groups:

```
. glm rate south [iweight=pop100k], link(identity) family(poisson) nolog
note: rate has noninteger values

Generalized linear models              No. of obs      =        168
Optimization     : ML                  Residual df     =        166
                                       Scale parameter =          1
Deviance         =  35580.37366        (1/df) Deviance =   214.3396
Pearson          =  42202.39912        (1/df) Pearson  =   254.2313

Variance function : V(u) = u           [Poisson]
Link function     : g(u) = u           [Identity]
```

```
                                       AIC           =     367.0684
Log likelihood  = -30831.74754         BIC           =      34729.8

---------------------------------------------------------------------
            |                OIM
      rate|     Coef.   Std. Err.       z    P>|z|    [95% Conf. Interval]
---------+-----------------------------------------------------------
    south|   5.981166   .0635338    94.14   0.000    5.856642    6.10569
    _cons|   3.470522   .0490169    70.80   0.000    3.374451   3.566594
---------------------------------------------------------------------
```

The Pearson dispersion statistic is a colossal 254, so the SE is too small. There is a lot of overdispersion, as the rates in the 168 records varied more than 100-fold from 0.33 to 38 per 100,000 person-years. The rate difference of 5.98 per 100,000 person-years is the same rate difference estimated by the Poisson regression rate ratio model:

. poisson deaths south, exp(pop100k) irr nolog
(output omitted)

```
---------------------------------------------------------------------
    deaths |      IRR   Std. Err.       z   P>|z|    [95% Conf. Interval]
---------+-----------------------------------------------------------
     south |  2.723419   .0401897   67.89  0.000    2.645777    2.80334
     _cons |  3.470522   .0490169   88.10  0.000    3.375769   3.567936
ln(pop100k) |        1  (exposure)
---------------------------------------------------------------------
```

From this model we can compute a rate difference of (2.723 × 3.471) – 3.471 = 5.98. The Poisson rate ratio and rate difference models estimate equivalent results. Now fit the negative binomial rate ratio model:

. nbreg deaths south, exp(pop100k) irr nolog

```
Negative binomial regression              Number of obs   =        168
                                          LR chi2(1)      =      63.67
Dispersion     = mean                     Prob > chi2     =     0.0000
Log likelihood = -1034.2138               Pseudo R2       =     0.0299

---------------------------------------------------------------------
    deaths|      IRR   Std. Err.       z   P>|z|    [95% Conf. Interval]
---------+-----------------------------------------------------------
    south|  3.180683   .4056579    9.07   0.000    2.477194   4.083955
    _cons|  3.267719    .317441   12.19   0.000     2.70119   3.953068
ln(pop100k)|        1  (exposure)
---------+-----------------------------------------------------------
  /lnalpha|  -.4260918  .1025346                  -.6270559  -.2251278
---------+-----------------------------------------------------------
    alpha|   .6530564   .0669609                   .5341621   .7984142
---------------------------------------------------------------------
LR test of alpha=0: chibar2(01) = 3.5e+04        Prob >= chibar2 = 0.000
```

This model (also see Table 17.3) estimates a rate ratio of 3.18, different from the rate ratio of 2.72 from Poisson regression, which weights observations by person-time. According to this model, the rate difference is $(3.181 \times 3.268) - 3.268 = 7.13$. Now fit the negative binomial rate difference model:

```
. glm rate south [iweight=pop100k], link(identity) family(nbinomial ml) nolog
note: rate has noninteger values
```

```
Generalized linear models                    No. of obs       =        168
Optimization      : ML                       Residual df      =        166
                                             Scale parameter =          1
Deviance          =  7283.819164             (1/df) Deviance =   43.87843
Pearson           =  8987.00819              (1/df) Pearson  =    54.1386

Variance function : V(u) = u+(.466)u^2       [Neg. Binomial]
Link function     : g(u) = u                 [Identity]

                                             AIC              =   259.6761
Log likelihood    = -21810.79127             BIC              =   6433.241
```

```
------------------------------------------------------------------------------
             |                 OIM
       rate  |      Coef.   Std. Err.      z    P>|z|     [95% Conf. Interval]
-------------+----------------------------------------------------------------
      south  |   5.981166    .122963    48.64   0.000     5.740163    6.222169
       _cons |   3.470522    .079302    43.76   0.000     3.315093    3.625952
------------------------------------------------------------------------------
```

Note: Negative binomial parameter estimated via ML and treated as fixed once
      estimated.

This model estimated the rate difference as 5.98, smaller than the estimate of 7.13 from the negative binomial rate ratio model, and identical to the rate difference from the Poisson ratio model and the Poisson difference model. This is because, unlike the negative binomial rate ratio model, the rate difference model weighted observations by person-time; the use of importance weights equal to person-time forced the model to do this. The SE of 0.12 for the rate difference is twice as large as the SE of 0.06 from the Poisson model, but there is still plenty of overdispersion; the Pearson dispersion statistic is 54.

Given the overdispersion evident for both Poisson and the negative binomial models, use of the robust variance seems a good choice:

```
. glm rate south [iweight=pop100k], link(identity) family(nb ml) nolog
vce(r) noheader
(output omitted)
```

```
------------------------------------------------------------------------------
             |               Robust
       rate  |      Coef.   Std. Err.      z    P>|z|     [95% Conf. Interval]
-------------+----------------------------------------------------------------
      south  |   5.981166   1.014411     5.90   0.000     3.992957    7.969375
       _cons |   3.470522   .5596389     6.20   0.000     2.37365     4.567394
------------------------------------------------------------------------------
```

The robust variance increased the SE from 0.12 to 1.01. If Poisson regression is used in the same way, with a robust variance estimator, the regression table output is exactly the same as that shown above. The use of negative binomial regression with person-time importance weights and a robust variance adds nothing compared with Poisson regression for the rate difference. The same applies to using importance weights in a negative binomial ratio model.

17.11 CONCLUSION

A summary of the important ideas in this chapter:

1. Negative binomial regression is one way of correcting the variance for a mean rate or rate ratio for the presence of overdispersion. But there may be no advantage over Poisson regression with a robust variance.
2. If (1) data are overdispersed and (2) fit a negative binomial distribution and (3) person-time is equal for all observations, negative binomial regression has an advantage over Poisson regression. It can fit not only valid estimates for mean rates and rate ratios, but can make valid predictions regarding probabilities, rates, and counts aside from means (Cameron and Trivedi 2013a p74).
3. If person-time varies across observations, estimated rates and rate ratios from negative binomial regression will usually differ from the person-time weighted estimates produced by Poisson regression.
4. When person-time varies, negative binomial regression weights records more equally, compared with person-time weighting. As counts become large, negative binomial regression tends to give equal weight to observations with different amounts of person-time.
5. If person-time varies, negative binomial regression tends to give more weight to less precise counts from smaller amounts of person time and less weight to larger counts from greater amounts of person-time.

Clustered Data

18

Studies of groups (or clusters) are common. Many analyses have assessed the effects of state traffic laws on crash rates of state residents. If we study several states in the same analysis, this becomes a study of groups, because the laws typically apply to all residents of each state. To test the effects of a new curriculum, it may be difficult to randomly assign students in the same classroom, or even the same school, to different curricula. It is easier to assign entire schools to the old and new teaching methods; the students are then grouped within school. To learn whether a new shoe can reduce the incidence of ankle injury among college baseball players, there are advantages to randomizing entire teams to shoe A or B, rather than trying to randomize individual players.

Customary statistical estimates of precision, such as confidence intervals (CI), assume that observations are independent. If we undertake a study that compares the outcomes of groups, or clusters, this assumption may not be true. Event rates for persons within groups, such as families, schools, teams, or people in a state, may be more alike than event rates between groups. Similarity of outcome occurrence within a group has been called within-cluster correlation. Between-group variation in outcome frequency is called between-cluster variability or heterogeneity. These terms describe the idea that events are more independent (diverse or spread out) between the clusters than they are within the clusters. The ankle injury rates of baseball players on the same team may be more alike (less independent) compared with other teams, because teammates share the same playing turf and weather in every game, have the same coach, and may imitate the base-stealing habits of their team members. Motorists within a state may have crash rates that are more alike than motorists in another state, because they use the same roads, are exposed to a similar level of drunk-driving, experience similar weather (snow, rain), and share other state-level factors that influence crash rates.

Clustering is a relative phenomenon. If there is only one group, there is no way to recognize or judge that event rates of persons within that group are more alike than rates between groups. If event rates in group A are compared with those in groups B and C, and if all groups have similar event rates, aside from any effect of covariates, then clustering is of no concern for the statistical comparison of the groups. If we compare the event rates of group A with groups D and E, and if there is considerable variation in outcome event rates between these three groups beyond variation due to covariates, then analytic methods are needed to account for the clustering. To some extent heterogeneity between groups corresponds to clustering within groups.

Clustering of data means that smaller units are within larger units, so clustered data is often described as hierarchical or multilevel data. There may be more than two levels of clustering. For example, observations may be on students, but students are clustered within classrooms and classrooms clustered within schools. Outcomes of students in a classroom may be similar compared with students in other classrooms, because students in the same classroom share the same teacher and the students may influence each other. Student outcomes in a school may be more alike, compared with students in other schools, because students in the same school have parents who selected that school, they share the same school budgets and principals and library facilities, and students learn from and play with fellow students within the same school.

A common type of clustered data arises if there are repeated observations on the same person or the same geographic area. For example, we may have state-level annual mortality rates for several years. The past event rate for an individual, community, or institution is often related to their current event rates. Repeated observations over time are often called longitudinal data. This is sometimes called cross-sectional panel data: the panels are the clusters that are followed over time, the cross-sections are the data at one point in time. Clustering of rates over time will be discussed in the next chapter.

Many books (Koepsell 1998, Murray 1998, Donner and Klar 2000, Hayes and Moulton 2009, Snijders and Bosker 2012, West, Welch, and Galecki 2015) and articles (Localio et al. 2001, Cummings and Koepsell 2002, Murray et al. 2004, Eldridge et al. 2004, Eldridge, Ashby, and Kerry 2006, Eldridge et al. 2008) provide advice about clustered data. This chapter reviews Stata commands that account for clustering in data. The terminology and taxonomy of methods for clustered data varies somewhat between authors. In this chapter we divide the methods into two broad categories: (1) variance adjustment methods that estimate associations using extensions of customary regression models and revise the variance estimates to account for the clustered nature of the data, and (2) mixed models that extend regression models by adding random effects.

18.1 DATA FROM 24 FICTITIOUS NURSING HOMES

To study an intervention meant to prevent falls among the elderly, an imaginary investigator recruited elderly women in 24 nursing homes. The goal was to enroll 20 subjects from each facility, but the number actually enrolled varied from 15 to 20. Participants were 65, 70, or 75 years and the age distribution varied across the homes: mean age was 67.8 years in 8 nursing homes, 70 years in another 8, and 71.8 in the rest. Twelve nursing homes were randomly assigned to the intervention. Three nursing homes opted out of the study after 0.3 years and 4 withdrew after 0.75 years. An additional 43 patients dropped out early, in a random manner, completing only half the person-time of other persons in the same nursing home.

Unknown to our mythical investigator, the true fall rate among control persons age 65 years was 0.5/year, at age 70 this doubled, and by age 75 it doubled again. Eight nursing homes (number 1 through 8) had no influence on these fall rates, in homes 9 through 16 the fall rate was doubled, and in homes 17 through 24 the rate quadrupled. This influence of nursing homes on falls arose because some nursing homes had slippery floors that promoted tripping, others had physicians who prescribed drugs that promoted falls, and some lacked sufficient staff to help feeble residents. In addition, the nursing homes with higher fall rates happened to have more elderly occupants. Finally, the true effect of the intervention was to reduce fall rates by 50%.

The rate variation by nursing home can be thought of as a heterogeneity problem; differences in the underlying rates by nursing home should be accounted for in our model. Or we can describe this as a clustering problem; rates are more similar among residents of the same nursing home. Heterogeneity and clustering are opposite sides of the same coin.

The rate and rate ratio values described were used, along with the person-time values, to create counts of fall events for each resident of 12 nursing homes using Expression 9.10 and a pseudo-random generator for Poisson counts. The remaining 12 nursing homes had expected fall counts produced in the same way, but the expected counts were then multiplied by a random value from a gamma distribution to simulate a random set of counts from a negative binomial distribution, using Expression 16.1. Alpha, the variance of the random variates for the negative binomial, was set at 0.6. The data generation programs used Stata's random variate functions, **rpoisson** and **rgamma**, and used code similar to that described by Hilbe (2010, 2011 pp136–137, 226).

18.2 RESULTS FROM 10,000 DATA SIMULATIONS FOR THE NURSING HOMES

Using the data generating process described earlier, the fall counts were generated 10,000 times. Each time this was done, the **rpoisson** and **rgamma** functions produced random variation in the counts. Twelve nursing homes were randomly assigned to the intervention in each simulation. Using Poisson regression for each of the 10,000 simulated sets of data, the mean crude rate ratio for falling, comparing patients who received the intervention with controls, was 0.5, just as expected. Adjusting for age using indicator variables for 70 and 75 years, the adjusted rate ratio for the intervention was still 0.5. Age was related to the fall rates, but thanks to randomization, age had no systematic relationship to the intervention and therefore age did not confound the association between the intervention and fall rates.

Using the 10,000 simulated data sets, the rate ratio for falling comparing persons 70 years to those 65, adjusted for the intervention, was 2.55 instead of the true value of 2. The rate ratio comparing those 75 with those 65 was estimated as 6.04 instead of the true value of 4. The bias in these estimates occurred because the nursing homes with the highest fall rates due to nursing home characteristics also happened to have the largest concentrations of older persons. This confounding of the age effects of individuals with the group level nursing home effects is a problem that can afflict any analysis of clustered data. Introducing this problem into the data was done deliberately, to demonstrate this difficulty. If indicator variables for the two nursing home groups with higher fall rates are added to the Poisson models, the correct age-related rate ratios of 2 and 4 appeared, along with the correct rate ratio for the intervention; the data were generated using two age-related and two nursing home related indicators, so this result was expected. However, this option would not be available in real data, as the analyst would not know from the data how true rates varied by nursing home. All the nursing homes could be added to the model as indicator variables, but that model could not correctly estimate the rate ratio for the intervention, because it is the nursing homes that were randomized to the intervention.

18.3 A SINGLE RANDOM SET OF DATA FOR THE NURSING HOMES

If the nursing home trial was done, there would be 1 set of data, not 10,000 sets. To better describe these data and related analyses, I picked a single set of data. I deliberately cherry-picked data with a somewhat erroneous rate ratio for the intervention. In these data, 12 nursing homes with 216 subjects received the intervention, and 12 homes with 200 persons were the controls. By chance, the mean age (69.2 years) in the intervention group was younger than the mean age (70.3) of the controls. Among intervention subjects 28% were age 75 years, compared with 38% of controls. This age imbalance illustrates a limitation of group level randomization studies; only 24 groups were randomized. Had the 416 subjects been individually randomized, this degree of age imbalance would be less likely. If Poisson regression is used to estimate the crude rate ratio for the intervention, indicated by the variable rx, the crude rate ratio is 0.34, a stronger association than the true rate ratio of 0.5:

```
Crude rate ratio model
. poisson falls rx, exp(ptime) irr nolog
(output omitted)
```

```
 ----------------------------------------------------------------------
      falls |        IRR   Std. Err.        z   P>|z|   [95% Conf. Interval]
 ------------+---------------------------------------------------------
         rx |     343845   .0288449    -12.73   0.000    .2917142    .405294
       _cons |   3.389002   .1356687      30.4   0.000     3.13326   3.665618
  ln(ptime) |          1  (exposure)
 ----------------------------------------------------------------------
```

Younger persons had lower fall rates and because of the age imbalance, the intervention association was confounded by age. Adjustment for age seems wise:

```
Age-adjusted rate ratio model
. poisson falls rx age70 age75, exp(ptime) irr nolog
(output omitted)
 ----------------------------------------------------------------------
      falls |        IRR   Std. Err.        z   P>|z|   [95% Conf. Interval]
 ------------+---------------------------------------------------------
         rx |   .4214672   .0355463    -10.24   0.000    .3572514   .4972258
      age70 |   3.047014   .4031136      8.42   0.000    2.351053   3.948996
      age75 |   6.640074   .8006096     15.70   0.000    5.242537   8.410161
       _cons |   .8996138   .1038231     -0.92   0.359    .7174972   1.127956
  ln(ptime) |          1  (exposure)
 ----------------------------------------------------------------------
```

Adjusting for age moved the intervention rate ratio to 0.42, closer to the true value of 0.5. When there is residual confounding despite randomization, adjustment for the potential confounder can correct this bias (Rothman 1977). This may be particularly true in group randomized trials, because randomization for a small number of groups may not remove all confounding by individual level characteristics. In the model above, the estimated rate ratios for age70 and 75 are both biased; 3.0 for age 70 instead of 2 and 6.6 for age 75 instead of 4. If we also adjust for the two nursing home groups that had higher rates (rate ratio 2 for the group labeled nh1, 4 for group nh2), all the rate ratio estimates move closer to their true values:

```
Age and nursing home category adjusted model
. poisson falls rx age70 age75 nh1 nh2, exp(ptime) irr nolog
(output omitted)
 ----------------------------------------------------------------------
      falls |        IRR   Std. Err.        z   P>|z|   [95% Conf. Interval]
 ------------+---------------------------------------------------------
         rx |   .5120587   .0447471     -7.66   0.000    .4314556   .6077198
      age70 |   2.493808   .3331035      6.84   0.000    1.919402   3.240111
      age75 |   4.625783   .5745441     12.33   0.000    3.626285   5.900768
        nh1 |     1.9291   .3189779      3.97   0.000    1.395109   2.667482
        nh2 |   3.901497   .6358947      8.35   0.000    2.834629   5.369902
       _cons |   .4428123   .0790692     -4.56   0.000    .3120527   .6283642
  ln(ptime) |          1  (exposure)
 ----------------------------------------------------------------------
```

Choosing the model above would be unlikely using actual data, as an analyst would have no way to identify the two nursing home groups labeled nh1 and nh2. These two groups were used to create the counts in this simulation, but in real data the true process that generated the data is unknown. Rates varied considerably from one nursing home to another (Figure 18.1), but random variation in this single

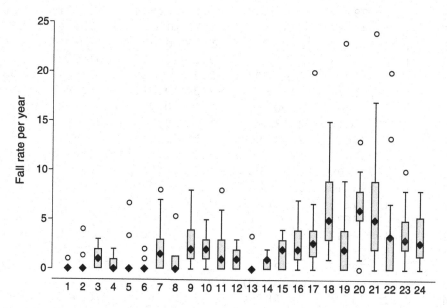

FIGURE 18.1 Boxplot showing rates of falling from 1 of 10,000 simulations for residents in 24 nursing homes. Black diamonds indicate the median rate for each home, boxes mark the 25th through 75th percentiles of the rates, the whiskers include the adjacent values (rates between the 25th percentile minus 1.5 times the 25th-75th percentile range and the 75th percentile plus 1.5 times the 25th-75h percentile range), and open circles are the extreme values beyond the whiskers. The nursing home identifiers, numbers 1–24, are on the horizontal axis.

set of data would make it hard to identify the three groups used to generate the data: homes 1–8 with the lowest rates, homes 9–16 with intermediate rates, and homes 17–24 with the highest rates. For example, home 13 looks as if it belongs in the lowest rate group and home 7 appears to have an intermediate rate. To deal with this variation, an analyst might be tempted to use indicator (dummy or factor) variables for all nursing homes, with the results shown below (the age indicator variables were omitted because this simplifies the following discussion.):

```
Age and nursing home indicators model
. poisson falls rx i.nhid, exp(ptime) irr nolog
note: 23.nhid omitted because of collinearity
```

```
Poisson regression                          Number of obs  =     416
                                            LR chi2(23)    =  545.57
                                            Prob > chi2    =  0.0000
Log likelihood = -706.7257                  Pseudo R2      =  0.2785
```

falls	IRR	Std. Err.	z	P>|z|	[95% Conf. Interval]
rx	.0593792	.0307137	-5.46	0.000	.0215453	.1636498
nhid						
2	2.052632	1.324968	1.11	0.265	.5792456	7.273765
3	.3065015	.0828685	-4.37	0.000	.1804239	.5206804
4	2.635135	1.558967	1.64	0.101	.8264665	8.401958
5	2.56579	1.959654	1.23	0.217	.5742555	11.46402

6	1.539474	.993726	0.67	0.504	.4344342	5.455323
7	.5644737	.1173031	-2.75	0.006	.3756261	.8482652
8	2.810811	1.721263	1.69	0.091	.846407	9.334348
9	.7719298	.1592195	-1.26	0.209	.5152377	1.156506
10	.5996241	.1367703	-2.24	0.025	.3834649	.9376323
11	.5789474	.1336079	-2.37	0.018	.3682995	.9100747
12	5.2	2.906888	2.95	0.003	1.73847	15.55391
13	3.25	2.482229	1.54	0.123	.7273902	14.52109
14	4.37069	2.499037	2.58	0.010	1.425138	13.40427
15	.4755639	.1174769	-3.01	0.003	.2930485	.7717529
16	.7719298	.1643352	-1.22	0.224	.5085885	1.171626
17	1.195246	.2341499	0.91	0.363	.8141532	1.754723
18	1.754386	.2911639	3.39	0.001	1.267234	2.42881
19	17.13636	8.858711	5.50	0.000	6.221379	47.20094
20	1.736842	.2887803	3.32	0.001	1.253814	2.405955
21	1.998302	.3276829	4.22	0.000	1.449041	2.755762
22	17.72727	9.799119	5.20	0.000	5.999604	52.37949
23	1	(omitted)				
24	16.35484	8.58654	5.32	0.000	5.844569	45.7657
_cons	3.454545	.4575657	9.36	0.000	2.664689	4.478528
ln(ptime)	1	(exposure)				

This model reports a strong association, rate ratio 0.059, between the intervention (rx) and fall rates. But the intervention did not vary within nursing homes and an estimate for the intervention is impossible if we adjust for all the nursing home groups. When a variable, nhid in this case, is factored into its categories, Stata automatically omits the level with the lowest number; nursing home 1 was omitted in this example. Nursing home 23 was also omitted because of collinearity. Stata omitted nursing home 23 because when all the indicator values for each nursing home were entered into the model, those values in combination were collinear with the effects of the intervention. At least one nursing home had to be omitted to get an estimate for the intervention. Stata selected nursing home 23 for omission because this was the highest numbered nursing home (last in numerical order from lowest to highest) among all the nursing homes in the control arm. In this model, the intercept rate of 3.45 is actually the fall rate for nursing home 23 (Figure 18.1). The rate ratio of 0.059, is simply the rate in nursing home 1 divided by the rate in nursing home 23: 0.205/3.45 = 0.06. So there is no useful estimate of the rate ratio for the intervention in this model. If we instruct Stata to fit the following model

```
. poisson falls i.nhid rx, exp(ptime) irr nolog
```

Stata would report no estimate for the intervention:

```
note: rx omitted because of collinearity
```

When there is perfect collinearity between regression variables, Stata's default is to omit the last term in the variable list that will remove the collinearity. Because the variable rx is collinear with the nursing home indicators in aggregate, if the indicators are entered into the model after the rx, one of the nursing homes will be dropped. The lesson here is that if the group level variable, rx in this case, does not vary within the groups, then we cannot simultaneously estimate the association for the group level variable and the association for all the groups with the model outcome. Complete adjustment for group is not possible.

18.4 VARIANCE ADJUSTMENT METHODS

Adjusted variance methods use customary regression models but adjust the variances to account for the clustered nature of the data. Adjusted variance procedures are described with terms such as quasi-likelihood, pseudo-likelihood, robust variance, clustered variance, generalized estimating equations, GEE, population averaged, or marginal methods. These methods estimate the regression coefficients in a model and separately estimate the variance for the model coefficients; two models are used and then folded into a single regression table (Young et al. 2007). Because the coefficient estimation process and the variance estimation are separated, this means that mistakes in the variance estimation have little or no influence on the coefficient estimation.

Many Stata regression commands allow a **vce(cluster cluster-name)** option. This uses a modified sandwich variance estimator which relaxes the assumption of independence within clusters defined by a variable name (Cameron and Trivedi 2009, Hardin and Hilbe 2012 pp36–37,384–385). This modified sandwich variance estimator can produce a variance that is larger or smaller than either the usual variance or the robust (usual sandwich) variance, depending upon the correlation of the data within the clusters; negative correlation shrinks the variance, positive correlation increases it.

Negative correlation within clusters means that there is more variation within the clusters than between the clusters. Imagine students are entering the 9th grade at a school where the philosophy is that students learn best in a classroom with students of diverse academic abilities. The school randomly assigns students to each classroom in a manner related to their average academic score in the previous year. Consequently each classroom has a similar proportion of students with As, Bs, Cs, and so on, in the 8th grade. In this situation the academic performance between classrooms could be more similar than performance within classrooms, resulting in negative correlation. In practice, this situation is so uncommon that it may be reasonable to assume for power calculations or an analysis that negative correlation is not possible (Donner and Klar 2000 p8).

Using the single set of simulated nursing home data described in the previous section, the age-adjusted rate ratio for the intervention using Poisson regression and the default Poisson variance is 0.421, SE 0.036 (Table 18.1, Model 1). If the **vce(cluster nhid)** option is used, with nursing homes identified by the variable nhid, the rate ratio remains unchanged, but the SE increases to 0.111 (Model 2), and the Z-statistic shrinks to 3.3. Stata has extensive commands for data from complex survey designs. The Stata **svyset** command can tell Stata that the primary sampling units, or groups, were the 24 nursing homes. Then the **svy: poisson** command with its usual variance will produce rate ratios and SEs (Model 3) identical to those from Poisson regression with the modified sandwich variance. These are the same model and this example shows that survey commands can sometimes be used to analyze multilevel data. The **svy: poisson** command will compare the Wald statistic (ratio of ln(rate ratio) to SE ln rate ratio) with a t-distribution instead of the normal (Z) distribution, and therefore the P-values and CIs will be larger than those from Poisson regression with the cluster variance option. Comparison with the t-distribution is a good choice if the number of groups is small, as in this example. For any of the models in Table 18.1 we can use the t-distribution, instead of the z-distribution, by extracting the ln rate ratio and SE estimate after regression, and using Stata's **ttail** and **invttail** functions with degrees of freedom equal to the number of groups minus 1 (Buis 2007).

The clustered variance option relaxes the assumption that the rates are independent within each nursing home, but it still assumes that the Poisson variance, albeit modified by the clustering, can be used. But the rate variations in these data are large, so the Poisson variance is probably too small. If we use the robust variance estimator (Model 4, Table 18.1), the usual sandwich variance, the SE for the rate ratio increases from 0.036 in model 1 to 0.068. But this is smaller than the SE of 0.111 in Models 2 and 3. So in this instance, accounting for clustering of rates within nursing homes does more to increase the variance than simply relaxing the assumption that the rates arose from three Poisson processes, one for each age group.

TABLE 18.1   Adjusted variance methods. Rate ratio from a group-randomized controlled trial comparing the fall rates of persons in nursing homes given a fall prevention intervention with persons in control nursing homes. The age-adjusted rate ratio, SE, and Z-statistics are shown from an ordinary Poisson regression model and several adjusted variance methods. The data are from just 1 of 10,000 simulations (Figure 18.1).

NO.	MODEL	STATA COMMAND	VARIANCE OPTION	CORRELATION OPTION [a]	RATE RATIO	SE	Z	P	95% CI
1	Poisson	poisson	default	none	0.421	0.036	10.2	<.0001	0.36, 0.50
2	Poisson	poisson	cluster	none	0.421	0.111	3.3	.0011	0.25, 0.71
3	Poisson	svy: poisson	cluster [b]	none	0.421	0.111	3.3	.0034	0.24, 0.73
4	Poisson	poisson	robust	none	0.421	0.068	5.4	<.0001	0.31, 0.58
5	Panel data Poisson (GEE)	xtpoisson, pa	default [c]	independent	0.421	0.036	10.2	<.0001	0.36, 0.50
6	Panel data Poisson (GEE)	xtpoisson, pa	robust	independent	0.421	0.111	3.3	.0011	0.25, 0.71
7	Panel data Poisson (GEE)	xtpoisson, pa	default [c]	exchangeable	0.446	0.060	6.0	<.0001	0.34, 0.58
8	Panel data Poisson (GEE)	xtpoisson, pa	robust	exchangeable	0.446	0.136	2.6	.0081	0.25, 0.81

SE = standard error

CI = confidence interval

[a] Models 1–4 have no correlation option; all assume independent observations, but variance adjustment is used to relax that assumption.

[b] The svy prefix indicates a command for survey data. There is no cluster variance option for the svy: poisson command. The syset command is used to designate the nursing homes (identified by variable nhid) as the primary sampling units. Then the svy: poisson command fits a model identical to that of the poisson, vce(cluster nhid) command. The survey commands use the t-distribution, not the normal (Z) distribution, and therefore the p-values and confidence intervals are larger than those from the equivalent poisson, vce(cluster) command.

[c] Population-averaged (PA) generalized estimating equation (GEE) models 5 and 7 used the default variance option. They differ in the chosen correlation structure. Models 5–8 required an xtset command to instruct the software that observations in nursing homes are not necessarily independent over time; this allows for clustering over time. In this example all the observations were made at the same time, so the clustering does not really involve time.

18.5 GENERALIZED ESTIMATING EQUATIONS (GEE)

Generalized estimating equations (GEE) were described by Liang and Zeger in 1986 (Zeger and Liang 1986). These regression commands use iteratively reweighted least squares to fit a wide variety of models. Detailed statistical formulae can be found in the Stata manual entry for **xtgee** and in a textbook (Hardin and Hilbe 2013). These models are sometimes referred to as quasi-likelihood models, population-averaged models, population-averaged generalized estimating equations (PA-GEE), or marginal models.

Hanley et al. (2003) wrote an excellent paper for readers who are not professional statisticians. Using simple numerical examples and clear wording, they described how GEE reweights the data to find the optimal variance estimates at the level of the clusters. This variance lies between the variance of an analysis that assumes all the observations are independent and a variance that ignores entirely the variation within clusters. The later approach is equivalent to assigning a single overall rate to each cluster.

Models 2, 3, and 4 estimate the same regression coefficients as Model 1, the ordinary Poisson model. Estimates from GEE may differ from ordinary Poisson model estimates, depending upon features of the data and the correlation structure that is assumed. GEE models average across clusters using the estimated cluster-level variance; this may result in coefficient estimates that differ from Model 1. GEE has been described as a semi-parametric approach, because it makes no use of random effects that are assumed to follow a parametric distribution. For this reason, I have included GEE among the variance adjusting methods. In discussions that contrast GEE and mixed model approaches, many authors treat the use of random effects by mixed models as the contrast of greatest importance; I have followed this practice by putting all the random effect estimates in their own Table 18.2.

GEE models are called population-averaged methods because they are estimates of the rate experienced by the average exposed person (residents of an intervention nursing home in this example) contrasted with the average non-exposed person (residents of control homes). A comparison is made between two populations, accounting for clustering within institutions. If we were to use GEE to study state-level laws across all 52 states, the result would be an estimate of how the law affected the average person in the entire United States. This is in contrast to a mixed-model, which estimates the exposure-related rate change for the average person within each nursing-home or state. This is sometimes called the subject-specific estimate of association (Hanley et al. 2003, Hubbard et al. 2010, Vittinghoff et al. 2012 p285). In a study of states, we might describe a GEE result as an estimate of what happened to the average person in the entire study region, while the mixed model estimates what we might expect to happen in the next state to adopt the law that was studied.

Many authors use the term marginal to indicate population-averaged estimates and use the term conditional to indicate subject-specific estimates. This terminology is well-accepted, but it can create confusion because there are also conditional models, such as conditional logistic and conditional Poisson regression, which estimate associations within clusters, but "condition" out the cluster effects. These conditional models are discussed in Chapter 20.

Stata's GEE commands have the prefix "**xt**", meaning that cross-sectional (the letter x) units have repeated measurements that are typically measured over time (the letter t). Stata has a generalized **xtgee** command, so a population-averaged Poisson GEE model can be fit using **xtgee, link(log) family-(poisson)**. An equivalent command is **xtpoisson, pa**, where the option **pa** means population-averaged. Both commands require that the user inform Stata, using the **xtset** command, about a variable that identifies the panels (clusters). The **xtset** command also identifies for Stata the repeated measures made over time (such as yearly rate data). Although Stata refers to this option as a measure of time, this variable could instead identify children within a family as child number 1, 2, and so on. Hanley et al. (2003) use an example of children clustered within families. The outcome of interest in their example was child height and all the children had their heights measured at the same time, but at different ages.

The fact that older children are usually taller was accounted for in their analysis by transforming the height measurements into differences, in standard deviation units, from the height of children of the same sex and age in a reference population. Thus, the outcomes were age-sex-adjusted heights, which they treated as repeated measurements within each family. In the nursing home data, the rate measurements for each resident can be thought of as repeated attempts to measure the same rate within each nursing home and age group. But these repeated measurements were all made over the same time period and they are not ordered in any way.

The GEE commands have options that allow the analyst to choose the correlation structure for the observations. There is no cluster variance option with the population-averaged GEE commands; instead, these commands let us pick a correlation structure that allows for certain types of clustering. Several correlation structures are possible, but since the rates of residents within each nursing home are not ordered and have no other expected structure, only two of the correlation options seem reasonable: **independent** or **exchangeable**. If we chose the independent correlation option, we are assuming that the rates within nursing homes are independent of each other; this results in GEE Model 5 (Table 18.1) with estimates identical to ordinary Poisson regression with Model 1 (Hardin and Hilbe 2013 p87). If the robust variance option is used, GEE Model 6 is identical to the cluster variance Poisson Model 4. Assuming independent correlation for these data, as in Model 5, cannot be justified, as the data generating process guaranteed that rates were more similar within nursing homes than between them.

Stata's default correlation choice for a GEE model is the exchangeable structure, which means that within a nursing home, we assume that the correlation of rates between any two pairs of records is the same. Exchangeable correlation is also called equal correlation, common correlation, or compound symmetry (Hardin and Hilbe 2013 pp63–64). This option makes sense in the nursing home example. The data were created in such a way that all persons in the same nursing home had their fall rate elevated by a multiplicative factor of 1 (no change), 2, or 4. These nursing home effects were the same, on a ratio scale and with some random variation, for all residents. On average the correlation should be the same between the fall rates of any two persons of the same age in the same nursing home. This correlation structure is relatively easy to estimate, as it requires only one additional correlation parameter. The exchangeable correlation structure changed the weighting so that the rate ratio changed by a modest amount from .421 to 0.446 (Model 7, Table 18.1). The SE for this estimate is 0.060, not too different from the robust SE of Model 4. If we use the robust variance option for this model, the SE increases to 0.136, similar to Models 2, 3, and 6 which all had SEs of 0.111.

In discussions of GEE models some authors distinguish between "model-based" or "data based" SEs. The former refers to SEs (or variances) from a GEE model without the robust variance option, the later refers to results when the robust variance is used (Hanley et al. 2003).

Which model is best in Table 18.1? Models 1 and 5 are surely poor choices, as they ignore the clustering of fall rates within nursing homes. Model 7 allows for exchangeable correlation between rates in nursing homes but fails to adjust the SE for the clustering; Model 8 is a better choice. But Model 8 changes the size of the rate ratio, albeit by a small amount; in this example, at least, there seems to be little reason not to prefer the rate ratio of 0.42, which is justified by the randomized trial design. Models 2, 3, and 6 are all the same model wrapped in different packaging. Should we prefer one of these or Model 4, which used the robust variance estimator?

Several authors suggest that when the number of clusters is small (Hubbard et al. 2010), say less than 40 (20 per trial arm) (Murray et al. 1998, Murray 1998, p126, Varnell et al. 2004) or 50 (Young et al. 2007) or 30 (Hayes and Moulton 2009 p200) the use of the robust sandwich variance may result in biased variance estimates. It is not always clear in these discussions whether the authors are referring to use of the fully robust sandwich variance, as in Model 4, or the cluster-robust (also called semirobust, empirical, or robust by various authors) variance, as in Models 2 and 6. The terminology of the literature about models for clustered data is not always transparent. Robust variance estimates are large-sample methods. Even though the nursing home data has 416 subjects, only 12 homes were assigned to each trial arm. It is common to see cluster randomized trials in which the number of clusters is small. Results are more reliable if there are many clusters with fewer subjects within each cluster. It is also best to use clusters of the same or similar size and use a randomization scheme that ensures the same number of clusters in each trial arm.

For the nursing home data, we can try to reason our way to the best model choice (Table 18.1). It is the clustering that is most important and therefore we should prefer Models 2, 3, and 6, which all deal with the clustered nature of the data. It is true that the data arose in part from a Poisson process and partly from a negative binomial process; therefore, we would like to relax the Poisson variance assumption. But use of the robust variance alone, as in Model 4, fails to deal with the clustered nature of the data; the clustering here is quite strong, with a lot of variation in rates from one nursing home to the next, while rates are more homogenous within nursing homes.

A re-randomization approach can be used for cluster-randomized trials (Gail et al. 1996, Murray 1998 pp115–117). This is particularly useful when the number of groups in each arm is balanced and there is not a lot of variation in the group size; both features are true for the nursing home data. Using the single data set for 24 nursing homes, the homes (not individuals) were rerandomized to the intervention and control group 199,999 times; in each replication 12 homes were assigned to the intervention. With each replication, Poisson regression was used to estimate the age-adjusted rate ratio for the intervention and these results were used, as discussed in Chapter 12, to estimate that the 95% CI for the rate ratio of 0.421 was 0.24, 0.74. This is close to the CI for models 2 and 6 and closest to the Model 3 CI (0.24, 073), the survey data model that compared the SE with the t-distribution. This result supports the argument that the variance should account for the clustering.

18.6 MIXED MODEL METHODS

Mixed models assume that the usual regression error terms are supplemented by quantities for random errors (Gardiner, Luo, and Roman 2009, Fitzmaurice, Laird, and Ware 2011 pp395–400, Cameron and Trivedi 2013a pp111–128). These hypothetical random errors are assumed to follow a statistical distribution, such as the Normal, Gamma, or inverse-Gaussian distribution. Mixed models are described as random effects, latent variable, generalized linear mixed models (GLMM), subject-specific, subject-specific GEE (SS-GEE), cluster-specific, and conditional methods.

When the nursing home data were analyzed by the methods in Table 18.1, a single intercept term was estimated for all 416 residents in the 24 nursing homes. In a Poisson model applied to one sample of the simulated data, shown earlier, with terms for the intervention (rx), age 70, and age 75 years, the intercept value was 0.90, which estimates the rate of falling among persons age 65 years who were not exposed to the intervention. This does not equal the true rate of 0.50 falls per year, but we would not know this in practice. The rate of falling varies between the nursing homes and it may be unreasonable for us to think that the rate of 0.90 applies equally to 65-year-olds in nursing home 1 and nursing home 20 (Figure 18.1). It might be nice if we could enter information about this variation in nursing home fall rates for 65-year-olds into the model.

As we saw earlier with the age and nursing home indicator model, we cannot enter dummy values for each nursing home and expect to estimate the intervention association as well. This is not possible because the intervention does not vary within each nursing home. Instead, let us assume that the 24 nursing homes were sampled from an infinite universe of nursing homes. These imagined nursing homes have underlying fall rates (the rate for those age 65 years) that follow a distribution; perhaps a Normal, Gamma, or inverse-Gaussian distribution. We do not know the fall rates of this endless nursing home population but using the known rates of the 24 nursing homes in our sample, we can assume that these rates approximate the true rates of the entire nursing home universe and add a random variable to the error terms of the regression model, as in Expression 17.2. This random variable is an estimate of the underlying rate in each nursing home. This means that the intercept rate is the average of the rates for 65-year-olds from each nursing home, but each nursing home is allowed to have its own random term for the deviation of its rate from this mean, following the chosen distribution. This idea is the basis for all mixed models that involve known variables (sometimes called fixed effects) and hypothesized random effects.

The mixed model approach enters information about the individual nursing homes rates into the model through a backdoor approach. Random error terms are used instead of explicit nursing home indicator terms. This means we do not have to enter each and every nursing home rate into the model, an approach that will not work. Instead we enter a single random effect that can vary from one nursing home to the next.

Since this random variable is added to the model error terms, it increases the variance for the model estimates. The increase is a function of the between-nursing-home rate variation, so this accounts for heterogeneity in rates by increasing the variance. To put this another way, the method accounts for the correlation of rates within, compared with between, nursing homes by allowing each nursing home to have its own intercept. This approach tends to account for any overdispersion in the rates.

The benefits of the mixed model approach come with a price. The method assumes that the random effects are unrelated to the explanatory variables (covariates) in the model (Gardiner, Luo, and Roman 2009, Hubbard et al. 2010, Wooldridge 2010, p286). When rates are analyzed, this zero correlation assumption extends to the person-time values. If this assumption is not true, the estimates and their variances can both be biased.

18.7 WHAT DO MIXED MODELS ESTIMATE?

Mixed models are sometimes described as conditional, meaning that the coefficient estimates are conditional upon the random effects. They are also described as being subject-specific; some authors refer to these as SS-GEE methods. The term subject-specific or individual-specific makes sense for longitudinal data with individuals who have repeated measurements made over time. This terminology does not describe the nursing home data well, as the clusters are nursing homes, not individuals; the term cluster-specific is a better fit for this example. The key idea is that mixed models estimate the associations within each cluster, whether that cluster is an individual with repeated observations or a nursing home with several residents.

The mixed model compares two subjects, one of whom received the fall intervention and another of the same age who did not receive the intervention, conditional on their being in the *same* nursing home. This comparison is not present in the data, because within each nursing home all the residents either received the intervention or none of them did. Nevertheless, that is what the mixed model is trying to estimate. This is in contrast to the marginal or population-averaged model, which compares the fall rates of two persons of the same age, who may be in the same or different nursing homes.

For a logistic model, which estimates odds ratios, the mixed model (cluster-specific or conditional) estimates will be further from 1 than the marginal (population-averaged) odds ratios. But for the Poisson rate ratio model with a single random effect (a random intercept) that has a mean of 0 on the ln scale, the population-averaged rate ratio and the mixed effects rate ratio are both attempts to estimate the same ratio (Ritz and Spiegelman 2004, Young et al. 2007, Gardiner, Luo, and Roman 2009, Fitzmaurice, Laird, and Ware 2011 p478). In other words, the mixed-model subject-specific ratio is equivalent to the population-averaged rate ratio. The same is true for a Poisson rate difference model that uses the identify link, as long as the random effect distribution has a mean of 0 on the additive scale (Ritz and Spiegelman 2004). If random coefficients are introduced, on top of the random intercept, then the subject-specific model and the population-averaged model are no longer the same.

Despite saying that conditional and marginal estimates of association for rates are equivalent in theory, the actual estimates from a population-averaged model and a mixed model may differ, to some degree, for several reasons. The two model methods will not necessarily produce identical estimates in actual data (Young et al. 2007, Gardiner, Luo, and Roman 2009). They are equivalent in theory, not necessarily in any single set of data.

18.8 MIXED MODEL ESTIMATES FOR THE NURSING HOME INTERVENTION

Stata has many mixed model commands, although sometimes the same model is disguised by different command names. The 18 models in Table 18.2 are variations on the age-adjusted rate ratio models shown earlier, but all involve a random effect. The rate ratios for the intervention are 0.35 to 0.41 in Table 18.2, pretty close to the estimates of 0.42 to 0.45 in Table 18.1. The log-linear models in Table 18.2 are all trying to estimate the same results as those in 18.1.

Models 9, 10, and 11 are negative binomial models. They assume that there is a random effect with a gamma distribution. Model 10, with a cluster-specific variance estimator, had the largest SE. This is similar to the situation in Table 18.1, where Poisson models with variance estimators for clusters (Models 2 and 3) had larger SEs compared with the robust variance method (Model 4 in Table 18.1, Model 11 in Table 18.2). Models 12 and 13 are mixed models for longitudinal (repeated-measures) panel data, but we can use them for clustered nursing-home data as well. These models also assume a gamma distribution for the random effects. All the models with gamma random effects (9–13) produce similar estimates of the intervention association, a rate ratio 0.40 or 0.41. But the negative binomial models (9, 11) with the default or robust variance methods had SEs that are too small. These models produced their estimates without accounting for the fact that residents were grouped in nursing homes. The panel data (**xt**) commands, however, required that we use the **xtset** command to tell the software about the clustering, before fitting the model. Thus, even with the default variance, the **xtpoisson** command (model 12) reported a SE of 0.092, almost the same as the SE (0.094) from negative binomial regression (model 10) with a cluster-variance estimator.

Some commands can be induced to produce results identical to those of other commands. For example, if we use **xtset** to designate the individuals as clusters (instead of the nursing homes), the **xtpoisson, re** command with the default variance (Model 12) will produce results identical to negative binomial Model 9. Similarly, Model 13a for panel data will mimic negative binomial Model 10. The same is true for Model 13b and Model 11. There is no reason we would designate the individuals as clusters, but these behaviors reveal the similarity between **xtpoisson** random effect methods and negative binomial methods.

Models 14–19 all assume the random effects are normally distributed. All the random intercept models (14–17) produce the same rate ratio estimate, but they differ somewhat in their SEs. All produce larger SEs, compared with negative binomial models 9 and 11, even with their default variance estimators, because all of them utilize information about the clustering. The SEs become larger when we specifically invoke the cluster or robust variance methods, but the increase is minimal.

Finally, models 18–19 are random coefficient models. They estimate a random effect for the intercept and an *additional* random effect for the intervention term. In the example this produces a small change in the rate ratio for the intervention.

18.9 SIMULATION RESULTS FOR SOME MIXED MODELS

Results in Tables 18.1 and 18.2 were for a single realization of the simulated nursing home data. The estimates differ from the true values to some degree, as they might be in real data. To better judge the performance of some of these models, I simulated the nursing home data 10,000 times, re-randomizing the person-time and intervention data, as described earlier. All of these models

TABLE 18.2 Mixed model methods. Rate ratio from a group-randomized controlled trial comparing the fall rates of persons in nursing homes given a fall prevention intervention with persons in control nursing homes. The age-adjusted rate ratio, SE, and Z-statistics are shown from several mixed model (random effect) methods. Data are the same as in Table 18.1, using just 1 of 10,000 simulations.

NO.[a]	MODEL	STATA COMMAND	VARIANCE OPTION	COVARIANCE OPTION[b]	RANDOM EFFECT OPTION	RATE RATIO	SE	Z	P	95% CI
9	Negative binomial	nbreg	default	none	gamma	0.402	0.045	8.1	<.0001	0.32, 0.50
10	Negative binomial	nbreg	cluster	none	gamma	0.402	0.094	3.9	.0001	0.25, 0.64
11	Negative binomial	nbreg	robust	none	gamma	0.402	0.054	6.8	<.0001	0.31, 0.52
12	Panel data Poisson	xtpoisson, re	default	none	gamma	0.408	0.092	4.0	.0001	0.26, 0.64
13 a,b	Panel data Poisson	xtpoisson, re	cluster or robust	none	gamma	0.408	1.00	3.7	.0002	0.25, 0.66
14 a,b	Mixed Poisson	mepoisson	default	independent or unstructured	normal, random intercept	0.365	0.086	4.3	<.0001	0.23, 0.58
15	Panel data Poisson	xtpoisson, re	default	none	normal	0.365	0.086	4.3	<.0001	0.23, 0.58
16 a,b,c,d	Mixed Poisson	mepoisson	cluster or robust	independent or unstructured	normal, random intercept	0.365	0.091	4.0	.0001	0.22, 0.60
17 a,b	Panel data Poisson	xtpoisson, re	cluster or robust	none	normal	0.365	0.091	4.0	.0001	0.22, 0.60
18 a,b	Mixed Poisson	mepoisson	default	independent	normal, random coefficient	0.347	0.087	4.2	<.0001	0.21, 0.57
19 a,b	Mixed Poisson	mepoisson	cluster or robust	independent	normal, random coefficient	0.347	0.085	4.3	<.0001	0.21, 0.56

SE = standard error
CI = confidence interval
[a] No. is the model number. The letters indicate that for some model numbers, more than one model option provided the same estimates.
[b] Models without a covariance option assume independence of the random effects, but variance adjustment is used to relax that assumption.

(Table 18.3) produced a rate ratio of 0.50 for the fall reduction program, because in the simulated data the intervention was randomly assigned and therefore had no systematic relationship to the age variables or the hypothesized random effects. The Poisson model (the second number 3 model in Table 18.3) with variables for the two nursing home groups was the only model that produced a nearly correct estimate for the intercept as well as nearly correct estimates for the rate ratios for nursing home groups 2 and 3. This model, as stated earlier, would be unlikely in a real analysis as we could not identify the correct nursing home groups. The SE for the intervention is smallest (SE = 0.05) for this model, demonstrating that having the right model improves efficiency because we have a closer fit to the data. We can estimate the same intervention effect of 0.50 with all the models, but we pay a price with a larger SE of 0.11 or 0.12.

The negative binomial model (Model 10, Table 18.3) produced estimates and SEs nearly identical to those of the Poisson model (the first Model 3, Table 18.3). The data were partly produced by a Poisson process and so the negative binomial model nearly reduced to the Poisson model. A panel data Poisson model with gamma-distributed random effects (Model 13), produced rate ratios of 2.1 and 4.3 for the two age groups, closer to the true rate ratios of 2.0 and 4.0 compared with the negative binomial model. Both models 10 (negative binomial) and 13 (panel data Poisson) assumed the random effects were gamma distributed. But the negative binomial model used a random effect for each of the 416 observations, whereas the panel data model used a random effect for each of the 24 nursing homes. Panel data model 13 has an advantage here. The

TABLE 18.3 Results from 10,000 simulations for each of several models. Rate ratios from a group-randomized controlled trial comparing the fall rates of persons in nursing homes given a fall prevention intervention with persons in control nursing homes. In each simulation the nursing-home data were recreated; person-time and treatment group were randomly reassigned. Robust SE shown in parentheses.

		EXPONENTIATED MODEL ESTIMATES (RATE RATIOS)					
NO.[a]	MODEL	INTERCEPT	INTERVENTION	AGE 70	AGE 75	NURSING HOME GROUP 1[b]	NURSING HOME GROUP 2[b]
3	Poisson	0.91 (0.17)	0.50 (0.11)	2.55 (0.40)	6.04 (0.96)	_[c]	_[c]
3	Poisson	0.49 (0.08)	0.50 (0.05)	2.01 (0.30)	4.02 (0.61)	2.01 (0.30)	4.03 (0.60)
3[d]	Poisson	0.32 (0.03)	_[c]	2.01 (0.31)	4.01 (0.61)	_[c]	_[c]
10	Negative binomial	0.91 (0.17)	0.50 (0.11)	2.55 (0.40)	6.05 (0.95)	_[c]	_[c]
13	Panel data Poisson, gamma random effect	1.11 (0.26)	0.50 (0.11)	2.09 (0.44)	4.27 (0.90)	_[c]	_[c]
16	Mixed Poisson, random intercept	0.98 (0.19)	0.50 (0.12)	2.09 (0.32)	4.27 (0.65)	_[c]	_[c]
19	Mixed Poisson, random coefficients	0.98 (0.19)	0.50 (0.12)	2.09 (0.32)	4.27 (0.65)	_[c]	_[c]

[a] No. corresponds to the model numbers in Tables 18.1 and 18.2.
[b] Nursing home group 1 (nh1) includes nursing homes 9–16; the rate ratio for falling in those homes, compared with nursing homes 1–8, was 2. Nursing home group 2 (nh2) includes homes 17–24; the rate ratio for falling in those homes, compared with homes 1–8, was 4.
[c] No estimate because this term was not in the model.
[d] This model included indicator terms for all the nursing homes.

model rate ratios for age were still biased because the data generating process put more old people with higher fall rates into the nursing homes with the highest underlying rates for those age 65 years. This means that the assumption that the random effects were independent of the covariates was violated in this example. Nevertheless, the mixed model approach (Models 13, 16, 19 in Table 18.3), produced rate ratios for ages 70 and 75 that were closer to the true values compared with the first Model 3 and Model 10 because the mixed models made some use of the rate information within each nursing home in the random effects.

If our main goal was to estimate the association between age and falls rates, we could use Model 3[d] (Table 18.3), a Poisson model that used the age groups as explanatory variables, adjusted for all the nursing homes using indicators, and omitted the treatment group indicator. This model correctly estimated the rate ratios for age 70 and age 75 years, but the intercept rate is too small because of confounding that resulted from omitting the treatment. As with all the models in Table 18.1, we cannot simultaneously estimate both the treatment association and the nursing home associations in the same model. The mixed model approach tries to have its cake and eat it too, but the age-related rate ratios have some bias due to confounding.

18.10 MIXED MODELS WEIGHT OBSERVATIONS DIFFERENTLY THAN POISSON REGRESSION

In Chapter 17, hypothetical data for five regions (Table 17.2) were used to show that Poisson regression uses person-time weighted averages of rates, whereas negative binomial regression weights rates more equally. The mixed model methods in Table 18.2 also weight rates more equally compared with Poisson regression. Consequently, results from Poisson and mixed model regression may differ substantially. The estimated rate ratios will almost surely differ if person-time varies between observations. In the example used here, there was minimal variation in person-time due to dropouts which were random.

18.11 WHICH SHOULD WE PREFER FOR CLUSTERED DATA, VARIANCE-ADJUSTED OR MIXED MODELS?

The mixed model approach offers potential advantages. Provided that the regression model is correct and the random effects part of the model is correctly specified, the mixed model approach can allow us to simultaneously estimate the nursing home effects, the treatment effects, and the age effects. In addition, mixed models provide information about how these effects are correlated. But this is not a free lunch. If the hypothesized random effects are incorrectly specified, the estimated associations can be severely biased. In contrast, the variance-adjusted methods of Table 18.1 rely on weaker assumptions; the estimated associations only depend on having the correct regression model.

Heagerty and Zeger (2000) discuss potential problems with mixed models. Their article is heavy with technical jargon and mathematical notation, but the crucial ideas appear in sections 4 and 5 of their paper, and in their discussion. The mixed models of Table 18.3 assume that a single estimate of variance for the random effects is sufficient. Heagerty and Zeger use simulated and actual data to show that if this assumption is incorrect, bias can arise in coefficient estimates or SEs. Mixed models try to estimate associations within clusters, even when there is no actual within-cluster variation in exposure. These are estimates that compare subjects who are not only alike regarding model covariates, but alike regarding "latent" variables which cannot be observed. Heagerty and Zeger show that these "extrapolations" are sensitive to model choices. They argue that if the goal is to estimate associations and account for data clustering, mixed-models are not needed and models such as those in Table 18.1 are less prone to bias. Their article was published with short commentaries by other statisticians. One of these, Neuhaus, takes the position that analysts should not even report mixed-model estimates for cluster level covariates that do not actually vary within the clusters. Raudenbush defends mixed models. And the authors respond to these comments.

In 2010, Hubbard et al. (Hubbard et al. 2010) published a clear review of the relative merits of population-averaged (GEE) and mixed-model methods. They argued that mixed model results should be regarded with some skepticism, as they rest on untestable assumptions about unobserved (latent) variables. Subramanian and O'Malley (2010) provided a robust defense of mixed models in the same journal issue. A vociferous rebuttal to that paper came from Van der Laan, Hubbard, and Jewell (2010); they used the phrase "faith-based inference" in their subtitle.

Helpful comparisons of these approaches appear in textbooks by Agresti (2002 pp500–502) and Fitzmaurice, Laird, and Ware (2011 pp473–486). These authors suggest that model choice can be made based on the goals of the research, a view shared by others (Heagerty and Zeger 2000). Van der Laan, Hubbard, and Jewell (2010), however, remark that

> ... this platitude ignores our main message – that the parameter of interest must also be connected to the data at hand. Thus, it is questionable to interpret within-neighborhood effects of a covariate change (such as crime rates) from mixed-effect models when the data do not include any variation of such attributes within neighborhoods. Such inference is based entirely on assumption and not on data ...

18.12 ADDITIONAL MODEL COMMANDS FOR CLUSTERED DATA

Stata has additional commands for clustered data. For the **xtpoisson** commands there are corresponding **xtnbreg** commands that use negative binomial regression as the underlying model. The random effects are for the distribution of the dispersion statistic. Similarly, there is a **menbreg** command for mixed models using the negative binomial distribution. The **meqrpoisson** command provides an alternative method for estimating mixed Poisson models. The **gllamm** (generalized linear latent and mixed model) command by Rabe-Hesketh can be installed in Stata and is described in textbooks (Skrondal and Rabe-Hesketh 2004, Rabe-Hesketh and Skrondal 2012), although it has been supplanted by the **xtpoisson** and **mepoisson** commands. Hilbe has written the **pigreg** command for a Poisson model with an inverse Gaussian (PIG) distribution for random effects (Hilbe 2011 pp341–343, Cameron and Trivedi 2013a pp123–124, Hilbe 2014 pp162–171). These additional commands are well described by their help files in Stata.

If you wish to fit a rate difference model with GEE methods, the **xtgee, pa** command can be used. A rate difference mixed-model can be estimated with **xtgee, re** or **meglm** with appropriate choices for the link, distribution family, and weights.

18.13 FURTHER READING

Many textbooks about clustered and longitudinal data have appeared. The book by West, Welch, and Galecki (2015) is limited to linear models for continuous outcomes, the mixed model equivalent of linear regression, and so there is no discussion of count or rate models. However the language is clear, the examples cover a range of clustered data problems, both clustered and longitudinal data are discussed, and there is helpful detail about several software packages. The book by Fitzmaurice, Laird, and Ware (2011) is focused on longitudinal data, but the same principles apply to any form of clustering and the writing is exceptionally clear. The encyclopedic volume by Wooldridge (2010) is heavy on mathematical notation, but this is accompanied by lucid writing. Only a small part of the book is about count models, but much information is given in that short space. Snijders and Bosker (2012) have written a fine discussion of multilevel modeling.

Longitudinal Data 19

Observations made on the same units (persons, government districts, hospitals, factories, etc.) over time are called longitudinal data, repeated measures, or cross-sectional panel data. This is a type of clustered data, in which the replicated measurements are clustered within the followed units. Statistical methods and Stata commands for clustered data were reviewed in Chapter 18. This chapter covers a few ideas that have not yet been discussed.

19.1 JUST USE RATES

A randomized controlled trial of an intervention to reduce falls among elderly persons (Shumway-Cook et al. 2007) was described in Chapter 12, with additional mention in Chapter 13. Most trial subjects were followed for a year and their fall events were recorded on monthly calendars. The main study outcome was each subject's total count of falls divided by their follow-up time; an incidence rate. Rates are a simple method for summarizing repeated events, especially when the exact timing of each event is not important. The data could have been treated as cross-sectional panel data, with a monthly fall rate for each subject. This would have offered little advantage in this study.

Rates for repeated events are a type of clustered data. If the rates fit a Poisson distribution well, we can assume a single Poisson process generated the falls and use Poisson assumptions to estimate the precision of the intervention effect on falls. But the spread of the observed fall rates was too great for a Poisson distribution. Methods for detecting this extra-Poisson dispersion were discussed in Chapter 12 and methods for dealing with this problem were reviewed in Chapter 13. Some people in the study had a propensity for falling that was much greater than that of others. This heterogeneity of rates is the flip-side of clustering. It arose because falls were heavily clustered within a few subjects. The methods of Chapter 13 were described as a way of correcting the variance when Poisson assumptions are insufficient, but they can also be thought of as methods for dealing with clustering when rates are analyzed.

19.2 USING RATES TO EVALUATE GOVERNMENTAL POLICIES

Investigators often evaluate governmental policies or laws by assessing how those policies are related to mortality rates, crash rates, or hospital admission rates. We might wish to know how graduated driving licensing policies are related to traffic crash mortality rates of teenagers, how firearm regulations are related to homicide rates, how anti-smoking policies are associated with cancer rates, or how smog regulations are associated with mortality. To simplify our discussion, let us assume that the geopolitical units are states and the policies are implemented at the state level.

These studies share certain limitations. First, the associations being measured are typically weak. Studying how a policy affects mortality often combines two or more steps in the causal pathway. A study of laws requiring smoke alarms in residences and fire-related mortality in homes combines two steps: (1) a possible effect of the law on the prevalence of working smoke alarms in homes and (2) a possible effect of smoke alarms on fire-related deaths. Many people are already doing what the law encourages; these goody-two-shoes have already installed smoke alarms. And others will not obey the law. If a law boosts smoke alarm prevalence from 40 to 80% and if smoke alarm presence reduces home fire deaths by 20%, the law would reduce deaths by 20% only in the 40% of the population that introduced new smoke alarms. Comparing populations with the law to those without would find a rate ratio of only [.6 × (rate without the law) + .4 × (rate without the law × .8)]/(.6 + .4) = 0.92.

A second limitation is that it may be hard to control for confounding by factors that influence mortality. Policy studies can usually only account for potential confounding factors at the group level. For example, a study may adjust for state unemployment levels or statewide alcohol consumption but cannot typically adjust for the employment status or drinking of individuals. Studies of geopolitical groups, such as states, are sometimes called ecological studies and many articles have discussed the bias that may arise because of lack of information about individual level confounders (Morgenstern 1998, Greenland 2001, 2002, Morgenstern 2008, Wakefield 2008, Weiss and Koepsell 2014 pp447–462). Although uncontrolled confounding is always possible, this concern may be mitigated if the study includes many states that implemented their laws at different times. Unemployment or alcohol use may affect mortality rates, but differences in these factors between geopolitical units or institutions can often be partly removed by making comparisons over time within the same units. Changes in these factors over time can only be confounders if any changes are related to the timing of law implementation in most states. If the study design can control for overall changes in rates over time, confounding may be minimized.

A third limitation is that if the policy has some effect, it is hard to know how quickly that effect will appear. We could assume that the total effect appears immediately after implementation. This would not be true for seat belt laws, as observational studies showed that belt usage increased slowly over many years. We could assume that the effect appears only after some lag time. Or that the effect gradually becomes stronger over time. We can use the data to try to model what happened, but there is a risk that this approach can mislead us. I was part of a group that tried to estimate how creating a state-wide trauma system affected traffic crash mortality (Nathens et al. 2000). Fractional polynomial methods (Royston and Altman 1994, Royston, Ambler, and Sauerbrei 1999) were used to model how the trauma system implementation was associated with mortality. A figure in that paper showed that initially mortality increased by about 3% after the new policies went into effect, mortality began to decrease only after 10 years, and mortality was reduced by 8% after 15 years. Do these results reflect reality or could it be that information in the tails of the data produced an unrealistic curve? One option is to limit the possible effects of an intervention to a few pre-specified possibilities. One study (Vavilala et al. 2004) of hospital admissions of children for trauma, limited the outcomes to four possibilities: (1) no change in admission rates; (2) a ratio change in rates that started immediately after the intervention and did not change further over time; (3) an immediate alteration in the linear trend (slope of rate change over time) in rates compared with the trend before the new policy; and (4) a combination of 3 and 4. This restricted approach was adopted to prevent overfitting.

Despite these limitations, studies of policies are important. It is worth trying to assess the possible effects of laws and regulations, while having some humility about our ability to estimate these effects.

19.3 STUDY DESIGNS FOR GOVERNMENTAL POLICIES

A simple design is a before-and-after study. A state implements a policy and the mortality rates in the year after implementation are compared with the rates in the year before. The obvious weakness of this design is that it fails to account for any secular trend in mortality that could have changed year-to-year rates regardless of the new policy. Any observed change might have occurred in the absence of the new policy. Absence of any change could arise if the policy had a salutary effect, but other factors caused rates to increase.

Another simple design is a cross-sectional approach that compares the mortality in a state with the intervention with the mortality in a state without the new policy. This design fails to account for the possibility that states may have differed already in their mortality rates prior to the new policy and that difference may bias the comparison.

We can improve on these study designs by adding more states to the analysis and adding many time periods before and after the new policy to the analysis. By doing this, we can control for trends in rates over time due to factors other than the new policy; yearly rates both before and after the policy change contribute to estimating rate changes unrelated to the policy. We can also control for the possibility that states have different rates for reasons unrelated to the policy, by including state rates before and after the time of the policy.

19.4 A FICTITIOUS WATER TREATMENT AND U.S. MORTALITY 1999–2013

To illustrate these ideas, I created a fictional data set and will show analyses for a few regression methods. U.S. all-cause mortality and population data were obtained from the Compressed Mortality Files of the National Center for Health Statistics for 15 years (1999–2013), 9 age groups (15–19, 20–24, 25–34, 35–44, 45–54, 55–64, 65–74, 75–84, and 85 years or older), and 50 states plus the District of Columbia: 15 x 9 x 51 = 6885 records (CDC WONDER). Using Poisson regression to model the linear change in rates, the crude mortality rate fell by 9% from 1999 to 2014 (Figure 19.1). During the 15-year interval, the proportion of the U.S. population that was elderly increased because of the boom in birthrates during 1946–1964 after World War II. The increasing prevalence of the elderly during 1999–2013 would tend to increase the crude mortality rates over time, so finding that the crude rates fell means that beneficial changes, such as reduced smoking, must be at work. The age-adjusted rate, adjusted for the age categories using the Standard 2000 population, fell by 18%, revealing the improved mortality within age categories.

The imaginary exposure for this example is a combination of substances added to the entire water supply of each state. This miraculous mixture contained a statin to lower cholesterol, a chemical that reduced the urge to smoke, and a compound that decreased the desire for alcohol. If states are ranked according to their mortality rates for persons 75–84 years in 1999, those with the lowest mortality, states ranked 1 through 5, were Hawaii, Florida, South Dakota, Arizona, and Utah. These low mortality states adopted the imaginary water treatment first, on January 1, 2001. States ranked 6–10 adopted the concoction in 2002. With each additional year, 5 more states opted for this policy, always according to their mortality ranking. By 2011 the last 6 states, with the highest mortality rates for ages 75–84 years, adopted this policy: Oklahoma, Louisiana, Alabama, Mississippi, Kentucky, and West Virginia.

If the intervention was real, it might not be surprising that states with the lowest mortality rates would adopt the potion first. Many people in these states already tend to have good health habits, access to advanced medical centers, and exposure to policies that foster longer life. Their populations and legislators might be more willing to use government power to promote health. The imaginary water treatment intervention reduced mortality by 5% and this effect began immediately after the mixture entered the water on January 1 of each year. To mimic this effect in the mortality data, the actual counts of deaths in all age categories were multiplied by 0.95 in the year the hypothetical intervention started for a state and in all subsequent years for that state.

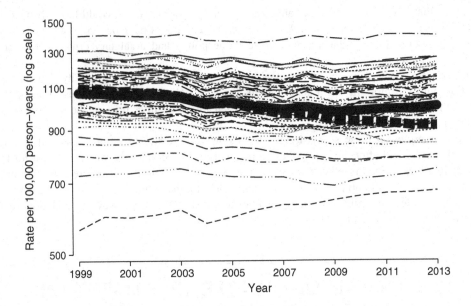

FIGURE 19.1 Crude all-cause mortality rates for persons age 15 years and older in the 50 states and the District of Columbia, 1999–2013. Each connected line is for a different state. The state with the highest rates was West Virginia, the lowest rates were for Alaska. The thick solid line connects the crude rates of the entire United States. The thick dashed line connects the age-adjusted rates for the United States.

19.5 POISSON REGRESSION

Plain vanilla Poisson regression with a robust or cluster variance can be used. Models 1 through 6 (Table 19.1) have notable bias (rate ratios 0.81 to 0.91) and they all have one feature in common; they omit a variable for state, a variable for time, or both. Failure to adjust for time means that the decrease in U.S. mortality from 1999 through 2013 will be entangled with the decrease due to the water treatment. Failure to adjust for state produced bias because the states with lowest mortality adopted the intervention earlier; adjusting for state means that the model compares populations in the same state, removing the confounding influence of between-state mortality differences. Once the models include both state, using categories, and time, using a continuous variable or year categories, the estimated rate ratios are close to the true value of 0.95 (models 7 through 12).

Model 5 with no variables aside from the chemical exposure produced a rate ratio of 0.86. But when age alone was added to the model, the rate ratio changed to 0.81 (model 1). This occurred because age-adjusted rates declined faster over time than crude rates, so introducing age categories into the model exaggerated the confounding effect of not controlling for time.

In the hypothetical nursing home example in Chapter 18, the goal was to account for clustering of rates within nursing home. Entering variables for all nursing homes into the model made it impossible to estimate the intervention effect, because the intervention did not vary within the nursing homes. In the water-treatment example, all the states *can* be in the model because the exposure varied over time within each state. Including the states in the model was necessary to remove confounding by between-state rate differences unrelated to the intervention. By including states, the model compared exposed and unexposed people in the same state, at different points in time.

TABLE 19.1 Rate ratios for all-cause mortality, from Poisson regression models, comparing states that used a fictional water treatment with the mortality expected without the water treatment. True rate ratio was 0.95. Variables used in each model are indicated by an X. Prefix "i." means indicator terms were used; for example, i. agecat signifies that 8 terms were used for the 9 age categories. The variable time was equal to (year-1999)/14. The term i.state##c.time produced indicators for each of the states (minus 1 state) and a second set of indicators for each state (minus 1) multiplied by a continuous time variable, allowing each state to have its own slope for rate changes over time. Models are listed in order from most biased to least biased.

		VARIABLES USED IN ADDITION TO A WATER TREATMENT VARIABLE				
MODEL NUMBER	RATE RATIO	i.AGECAT	TIME	i..YEAR	i..STATE	i..STATE##C.TIME
1	0.8073	X				
2	0.8160	X	X			
3	0.8446		X			
4	0.8524	X			X	
5	0.8636					
6	0.9065				X	
7	0.9443	X	X			X
8	0.9547			X	X	
9	0.9458		X		X	
10	0.9465	X	X		X	
11	0.9517	X		X	X	
12	0.9497	X		X		X
13	0.9499	X	X[a]			X

a In Model 13, time was expressed using a fractional polynomial term with two dimensions.

Age is powerfully related to mortality. But models 8 and 9 produced estimated associations close to the true value of 0.95, despite failure to adjust for age. Age was ultimately not important as a confounder because it had no systematic relationship with the water treatment intervention. After controlling for state and time, the minor differences in age distributions between the states were not important.

This example used real counts of deaths and population estimates for the United States over a 15-year period. The fabricated part of the example was the change in rate numerators related to the water treatment. It was easy to estimate the expected rate ratio of 0.95, without adjusting for any of the multitude of other factors that influenced U.S. mortality rates. Information about the economy, personal health habits, and other state policies was omitted from the analysis. Unless a new policy happens to be implemented in many states at the same time that other important mortality risk factors change, bias related to these factors may be minimal. The power of cross-sectional panel data is that the mortality propensity of each state is repeatedly measured both before and after the intervention. For example, in these data, the state of Nebraska contributed data for 1999–2003 with no special water treatment and data from 2004 to 2013 with water treatment. This is different from cohort studies of death or the onset of cancer, with an outcome that is only measured at a single point in time. We may adjust for several risk factors, but this still leaves a lot of room for variation in each subject's propensity for the outcome.

Table 19.1 ignores several modeling possibilities. Interactions between time and age and between state and age could be considered. Age could be transformed by assigning a value for age roughly midway through each age category and then use those values as a linear term for age or in a more flexible manner. I tried this and found no reason to prefer this approach for these data. Table 19.1 suggests that these additions are unnecessary, but they might be worth considering in a real analysis.

In this example we know that the true rate ratio is 0.95, so any model that produces an estimate close to 0.95 seems reasonable. In a real analysis the true rate ratio would not be known. In that situation, we could add and remove variables from the model and examine their influence on the rate ratio for exposure. We would surely want to include both time (as a continuous or categorical variable) and state indicators. Even if these variables did not change the estimated rate ratio to any notable degree, including these variables would be reassuring to readers. Additional adjustment for age would be made only if it produced a notable change in the rate ratio for the exposure(s) of interest. This change in estimate approach is nicely described elsewhere (Greenland and Rothman 2008c pp261–263). Statistical significance is not involved in these choices. Stepwise methods that rely upon statistical significance should be avoided, as they are known to produce bias (Harrell 2001 pp56–58, Greenland 2008b p419).

Which model is best in Table 19.1? I see no clear best choice, but a good pick is Model 11, with indicator terms for age, year, and state. This choice is more parsimonious than models 7, 12, and 13. Model 11 may be more robust than models that use time as a linear variable or those that omit age. Using model 11, the rate ratio for the exposure is 0.9517. The usual Poisson standard error (SE) is 0.0006, the robust SE is 0.0037, and the SE adjusted for clustering on state is 0.0043 (Z = 10.9) (Table 19.2). So the clustered variance option seems reasonable. It would be ideal if we could simultaneously account for the clustered nature of the rates within each state and the extra-Poisson variation in the rates. A bootstrap approach could be used, sampling states to account for the clustering within state. The percentile bootstrap 95% confidence interval was 0.941, 0.959, close to the interval of 0.943, 0.960 using Poisson regression and the cluster variance option (Table 19.2).

Although I will focus on Model 11 for now, I will return to Model 12 later. Model 12 not only included indicator terms for each state, but it added terms for the interaction between each state and the linear change in rates over time. This model allowed each state to have its own temporal trend in mortality rates.

19.6 POPULATION-AVERAGED ESTIMATES (GEE)

The water-treatment data are cross-sectional panel data. The panels are the states and the data are cross-sectional within each year. Stata's **xtpoisson** command is intended specifically for this type of data. If we use the **xtset** command to designate the panels and the times at which measurements were made, Stata will do a lot of bookkeeping for us. The typical command is

TABLE 19.2 Rate ratios and other statistics for all-cause mortality comparing states that used a fictional water treatment with the mortality expected for the same states absent the water treatment. True rate ratio was 0.95. Models used 14 indicator variables for the year (years 1999–2013), 8 indicators for 9 age categories, and 50 indicators for the 50 states and District of Columbia. Panel data (xtpoisson) models used 459 panels for each state-age category. Robust or cluster variance estimators were used, whichever produced a larger SE.

NO.	MODEL	STATA COMMAND	VARIANCE OPTION	RATE RATIO	SE	Z	95% CI
1	Poisson	poisson	cluster	0.9517	0.0043	10.9	0.943, 0.960
2	Panel data Poisson (GEE)	xtpoisson, pa	robust	0.9517	0.0028	16.6	0.946, 0.957
3	Panel data Poisson (GEE)	xtpoisson, fe	robust	0.9523	0.0028	16.6	0.947, 0.958
4	Negative binomial	nbreg	cluster	0.9373	0.0054	11.2	0.929, 0.948

SE = standard error
CI = confidence interval

"**xtset** panel variable time variable". We can then use **xt** commands to describe, summarize, and tabulate the data, and even create a plot similar to Figure 19.1

There is a fly in the **xt** ointment. The **xt** commands only allow for one level of clustering. The water-treatment data have two levels; there is clustering within age-categories which are clustered within state. We would like to tell Stata this so that the software "knows" that people in age category 65–74 years in West Virginia have rates more similar to those of people 55–64 years in West Virginia compared with people age 55–64 in Utah. If we use a numeric value for each state (stcode is such a variable), we can tell Stata that stcode and year are the panel and time variables with the command "**xtset** stcode year". But Stata will come to a halt and deliver the message "repeated time values within panel". Stata's **xt** commands want a panel variable that has only one set of repeated rates at each point in time. In these data, there are nine rates, one for each age group, for each year within each state. To get around this problem, we can create a new panel variable with a unique code for each state and age category: a total of 9 x 51 = 459 panels. But if we use these panels with **xtpoisson**, Stata will not know if two age groups are within the same state.

If we create 459 panels and use **xtpoisson** with an independent correlation structure, the estimated rate ratios for the water treatment are the same as the rate ratios in Table 19.1, even though **xtpoisson** uses GEE instead of maximum likelihood to fit the model. The estimated rate ratio for the water treatment intervention is 0.9517 with a SE of 0.0006; this is what we obtained from Poisson regression with the usual variance estimator. The **xtpoisson** command failed to account for the within-state clustering because we provided it with inadequate panel information. If we use the robust variance estimator the SE increases to 0.0028, which is smaller than the robust SE from Poisson regression (0.0037) and smaller than the SE from Poisson regression with the **vce(cluster** state) option (.0043) (Table 19.2). Because we cannot provide the ideal clustering information, the **xtpoisson** command is an inferior choice compared with ordinary Poisson regression for the water-treatment data.

We could collapse the data on state and year; ignore the age categories and create a single record for the count of deaths and population total of each state in each year. Then declare the states as panels, adjust for all state year indicators, and use **xtpoisson** to estimate the water-treatment rate ratio: 0.9547 with SE .0006 and a robust SE of .0042 (Z = 10.4). This result is slightly biased by failure to adjust for age, but the SE and Z-statistic are similar to those from Poisson regression with age-adjustment and clustering on state (Table 19.2).

Collapsing the data on state and year will omit the age-related heterogeneity of rates. This may shrink the SE, although not by much in this example. As we do not really need to adjust for confounding by age in these data, is this approach reasonable? This question raises a host of additional questions. If it is *not* reasonable to collapse the data on age, should we use mortality data grouped by sex and race (Black, White, other) in addition to age? These additional categories are available in the compressed mortality files. Should we declare as a limitation of any analysis our failure to account for heterogeneity of rates by religion, income, education level, occupation, and an infinite number of other characteristics? I do not have firm answers to these questions, but it seems to me that our ability to account for heterogeneity in rates, or any outcome statistic, will always face practical limitations.

19.7 CONDITIONAL POISSON REGRESSION, A FIXED-EFFECTS APPROACH

The terminology for clustered-data models is sometimes cryptic. A random-effects model introduces random effect variables in addition to the usual, fixed-effects, regression variables. You might think, therefore, that a model without random effects is a fixed-effects model; for example, ordinary Poisson regression. But the term fixed-effects model is used for a model in which the clustering variable is "conditioned" out of the model. The regression model estimates associations within the clusters (states in the water-treatment data), but estimated associations for the states themselves are not made by the fixed-effects regression model.

There is an obvious parallel between this fixed-effects approach and the use of conditional logistic regression, which estimates odds ratios within matched-sets but does not estimate the associations for the sets themselves; the indicators for the matched sets do not appear in the model output. This is what a fixed-effects model does. So you might think that a fixed-effects Poisson model should be called a conditional model. This name is used, but this is not the same as a random-effects model, which is sometimes called a conditional model because it produces estimates conditional on the random effects (as opposed to a marginal model). Wooldridge gives a short account of the convoluted terminology of clustered data models (Wooldridge 2010 pp285–287). Glymour and Greenland describe the differences between conditional and marginal probabilities (Glymour and Greenland 2008 pp184–185), and Greenland and Rothman discuss the distinctions between conditional and unconditional estimation (Greenland and Rothman 2008c pp272–273). The confusion arises because the word "conditional" is used to describe two different modeling approaches.

The fixed-effects approach to correlated data was not discussed in Chapter 18 because it can only estimate associations for exposures that vary within the clusters. The fall intervention in Chapter 18 did not vary within the nursing homes and so the fixed-effects method could not be used. When the exposure varies within the clusters, as it does in the water-treatment example, the fixed-effects approach has the advantage of controlling (or adjusting) for all variables that are constant within clusters. This means that state-level characteristics that were unchanged, or little changed, over time were removed as potential confounders. The large differences in rates between the states are of no concern to a fixed-effects model, because estimation occurs within states.

The Stata command for a fixed-effects Poisson model is **xtpoisson, fe**. This is also called conditional Poisson regression or conditional Poisson fixed-effects regression. It is the Poisson equivalent of conditional logistic regression. The model is fit using maximum likelihood. When many strata contain small numbers of observations, as is often true in matched case-control data, the odds ratio from unconditional logistic regression may be biased and the odds ratio from conditional logistic regression is preferred. But for rate ratios, the conditional and unconditional methods will produce the same estimates (Greenland and Rothman 2008c pp272–273). If there are 500 small strata, the unconditional (ordinary) Poisson model can estimate 499 rate ratios for strata entered as indicator terms. Or the stratum rate ratios can be omitted by using **xtpoisson, fe**. The rate ratios for the variables that vary within the strata will be the same using either approach. Conditional methods cannot be used for estimating rate differences; they work only for rate ratios and odds ratios (Greenland and Rothman 2008c pp272–273).

When conditional Poisson regression (**xtpoisson, fe**) was applied to the 13 models in Table 19.1, the rate ratios were never smaller than 0.85. The fixed effects command created rate ratios for water treatment within 459 strata defined by age and state, so all models effectively used "indicators" for the age and state categories. All models included the terms in Model 4 of Table 19.1, regardless of whether or not i.agecat and i.state were explicitly entered into the model variable lists. The output for Model 11 is shown here with most of the useless i.agecat and i.stcode results omitted:

```
. xtpoisson deaths waterrx i.year i.agecat i.stcode, exposure(pop) irr fe
nolog
note: you are responsible for interpretation of non-count dep. variable

Conditional fixed-effects Poisson regression    Number of obs    =    6,885
Group variable: panel                            Number of groups =      459
                                                 Obs per group:
                                                             min =       15
                                                             avg =     15.0
                                                             max =       15
```

```
                                          Wald chi2(15)   =        .
Log likelihood = -54917.565               Prob > chi2     =        .
------------------------------------------------------------------------
   deaths |      IRR   Std. Err.        z    P>|z|    [95% Conf. Interval]
----------+-------------------------------------------------------------
  waterrx | .9522642   .0005925    -78.62    0.000    .9511037   .9534261
          |
     year |
     2000 | .9927372   .0009146     -7.91    0.000    .9909463   .9945314
     2001 | .9810514   .0009054    -20.73    0.000    .9792784   .9828276
     2002 | .9769585   .0009088    -25.06    0.000     .975179   .9787413
     2003 | .9624892   .0009071    -40.57    0.000    .9607129   .9642688
     2004 | .9281589   .0008872    -77.99    0.000    .9264216   .9298994
     2005 | .9295282   .0008948    -75.91    0.000     .927776   .9312837
     2006 | .9026552   .0008954   -103.25    0.000     .900902   .9044118
     2007 | .8833858    .000904   -121.17    0.000    .8816158   .8851594
     2008 | .8838337   .0009252   -117.97    0.000    .8820223   .8856489
     2009 | .8547334   .0009293   -144.37    0.000     .852914   .8565567
     2010 | .8531141   .0009487   -142.86    0.000    .8512568   .8549755
     2011 | .8480469   .0009424   -148.32    0.000    .8462019    .849896
     2012 | .8377246   .0009291   -159.65    0.000    .8359056   .8395476
     2013 | .8365908   .0009244   -161.47    0.000    .8347809   .8384046
          |
   agecat |
    20-24 |        1  (omitted)
 (output omitted)
    75-84 |        1  (omitted)
      85+ |        1  (omitted)
          |
   stcode |
        2 |        1  (omitted)
 (output omitted)
       56 |        1  (omitted)
  ln(pop) |        1  (exposure)
-------------------------------------------------------------------------
```

The same estimate for waterrx, the water treatment variable, would be produced by a shorter command:

```
. xtpoisson deaths waterrx i.year, exp(pop) irr fe nolog
note: you are responsible for interpretation of non-count dep. variable

Conditional fixed-effects Poisson regression   Number of obs    =      6,885
Group variable: panel                          Number of groups =        459
                                               Obs per group:
                                                           min =         15
                                                           avg =       15.0
                                                           max =         15

                                               Wald chi2(15)    = 237708.13
Log likelihood = -54917.565                    Prob > chi2      =     0.0000
```

```
--------------------------------------------------------------------
  deaths |     IRR    Std. Err.       z     P>|z|    [95% Conf. Interval]
---------+----------------------------------------------------------
 waterrx | .9522642    .0005925    -78.62    0.000    .9511037    .9534261
         |
    year |
    2000 | .9927372    .0009146     -7.91    0.000    .9909463    .9945314
    2001 | .9810514    .0009054    -20.73    0.000    .9792784    .9828276
    2002 | .9769585    .0009088    -25.06    0.000     .975179    .9787413
    2003 | .9624892    .0009071    -40.57    0.000    .9607129    .9642688
    2004 | .9281589    .0008872    -77.99    0.000    .9264216    .9298994
    2005 | .9295282    .0008948    -75.91    0.000     .927776    .9312837
    2006 | .9026552    .0008954   -103.25    0.000     .900902    .9044118
    2007 | .8833858     .000904   -121.17    0.000    .8816158    .8851594
    2008 | .8838337    .0009252   -117.97    0.000    .8820223    .8856489
    2009 | .8547334    .0009293   -144.37    0.000     .852914    .8565567
    2010 | .8531141    .0009487   -142.86    0.000    .8512568    .8549755
    2011 | .8480469    .0009424   -148.32    0.000    .8462019     .849896
    2012 | .8377246    .0009291   -159.65    0.000    .8359056    .8395476
    2013 | .8365908    .0009244   -161.47    0.000    .8347809    .8384046
 ln(pop) |        1 (exposure)
--------------------------------------------------------------------
```

Although state variables and age variables do not appear in the model variable list or this regression table output, they were used to create the estimates, because the model created estimates *within* the 459 age-state panels. We could produce the same estimates using a Poisson regression command that includes the 459 panels as indicator variables: poisson deaths waterrx i.year i.panel i. agecat, exp(pop) irr nolog. Printing the output would waste a lot of paper. The conditional SE for the waterrx variable is 0.0006, which is too small (Table 19.2). The robust SE is 0.0028, smaller than the SE from Poisson regression.

19.8 NEGATIVE BINOMIAL REGRESSION

Negative binomial regression has been used to study state-level policies (Levy, Vernick, and Howard 1995, Cummings et al. 1997, Grabowski, Campbell, and Morrisey 2004, Webster et al. 2004). As discussed in Chapter 17, results from Poisson and negative binomial regression may differ because they weight observations differently. When negative binomial regression was used to fit the 13 models in Table 19.1, only Model 8 produced a rate ratio that rounded to 0.95; all the others had smaller rate ratios. Model 11 produced a rate ratio of 0.9373 with a Z-statistic that was actually larger than the statistic from Poisson regression (Tables 19.1 and 19.2). In this instance, negative binomial regression produced a somewhat biased rate ratio and was no more "conservative" than Poisson regression. The differences in the rate ratios from Poisson and negative binomial regression in real data are often small, as was the case in this example. But occasionally one will find estimates that differ to a notable degree. If there is substantial variation in person-time and the counts are not small, the estimated rate ratios can differ due to the different weighting schemes. There seems to be little advantage to using negative binomial regression for this kind of analysis.

19.9 WHICH METHOD IS BEST?

So which method of analysis is best? I have not exhaustively pursued all possible methods and models. Many models produced results that were similar. All methods had some limitations. None was clearly superior to ordinary Poisson regression with a robust (sandwich) variance.

19.10 WATER TREATMENT IN ONLY 10 STATES

In the water-treatment example, all 51 regions adopted the fictional new policy. Now imagine that the treatment was adopted only by the 10 states (Hawaii, Florida, South Dakota, Arizona, Utah, Connecticut, North Dakota, Rhode Island, California, Minnesota) with the lowest mortality rates in 1999 for persons aged 75–84 years. In each year from 2001 through 2010, one of these states started treating their water. All of these states had decreases in their age-adjusted mortality rates using the actual rates, modified by the additional 5% mortality reductions due to the imaginary water treatment (Figure 19.2). These decreases were greater than the decline among the 41 regions that did not initiate water treatment. We can use the actual mortality data, without any hypothetical water treatment, to estimate the average slope of the ln rates over time. The model shown here (time = (year-1999)/14) estimated that the actual average mortality change over 14 years, adjusted for age, was a 17% decrease (rate ratio 0.828) in 41 regions that were not assigned to water treatment, and a 21% decrease (rate ratio 0.794) in the 10 states that were selected for water treatment:

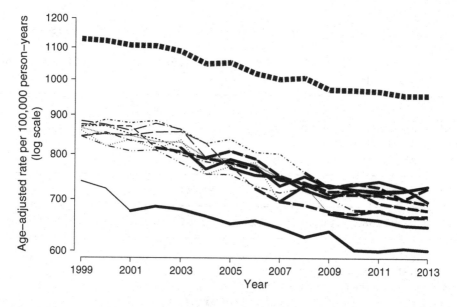

FIGURE 19.2 Age-adjusted all-cause mortality rates for persons age 15 years and older in 10 states that had the lowest mortality rates among persons age 75–84 years. Each connected line is for a different state and the thick dashed line at the top of the graph is for the 40 states and the District of Columbia, which never adopted the hypothetical water treatment described in the text. Actual rates in the 10 water-treatment states were changed by decreasing the crude age-specific rate numerators by 5% for one state in each of the years 2001–2010; rates in subsequent years were also reduced after the first reduction. Thick solid or dashed lines show the age-adjusted rates for the periods with this 5% reduction.

```
. poisson deaths i.agecat c.time##i.waterstate i.agecat, /*
>       */ exp(pop) irr vce(cluster stcode) nolog

Poisson regression                          Number of obs   =       6,885
                                            Wald chi2(11)   =   177738.88
                                            Prob > chi2     =      0.0000
Log pseudolikelihood = -223190.63           Pseudo R2       =      0.9947
                        (Std. Err. adjusted for 51 clusters in stcode)
```

```
------------------------------------------------------------------------------
                 |               Robust
          deaths |      IRR   Std. Err.      z    P>|z|    [95% Conf. Interval]
-----------------+------------------------------------------------------------
          agecat |
           20-24 | 1.570657   .0195692    36.24   0.000    1.532767    1.609484
           25-34 | 1.786925   .0334979    30.97   0.000    1.722462    1.853801
           35-44 |  3.19444   .0526797    70.43   0.000     3.09284    3.299377
           45-54 | 7.153866   .1195689   117.73   0.000    6.923312    7.392097
           55-64 | 15.33299   .2790727   149.99   0.000    14.79566    15.88984
           65-74 | 35.16947   .8489669   147.48   0.000    33.54427     36.8734
           75-84 | 87.54289    2.29748   170.41   0.000    83.15376    92.16369
             85+ | 248.6146   6.610211   207.46   0.000    235.9906    261.9138
                 |
            time |  .827581   .0070975   -22.07   0.000    .8137864    .8416094
   1.waterstate |  .8912931  .0128816    -7.96   0.000       .8664    .9169015
                 |
 waterstate#c.time |
               1 | .9597636   .0159597    -2.47   0.014    .9289874    .9915593
                 |
           _cons | .0006673  .0000208  -234.99   0.000    .0006278    .0007093
         ln(pop) |        1  (exposure)
------------------------------------------------------------------------------
```

```
. * trend in no-water-treatment states
. lincom time, irr
 ( 1) [deaths]time = 0
---------------------------------------------------------------------
   deaths |     IRR  Std. Err.      z    P>|z|   [95% Conf. Interval]
----------+----------------------------------------------------------
      (1) | .827581  .0070975   -22.07   0.000   .8137864   .8416094
---------------------------------------------------------------------
```

```
. * trend in water treatment states
. lincom time + 1.waterstate#c.time, irr
 ( 1) [deaths]time + [deaths]1.waterstate#c.time = 0
---------------------------------------------------------------------
   deaths |     IRR   Std. Err.      z    P>|z|   [95% Conf. Interval]
----------+----------------------------------------------------------
      (1) | .7942821  .0115338   -15.86   0.000    .771995   .8172126
---------------------------------------------------------------------
```

Once again, Models (1–6) that failed to include both state and time provided biased estimates (Table 19.3). This was true whether the analysis included all states or was limited to states that changed their water-treatment status. For model 3, which adjusted only for the linear trend in time for all states combined, the rate ratio was 0.90, biased downward because rates were already lower in the water-treatment states (Figure 19.2). When model 3 was limited to the 10 treatment states, the rate ratio was biased upward to 1.17. This arose because the average decline in crude rates, including water treatment, was greatest in the 2 largest states, Florida and California. This resulted in a time trend estimate of change that was too large for all 10 states: adjusted for water treatment, the model estimated that crude rates declined by 30%. If we add adjustment for age-categories, the decline was 23% and the water-treatment rate ratio changed to 0.97. This is partly because the trend over time in age-adjusted rates is much less than the change in crude rates, and partly because Florida's age-adjusted rate change was near the middle of the pack. If Florida and California are omitted, the time adjusted rate ratio is 0.93. If we adjust for state (Model 9) the rate ratio was 0.94.

Table 19.3 reenforces the view that we should adjust for state and time, at a minimum. The state-time adjusted models, 7–13, have rate ratios ranging from 0.93 to 0.95. Model 11 produced a slightly biased estimate of 0.93 when all states were used. This bias was rectified in models 7 and 12, which included state × time interaction terms: i.state##c.time. These terms allowed each state to have its own secular trend in rates, relaxing the assumption that the change over time had the same average value for all states.

TABLE 19.3 Rate ratios for all-cause mortality, from Poisson regression models, comparing states that used a fictional water treatment with expected mortality without the treatment. Only 10 of the states treated their water. First column of rate ratios used data for all 50 states and the District of Columbia. Second column used only the 10 states that adopted the water treatment. True rate ratio was 0.95. Variables used in each model are indicated by an X. Models used were the same as those in Table 19.1

MODEL NUMBER	ALL 51 STATES RATE RATIO	10 STATES THAT TREATED THEIR WATER. RATE RATIO	VARIABLES USED IN ADDITION TO A WATER TREATMENT VARIABLE				
			i.AGECAT	TIME	i.YEAR	i.STATE	i.STATE##C.TIME
1	0.8040	0.8675	X				
2	0.8353	0.9707	X	X			
3	0.9033	1.1720		X			
4	0.8391	0.8380	X			X	
5	0.8871	1.0010					
6	0.8885	0.8885				X	
7	0.9508	0.9509	X	X			X
8	0.9270	0.9451			X	X	
9	0.9260	0.9441		X		X	
10	0.9308	0.9490	X	X		X	
11	0.9315	0.9505	X		X	X	
12	0.9529	0.9528	X		X		X
13	0.9522	0.9528	X	X[a]			X

[a] In Model 13, time was expressed using a fractional polynomial term with two dimensions.

19.11 CONDITIONAL POISSON REGRESSION FOR THE 10-STATE WATER-TREATMENT DATA

Using these data in which 10 states changed their water treatment, rate ratios for models 7–12 were estimated using conditional (fixed-effects) Poisson regression (Table 19.4). Because the conditional models create estimates within the panels, they all include age and state effects without any need to enter i.agecat or i.state. This makes some models redundant; Models 8 and 11 are identical, as are Models 9 and 10. Models 8–11 all produced somewhat biased estimates, rate ratios of 0.93, because they used a single time estimate or a single set of dummy variable year (i.year) estimates to account for the changes in rates over time due to factors aside from the water treatment. This single estimate was less than ideal because the changes over time differed in the states that treated their water compared with the remaining 41 regions (Figure 19.2). The conditional models fixed this problem by restricting the analysis to the 10 water-treatment states. Models 7 and 12 produced nearly unbiased estimates whether all states or 10 states were used, because these models allowed each state to have its own trend in rates over time, aside from any influence of water treatment.

In an actual analysis it may be useful to compare results from conditional and unconditional analyses, and results from models that use all available regions and models restricted to regions that changed their exposure status. Differences in model estimates may reveal the need for interaction terms between regions and time, or other modifications.

19.12 A PUBLISHED STUDY

Rosengart et al. (2005) used these cross-sectional panel data methods and Poisson regression with a robust variance estimator to study the association between state-level handgun purchase or ownership policies and rates of homicide and suicide. Full disclosure: I was involved in this study. I hesitate to cite this paper, as many people have strong feelings about gun laws; I do not want the methods to be judged

TABLE 19.4 Rate ratios for all-cause mortality, from conditional (fixed-effects) Poisson regression models, comparing states that used a fictional water treatment with expected mortality without treatment. Only 10 of the states treated their water. First column of rate ratios used data for all 50 states and the District of Columbia. Second column used only the 10 states that adopted water treatment. True rate ratio was 0.95. Variables used in each model are indicated by an X. Models used were the same as those in Table 19.1

MODEL NUMBER	ALL 51 STATES RATE RATIO	10 STATES THAT TREATED THEIR WATER. RATE RATIO	VARIABLES USED IN ADDITION TO A WATER TREATMENT VARIABLE				
			i.AGECAT	TIME	i.YEAR	i.STATE	i.STATE##C.TIME
7	0.9498	0.9498	X	X			X
8	0.9299	0.9494			X	X	
9	0.9293	0.9481		X		X	
10	0.9293	0.9481	X	X		X	
11	0.9299	0.9494	X		X	X	
12	0.9519	0.9516	X		X		X

by the results. Regardless of the results, the paper uses many of the ideas discussed in this chapter, applying them to actual data. The paper used model 12 (Tables 19.1 and 19.2). Interactions between state and time allowed each state to have its own trend in rates over the study interval. Indicator variables were used for state and year and additional variables were included in the regression model. State-specific rate ratios were estimated by adding model terms between each law and each state. These state-specific law estimates were extracted from the regression results and studied further using meta-analytic methods for heterogeneity, forest plots, and summary rate ratios using fixed and random effects. Stata has an extensive array of meta-analysis commands that can be applied to rate ratios or rate differences (Palmer and Sterne 2015). I am not suggesting that the methods used in this paper are the best approach, but the paper illustrates what is possible for an analysis of mortality rates.

Further information about policy studies, cross-sectional panel data, and longitudinal data can be found in several textbooks (Wooldridge 2010, Fitzmaurice, Laird, and Ware 2011, Weiss and Koepsell 2014 pp447–462).

Matched Data

20

This chapter reviews statistical methods for matched data, especially for randomized trials and cohort studies. In addition to methods that can be used for rate ratios, I cover methods for odds, risk, and hazard ratios, partly because these methods illustrate important points about matched data and partly because examples with binary outcomes are simpler to discuss.

20.1 MATCHING IN CASE-CONTROL STUDIES

Matching is common in case-control studies and matching is so often described with regard to this study design that a short review is justified. Cases, typically a group of limited size, are used to estimate the prevalence of exposure among those with the outcome. Controls are sampled to estimate the prevalence of exposure in the larger population from which the cases arose. If controls are matched to cases on a confounding variable X, this will produce a set of controls more like the cases regarding X (and possibly other variables), but less like the original unmatched control population, resulting in a biased estimate of control exposure prevalence (Rothman, Greenland, and Lash 2008b). This bias can be removed by accounting for the matching strata in the analysis, using stratified Mantel-Haenszel methods, logistic regression stratified on the matched sets, or conditional logistic regression if there are many matched strata with sparse data.

The virtue of matching on a confounding variable for a case-control study is that it may enhance efficiency. For example, if the average case is much older than persons in the larger population of noncases, sampling controls randomly and adjusting for age can remove age-related confounding bias, but the estimated odds ratios may be imprecise because the elderly cases are compared with only a few elderly controls and many younger controls may have no corresponding young cases. Matching on age and conducting a matched analysis can result in more precise estimates. However matching on a variable that is not a confounder will usually reduce efficiency (Rothman, Greenland, and Lash 2008b).

The salient features of matching in a case-control study are: (1) those with the study outcome (cases) are matched to others without the outcome (controls) on levels of a confounding variable, without regard to exposure status; (2) matching can improve statistical precision; (3) a matched-analysis is required to remove bias introduced by the matching. Details about matching in a case-control study are provided by Rothman, Greenland, and Lash (2008b). Case-control studies will be ignored in the rest of this chapter, as they do not use incidence rates.

20.2 MATCHING IN RANDOMIZED CONTROLLED TRIALS

Matching is often called blocking in the literature about randomized trials. Using randomized blocks of small size prevents large imbalances between the number of treated and control subjects. Treatment and control groups of equal size, or some constant ratio, is usually most efficient in terms of statistical precision for a given cost. Blocking also ensures that the ratio of treated to untreated subjects varies little with calendar time, preventing bias that could arise if the treatment effect or characteristics of the recruited subjects varies with time (Greenland 1987c, Altman and Royston 1988). In a multicenter trial, blocking within each center is often done because of concern that patient characteristics or treatment effectiveness may vary between centers.

Blocking on covariates related to the outcome is not often done, as randomization can often create the necessary balance. Even if adequate balance is not achieved for some measured characteristics, this imbalance can be removed by a stratified or adjusted analysis (Rothman 1977, Rosenberger and Lachin 2002 pp53–55). Blocking on a risk factor can increase statistical precision if the outcome is continuous, mean differences are estimated, and the analysis is stratified on the blocks (Greenland and Morgenstern 1990, Rosenberger and Lachin 2002 pp124–126, Rothman, Greenland, and Lash 2008b p175). But the efficiency gain is often too small to justify the added expense or difficulty related to matching (Rosenberger and Lachin 2002 pp124–126). For outcomes that are risks or rates, there may be no gain in efficiency (Greenland and Morgenstern 1990, Rosenberger and Lachin 2002 pp124–126, Rothman, Greenland, and Lash 2008b p175).

Unlike the situation in a case-control study, a matched (or blocked) randomized trial may not require a matched analysis to eliminate bias related to the matching variable. The overall comparison of treated and control subject outcomes, ignoring any matching factors, will be unbiased and the same as the matched comparison provided that (1) the matching ratio is constant within the matched sets, (2) follow-up is sufficiently complete that imbalance on the matching factors is absent or minimal, and (3) missing data does not create imbalance regarding the matching factors. Doing a matched analysis of a matched (or blocked) trial, may alter the size of P-values and confidence intervals (CI), compared with an unmatched analysis. Differences in these statistics is often inconsequential and therefore it is common to see analyses in which blocking of treatment assignment is ignored in the analysis.

In summary, important features of matching (blocking) in a randomized trial include: (1) those assigned to treatment are matched to others (controls) who are not treated (or differently treated), (2) the matching usually results in matched sets of subjects enrolled at about the same time, (3) matching may sometimes be on levels of an outcome risk factor, such as enrollment site, (4) matching should be unrelated to final outcome status, (5) matching may or may not improve statistical precision, (6) a matched-analysis is not always required to remove bias related to the matching characteristics, (7) standard errors (SE) from a matched analysis will not usually be greatly different from those in an unmatched analysis.

20.3 MATCHING IN COHORT STUDIES

Matching is not common for cohort studies. Matching exposed subjects to those not exposed (or vice versa) can be expensive and cumbersome. Doing this can increase or decrease statistical precision for ratios or differences of both risks and rates (Greenland and Morgenstern 1990). Removing confounding bias, alone, will not justify matching in most cohort studies, as other methods (stratification, regression adjustment) can achieve the same goal.

When matching is used and the ratio of exposed to unexposed subjects is constant in each matched set, there will be no systematic relationship between the exposure status that the matching variables. If each exposed man is always matched to three unexposed men and each exposed woman is always matched to three unexposed women, then 25% of both sexes will be exposed, eliminating sex as a potential confounder in the data. A crude comparison of the exposed and unexposed subjects that ignores the matching will not be biased by confounding related to the matching factor, provided follow-up and data collection are complete enough to avoid imbalance in the matching factors. But in cohort studies it is usually necessary to adjust for factors other than the matching factors. When this is done, the matching factor may not be balanced within levels of the adjusting variables. Consequently, if the analysis of a cohort study involves adjustment for confounders that were not matching variables, it may be necessary to account for the matching variables in the analysis (Sjölander and Greenland 2013).

In comparison with a case-control study, the key features of matching in a cohort study are that (1) matching may improve or degrade statistical precision, (2) a crude comparison of the exposed and unexposed subjects will not usually require a matched analysis (Rothman, Greenland, and Lash 2008b), but (3) in many studies the analysis will need to adjust for or stratify on the matching variables after adjusting for other confounding variables (Sjölander and Greenland 2013).

20.4 MATCHING TO CONTROL CONFOUNDING IN SOME RANDOMIZED TRIALS AND COHORT STUDIES

Matching is not used in many randomized controlled trials or cohort studies because it requires extra expense and effort. However, matching in some situations can be both convenient and effective as a method for minimizing possible confounding. Some randomized trials make comparisons within the same person to eliminate confounding by genetic factors, age, sex, and behaviors. To test laser treatment of retinal disease, one eye of each subject can be randomized to treatment and the other to control status. Similarly, some dental treatments can be evaluated by randomizing some teeth to treatment and some to control status within the same person. Hip protectors are cushioning pads intended to prevent hip fractures. To estimate the efficacy of protectors, the hips of each study participant could be randomly assigned to use of the protector or not (Cummings, McKnight, and Greenland 2003, Cummings and Weiss 2003, Cummings 2007a). Randomizing the two hips of each individual, one to a hip protector and the other not, would control for bone density, propensity to fall, and other risk factors. A matched design and matched analysis would avoid imbalance due to dropouts or missing data, because those factors would always eliminate both hips in a pair.

Matching can be used to reduce confounding in some cohort studies. To estimate the effects of discrimination, the Department of Housing and Urban Development used test pairs of individuals, one black and one white, and had them separately try to rent or buy from the same landlord or realtor. These test individuals were trained to provide the same financial history and other information, so that any difference in the behavior of the landlord or realtor could be reasonably attributed to racial discrimination. Page used these data (Page 1995) and a matched analysis method (conditional Poisson regression) to estimate that the number of rental units or houses shown to black test subjects was smaller than the number shown to white subjects: unadjusted count ratio 0.82. In this example the matching variable is the landlord or realtor.

Matching may be useful for a cohort study if it is possible to match exposed and unexposed subjects on variables that are otherwise difficult to measure (Cummings, McKnight, and Greenland 2003, Cummings, McKnight, and Weiss 2003). Matching exposed to unexposed subjects on variables that are difficult to measure may eliminate confounding by those variables, or at least reduce confounding compared with an unmatched design. The use of twins for cohort studies is an example. Comparison of identical twins eliminates confounding by genetic factors and possibly by other childhood exposures if the twins grew up in the same household, compared with a study of persons who are not twins.

To estimate the association of seat belt use with death when a crash occurs, investigators would like to compare belted and unbelted vehicle occupants in crashes of similar severity. It is hard to measure crash forces, which are related to vehicle speed, the resistance of any object that the vehicle strikes, and the ability of the vehicle to absorb energy. Even if reasonably accurate measurements are possible, obtaining this information is expensive. An alternative is to compare belted and unbelted occupants who were in the same vehicle, adjusting for factors such as seat position (driver or passenger, front or rear), age, sex, and presence of an air bag (Evans 1986, Cummings, McKnight, and Greenland 2003, Cummings, McKnight, and Weiss 2003). Comparing people in the same vehicle means they are matched on vehicle speed, crash angle, whether or not the vehicle rolled over, distance to the nearest hospital, ambulance response time, vehicle make and model, and a myriad of other factors. The merits of matching in crash studies was been debated in a set of papers (Cummings and McKnight 2010, Elliott 2010, Rice and Anderson 2010).

Life vests are thought to prevent drowning, but reliable estimates of their effectiveness are not available. Cummings, Mueller, and Quan (2010) used Coast Guard data to compare the outcomes of persons in the same vessel: the matched-set risk ratio for drowning among boaters wearing a life vest, compared with those who did not, was 0.5. The authors cautioned that deficiencies in the data, including unmeasured confounders such as swimming ability, may have been a source of bias in this estimate.

In another example, Rivara et al. (2007) studied reviewers for a pediatrics journal. Each of 140 manuscripts submitted to the journal were assigned to a reviewer suggested by the authors and also to another reviewer selected by the editor only. Thus, pairs of reviewers were matched on the paper they reviewed; any differences found between reviewers could not be ascribed to the quality of the reviewed paper. There were only small differences in the quality of the reviews by the two reviewer types, but reviewers picked by the editor were less likely to recommend acceptance or revision (versus rejection) compared with reviewers suggested by the article authors: matched-pair risk ratio for acceptance or revision 0.88 (95% CI 0.78 to 0.98).

The potential benefits of matching for an observational cohort study have been emphasized by Rubin (Rubin 1973, 1997, 2006) and Rosenbaum (Rosenbaum 2010). They point out that matching can often be used in computerized data with little additional cost or effort. Matching, either at the individual level or using broad strata, can ensure that there is sufficient overlap between the exposed (treated) and unexposed (control) groups with regard to the matching variables. If a propensity score is created to estimate the probability of being in the treated group, the analyst can examine whether there are many treated subjects with scores higher than the highest score in the control group, and also whether there are many control subjects with scores lower than any score in the treated group. It may be best to omit those who have propensity scores so extreme that they fail to overlap the score distribution of the comparison group (Cummings 2008). Otherwise the analysis may be biased by comparisons between subjects who are so profoundly different that the estimates involve unjustified extrapolations.

20.5 A BENEFIT OF MATCHING; ONLY MATCHED SETS WITH AT LEAST ONE OUTCOME ARE NEEDED

If matching is done and a matched analysis is used, only those matched sets with at least one outcome are needed to produce unbiased estimates of odds, risk, rate or hazard ratios for the entire cohort. Matched sets without any outcomes can be omitted, as they will not contribute to the ratio estimates for discrete outcomes.

Consider hypothetical matched data for 150 vehicles that crashed (Table 20.1). The risk of death for unbelted drivers and passengers was enormous; 0.2 in cars that crashed at fast speed, 0.6 in cars that crashed at very fast speed. This risk was not affected by seat position (driver versus front passenger), but it was reduced by half among those who wore a seat belt. All the drivers in the fast crashes wore seat belts, as did half the drivers in the very fast crashes. Passengers never used seat belts. Because belt use was less common in very fast crashes, compared with fast crashes, crash speed was a confounder of the association between belt use and death. Failure to account for speed produces a rate ratio that exaggerates the benefits of seat belts.

The vehicle counts in the last column of Table 20.1 can be used to calculate the risk ratios within strata defined by speed and driver belt use. In the fast cars the risk of death for drivers, who were all

TABLE 20.1 Hypothetical data for driver-passenger pairs in 150 vehicles that crashed. The risk of death did not vary by seat position. For vehicles that crashed at fast speed, the risk of death for an unbelted occupant was 0.2. Seat belts reduced that risk to 0.1, for a belt use risk ratio of 0.5. In very fast cars the risk of death for an unbelted person was 0.6, the risk when belted was 0.3, and the risk ratio for death if belted, compared with unbelted, was again 0.5. In these data no passengers were belted. In fast cars all drivers were belted and in very fast cars half of the drivers were belted.

SPEED	DRIVER BELTED	DRIVER UNBELTED	OUTCOME	NUMBER OF CARS
Fast	X		Both died	1
Fast	X		Passenger died	9
Fast	X		Driver died	4
Fast	X		No one died	36
Very fast	X		Both died	9
Very fast	X		Passenger died	21
Very fast	X		Driver died	6
Very fast	X		No one died	14
Very fast		X	Both died	18
Very fast		X	Passenger died	12
Very fast		X	Driver died	12
Very fast		X	No one died	8

belted, was $(1 + 4)/(1 + 9 + 4 + 36) = 5/50 = 0.1$. The risk for the passengers (all unbelted) was $(1 + 9)/(1 + 9 + 4 + 36) = 10/50 = 0.2$. Since these are matched sets, the denominators for the belted and unbelted risks are identical, 50. So the risk ratio comparing those belted with those unbelted is $[(1 + 4)/(1 + 9 + 4 + 36)]/[(1 + 9)/(1 + 9 + 4 + 36)] = (1 + 4)/(1 + 9) = 0.5$. The counts of 1, 4, and 9 can all be obtained from the pairs with at least one death; we don't need the 36 fast vehicles with no deaths to calculate the risk ratio. A similar calculation can be applied to the very fast vehicles in which drivers were belted and passengers were not.

Matched-pair data for a dichotomous exposure and dichotomous outcome can be arranged in a 2 x 2 contingency table for the counts of the matched pairs. This is shown in Table 20.2 for the counts of vehicles in Table 20.1. The matched-pair odds ratio, described in many textbooks and articles, makes use of the pairs discordant on the outcome: odds ratio = $B/C = 10/30 = 0.33$. The matched-pair risk ratio makes use of pairs with at least one outcome: risk ratio = $(A + B)/(A + C) = 20/40 = 0.5$. Neither the odds ratio or the risk ratio use the pairs with no outcomes, the 50 vehicles in cell D. Table 20.2 shows counts for 100 vehicles, but there were 150 vehicles in Table 20.1. For a simple matched-pair analysis that assumes there is no confounding by seat position (or any other variable), the 50 vehicles with only unbelted occupants contribute nothing to estimating the effects of seat belt use and they do not appear in

TABLE 20.2 Reformatted data for the driver-passenger pairs in 150 vehicles described in Table 20.1. Cell counts for number of vehicles. Cells are designated A, B, C, and D.

	NOT BELTED		
BELTED	DIED	SURVIVED	TOTAL
Died	A 10	B 10	20
Survived	C 30	D 50	80
Total	40	60	100

Table 20.2. Later I will discuss more flexible methods which can use the unbelted pairs to estimate a possible association between seat position and death, and then adjust the belt association for the possible confounding effects of seat position.

Because only matched sets with an outcome are required for a valid matched analysis, the use of a matched analysis can provide unbiased estimates in some situations in which other analyses would be biased. Crash data is one example. The National Highway Traffic Safety Administration collects data regarding all crashes with a death on public roads into a data set called the Fatality Analysis Reporting System. Crashes without a death are not included; thus most vehicles that crashed, more than 99%, are not in these data (National Highway Traffic Safety Administration 2004). An analysis which accounts for the matching of vehicle occupants can provide valid risk ratio estimates of seat belt effects on the risk of death for *all* crashes with two or more vehicle occupants. (The estimates may also be valid for vehicles that crashed with one occupant, because those crashes are not systematically different, in ways that would influence the size of the seat belt risk ratio, from vehicles with two or more occupants (Cummings, Wells, and Rivara 2003).)

The use of matched methods not only makes possible some analyses of crash data, but it can save time and money because matched analyses only need data for those matched sets with an outcome. A good example of how matched methods can save time and money was described by Walker and colleagues (Walker et al. 1981, Walker 1982, Walker et al. 1983). Those investigators wished to estimate any association between vasectomy and later non-fatal myocardial infarction. They used data for members of Group Health Cooperative of Puget Sound for the period 1963 through the end of 1978. First they identified men (4,830) who had a vasectomy during this period and were still plan members in 1978. They used electronic data to match each of these men to five men without vasectomies who were still in the plan in 1978; they matched on year of birth and membership in the plan at the time of the vasectomy. The rate of non-fatal infarction among the vasectomized men was 23/24420 = 0.94 per 1,000 man-years, compared with a rate of 120/122100 = 0.98 per 1,000 man-years among men without vasectomy: rate ratio 1.0 (95% CI 0.6, 1.5) comparing vasectomized men to other men.

To determine whether the estimated rate ratio of 1.0 might be biased by unmeasured confounders, Walker and coauthors first randomly selected just one of the five unexposed men for each man with a vasectomy. They recognized that only those pairs with one or more outcomes (a non-fatal myocardial infarction) were needed, so they limited further attention to those pairs only. After a few additional exclusions, they ended up with 36 matched pairs and extracted data from the paper records of these 72 patients. They found that adjustment for confounders in this subset of their data produced little change in the hazard ratio for the matched pairs and concluded that the rate ratio of 1.0, estimated from the 4,830 vasectomized men and 24,150 not vasectomized men, was not likely to be biased by unmeasured confounders.

20.6 STUDIES DESIGNS THAT MATCH A PERSON TO THEMSELVES

In a crossover study of two (or more) treatments, each subject receives both treatments and their outcomes under the two treatments are compared (Hills and Armitage 1979, Senn 2002, Jones and Kenward 2003, Mills et al. 2009). If treatment order is randomized, this is a type of randomized controlled trial. The design controls for confounding by any factor which is invariant within a person; genetic make-up, for example. A factor that changes over time, from the first treatment to the second, can be a potential confounder, although randomizing the order of the treatments may control for some of these factors. In these studies there is often concern about carryover bias (Cummings 2010), worry that the effect of the first treatment may persist long enough to influence the results of the second treatment. This is a matched design trial, in which each person given a treatment is matched to themselves when not given the treatment (or a different treatment) at another time.

The case-crossover study design is a type of case-control study in which the exposure status of the case is compared with their own exposure status at some other, typically earlier, point in time (Maclure 1991). The design matches a person-time period during which the case outcome occurred with a control time period for the same individual. This method only works for exposures that vary over time and it is best used for short-term exposures. If the exposure does not vary, or varies only after long time intervals, it would be unwise to use this design. For example, if the exposure was smoking, this design would be nearly useless, as most people who smoke during one time interval also smoked during other recent time intervals. In a study by Mittleman et al. (1993) the cases were 1,228 persons with a nonfatal myocardial infarction: (1) 50 had experienced heavy exertion in the hour prior to their symptoms, but not during the same hour of the prior day, (2) 9 had exerted in their control hour only, (3) and 4 exerted in both periods. The matched-pair odds ratio for infarction when exerting heavily, compared with not exerting, was 50/9 = 5.6. Another case-crossover study estimated that use of a cell phone increased the risk of a traffic crash: risk ratio 4.3 for a crash when a phone was used, compared to when it was not (Maclure and Mittleman 1997, Redelmeier and Tibshirani 1997a). This design has been discussed in review articles (Redelmeier and Tibshirani 1997b, Maclure and Mittleman 2000).

The idea of comparing two time periods from the same individual was extended to rates with multiple outcome events in papers by Farrington and others (Farrington 1995, Farrington, Nash, and Miller 1996, Whitaker et al. 2006, Whitaker 2008, Whitaker, Hocine, and Farrington 2009). The authors called this the case series method or the self-controlled case series. Their methods arose from investigations of vaccine side-effects. For example, investigators studied whether the rate of seizures after receiving a vaccine differed from the rate in some prior interval for the same person. These studies used matched-pair cohort methods for rates which match a time period soon after the exposure (a vaccination, for example) to another time period before the exposure.

If the outcome is dichotomous or a count, the matched methods described later in this chapter may be used for all three of the study designs I have just discussed.

20.7 A MATCHED ANALYSIS CAN ACCOUNT FOR MATCHING RATIOS THAT ARE NOT CONSTANT

When the matched sets maintain a constant ratio of exposed to unexposed subjects, an unmatched analysis can produce estimates unconfounded by the matching factors. But if the ratio of exposed and unexposed subjects varies within the matched sets, an unmatched analysis may still be biased by confounding related to the matching factors. Imagine we match each of 100 exposed men to a single unexposed man. And we match each of 100 exposed woman to 3 unexposed women. If an unmatched analysis is done, sex may still confound the association of interest, as 50% of the exposed will be male compared with 25% of the unexposed. This bias is removed by a matched analysis, because the comparisons are made within the matched sets; because the matching factors, sex in this example, do not vary within those sets, they cannot confound the comparisons.

Non-constant matching ratios can arise in data by design or for other reasons. In vehicle crash data, vehicles can have more than two occupants and so the ratio of belted to unbelted occupants can vary. Flexible matched analysis methods can account for any number of occupants with any combination of belt use. Earlier I mentioned a study of life vests and drowning (Cummings, Mueller, and Quan 2010); the number of boaters in each vessel varied, as did the proportion using life vests. A matched analysis accounted for these variations.

20.8 CHOOSING BETWEEN RISKS AND RATES FOR THE CRASH DATA IN TABLES 20.1 AND 20.2

The data in Tables 20.1 and 20.2 can be used to estimate risks and risk ratios. Chapters 2 and 5 discussed reasons for choosing between risks and rates. Here I discuss why risks, rather than rates, may be preferred for a study of mortality after a traffic crash.

The Fatality Analysis Reporting System data includes information about all vehicles and persons involved in a crash with at least one death within 30 days. About half of crash deaths occur at the scene, 90% within the first day, and 99% within 10 days. The 30-day cutoff captures most crash-related deaths and saves money by avoiding searches for the few additional deaths that occur later. The data includes information about time to death (although this is often missing) but using this information to estimate a rate ratio could be misleading for two reasons.

Let us imagine that the true risk ratio for death, comparing belted with unbelted vehicle occupants, is 0.5 as in Tables 20.1 and 20.2. Also imagine that unbelted persons who die do so 2 days after the crash and belted persons who die do so 4 days after the crash. If this is so, then the rate ratio estimate for belt effects will be further from 1.0 than the risk ratio of 0.5, because (1) death would be less frequent when belted and (2) death would come later if a belt was worn. But would delaying death by 2 days be advantageous? Deaths at 2, 3, or 4 days after a crash often occur among persons on a ventilator in an intensive care unit. Would 2 extra days of life on a ventilator, perhaps in great discomfort, be beneficial or harmful? Using the risk ratio avoids this question by ignoring the actual time to death.

There is a second reason not to use rates. An analysis based on rates assumes that the rate remains constant over time; doubling follow-up time doubles the count of events. This assumption is often not true and so we adjust for age and other variables that may explain changes in rates with additional follow-up time. The assumption of a constant rate over 30 days of follow-up is unrealistic for deaths after a crash; the rate is highest immediately after the crash and quickly declines to nearly zero at 30 days. If the average time to death is as described in the previous paragraph, simply changing the length of follow-up time from 30 to 60 days would change the rates and the rate ratio, because the person-time denominators of the rates among belted and unbelted survivors would double, while the rate numerators would remain about the same. The ratio of these lower rates would change in this example.

A third reason to eschew rates is that they are not collapsible for crash mortality. This problem arises when outcomes are common. The difficulties produced by noncollapsibility were discussed in Chapter 8. While death is rare in *all* traffic crashes, it is sufficiently common in a notable subgroup of crashes that lack of collapsibility will be an issue.

20.9 STRATIFIED METHODS FOR ESTIMATING RISK RATIOS FOR MATCHED DATA

Although this is a book about rates, I will first discuss Stata commands which can be used to estimate risk ratios for matched sets. These commands can also estimate rate ratios for single events, and recurrent events for some of these commands, if the follow-up person-time for all subjects is the same, because follow-up time can then be ignored. For these examples I will use the data in Tables 20.1 and 20.2.

Start with Stata's **cs** (<u>c</u>ohort <u>study</u>) command. This command is handy for tabulating and examining data. With the or option, it will produce the odds ratio as well as the risk ratio and risk difference for the data in Tables 20.1 and 20.2:

```
. cs died belt, or

                  | Belted                  |
                  | Exposed  Unexposed  |    Total
- - - - - - - - - +- - - - - - - - - - - - - +- - - - - - -
         Cases |      20         100  |      120
      Noncases |      80         100  |      180
- - - - - - - - - +- - - - - - - - - - - - - +- - - - - - - -
         Total |     100         200  |      300
                  |                         |
          Risk |      .2          .5  |       .4
                  |                         |
                  | Point estimate      |  [95% Conf. Interval]
                  |- - - - - - - - - - - - - +- - - - - - - - - - - - - -
Risk difference |        -.3           | -.4046334   -.1953666
    Risk ratio |         .4           |  .2639325    .6062156
  Prev. frac. ex. |       .6           |  .3937844    .7360675
 Prev. frac. pop |        .2           |
    Odds ratio |        .25           |  .1430274    .4373353  (Cornfield)
                  +- - - - - - - - - - - - - - - - - - - - - - - - - - -
            chi2(1) =   25.00       Pr>chi2 = 0.0000
```

The risk ratio in this output is 0.4 instead of the true value of 0.5, because the analysis failed to account for confounding by speed. The odds ratio of 0.25 is further from 1 than the risk ratio, because the outcome is common, especially in cars that crashed when going very fast. If speed was measured, we could adjust for it and get the correct risk ratio using Mantel-Haenszel weights:

```
. cs died belt, by(speed)

  Crash speed |     RR    [95% Conf. Interval]   M-H Weight
- - - - - - - - - - +- - - - - - - - - - - - - - - - - - - - - - - - - - -
            0 |     .5   .1840521   1.358311              5
            1 |     .5   .3210202   .7787672           22.5
- - - - - - - - - - +- - - - - - - - - - - - - - - - - - - - - - - - - - -
        Crude |     .4   .2639325   .6062156
  M-H combined |     .5   .3333125   .7500468
- - - - - - - - - - - - - - - - - - - - - - - - - - - - - - - - - - - - - - -
Test of homogeneity (M-H)    chi2(1) =   0.000  Pr>chi2 = 1.0000
```

Adjusting for speed is not possible in this example, because crash speed is so hard to measure after a crash. Another way to get an unbiased estimate for matched-pair data is to only use belted subjects who were matched to unbelted subjects; the discordant pairs. This analysis ignores the driver-passenger pairs in which both were unbelted. The variable nobelts is equal to 1 for the pairs without any seat belt use, 0 if anyone was belted. Recall that passengers were never belted. This analysis uses only 100 pairs:

```
. cs died belt if nobelts==0, or

                | Belted              |
                | Exposed  Unexposed  |    Total
   -------------+---------------------+---------
       Cases |      20          40   |       60
    Noncases |      80          60   |      140
   -------------+---------------------+---------
       Total |     100         100   |      200
             |                       |
        Risk |      .2          .4   |       .3
             |                       |
             |  Point estimate       |  [95% Conf. Interval]
             |-----------------------+----------------------
 Risk difference |      -.2          |  -.323959   -.076041
      Risk ratio |       .5          |   .3157516   .7917616
  Prev. frac. ex. |      .5          |   .2082384   .6842484
 Prev. frac. pop |      .25          |
      Odds ratio |      .375         |   .2001517   .7030455 (Cornfield)
             +-----------------------------------------------
                   chi2(1) =    9.52   Pr>chi2 = 0.0020
```

In this analysis, the risk ratio of 0.5 is correct, even though we did not use a matched analytic method. This shows that a matched cohort study with a constant matching ratio does not always require a matched analysis to get an unbiased result. Confounding by the matching variable is eliminated by the matched design.

If we limit the data to those matched sets with at least one dead person (sumdied≥1), but fail to use a matched analysis, the results are biased:

```
. cs died belt if sumdied>=1, or

                | Belted              |
                | Exposed  Unexposed  |    Total
   -------------+---------------------+---------
       Cases |      20         100   |      120
    Noncases |      30          34   |       64
   -------------+---------------------+---------
       Total |      50         134   |      184
             |                       |
        Risk |      .4      .7462687 |   .6521739
             |                       |
             |  Point estimate       |  [95% Conf. Interval]
             |-----------------------+----------------------
 Risk difference |  -.3462687        |  -.500759   -.1917783
      Risk ratio |      .536         |   .376378    .7633178
  Prev. frac. ex. |     .464         |   .2366822    .623622
 Prev. frac. pop |    .126087        |
      Odds ratio |   .2266667        |   .1145971   .4482905 (Cornfield)
             +-----------------------------------------------
```

All the odds ratios in these tables are biased. To get the correct odds ratio of 0.33, we can use the mhodds command, which can compute an odds ratio stratified on the matching variable, vehid (vehicle identifier) in this example. This analysis uses only the 40 pairs in which subjects are discordant on both the exposure (seat belt use) and the outcome (died):

```
. mhodds died belt vehid

Mantel-Haenszel estimate of the odds ratio
Comparing belt==1 vs. belt==0, controlling for vehid

note: only 40 of the 150 strata formed in this analysis contribute
      information about the effect of the explanatory variable

  ----------------------------------------------------------
   Odds Ratio   chi2(1)     P>chi2     [95% Conf. Interval]
  ----------------------------------------------------------
    0.333333    10.00      0.0016     0.162954   0.681857
  ----------------------------------------------------------
```

Next we use a command, **csmatch**, which a colleague and I wrote for matched-pair cohort data (Cummings and McKnight 2004):

```
. csmatch died belt, group(vehid)

                 | Not exposed               |
Exposed          |  Outcome=1   Outcome=0    |   Total
-----------------+--------------------------+--------
Outcome = 1      |      10          10       |     20
Outcome = 0      |      30          50       |     80
-----------------+--------------------------+--------
         Total   |      40          60       |    100

Cohort matched-pair risk ratio        [95% Conf. Interval]
                      0.50000       0.32258    0.77500
```

The **csmatch** command classifies pairs according to exposure and outcome to produce the counts of pairs for cells A, B, C, and D that were shown in Table 20.2. The matched-pair risk ratio is (A+B)/(A+C) = 20/40 = 0.5. The variance of the ln(risk ratio) is (B+C)/[(A+B) × (A+C)] (Greenland and Robins 1985), which is used to estimate the CI. Cell D contributes nothing to these estimates, so the command will produce the same risk ratio and CI if the data are limited to the pairs with one or two dead occupants (Cummings, McKnight, and Greenland 2003). To show that cell D is not needed, we can apply **csmatch** to those pairs with 1 or more deaths:

```
. csmatch died belt if sumdied>=1, group(vehid)

                 | Not exposed               |
Exposed          |  Outcome=1   Outcome=0    |   Total
-----------------+--------------------------+--------
Outcome = 1      |      10          10       |     20
Outcome = 0      |      30           0       |     30
-----------------+--------------------------+--------
         Total   |      40          10       |     50


Cohort matched-pair risk ratio        [95% Conf. Interval]
                      0.50000       0.32258    0.77500
```

If we only have the pairs with a death, it is no longer possible to correctly estimate the risk of death separately for those belted and unbelted, using the available data. But we can estimate the risk ratio.

Stata has a command called **mcci**, which is the immediate version of the **mcc** (matched case-control) command, and this can be used for the counts produced by csmatch:

```
. mcci 10 10 30 50

                | Controls              |
Cases           | Exposed  Unexposed    |    Total
----------------+-----------------------+---------
     Exposed |       10         10  |       20
   Unexposed |       30         50  |       80
----------------+-----------------------+---------
       Total |       40         60  |      100

McNemar's chi2(1) =    10.00   Prob > chi2 = 0.0016
Exact McNemar significance probability       = 0.0022

Proportion with factor
      Cases              .2
      Controls           .4      [95% Conf. Interval]
                     --------     ----------------
      difference        -.2      -.3275978  -.0724022
      ratio              .5       .3225786   .7750049
      rel. diff.  -.3333333      -.5718926  -.0947741
      odds ratio   .3333333       .1453636   .7005703  (exact)
```

The mcci command produces both the same rate ratio and CI as the **csmatch** command and also produces the same odds ratio as the **mhodds** command, but the labeling of the rows and columns is confusing; the words "cases" and "controls" are used instead of "exposed" and "not exposed". The table says that there were 10 pairs with occupants both exposed to seat belts, when in fact there were no such pairs. Stata's **mcc** command can also be used for these data. The **mcc** command requires us to create new variables, a chore which I will not show here. Instead, we can use the **mcci** command to produce the output table and results that would be produced by the **mcc** command:

```
. mcci 0 10 30 60

                | Controls              |
Cases           | Exposed  Unexposed    |    Total
----------------+-----------------------+----------
     Exposed |        0         10  |       10
   Unexposed |       30         60  |       90
----------------+-----------------------+----------
       Total |       30         70  |      100

McNemar's chi2(1) =    10.00    Prob > chi2 = 0.0016
Exact McNemar significance probability       = 0.0022
```

```
Proportion with factor
    Cases              .1
    Controls           .3    [95% Conf. Interval]
                     -------  ----------------
    difference        -.2    -.3275978  -.0724022
    ratio         .3333333    .1629536   .6818575
    rel. diff.   -.2857143    -.486509  -.0849196
    odds ratio   .3333333     .1453636   .7005703  (exact)
```

Cell A is empty in the output above, so the matched-pair risk ratio (A+B)/(A+C) and the matched-pair odds ratio, B/C, are both 0.33 in this example.

20.10 ODDS RATIOS, RISK RATIOS, CELL A, AND MATCHED DATA

This difference between tables with and without an empty cell A (no pairs with two deaths) is important. It is the presence of some matched-pairs with two outcomes that makes the risk ratio differ from the odds ratio.

When an outcome is rare, the risk ratio and the odds ratio will be approximately equal. Deaths are rare in vehicle crashes. In 2002 there were about 10,594,000 passenger cars and light trucks in crashes and 37,232 vehicle occupant deaths: 0.0035 deaths per vehicle that crashed (National Highway Traffic Safety Administration 2004). Because deaths were rare, one might expect that the odds ratio for death among belted occupants, compared with not belted occupants, would be similar to the risk ratio. But a matched analysis of crash data will produce a odds ratio for seat belt use that is further from 1 than the risk ratio. Olson et al used Fatality Analysis Reporting System data and a matched analysis to estimate associations between air bags and death in a crash (Olson, Cummings, and Rivara 2006). Using a subset of these data for front seat occupants age 16 years and older, there were 45,796 drivers paired in the same vehicle with 45,796 front seat passengers. Using the 7,848 pairs discordant on seat belt use, and ignoring any possible confounding by age and sex, the seat belt use risk ratio for death was 0.40:

```
. csmatch dead belted, group(idn)

                  | Not exposed               |
Exposed           | Outcome=1   Outcome=0      |   Total
------------------+---------------------------+--------
Outcome = 1       |    1161        1298        |   2459
Outcome = 0       |    4915         474        |   5389
------------------+---------------------------+--------
      Total       |    6076        1772        |   7848

Cohort matched-pair risk ratio      [95% Conf. Interval]
                       0.40471       0.38885    0.42121
```

The odds ratio, which ignores the 1,161 pairs in cell A, was 1298/4915 = 0.26, which we can calculate from the table or with the **mhodds** command (idn is a vehicle identifier code):

```
. mhodds dead belted idn

Mantel-Haenszel estimate of the odds ratio
Comparing belted==1 vs. belted==0, controlling for idn

note: only 6213 of the 45796 strata formed in this analysis contribute
      information about the effect of the explanatory variable


 -----------------------------------------------------
  Odds Ratio    chi2(1)    P>chi2     [95% Conf. Interval]
 -----------------------------------------------------
   0.264090    2105.70    0.0000     0.248421    0.280747
 -----------------------------------------------------
```

Although the risk of death was small in *all* crashes, the odds ratio of 0.26 is not a good approximation of the risk ratio of 0.40. The odds ratio will approach the risk ratio only if the outcome is sufficiently *rare in all noteworthy strata* of the data used in the analysis. If we adjust for a variable that defines a segment of the crash population in which death is common, and if this segment is large enough to influence the ratio estimate, then the odds ratio will be further from 1 than the risk ratio. The matched risk and odds ratios are not crude (unadjusted) estimates. They are both "adjusted" for all those matching factors that are shared by occupants of the same vehicle; this includes many factors that define smash-ups with a high risk of death. For example, death will be common in vehicles that were traveling at 60 miles per hour and collided head-on with another vehicle. Since speed and head-on collision were not explicitly used to produce the matching adjusted ratio estimates (those variables were not even in the data I used), how did the matched analysis "know" that death was common in a nontrivial group of crashes? The answer lies in cell A, the 1,161 pairs with two deaths.

There were about .0035 deaths per crashed vehicle among about 10 million vehicles that crashed in 2002 (National Highway Traffic Safety Administration 2004). Imagine that 5 million of those vehicles had front-seat pairs with one belted and one not. Assume that the risk of death for each belted person was .003 and the risk for each unbelted person was .006, with no variation in these risks. If that were so, then the expected number of front-seat pairs with 2 deaths would be .003 x .006 x 5 million = 90. The cross-tabulated matched-pair data for all 5 million vehicles crashes would look like this:

```
. csmatch died belted, group(pairid)

                  | Not exposed                |
Exposed           | Outcome=1    Outcome=0  |    Total
 -----------------+-----------------------+--------
Outcome = 1       |       90        14910  |    15000
Outcome = 0       |     29910      4955090  |  4985000
 -----------------+-----------------------+--------
      Total       |     30000      4970000  |  5000000


Cohort matched-pair risk ratio      [95% Conf. Interval]
                     0.50000        0.49031    0.50988
```

In the table, the number of pairs with two deaths is small, 90, relative to the counts of pairs with 1 death in cells B and C of the table. The rare occurrence of two deaths in cell A would occur in a large population where the risk of death was small and constant. The odds ratio is 14910/29910 = 0.498, close to the risk ratio of 0.5. But in real crash data, as shown earlier, the number of belted-unbelted pairs with two deaths was 1,161, which is large relative to the 1,298 belted-unbelted pairs with a belted occupant death and the 4,915 belted-unbelted pairs with an unbelted occupant death. The relatively large count in cell A arose because the risk of death varies greatly in crashes; while that risk is small overall in all crashes, the risk is very high in some crashes, resulting in the divergence of the odds ratio from the risk ratio. The large number of pairs in cell A, compared with cells B and C, of the matched analysis reveals that a notable number of crashes must have a high risk for death.

The real crash data used above differs from the example used in Tables 20.1 and 20.2, because the counts for those tables were created so that the risk of death was homogeneous within each of the four categories defined by crash speed and seat belt use. This was done to demonstrate how a matched analysis works. But risk homogeneity does not exist in real crash data and no assumption of homogeneity of risk is needed to analyze these data.

20.11 REGRESSION ANALYSIS OF MATCHED DATA FOR THE ODDS RATIO

Logistic regression can be used to estimate the odds ratio for death if belted, compared with not belted. This odds ratio was 0.33 in the matched-pair analyses of Tables 20.1 and 20.2. The results from logistic regression are shown here:

```
. logistic died belt, or nolog
```

Logistic regression

Number of obs   =   300
LR chi2(1)   =   26.47
Prob > chi2   =   0.0000

Log likelihood = -188.66968

Pseudo R2   =   0.0655

died	Odds Ratio	Std. Err.	z	P>|z|	[95% Conf. Interval]
belt	.25	.071807	-4.83	0.000	.1423807	.4389642
_cons	1	.1414214	0.00	1.000	.7579175	1.319405

The estimated odds ratio 0.25 is biased by confounding related to crash speed. Adjusting for speed, a variable unknown to us in these hypothetical data, most of the bias is removed:

died	Odds Ratio	Std. Err.	z	P>|z|	[95% Conf. Interval]
belt	.3191093	.0964236	-3.78	0.000	.1764967	.5769557
speed	5.240068	1.683204	5.16	0.000	2.792002	9.834632
_cons	.2791226	.0837052	-4.26	0.000	.1550711	.5024109

The new estimate of 0.319 is still slightly different from the matched-pair odds ratio of 0.3333. If we limit the logistic regression analysis to the 100 belted-unbelted pairs only, the estimate becomes 0.3303. The difference between these two estimates is trivial, but the correct estimate is 0.3333.

We can enter each vehicle identifying number as an indicator variable into a logistic model. This results in pages of output, some of it shown here:

```
. logistic died belt i.vehid, nolog
note: 4401.vehid != 0 predicts success perfectly
      4401.vehid dropped and 2 obs not used

. . .

(pages of output omitted for pairs not discordant on the outcome or exposure)
. . .

note: 16014.vehid != 0 predicts failure perfectly
      16014.vehid dropped and 2 obs not used
note: 15006.vehid omitted because of collinearity
```

Logistic regression				Number of obs	=	128
				LR chi2(64)	=	20.93
				Prob > chi2	=	1.0000
Log likelihood = -78.257876				Pseudo R2	=	0.1180

died	Odds Ratio	Std. Err.	z	P>|z|	[95% Conf. Interval]	
belt	.1111111	.0573775	-4.25	0.000	.040383	.3057145
vehid						
4401	1	(empty)				
4801	1	2.309401	-0.00	1.000	.0108202	92.41996

```
. . .
```

(pages of output omitted for vehicles that all have odds ratios of 1 or 0.3333)

```
. . .
```

6432	1	(empty)				
_cons	3	4.959839	0.66	0.506	.1174484	76.62939

In this output, the odds ratio of 0.11 is biased because unconditional logistic regression performs poorly when data are sparse, meaning that there are many small strata with few outcomes in each (Breslow and Day 1980 pp149–151, Greenland 2008c p433, Greenland and Rothman 2008c p263, Kleinbaum and Klein 2010 pp107–111, Greenland, Mansournia, and Altman 2016). Sparse data bias pushes the odds ratio further from 1. For a matched-pair odds ratio the biased estimate from ordinary logistic regression is the square of the true odds ratio (Breslow and Day 1980 pp149–151): $0.33333333^2 = 0.11111$, which is the estimate shown here. In general, logistic regression requires about 10 outcome events for each regression variable, although in some situations a smaller number of events, in the range of 5 to 9, may be sufficient (Pike, Hill, and Smith 1980, Robinson and Jewell 1991, Peduzzi et al. 1996, Vittinghoff and McCulloch 2007). In this example, there were 150 vehicles entered into the model, plus a variable for belted, for a ratio of about 120 deaths per variable = .8 outcomes per variable. Sparse data indeed.

To flexibly estimate odds ratios from matched data and avoid sparse data bias, conditional logistic regression is typically used. The estimates for each pair are not estimated, but "conditioned" out of the analysis:

```
. clogit died belt, or group(vehid) nolog
note: multiple positive outcomes within groups encountered.
note: 86 groups (172 obs) dropped because of all positive or
      all negative outcomes.
```

```
Conditional (fixed-effects) logistic regression

                                          Number of obs    =        128
                                          LR chi2(1)       =      10.46
                                          Prob > chi2      =     0.0012
Log likelihood = -39.128938               Pseudo R2        =     0.1180
------------------------------------------------------------------------
    died | Odds Ratio  Std. Err.     z    P>|z|     [95% Conf. Interval]
-------+----------------------------------------------------------------
    belt |  .3333333   .1217161   -3.01   0.003      .1629536   .6818575
------------------------------------------------------------------------
```

The Cox proportional hazard model, stratified on vehicle, can be used to exactly reproduce the odds ratios and CIs obtained from conditional logistic regression, by using the exact partial-likelihood method for tied survival times (Cummings, McKnight, and Weiss 2003). In the past, some software packages used this approach to implement conditional logistic regression, because the two models are mathematically identical:

```
. gen byte time = 1

. stset time, failure(died==1)

     failure event:  died == 1
obs. time interval:  (0, time]
  exit on or before:  failure


- - - - - - - - - - - - - - - - - - - - - - - - - - - - - - - - - - - - -
    300  total observations
      0  exclusions
- - - - - - - - - - - - - - - - - - - - - - - - - - - - - - - - - - - - -
    300  observations remaining, representing
    120  failures in single-record/single-failure data
    300  total analysis time at risk and under observation
                                       at risk from t =         0
                              earliest observed entry t =         0
                                 last observed exit t =         1

. stcox belt, hr strata(vehid) exactp nolog
        failure _d: died == 1
  analysis time _t:  time
Stratified Cox regr. – exact partial likelihood

No. of subjects =        300            Number of obs  =        300
No. of failures =        120
Time at risk    =        300
                                        LR chi2(1)     =      10.46
Log likelihood  = -39.128938            Prob > chi2    =     0.0012
```

```
---------------------------------------------------------------------
     _t | Haz. Ratio   Std. Err.        z    P>|z|    [95% Conf. Interval]
--------+------------------------------------------------------------
   belt |  .3333333    .1217161     -3.01    0.003    .1629536    .6818575
---------------------------------------------------------------------
                                                           Stratified by vehid
```

20.12 REGRESSION ANALYSIS OF MATCHED DATA FOR THE RISK RATIO

If Poisson regression is used for the data in Table 20.1 and speed omitted from the regression model, the ratio estimate is 0.4, biased from 0.5 because we have not adjusted for speed. This ratio can be interpreted as a risk ratio, because everyone was followed for 30 days:

```
. poisson died belt, irr nolog

Poisson regression                       Number of obs  =        300
                                         LR chi2(1)     =      16.90
                                         Prob > chi2    =     0.0000
Log likelihood = -221.50348              Pseudo R2      =     0.0368

---------------------------------------------------------------------
   died |    IRR    Std. Err.       z    P>|z|     [95% Conf. Interval]
--------+------------------------------------------------------------
   belt |     .4    .0979796    -3.74    0.000     .2474908    .6464887
  _cons |     .5         .05    -6.93    0.000     .4110076    .6082613
---------------------------------------------------------------------
```

If each vehicle identifier (vehid) is entered as an indicator variable, the risk ratio will account for the matching on vehicle. The method is clumsy, because it inserts 149 indicator terms into the model, but it works:

```
. poisson died belt i.vehid, irr nolog

Poisson regression                       Number of obs  =        300
                                         LR chi2(150)   =     137.98
                                         Prob > chi2    =     0.7500
Log likelihood = -160.96344              Pseudo R2      =     0.3000

---------------------------------------------------------------------
   died |    IRR    Std. Err.       z    P>|z|     [95% Conf. Interval]
--------+------------------------------------------------------------
   belt | .5000017    .1369287    -2.53    0.011     .292324    .8552214
        |
  vehid |
   4801 |  .500018     .612384    -0.57    0.571    .0453418    5.514074
   4802 |  .500018     .612384    -0.57    0.571    .0453418    5.514074
```

```
 4803 |   .500018    .612384    -0.57   0.571    .0453418    5.514074
 4804 |   .500018    .612384    -0.57   0.571    .0453418    5.514074
 4805 |   .500018    .612384    -0.57   0.571    .0453418    5.514074

(output omitted for over one hundred indicators)

16014 |  6.71e-09   .0000579    -0.00   0.998        0          .
       |
 _cons | 1.333345   .9506368     0.40   0.687    .3296555    5.392931
------------------------------------------------------------------
```

Unlike the situation with ordinary logistic regression, ordinary Poisson regression will get correct estimates despite using many sparse strata (Greenland and Rothman 2008c pp272–273). This idea was introduced in Chapter 19. In a large set of data this method will be time-consuming, can produce pages of output, and may overwhelm computer memory with all the estimated terms. The computing chore can be reduced by limiting the data to the pairs with at least one death, but the method is still clumsy.

A more convenient approach, mentioned in Chapter 19, is conditional Poisson regression, implemented by the **xtpoisson, fe** command, which implements a conditional or fixed effects model. The confusing name for this command was discussed in Chapter 19:

```
. xtset vehid
     panel variable: vehid (balanced)

. xtpoisson died belt, fe irr nolog
note: 58 groups (116 obs) dropped because of all zero outcomes

Conditional fixed-effects Poisson regression    Number of obs   =     184
Group variable: vehid                            Number of groups =      92

                                                 Obs per group:
                                                            min =       2
                                                            avg =     2.0
                                                            max =       2

                                                 Wald chi2(1)    =    6.41
Log likelihood = -60.37156                       Prob > chi2     =  0.0114

------------------------------------------------------------------
    died |    IRR   Std. Err.      z    P>|z|    [95% Conf. Interval]
---------+--------------------------------------------------------
    belt |     .5   .1369306    -2.53   0.011    .2923202    .8552265
------------------------------------------------------------------
```

The conditional Poisson model does not create any estimates for each of the pair indicator variables; they are "conditioned" out of the model. This model cannot estimate associations between the outcome and any variable used for the matching. The model can only estimate associations for exposures that vary within each vehicle. This convenient command is just what is needed to estimate risk ratios when matching is used (Cummings et al. 2002, Norvell and Cummings 2002, Cummings, McKnight, and Greenland 2003, Cummings, McKnight, and Weiss 2003, Cummings, Wells, and Rivara 2003, Cummings and McKnight 2004, Cummings and Rivara 2004, Cummings and McKnight 2010, Cummings 2011). The estimated association between seat belt use and death, 0.5, is the same in the conditional Poisson model as it is in the ordinary Poisson model with many indicator variables. Not only is the estimate the same, but the SEs, P-values, and CIs are the same. These models are mathematically equivalent. The conditional model is more convenient, and faster, because it omits all the indicator terms from the output.

The CIs and P-values for risk ratios will be too large with this model, because the binary outcomes do not fit a Poisson distribution. Compared with the Poisson distribution, these data are underdispersed. This can be remedied by using the robust variance option or bootstrap methods. Stata introduced a robust (sandwich) variance option for the **xtpoisson, fe** command in June of 2010 (Cummings 2011). But this variance estimator is not exactly the same as that used by ordinary Poisson regression. Using ordinary Poisson regression and indicator variables for each vehicle, the SE for the belt variable shrinks from 0.14 to 0.08 with the robust variance option. Using conditional Poisson regression with the robust variance, the SE is 0.11. This behavior is typical; the estimated robust variance will be larger using conditional, compared with ordinary, Poisson regression.

The **xtpoisson, fe** command allows the analyst to adjust for variables that vary within the pairs. One could limit an analysis of the association of seat belt use with death by just using the pairs that were discordant on seat belt use. But it may be important to adjust for variables such as sex, age, seat position, or the presence of an air bag, factors that may vary within a vehicle even when the occupants are concordant on seat belt use. If so, the use of all available data may be best, so the associations of these confounders with death may be estimated as precisely as possible; statistical power can be gained. To illustrate this, consider again the crash data from the study by Olson, Cummings, and Rivara (2006), used earlier to demonstrate the use of the csmatch command. There were 45,796 front-seat pairs. Of these, 42,227 pairs had one or two deaths, so those pairs can contribute to a matched analysis. Among the pairs with a death, the 7,374 pairs discordant on seat belt use can contribute to an estimate for the seat belt use risk ratio. Within the pairs with a death, 21,787 pairs had one male and one female occupant; those pairs can contribute to an estimate of the association of male sex, compared with female sex, with the outcome of death. There was overlap between these groups; 3,607 pairs had at least one death and were discordant on both belt use and sex. The total number of pairs that can contribute jointly to estimates for seat belt use and male sex in a matched analysis was 25,554.

If we enter only a term for seat belt use into the model, the regression output is shown below. The sample was limited to the pairs with a death (**sumdead > 0**) and discordant on belt use (**sumbelted==1**). If all pairs had been used, the regression table output would be identical:

```
. xtpoisson dead belted if sumdead>0 & sumbelted==1, irr fe nolog

Conditional fixed-effects Poisson regression    Number of obs    =   14,748
Group variable: idn                             Number of groups =    7,374

                                                Obs per group:
                                                             min =        2
                                                             avg =      2.0
                                                             max =        2

                                                Wald chi2(1)     =  1432.45
Log likelihood = -4320.086                      Prob > chi2      =   0.0000

------------------------------------------------------------------------------
    dead |      IRR    Std. Err.       z    P>|z|     [95% Conf. Interval]
---------+--------------------------------------------------------------------
  belted |  .4047071   .0096728   -37.85    0.000     .3861858     .4241166
------------------------------------------------------------------------------
```

Here is a similar analysis with male sex as the only exposure variable, limited to the pairs discordant on sex:

```
. xtpoisson dead msex if sumdead>0 & summale==1, irr fe nolog

Conditional fixed-effects Poisson regression    Number of obs   =    43,574
Group variable: idn                             Number of groups =    21,787

                                                Obs per group:
                                                         min =         2
                                                         avg =       2.0
                                                         max =         2

                                                Wald chi2(1)    =     93.64
Log likelihood = -15054.691                     Prob > chi2     =    0.0000

------------------------------------------------------------------------------
    dead |       IRR   Std. Err.      z    P>|z|     [95% Conf. Interval]
---------+--------------------------------------------------------------------
    msex |  .8864084   .0110449    -9.68   0.000     .8650229    .9083226
------------------------------------------------------------------------------
```

Next is an analysis limited to pairs with a death and discordant on belt use, sex, or both:

```
. xtpoisson dead belted msex if sumdead>0 /*
>       */ & (sumbelt==1 | summale==1), irr fe nolog

Conditional fixed-effects Poisson regression    Number of obs   =    51,108
Group variable: idn                             Number of groups =    25,554

                                                Obs per group:
                                                         min =         2
                                                         avg =       2.0
                                                         max =         2

                                                Wald chi2(2)    =   1556.65
Log likelihood = -16854.145                     Prob > chi2     =    0.0000

------------------------------------------------------------------------------
    dead |       IRR   Std. Err.      z    P>|z|     [95% Conf. Interval]
---------+--------------------------------------------------------------------
  belted |  .3992509   .0095682   -38.31   0.000     .3809312    .4184516
    msex |  .8634049   .0109415   -11.59   0.000     .8422242    .8851184
------------------------------------------------------------------------------
```

In this output, the estimated associations for both belt use and male sex are slightly different compared with the unadjusted analyses. In addition, the SEs are smaller and Z-statistics larger, so both estimates were more precise when 25,554 pairs were used. The gain in precision is small here, but the message is clear; use all the available pairs provided this fits the planned study design and doing this is not costly.

Just as a version of the Cox proportional hazards model is mathematically equivalent to a conditional logistic model, so a version of the Cox model is mathematically identical to the conditional Poisson model. We can estimate risk ratios with a stratified Cox proportional hazards model which deals with tied survival times by using the Breslow method (Cummings, McKnight, and Greenland 2003, Cummings, McKnight, and Weiss 2003, Cummings and McKnight 2004, Cummings 2011):

```
. gen byte time = 1

. stset time, failure(died==1)
     failure event:  died == 1
obs. time interval:  (0, time]
  exit on or before:  failure


------------------------------------------------------------------
      300  total observations
        0  exclusions
------------------------------------------------------------------
      300  observations remaining, representing
      120  failures in single-record/single-failure data
      300  total analysis time at risk and under observation
                                          at risk from t =         0
                               earliest observed entry t =         0
                                   last observed exit t =         1


. stcox belt, hr strata(vehid) breslow nolog
        failure _d: died == 1
  analysis time _t: time

Stratified Cox regr. - Breslow method for ties
No. of subjects =        300                  Number of obs  =          300
No. of failures =        120
Time at risk    =        300
                                              LR chi2(1)     =         6.80
Log likelihood  =  -79.779681                 Prob > chi2    =       0.0091


------------------------------------------------------------------
     _t | Haz. Ratio   Std. Err.        z   P>|z|    [95% Conf. Interval]
--------+---------------------------------------------------------
   belt |         .5    .1369306    -2.53   0.011    .2923202    .8552265
------------------------------------------------------------------
                                                  Stratified by vehid
```

In the command line for this output, the **breslow** option was used, but since this is the default option in Stata, it is not necessary to explicitly invoke this option. The results for all estimated statistics are exactly those from the **xtpoisson, fe** command. As noted earlier, fixed-effects conditional Poisson regression with a robust variance estimator will produce a smaller SE (0.11) compare with the usual variance estimator (.14), but the SE will be even smaller (0.08) with ordinary Poisson regression, vehicle indicator terms, and the robust variance. Adding the robust variance option to the Cox model used will produce the SE of (0.08).

Colleagues and I have used this matched study design to estimate risks ratios for death related to seat belts (Cummings et al. 2002, Cummings, Wells, and Rivara 2003, Schiff and Cummings 2004), airbags (Olson, Cummings, and Rivara 2006), and motorcycle helmets (Norvell and Cummings 2002). Others have used it to study the association between vaccine administration and febrile seizures (Barlow et al. 2001).

20.13 MATCHED ANALYSIS OF RATES WITH ONE OUTCOME EVENT

Creating and describing hypothetical matched data for risks is fairly simple, as the outcomes are just 0 or 1. Creating rate data is more complex. To generate hypothetical data with a constant rate, I assigned a subject number from 1 to N to each imaginary person and used a variation of Expression 2.4 to generate the time to death for those who died before the end of follow-up: time to death = ln(initial number of subjects/(initial number of subjects − subject number))/rate. This method is only approximately correct in a finite sample and produces counts and person-time estimates that are not exactly those predicted by Expressions 2.1 or 2.7. But in a large sample this approach is sufficiently accurate. Using this method, time to death was estimated for 2,000 hypothetical unexposed subjects with a constant mortality rate of 0.01 per person-year and follow-up limited to 10 years: the shortest time to death was .050 years, the longest was 9.98 years, 190 subjects died, and the total person-time was 19037.5 years. Data were also generated for 2,000 exposed subjects with a mortality rate of 0.02 and 10 years of follow-up. These data for 4,000 people are described by the **ir** command here, where the estimated rate ratio of 2.0 is equal to the true rate ratio:

```
. ir died exposed time
                 | Exposed               |
                 | Exposed   Unexposed   |      Total
-----------------+-----------------------+---------
          Died |     362         190   |        552
Time to death or |  18131.92    19037.51 |   37169.43
-----------------+-----------------------+---------
                 |                       |
Incidence rate |  .0199648    .0099803  |   .0148509
                 |                       |
                 |  Point estimate       |  [95% Conf. Interval]
                 |-----------------------+-----------------------
Inc. rate diff. |      .0099845         |  .0074858    .0124832
Inc. rate ratio |      2.000421         |  1.673678    2.397147 (exact)
Attr. frac. ex. |      .5001051         |  .4025136    .5828374 (exact)
Attr. frac. pop |      .3279675         |
                 +-----------------------------------------------
               (midp)   Pr(k>=362) =                 0.0000 (exact)
               (midp) 2*Pr(k>=362) =                 0.0000 (exact)
```

To create matched pairs, I matched each exposed person to a randomly chosen unexposed person. This is equivalent to matching on a variable that not a confounder. This would usually be unwise in a real study, but here it helps create a simple data set that can be used to illustrate various regression commands. Data like this might arise in a randomized trial that assigned people to treatment or control status in randomized blocks of size 2. To carry out the matching I used Stata's pseudo-random number generator and assigned each matched-pair an identifier called "pairid". Because of this random process, the rate ratios from matched and unmatched analyses will differ somewhat, just as they would in real data. Both matched and unmatched methods can produce unbiased rate ratio estimates, but in real data those estimates will vary due to what we call sampling variation or "chance." The larger the sample size, the more likely it is that the rate ratios from matched and unmatched analyses will agree; in statistical jargon, they are asymptotically equivalent. Data for two pairs are shown here:

```
+-------------------------------+
| pairid  exposed   died    time |
|-------------------------------|
|    45      No     No        10 |
|    45      Yes    No        10 |
|-------------------------------|
|    46      No     Yes  4.8665172 |
|    46      Yes    Yes  2.8020695 |
+-------------------------------+
```

Pair 45 will contribute nothing to a matched analysis, as no one died. Pair 46 had two deaths; the exposed person who died after 2.8 years will be compared with the unexposed person who died at 4.9 years.

The **cs** command and the **csmatch** command both produce risk ratios of 1.905. This ratio can be computed from Expression 2.9, which relates risks to rates: $(1 - \exp(-.02 \times 10))/(1 - \exp(-.01 \times 10)) = 1.905$. After three decimal places the risk ratios from Expression 2.9 and from the data for 2,000 pairs differ somewhat, because of rounding error in finite data for rates. This risk ratio is correct if we want the risk ratios for 10 years of follow-up, not the rate ratios. These commands do not estimate rate ratios.

Ordinary Poisson regression can estimate the rate ratio of 2.0 using an unmatched analysis; this is the same rate ratio estimated above by the **ir** command. If the Poisson model is limited to the pairs with one or two deaths, but ignores the matching, the rate ratio estimate is biased at 2.41. When data are restricted to the matched-pairs with an outcome, an unmatched analysis of rates will usually be biased.

If Poisson regression is used with pairid as an indicator variable, the model would create 2,000 estimates; this is a clumsy approach. Conditional Poisson regression can produce the same result with less output:

```
. xtset pairid
      panel variable:  pairid (balanced)

. xtpoisson died exposed, exp(time) fe irr nolog
note: 1473 groups (2946 obs) dropped because of all zero outcomes

Conditional fixed-effects Poisson regression    Number of obs    =    1,054
Group variable: pairid                           Number of groups =      527

                                                 Obs per group:
                                                              min =        2
                                                              avg =      2.0
                                                              max =        2

                                                 Wald chi2(1)     =   130.47
Log likelihood = -670.46524                      Prob > chi2      =   0.0000

------------------------------------------------------------------------------
       died |      IRR    Std. Err.      z    P>|z|     [95% Conf. Interval]
------------+-----------------------------------------------------------------
    exposed |  3.199792   .3258224    11.42   0.000     2.620881    3.906576
   ln(time) |        1   (exposure)
------------------------------------------------------------------------------
```

The result, a rate ratio of 3.2, is biased. Why? In this analysis, conditional Poisson regression is comparing each exposed subject with their randomly matched unexposed person, using all follow-up time. For a paired analysis of rate ratios for single outcome events, such as death, this is not the comparison we want. Imagine that the exposed person died at 2.1 years and the unexposed person lived to 7.1 years. Within that pair, the exposed person who died at 2.1 years can be compared with their matched unexposed person who was still alive at 2.1 years. The fact that the unexposed person lived for another 5 years is not relevant, because after 2.1 years they are the only person remaining alive in the matched set and their outcome during this additional survival time cannot be compared with that of anyone else. Only the comparison at 2.1 years is pertinent. In a matched-pair with two deaths, the person-time of the first person to die is used for the comparison and the additional survival time of the other person is not pertinent.

Think of this another way. The matched pair comparison only used the pairs with 1 or more deaths. Everyone who died is in one of these pairs, so the dead and their person-time were fully represented in the matched analysis. However, only 165 (10%) of the 1,638 exposed people who survived were used in the matched analysis, compared with 337 (19%) of the 1,810 unexposed survivors. So relatively more person-time from unexposed survivors, compared with exposed survivors, was included in the pairs with one death. This can be characterized as a type of selection bias, in which more person-time from unexposed subjects was brought into the analysis. This bias arose because people were selected into the pairs based upon their outcome or the outcome of their matched person. We can see this differential selection of person-time using the **ir** command:

```
. ir died exposed time if sumdied>0
                 | Exposed                |
                 | Exposed   Unexposed  |   Total
-----------------+----------------------+-----------
          Died |     362         190  |      552
  Time to death or | 3401.921    4307.511  |  7709.432
-----------------+----------------------+-----------
                 |                      |
  Incidence rate | .1064105    .044109  |  .0716006
                 |                      |
                 |   Point estimate     |  [95% Conf. Interval]
                 |----------------------+------------------------
  Inc. rate diff. |      .0623015        |  .0496723    .0749306
  Inc. rate ratio |     2.412443        |  2.018402    2.890882 (exact)
  Attr. frac. ex. |      .5854824        |  .5045587    .6540848 (exact)
  Attr. frac. pop |      .3839577        |
                 +-----------------------------------------------
```

In the stratified analysis the rate ratio is 2.4, biased upward compared with the true rate ratio of 2. But the biased rate ratio from the matched **xtpoisson, fe** analysis was even larger, 3.2. The matched analysis further exaggerated the effect of the selection bias by more frequently pairing dead exposed persons who had short survival intervals with unexposed 10-year survivors, compared to the opposite comparison of dead unexposed persons with long-term exposed survivors.

The Cox proportional hazards model can make the desired comparison. In the jargon of survival analysis, the matched sets are called risk sets. When only one living person remains in a risk set, their additional follow-up time is correctly ignored; this is what the Cox model does. The use of the Cox model for paired data was described by Walker and colleagues (Walker et al. 1981, Walker 1982, Walker et al. 1983) in articles about vasectomy and myocardial infarction. To use this model, we had to provide Stata information about time and the failure variable:

```
. stset time, failure(died) id(id)

                id:  id
     failure event:  died != 0 & died < .
obs. time interval:  (time[_n-1], time]
 exit on or before:  failure


- - - - - - - - - - - - - - - - - - - - - - - - - - - - - - - - - - - - - - - - -
        4000  total observations
           0  exclusions
- - - - - - - - - - - - - - - - - - - - - - - - - - - - - - - - - - - - - - - - -
        4000  observations remaining, representing
        4000  subjects
         552  failures in single-failure-per-subject data
   37169.432  total analysis time at risk and under observation
                                           at risk from t =        0
                                  earliest observed entry t =        0
                                      last observed exit t =       10
```

Using all the data and ignoring the matching, the Cox model can get the unbiased rate ratio:

```
. stcox exposed, nolog
        failure _d:  died
  analysis time _t:  time
               id:  id


Cox regression – no ties
No. of subjects =          4,000          Number of obs   =       4,000
No. of failures =            552
Time at risk    = 37169.43213
                                          LR chi2(1)      =       63.19
Log likelihood =   -4506.8209            Prob > chi2     =      0.0000


- - - - - - - - - - - - - - - - - - - - - - - - - - - - - - - - - - - - - - - - -
      _t | Haz. Ratio   Std. Err.      z    P>|z|     [95% Conf. Interval]
- - - - - - - + - - - - - - - - - - - - - - - - - - - - - - - - - - - - - - - - -
 exposed |   2.000408    .1792247    7.74   0.000     1.678247    2.384411
- - - - - - - - - - - - - - - - - - - - - - - - - - - - - - - - - - - - - - - - -
```

This output used all the data. This is not terribly useful, as we can get the same rate ratio from ordinary Poisson regression or the **ir** command. More useful is the fact that we can do a matched (or stratified) analysis limited to the pairs with an outcome, as shown here:

```
. stcox exposed if sumdied>0, strata(pairid) nolog
        failure _d:  died
  analysis time _t:  time
               id:  id
Stratified Cox regr. – no ties

No. of subjects =          1,054          Number of obs   =       1,054
No. of failures =            552
Time at risk    = 7709.432127
```

```
                                          LR chi2(1)       =     59.23
Log likelihood =    -335.67354            Prob > chi2      =    0.0000

------------------------------------------------------------------------
     _t | Haz. Ratio   Std. Err.      z    P>|z|    [95% Conf. Interval]
--------+---------------------------------------------------------------
exposed |   1.994318    .1842001    7.47   0.000     1.664085    2.390086
------------------------------------------------------------------------
                                                   Stratified by pairid
```

The regression model here used data from only 1,054 of the 4,000 records. The rate ratio of 1.9943 is an excellent estimate of the true rate ratio of 2.0. Due to sampling variation (or "chance" if you like) this differs slightly from the rate ratio of 2.0004 produced when all 4,000 records were used. The SE is only slightly larger and the Z-statistic slightly smaller.

The Poisson and Cox models are mathematically equivalent (Whitehead 1980, Laird and Olivier 1981, Royston and Lambert 2011 pp47–62) if they are parameterized in the same way. The output from a stratified Cox model with the Breslow method for tied survival times, shown above, can be exactly replicated by a conditional Poisson model. To do this, and show that it works using only matched sets with a death, start by keeping only the pairs with a death, designate the time variable, and tell Stata that we have one record only for each person in the data, indicated by the variable "id":

```
. keep if sumdied>0
(2,946 observations deleted)

. stset time, failure(died) id(id)

              id:  id
   failure event:  died != 0 & died < .
obs. time interval:  (time[_n-1], time]
 exit on or before:  failure

------------------------------------------------------------------------
    1054  total observations
       0  exclusions
------------------------------------------------------------------------
    1054  observations remaining, representing
    1054  subjects
     552  failures in single-failure-per-subject data
7709.432  total analysis time at risk and under observation
                                        at risk from t =         0
                                earliest observed entry t =         0
                                 last observed exit t =        10
```

Next invoke the **stsplit** command (meaning survival time split) to divide survival time into separate intervals at each failure time within the pairs. The command creates a new variable, riskset, which identifies the risk sets that we wish to compare:

```
. stsplit, at(failures) strata(pairid) riskset(riskset)
(552 failure times)
(527 observations (episodes) created)
```

```
. replace died=0 if died==.
(527 real changes made)
```

To show the new risk set data, I list below the records for pairid 5. The exposed person died at 7.833 years. This pair is now in risk set number 1. The time for both subjects has been set to 7.833 years, corresponding to the time of the first death in pairid 5. The unexposed person actually lived to the end of the 10-year follow-up. That person's data is shown in the list, but they are now assigned a missing riskset number. In a conditional Poisson analysis stratified on riskset, this record with 10 years of follow-up will contribute nothing:

```
+--------------------------------------------+
| pairid  riskset  exposed   died       time |
|--------------------------------------------|
|      5        1      No      No   7.8326905 |
|      5        1      Yes    Yes   7.8326905 |
|      5        .      No      No          10 |
+--------------------------------------------+
```

Below I list records for pair 29 in which both persons died. The exposed person died at 3.468 years. The unexposed person lived and they are now assigned the same follow-up time, 3.468 years. The unexposed person actually died at 4.239 years, but they are now alone in risk set number 9; because they are alone in this risk set, their actual time of death will be ignored in the matched analysis:

```
+--------------------------------------------+
| pairid  riskset  exposed   died       time |
|--------------------------------------------|
|     29        8      No      No   3.4675039 |
|     29        8      Yes    Yes   3.4675039 |
|     29        9      No     Yes   4.2385716 |
+--------------------------------------------+
```

Next I defined the stratifying (matching) variable for the conditional Poisson model and then produce the regression results here:

```
. xtset riskset
     panel variable:  riskset (unbalanced)

. xtpoisson died exposed, exp(time) fe irr nolog
note: 25 groups (25 obs) dropped because of only one obs per group

Conditional fixed-effects Poisson regression      Number of obs     =      1,054
Group variable: riskset                            Number of groups  =        527

                                                   Obs per group:
                                                                 min =          2
                                                                 avg =        2.0
                                                                 max =          2

                                                   Wald chi2(1)      =      55.86
Log likelihood = -335.67354                        Prob > chi2       =     0.0000
```

```
----------------------------------------------------------------
     died |      IRR    Std. Err.      z    P>|z|    [95% Conf. Interval]
---------+------------------------------------------------------
  exposed |  1.994318   .1842001    7.47   0.000    1.664085    2.390086
 ln(time) |        1   (exposure)
----------------------------------------------------------------
```

The output reports that 25 observations were dropped. Those were the additional hypothetical persons who were assigned alone to their own risk set when there were two deaths in a pair and they were the second person to die. An example for riskset 9, pairid 29, was shown earlier. The conditional Poisson model produces rate ratio estimates that are identical to the hazard ratios from the Cox model. This shows the equivalence of Cox and Poisson models when similarly parameterized and shows that both can estimate unbiased rate (or hazard) ratios from matched sets with at least one outcome. If we use the **stcox** command again but stratify on the riskset variable, the resulting estimates will be the same as those above (output not shown).

A key point in this section is that when person-time varied, as it did in this example, the unmatched analysis was unbiased, but a matched analysis produced a biased estimate unless steps were taken to compare persons within the matched sets (or risk sets) who had equal amounts of follow-up time.

20.14 MATCHED ANALYSIS OF RATES FOR RECURRENT EVENTS

Imagine data for a cohort study with 20,000 subjects who were followed for an outcome that could recur. All persons were followed for 2 years. Half the group had an outcome rate of 0.1 per year. The other half was exposed to a factor that doubled this event rate. The distribution of event outcomes for the cohort members were generated from Poisson processes for rates of 0.1 and 0.2, using Expression 4.1; some rounding was necessary for this finite sample. The event counts are shown according to exposure status:

```
Outcome |
  event |    Exposed
  count |    No      Yes |    Total
--------+----------------+-------
      0 |  8,187   6,703 |   14,890
      1 |  1,637   2,681 |    4,318
      2 |    164     536 |      700
      3 |     11      72 |       83
      4 |      1       7 |        8
      5 |      0       1 |        1
--------+----------------+-------
  Total | 10,000  10,000 |   20,000
```

A summary of the counts, person-time of observation, and the rate ratio are shown here using the **ir** command:

```
. ir events exposed time

                | Exposed            |
                | Exposed  Unexposed |      Total
----------------+--------------------+---------
Outcome event co |    4002      2002  |      6004
    Person-time  |   20000     20000  |     40000
----------------+--------------------+---------
                |                    |
 Incidence rate |   .2001      .1001 |     .1501
                |                    |
                | Point estimate     | [95% Conf. Interval]
                |--------------------+----------------
Inc. rate diff. |         .1         | .0924066   .1075934
Inc. rate ratio |     1.999001       | 1.894093   2.110232   (exact)
                +------------------------------------------
```

The rate ratio differed from 2.0 only because of rounding in the counts, which produced an excess of four deaths in these data. A pseudo-random number generator was used to match each exposed person to someone not exposed. This mimics what could occur in a randomized trial with block sizes of 2. The matching variable is not a confounder in this example.

If we ignore the matching, ordinary Poisson regression will produce these results:

```
. poisson events exposed, exp(time) irr nolog

Poisson regression               Number of obs   =   20,000
(output omitted)


------------------------------------------------------------------------
   events |    IRR     Std. Err.      z    P>|z|    [95% Conf. Interval]
---------+--------------------------------------------------------------
 exposed | 1.999001   .0547221    25.30   0.000    1.894574    2.109184
   _cons |    .1001   .0022372  -102.98   0.000    .0958098    .1045823
ln(time) |        1   (exposure)
------------------------------------------------------------------------
```

A matched analysis of the pairs with an outcome can produce the same results:

```
. xtset pairid
      panel variable: pairid (balanced)


. xtpoisson events exposed, exp(time) fe irr nolog
note: 5507 groups (11014 obs) dropped because of all zero outcomes

Conditional fixed-effects Poisson regression   Number of obs    =   8,986
Group variable: pairid                         Number of groups =   4,493
(output omitted)
```

```
-------------------------------------------------------------------
    events |      IRR  Std. Err.       z    P>|z|    [95% Conf. Interval]
--------+----------------------------------------------------------
   exposed |  1.999001  .0547221    25.30   0.000    1.894574    2.109184
 ln(time) |        1  (exposure)
-------------------------------------------------------------------
```

The output above is based on 4,493 of the original 10,000 matched-pairs. This example shows that a matched analysis limited to pairs with the outcome can reproduce the rate ratio estimates of an unmatched analysis, with the same SEs. Because of this equivalence, investigators often ignore any blocking in the analysis of a randomized trial.

Because the matching variable was not a confounder of the exposure-event association, ordinary Poisson analysis limited to the matched pairs with at least one outcome can also produce the same rate ratio and SE:

```
. poisson events exposed if sumevents>0, exp(time) irr nolog
Poisson regression                              Number of obs   =    8,986
(output omitted)
```

```
-------------------------------------------------------------------
    events |      IRR  Std. Err.       z    P>|z|    [95% Conf. Interval]
--------+----------------------------------------------------------
   exposed |  1.999001  .0547221    25.30   0.000    1.894574    2.109184
     _cons |   .222791  .0049793   -67.18   0.000    .2132425    .2327671
 ln(time) |        1  (exposure)
-------------------------------------------------------------------
```

Now imagine that the matching was done on a potential confounding characteristic which doubled the event rates, a variable called "confounder." The yearly event rates for the exposed (0.2) and unexposed (0.1) are just as before, but the matched pairs can now be classified as follows: (1) 1,000 pairs in which all had the confounding characteristic and all were exposed, (2) 3,000 pairs with the confounding characteristic and 1 member of each pair exposed; (3) 1,000 pairs without the confounding characteristic and 1 member exposed; and (4) 5,000 pairs without the confounder and no one exposed. The confounding characteristic is found more often in the exposed than those unexposed. Consequently, a Poisson regression model that fails to include the confounder produces a biased estimate of the exposure association:

```
. poisson events exposed, exp(time) irr nolog
```

```
Poisson regression                              Number of obs   =    20,000
(output omitted)
```

```
-------------------------------------------------------------------
    events |      IRR  Std. Err.       z    P>|z|    [95% Conf. Interval]
--------+----------------------------------------------------------
   exposed |  3.026117  .0691167    48.48   0.000    2.893638    3.164661
     _cons |    .12125   .002081  -122.94   0.000    .1172392     .125398
 ln(time) |        1  (exposure)
-------------------------------------------------------------------
```

If the confounder is added to the Poisson model, the unbiased estimate of 2.0 is produced:

```
   ----------------------------------------------------------------
     events |      IRR   Std. Err.       z   P>|z|    [95% Conf. Interval]
   ---------+------------------------------------------------------
    exposed |  2.003296  .0564155    24.67   0.000     1.89572    2.116977
 confounder |  2.001822   .059311    23.43   0.000    1.888886    2.121511
      _cons |  .0998208  .0020065  -114.64   0.000    .0959647    .1038319
   ln(time) |         1  (exposure)
   ----------------------------------------------------------------
```

But if the data are limited to the 5,005 matched pairs with at least one outcome event, the ordinary Poisson model produces biased estimates:

```
   ----------------------------------------------------------------
     events |      IRR   Std. Err.       z   P>|z|    [95% Conf. Interval]
   ---------+------------------------------------------------------
    exposed |  1.827531  .0417409    26.40   0.000    1.747525    1.911201
      _cons |  .2899231  .0049758   -72.14   0.000     .280333    .2998414
   ln(time) |         1  (exposure)
   ----------------------------------------------------------------
```

If we adjust for the confounding variable in the 5,005 pairs with an outcome, the Poisson regression rate ratio is still biased: 1.78. This bias arises because person-time is removed from the analysis in a differential manner related to the confounding variable. Conditional Poisson regression can give us the unbiased estimate using only the 5,005 pairs with an outcome:

```
. xtpoisson events exposed if sumevents>0, exp(time) fe irr nolog

Conditional fixed-effects Poisson regression   Number of obs    =   10,010
Group variable: pairid                          Number of groups =    5,005
(output omitted)
```

```
   ----------------------------------------------------------------
     events |      IRR   Std. Err.       z   P>|z|    [95% Conf. Interval]
   ---------+------------------------------------------------------
    exposed |  2.002144  .0655473    21.20   0.000    1.877709    2.134826
   ln(time) |         1  (exposure)
   ----------------------------------------------------------------
```

You probably noticed that the ordinary Poisson model that used all the data and adjusted for the confounder produced a rate ratio for the exposed of 2.0033 (SE 0.056) that was slightly different from the conditional Poisson regression estimate of 2.0021 (SE 0.066). If we use only the 8,000 pairs discordant on exposed status, the ordinary Poisson model produces exactly the same estimates as the conditional model:

```
. poisson events exposed confounder, exp(time) irr nolog

Poisson regression                              Number of obs    =    8,000
(output omitted)
```

```
    events |     IRR Std. Err.     z    P>|z|   [95% Conf. Interval]
-----------+------------------------------------------------------------
   exposed | 2.002144 .0655473  21.20  0.000    1.877709    2.134826
confounder |        2 .0881917  15.72  0.000    1.834406    2.180542
     _cons | .0999286 .0046263 -49.75  0.000    .0912603    .1094202
  ln(time) |        1 (exposure)
-----------+------------------------------------------------------------
```

The **xtpoisson, fe** command produced the unbiased rate ratio using only the matched pairs with at least one outcome. It can do this even if we cannot measure the size of the potential confounder; only matching on the confounder is needed. The conditional fixed-effects Poisson analysis is the method Farrington and others used for studies of rates using the self-controlled case series design (Farrington 1995, Farrington, Nash, and Miller 1996, Whitaker et al. 2006, Whitaker 2008, Whitaker, Hocine, and Farrington 2009). Those studies compared different time intervals with exposure and outcome information for the same person. The design has been helpful in examining the safety of vaccines; for example, by estimating the rate ratio of febrile seizures during time intervals after vaccination, compared with time intervals without vaccination. The design limits data collection to cases only, those who have had the outcome event, thereby greatly decreasing the cost of these studies.

20.15 THE RANDOMIZED TRIAL OF EXERCISE AND FALLS; ADDITIONAL ANALYSES

Recall the randomized trial of exercise and falls, described in Chapters 12 (Table 12.1) and 13 (Table 13.1). Some would argue that since blocking was used in the randomization, the blocking should be part of the analysis. None of the results in Table 13.1 did this, except for the last analysis which re-randomized both the block sizes and the subjects within each block. Even in that analysis the rate ratio estimate after each set of treatment re-assignments was a simple comparison of those treated with those not, not an analysis that incorporated the blocks.

The investigators used blocking to promote balance between the two treatment arms, hoping this would increase statistical efficiency. Blocking ensured that exercise and control subjects were enrolled at similar times and blocking was done within each center. Because of the blocking, possible confounding by center and calendar time was effectively removed, regardless of whether blocking was formally incorporated into the analysis. As mentioned previously, there was little reason to think that blocking would influence the SEs for a rate ratio outcome (Greenland and Morgenstern 1990, Rosenberger and Lachin 2002 pp124–126, Rothman, Greenland, and Lash 2008b p175). Nevertheless, some may argue that the blocks should have been used in the analysis.

Using ordinary Poisson regression with a robust variance, the rate ratio for falling, comparing the exercise group with the control group, was 0.752, with SE 0.139, P-value 0.125. Using Poisson regression with indicator variables for each block and a robust variance, the rate ratio was 0.743, SE 0.119, P-value 0.063. Using conditional Poisson regression with conditioning on blocks and the robust variance, the rate ratio was 0.743, SE 0.120, P-value 0.067. Both analyses that used the blocking produced identical rate ratios, but slightly different SEs and P-values. This was because, as explained in Section 20.12, the two methods use slightly different formulae for the robust variance.

I previously claimed that when the data are complete, unmatched and matched analyses will produce the same results. So why did ordinary Poisson regression estimate a rate ratio of 0.752 and conditional Poisson regression estimated 0.743? These data are not complete in two respects. First, at one study site the last block enrolled only 1 person. The data from that person was used in the ordinary Poisson model, but contributed nothing to the matched analyses. Second, 13 people dropped out early, creating imbalance regarding person-time within some of the blocks. If the time for these 13 persons is reset to 1 and the unmatched person in the last block is omitted, then the matched and unmatched analyses produce identical rate ratios.

Since the blocked analyses produced a somewhat smaller SE and P-value, should that be preferred? I repeated the rerandomization using the blocking methods of the original trial and this time I used conditional Poisson regression, conditioned on the block identifiers, to analyze each of the 199,999 rerandomized datasets. The final result was a rate ratio of 0.74, a P-value of 0.13, and a 95% CI of 0.51 to 1.08, little different from most results in Table 13.1. Perhaps the most important lesson here is that matched and unmatched analyses may differ due to dropouts and missing data.

20.16 FINAL WORDS

In a cohort study or randomized controlled trial, matching may sometimes be a good choice for reducing confounding bias. A matched design and analysis may or may not be more statistically efficient. If matching is used, a matched analysis may be required to remove bias due to the matching factors. If data are only available for matched sets with 1 or more outcomes, by design or for other reasons, a matched analysis can produce unbiased odds, risk, rate, or hazard ratios. In data limited to matched sets with an outcome, an unmatched analysis will usually be biased.

Marginal Methods

21

Stata has **postestimation** commands for extracting information from a regression model. Especially useful are **lincom** (for linear comparisons of estimated coefficients), **nlcom** (for non-linear comparisons), and **predict** (to estimate predicted means, probabilities, rates, and other statistics). Typing "help poisson postestimation" in Stata's command window will produce a list of commands that can be used after Poisson regression. Among these are **margins, margins contrast**, and **marginsplot**, commands that can manipulate predicted means, probabilities, counts, or rates from a regression model. Several authors have discussed aspects of marginal methods (Lane and Nelder 1982, Flanders and Rhodes 1987, Greenland and Holland 1991, Localio, Margolis, and Berlin 2007, Greenland, Rothman, and Lash 2008b pp67–68, Greenland 2008c pp386–388). This chapter illustrates some uses for marginal methods.

21.1 WHAT ARE MARGINS?

Statisticians distinguish between marginal and conditional probabilities (Lindsey 1995 pp9–10, Wikipedia). Suppose we have data for men and women, age 40 and 60 years, who are followed for 1 year for the occurrence of death. What is the probability (risk within 1 year) of death for a man? The answer surely depends on whether the man is age 40 or 60. We could separately calculate the proportion that died for men age 40 and men age 60. Those two proportions would be a good first guess at the *conditional* probabilities; probabilities for death conditional on whether the man is 40 or 60. If we prefer an answer that ignores age, we could just calculate the proportion of all men who died. That would be a good first guess at a *marginal* probability, because the ages of the men are not part of the probability estimate.

A statistician could improve on the rough proportions in the previous paragraph. The statistician might reason that the probability of death for 60-year-olds, divided by the probability for 40-year-olds, may be alike for men and women. Similarly, the probability of death for men, divided by that for women, may be the same for persons age 40 and persons age 60. Using stratified or regression methods, joint probabilities can be estimated for men age 40, men age 60, women age 40, and women age 60. In the past, statisticians used to put joint probabilities into a table and sum or average them in the table margins; the term *marginal* probability came into use. To calculate the probability of death for a man, add up the *predicted* probabilities for all men and divide by the number of men to get the average marginal probability across the age distribution of the men. Marginal probabilities, marginal rates, and other marginal statistics are quantities estimated using the joint distribution of the variables in a regression model.

21.2 CONVERTING LOGISTIC REGRESSION RESULTS INTO RISK RATIOS OR RISK DIFFERENCES: MARGINAL STANDARDIZATION

Start with a simple case: a short description of how marginal commands work for probabilities estimated by logistic regression. Suppose we have cohort data for death within a year. Assume we fit a logistic model for the outcome of death with two explanatory variables: male sex and age (40 or 60 years). Maximum likelihood is used to fit the model, which can then estimate four joint probabilities; one each for females 40, females 60, males 40 and males 60. We can use **margins** to extract the average predicted probabilities of death for males, "adjusted" for age. The software will first treat everyone in the data as if they were male. The joint probabilities used for each subject will be those for males only at each age, but the age distribution for the marginal average probability will be that of *all* persons in the data, males and females. The method sums up joint probabilities and divides by the number of persons (or records) in the data. The resulting average probability is *standardized* to the age distribution of the entire regression sample, regardless of sex. Unless males and females happen to have the same age distribution, or age is unrelated to death, this age-standardized probability for males will differ from the average probability computed from male subjects alone. To estimate the average age-standardized probability, or risk, for females, the software will use the model predicted joint probabilities of death for females at each age and the same age distribution, which includes the ages of the males.

The marginal average probabilities for men and women are standardized to the same age distribution and a ratio or difference comparison of these predicted risks will be free of confounding bias related to age, provided the adjustment for age in the logistic model was adequate. This method is sometimes called *marginal standardization* and it has been used to obtain adjusted risk ratios and risk differences from logistic regression models (Greenland and Holland 1991, Greenland 2004, Localio, Margolis, and Berlin 2007, Cummings 2009a, 2011). This is also called the counterfactual mean marginal prediction, because the marginal rate for males treats the records for females as if they were for males, counter to the fact that they were for females.

21.3 ESTIMATING A RATE DIFFERENCE FROM A RATE RATIO MODEL

Marginal standardization of rates is similar to what has just been described for risks. The **margins, predict(ir)** command creates a weighted-average of rates, weighted by the distribution of the data records according to their classification by the regression variables.

Chapter 10 discussed regression models which can produce adjusted rate differences. But I pointed out that rate difference models often fail to converge and rates may be more homogeneous on a multiplicative scale compared with an additive scale. Fitting a rate ratio model and then using **margins** to estimate an adjusted rate difference can be useful in two situations. First, if an adjusted rate difference is desired but there is difficulty fitting the rate difference regression model, the **margins** command may be used to obtain the adjusted rate difference from a rate ratio model. Second, there may be evidence that the rate ratio model is preferred because it has a superior fit to the data. If an adjusted rate difference is still desired, it may be best to extract information from the ratio model to produce the adjusted rate difference. The following examples show how this is done.

21.4 DEATH BY AGE AND SEX: A SHORT EXAMPLE

Women (12,000) and men (6,000), classified by age (40 or 60 years) were followed until death or for 1 year, whichever interval was shortest (Table 21.1). Mortality was lowest, 1 per 100 person-years, among women age 40 and was twice as great among women age 60. At age 40 the male rate was twofold that of females at the same age, but at age 60 the male rate was only 1.8-fold greater than that of females age 60. Assuming these true rates did not change as age increased during follow-up, the observed "counts" (not rounded to an integer) of deaths can be calculated from Expression 2.6 and observed person-years from Expression 2.7. A Poisson rate ratio model applied to these data is below:

```
. poisson deaths i.male i.age, exp(time100) irr nolog
note: you are responsible for interpretation of noncount dep. variable

Poisson regression                        Number of obs  =         4
                                          LR chi2(2)     =      7.28
                                          Prob > chi2    =    0.0263
Log likelihood = -7.8612002               Pseudo R2      =    0.3164

------------------------------------------------------------------------
     deaths |      IRR    Std. Err.      z    P>|z|    [95% Conf. Interval]
------------------------------------------------------------------------
       male |
       Male | 1.920011    .6138561    2.04   0.041    1.026035   3.592903
            |
        age |
         60 | 1.950015    .7731289    1.68   0.092     .8965181   4.241472
      _cons | 1.0204      .3946764    0.05   0.958     .4781208   2.177726
ln(time100) |        1   (exposure)
------------------------------------------------------------------------
```

This Poisson model constrained the rates for men, divided by those for women, to be the same at both age 40 and 60: the maximum likelihood estimate was a ratio of 1.92. The true ratio of male to female rates at age 40 was 2.0 and at age 60 it was 1.8 (Table 21.1), but the true rates would not be known. Without that knowledge, we usually assume that the variation in the ratios is what we expect in finite samples. Similarly, the rate ratio of 1.95 for age 60 versus 40 falls between the true age ratios of 2.0 for women and 1.8 for men. The Poisson model used an iterative algorithm to find the two coefficients, ln(1.92) and ln(1.95), that fit best into Expression 9.3. (In this example, an interaction term between age and sex had a rate ratio of 0.95 and a P-value of 0.9. This suggests that the reduced, or constrained, model, without the interaction term, is sufficient.)

TABLE 21.1 Women (12,000) and men (6,000) were followed for 1 year or until death, whichever came first. Death "counts" and person-years rounded to three decimals. Rates shown per 100 person-years, person-years in units of 100.

SEX	AGE (YEARS)	COUNT OF PERSONS	DEATHS	PERSON-YEARS (100)	MORTALITY RATE
Female	40	4000	3.998	3.998	1.0
Female	60	8000	15.984	7.992	2.0
Male	40	2000	3.966	1.998	2.0
Male	60	4000	15.171	3.992	3.8

Stata commands can be used to obtain jointly predicted rates and marginal rates:

```
. poisson deaths i.male i.age, exp(time100) irr nolog
(output omitted)

. * create a variable that preserves the original coding for males
. gen oldmale = male

. * recode all records as if they were for females
. replace male = 0
(2 real changes made)

. * predict the joint age-sex rates for each record as if all were female:
ratef
. predict double ratef, ir

. * Now get the predicted rates treating all records as male: ratem
. replace male = 1
(4 real changes made)

. predict double ratem, ir

. /* get the average of the female only and male only rates. These are
> marginal rates, so we will dub these mratef and mratem */
. summ ratef, meanonly

. scalar mratef = r(mean)

. summ ratem, meanonly

. scalar mratem = r(mean)

. * reset male back to the original coding:
. replace male = oldmale
(2 real changes made)

. * list true (trate) and predicted rates
. list male age trate ratem ratef, sepby(male)

    +-------------------------------------+
    | male   age   trate      ratem       ratef   |
    |-------------------------------------|
 1. | Female   40   .001   1.9591795      1.0204   |
 2. | Female   60   .002   3.8204286   1.9897949   |
    |-------------------------------------|
 3. |   Male   40   .002   1.9591795      1.0204   |
 4. |   Male   60   .0038  3.8204286   1.9897949   |
    +-------------------------------------+

. * display the marginal rates
. di "Marginal male rate = " mratem _skip(4) "Marginal female rate = " mratef
Marginal male rate = 2.8898041   Marginal female rate = 1.5050975
```

. /* show that the ratio of marginal rates is the rate ratio for males vs
females
> which was estimated by the Poisson regression model */
. di "Age-adjusted rate ratio for males vs females: " mratem/mratef
Age-adjusted rate ratio for males vs females: 1.9200113

Instead of all of these commands, it is easier to let the margins command do all this and produce
other statistics as well:

. margins male, predict(ir)

```
Predictive margins                              Number of obs   =      4
Model VCE    : OIM

Expression   : Predicted incidence rate, predict(ir)
-----------------------------------------------------------------------
             |            Delta-method
             |   Margin  Std. Err.      z    P>|z|   [95% Conf. Interval]
----------- +----------------------------------------------------------
      male |
    Female |  1.505097  .3461795    4.35   0.000    .826598   2.183597
      Male |  2.889804  .6778854    4.26   0.000   1.561173   4.218435
-----------------------------------------------------------------------
```

. * calculate the difference of the marginal rates
. margins r.male, predict(ir)

```
Contrasts of predictive margins
Model VCE    : OIM

Expression   : Predicted incidence rate, predict(ir)

--------------------------------------
             |   df    chi2   P>chi2
------- +-----------------------------
      male |    1    3.46   0.0630
--------------------------------------


------------------------------------------------------
             |            Delta-method
             |  Contrast   Std. Err.   [95% Conf. Interval]
------------- +----------------------------------------
          male |
(Male vs Female) |  1.384707  .7446655   -.0748109  2.844224
------------------------------------------------------
```

These commands give a quick overview of what predict and margins can do. More details follow in
the next example.

21.5 SKUNK BITE DATA: A LONG EXAMPLE

Bites due to striped skunks are common in Hediondo, New Mexico. Women and the elderly are fanged more often because they cannot flee as fast as young men. Many Hediondo residents have recently started taking a vitamin pill that causes their sweat to emit an odor which attracts skunks, resulting in more skunk bites for vitamin users.

The Hediondo Department of Health has data for a random sample of 7,500 residents who took the vitamin daily and similar data for 7,500 vitamin-abstainers (Table 21.2). All were followed for 1 year or until their first skunk bite, whichever interval was shorter. Members of both cohorts were age 40, 45, 50, 55, or 60 years. The following are true: (1) the lowest skunk bite rate was 1 per 1,000 person-years among 40-year-old abstainer males, (2) the rate doubled for each 5-year age increment, (3) female rates were twice those of males, and (4) pill-taking was associated with a two-fold rate increase. Pill-takers were more often female (78% vs. 21%) and younger (mean age 47 vs. 53 years) compared with

TABLE 21.2 Hypothetical data for 15,000 persons followed to a skunk-bite or for 1 year, whichever came first. Bite rate lowest among 40-year-old men who did not take a vitamin pill. Rates twofold higher for men, multiplied by two for each 5-year increment in age, and doubled by taking the pill. Rates shown per 1,000 person-years, person-years in units of 1,000. Bite "counts" rounded to the nearest decimal, person-years rounded to nearest three decimals, but calculations in the text, from Expressions 2.6 and 2.7, used maximum computer precision.

PILL USE	SEX	AGE (YEARS)	COUNT OF PERSONS	BITES	PERSON-YEARS (1,000)	BITE RATE
Abstainer	Male	40	200	0.2	0.200	1
Abstainer	Male	45	200	0.4	0.200	2
Abstainer	Male	50	300	1.2	0.299	4
Abstainer	Male	55	400	3.2	0.398	8
Abstainer	Male	60	500	7.9	0.496	16
Abstainer	Female	40	400	0.8	0.400	2
Abstainer	Female	45	800	3.2	0.798	4
Abstainer	Female	50	1,200	9.6	1.195	8
Abstainer	Female	55	1,600	25.4	1.587	16
Abstainer	Female	60	1,900	59.8	1.870	32
Pill-taker	Male	40	1,900	3.8	1.898	2
Pill-taker	Male	45	1,600	6.4	1.597	4
Pill-taker	Male	50	1,200	9.6	1.195	8
Pill-taker	Male	55	800	12.7	0.794	16
Pill-taker	Male	60	400	12.6	0.394	32
Pill-taker	Female	40	500	2.0	0.499	4
Pill-taker	Female	45	400	3.2	0.398	8
Pill-taker	Female	50	300	4.8	0.298	16
Pill-taker	Female	55	200	6.3	0.197	32
Pill-taker	Female	60	200	12.4	0.194	64

abstainers. Assuming these true rates did not change as age increased during follow-up, the observed bite counts were calculated from Expression 2.6 and bite-free person-years from Expression 2.7. Bite counts and person-years (units of 1 thousand) were rounded for Table 21.1, but calculations for this example used bites and person-time with maximum computer precision.

21.6 OBTAINING THE RATE DIFFERENCE: CRUDE RATES

Our goal is to estimate the bite rate difference comparing vitamin pill-takers with abstainers. Rates per 1,000 person-years were used (indicated by rate1k) and person-time was in 1,000-year units (time1k). The **ir** command can calculate the crude rate ratios and differences; however, it rounds the number of bites to the nearest integer:

```
. ir bites pill time1k
                    |  Pill-taker
                    |    Exposed    Unexposed  |   Total
--------------------+--------------------------+--------
             Bites  |        74           112  |      186
  Person-time,1000  |  7.463007      7.443931  | 14.90694
--------------------+--------------------------+--------
                    |                          |
  Incidence rate    |  9.915575      15.04581  | 12.47741
                    |                          |
                    |    Point estimate        | [95% Conf. Interval]
                    |--------------------------------------------------
  Inc. rate diff.   |     -5.130238            | -8.717481   -1.542996
  Inc. rate ratio   |      .6590255            |  .4845609    .8918204
                    |                          |              (exact)
  Prev. frac. ex.   |      .3409745            |  .1081796    .5154391
                    |                          |              (exact)
  Prev. frac. pop   |      .1707054            |
                    +--------------------------------------------------
                       (midp)  Pr(k<=74)  =                   0.0025
                                                              (exact)
                       (midp) 2*Pr(k<=74) =                   0.0050
                                                              (exact)
```

Because the rates were small and follow-up short, both rate denominators, shown here, were close to the 7.5-thousand-person-years that would have been observed if no one was bitten.

Now fit a rate ratio model with only the pill (pill-taker=1, abstainer=0) variable:

```
. poisson bites i.pill, exp(time1k) irr nolog
note: you are responsible for interpretation of noncount dep. variable

Poisson regression                        Number of obs   =         20
                                          LR chi2(1)      =       7.95
                                          Prob > chi2     =     0.0048
Log likelihood = -102.31106               Pseudo R2       =     0.0374
```

```
------------------------------------------------------------------
      bites |     IRR   Std. Err.     z    P>|z|   [95% Conf. Interval]
-----------+------------------------------------------------------
       pill |
Pill-taker | .6579152  .0987386   -2.79   0.005   .4902564   .8829103
      _cons | 15.00672  1.419847   28.63   0.000   12.46666   18.06431
ln(time1k) |        1  (exposure)
------------------------------------------------------------------
```

In the model command, the prefix **i.** was placed in front of the pill variable. Stata uses **i.** to designate a variable as an indicator or factor variable. If **i.** is omitted, subsequent marginal commands will issue an error message that says "factor 'pill' not found in list of covariates". Stata means something like: "if 'pill' is a factor variable, the **i.** prefix is needed so marginal commands will know this".

The estimated rate ratio of 0.66 is biased away from the true rate ratio of 2.0 because pill-takers were often young and male, characteristics associated with lower bite rates. The bias is so great that the rate ratio suggests the vitamin prevented bites. Marginal commands can use the regression results to estimate the crude rates for pill-takers and controls:

```
. margins pill, predict(ir)

Adjusted predictions                      Number of obs    =      20
Model VCE    : OIM

Expression   : Predicted incidence rate, predict(ir)

------------------------------------------------------------------
           |           Delta-method
           |   Margin   Std. Err.     z    P>|z|   [95% Conf. Interval]
-----------+------------------------------------------------------
      pill |
 Abstainer | 15.00672  1.419847   10.57   0.000   12.22387   17.78957
Pill-taker | 9.873147  1.150193    8.58   0.000   7.618809   12.12748
------------------------------------------------------------------
```

The **predict(ir)** option produced incidence rates, rather than counts or probabilities. These rates are a bit different from those produced by the **ir** command, because **ir** rounded the counts of bites to the nearest integer. The Poisson model and **margins** used the fractional counts of bites. The crude rate for the abstainers, 15.0 can be estimated using rates for the abstainers only; the age and sex distribution of the pill-takers need not enter into the calculations. It is easy to see that this is true from the **ir** command output. You could estimate this rate without rounding error by using a Poisson model limited to abstainers only. This rate was already reported by the Poisson model shown above; it is the rate for the constant or intercept term. The same remarks apply to the crude rate for the pill-takers, 9.9. Any comparison of these crude rates is biased because nothing was been done to account for the different age and sex distributions of the pill-taking and abstainer cohorts.

We can use **margins, contrast** to get the crude rate difference, 15.0 − 9.9 = -5.1, along with a P-value, standard error (SE), and confidence interval (CI):

```
. margins r.pill, predict(ir) contrast

Contrasts of adjusted predictions
Model VCE    : OIM
```

Expression : Predicted incidence rate, predict(ir)

```
-------------------------------------
          |    df    chi2   P>chi2
----------+--------------------------
     pill |     1    7.89   0.0050
-------------------------------------
```

```
----------------------------------------------------------------------
                    |              Delta-method
                    |  Contrast  Std. Err.   [95% Conf. Interval]
--------------------+-------------------------------------------------
               pill |
(Pill-taker vs Abstainer) |  -5.13357  1.827269   -8.714951  -1.552189
----------------------------------------------------------------------
```

The **r.** prefix in the **margins, contrast** command tells Stata that the reference or baseline level for pill use should be used for the comparison: this is 0 = abstainers. We can get the same results by telling **margins** to **post** the rates, which puts the rates and related information into memory, and then use **lincom** to estimate the rate difference, as shown here:

```
. margins pill, predict(ir) post
```

```
Adjusted predictions                          Number of obs   =      20
Model VCE    : OIM
```

Expression : Predicted incidence rate, predict(ir)

```
-------------------------------------------------------------------------
           |         Delta-method
           |  Margin  Std. Err.      z    P>|z|    [95% Conf. Interval]
-----------+-------------------------------------------------------------
      pill |
 Abstainer | 15.00672  1.419847   10.57   0.000    12.22387   17.78957
Pill-taker |  9.873147 1.150193    8.58   0.000     7.618809  12.12748
-------------------------------------------------------------------------
```

```
. lincom _b[1.pill] - _b[0.pill]
```

```
( 1)  - 0bn.pill + 1.pill = 0
```

```
-------------------------------------------------------------------------
       |    Coef.    Std. Err.      z     P>|z|    [95% Conf. Interval]
-------+-----------------------------------------------------------------
   (1) |  -5.13357   1.827269    -2.81    0.005    -8.714951  -1.552189
-------------------------------------------------------------------------
```

The rate difference, SE, and other statistics here are identical to those reported previously by **margins r.pill, predict(ir)**. A rate difference regression model can estimate the same rate difference statistics:

```
. glm rate pill [iweight=time1k], link(identity) family(poisson) nolog
note: rate1k has noninteger values
```

Generalized linear models	No. of obs = 20
Optimization : ML	Residual df = 18
	Scale parameter = 1
Deviance = 136.3405566	(1/df) Deviance = 7.574475
Pearson = 170.2905154	(1/df) Pearson = 9.460584
Variance function: V(u) = u	[Poisson]
Link function : g(u) = u	[Identity]
	AIC = 9.957139
Log likelihood = -97.57139395	BIC = 82.41738

```
------------------------------------------------------------------------
             |               OIM
      rate1k |   Coef.    Std. Err.     z    P>|z|    [95% Conf. Interval]
-------------+----------------------------------------------------------
        pill |  -5.13357  1.827269   -2.81   0.005   -8.714951   -1.552189
       _cons |  15.00672  1.419847   10.57   0.000   12.22387    17.78957
------------------------------------------------------------------------
```

All of this output shows that the crude rate difference from the simplest rate ratio model, assisted by marginal commands, can produce the same results as the simplest rate difference model. These models are equivalent expressions, or reparameterizations, of the same information when only a single binary explanatory variable is used.

21.7 USING THE ROBUST VARIANCE

The robust variance estimator can be used for the rate difference model:

```
. glm  rate  pill  [iw=time1k],  link(identity)  family(poisson)  nolog
vce(robust)
(output omitted)
```

```
------------------------------------------------------------------------
             |             Robust
      rate1k |   Coef.    Std. Err.     z    P>|z|    [95% Conf. Interval]
-------------+----------------------------------------------------------
        pill |  -5.13357  5.805842   -0.88   0.377   -16.51281    6.245671
       _cons |  15.00672  4.814238    3.12   0.002    5.570983   24.44245
------------------------------------------------------------------------
```

Using the robust variance changed the SE for pill exposure from 1.8 to 5.8. Exactly the same results can be produced by Poisson ratio regression with a robust variance estimator, followed by marginal commands with an unconditional variance:

```
. poisson bites i.pill, exp(time1k) irr nolog vce(robust)
(output omitted)
```

```
----------------------------------------------------------------------
             |                Robust
       bites |    IRR     Std. Err.     z    P>|z|   [95% Conf. Interval]
-------------+--------------------------------------------------------
        pill |
 Pill-taker  | .6579152   .3021749   -0.91   0.362   .2674362   1.618526
       _cons | 15.00672   4.814238    8.44   0.000   8.002312   28.14206
   ln(time1k)|        1   (exposure)
----------------------------------------------------------------------
```

```
. margins r.pill, predict(ir) vce(unconditional)
```

Contrasts of adjusted predictions

Expression   : Predicted incidence rate, predict(ir)

```
------------------------------------
        |    df    chi2   P>chi2
--------+---------------------------
   pill |     1    0.78   0.3766
------------------------------------
```

```
----------------------------------------------------------------------
                            |         Unconditional
                            | Contrast  Std. Err.    [95% Conf. Interval]
----------------------------+-----------------------------------------
                       pill |
  (Pill-taker vs Abstainer) | -5.13357  5.805842    -16.51281   6.245671
----------------------------------------------------------------------
```

21.8 ADJUSTING FOR AGE

In earlier output, both the rate ratio (0.66) and the rate difference (–5.1) were biased. Adjusting for age can remove some of this confounding bias. In the models shown here, the variable age5 = (age–40)/5 expresses age as a linear term using units equal to 5 years:

```
. poisson bites i.pill age5, exp(time1k) irr nolog
note: you are responsible for interpretation of noncount dep. variable
```

```
Poisson regression                        Number of obs   =         20
                                          LR chi2(2)      =     129.95
                                          Prob > chi2     =     0.0000
Log likelihood = -41.312107               Pseudo R2       =     0.6113
```

```
--------------------------------------------------------------------------
      bites |      IRR   Std. Err.      z    P>|z|     [95% Conf. Interval]
------------+-------------------------------------------------------------
       pill |
Pill-taker |  1.403691   .2251515    2.11   0.035     1.025036    1.922224
      age5 |  2.033825   .1440018   10.03   0.000     1.770295    2.336585
      _cons |   1.69259   .4412517    2.02   0.044     1.015422    2.821349
ln(time1k) |         1  (exposure)
--------------------------------------------------------------------------
```

The age-adjusted rate ratio for pill-taking (1.4) is closer to the true rate ratio (2.0), compared with the crude rate ratio, so adjustment for age in years as a linear term removed some confounding bias. Age as a linear term makes sense, because the data were created so that rates would increase by 2 for each additional 5 years of age. If we adjust for age using indicators for each level of age5 (not shown), the pill-taker rate ratio is nearly the same as in the model with age5 as a linear term. Now obtain the age-adjusted rates and rate difference for pill-use using marginal commands:

```
. margins pill, predict(ir)

Predictive margins                              Number of obs   =       20
Model VCE    : OIM

Expression   : Predicted incidence rate, predict(ir)

-----------------------------------------------------------------------------
            |            Delta-method
            |   Margin   Std. Err.      z    P>|z|     [95% Conf. Interval]
------------+----------------------------------------------------------------
       pill |
  Abstainer | 11.06726   1.065325   10.39   0.000     8.979256    13.15525
 Pill-taker | 15.53501   1.907959    8.14   0.000     11.79548    19.27454
-----------------------------------------------------------------------------

. margins r.pill, predict(ir)

Contrasts of predictive margins
Model VCE    : OIM

Expression   : Predicted incidence rate, predict(ir)

---------------------------------------
            |   df    chi2   P>chi2
------------+--------------------------
       pill |    1    3.98   0.0460
---------------------------------------


----------------------------------------------------------------------------
                         |           Delta-method
                         |  Contrast   Std. Err.    [95% Conf. Interval]
-------------------------+--------------------------------------------------
                    pill |
(Pill-taker vs Abstainer) |  4.467752   2.238791    .0798022    8.855702
----------------------------------------------------------------------------
```

The age-adjusted pill-taker rate is 15.5, larger than the crude rate of 9.9. To calculate this age-adjusted (or marginal or standardized) pill-taker rate, marginal commands obtained the joint predicted bite rates for each record in the data, using pill-use and age only, and assigned these to all the records by age level. There were two predicted rates for pill-users age 40, one for females and the other for males. These were assigned to all four of the records for persons age 40, regardless of age and actual pill-use status. The same was done for age 45, 50, and so on. The average of these 20 rates is the marginal rate for pill-takers, standardized to the distribution of all records by age. The same procedure was used to produce the marginal rate for abstainers. A ratio or difference (4.5 per 1,000 person-years) comparison of these two rates can be described as age-adjusted or age-standardized. We can show these details using Stata commands,

```
. poisson bites i.pill age5, exp(time1k) irr nolog
(output omitted)

. * next command just allows us to keep the old values for the pill variable
. gen opill = pill

. label var opill "Original pill use coding"
. label val opill pill

. * Now treat every record as an abstainer and get predicted rates for
pill==0
. replace pill = 0
(10 real changes made)

. * get the predicted rates for abstainers at each level of age
. predict double rate0, ir

. label var rate0 "Rates for abstainers at each age level"

. sort opill female age

. list opill pill female age rate1k rate0
```

```
     +-----------------------------------------------+
     |    opill        pill   female   age   rate1k      rate0 |
     |-----------------------------------------------|
  1. | Abstainer   Abstainer    Male    40        1   1.6925899 |
  2. | Abstainer   Abstainer    Male    45        2   3.4424321 |
  3. | Abstainer   Abstainer    Male    50        4   7.0013054 |
  4. | Abstainer   Abstainer    Male    55        8   14.239432 |
  5. | Abstainer   Abstainer    Male    60       16   28.960516 |
     |-----------------------------------------------|
  6. | Abstainer   Abstainer  Female    40        2   1.6925899 |
  7. | Abstainer   Abstainer  Female    45        4   3.4424321 |
  8. | Abstainer   Abstainer  Female    50        8   7.0013054 |
  9. | Abstainer   Abstainer  Female    55       16   14.239432 |
 10. | Abstainer   Abstainer  Female    60       32   28.960516 |
     |-----------------------------------------------|
 11. | Pill-taker  Abstainer    Male    40        2   1.6925899 |
 12. | Pill-taker  Abstainer    Male    45        4   3.4424321 |
 13. | Pill-taker  Abstainer    Male    50        8   7.0013054 |
```

```
14. | Pill-taker  Abstainer    Male   55    16  14.239432 |
15. | Pill-taker  Abstainer    Male   60    32  28.960516 |
    |------------------------------------------------|
16. | Pill-taker  Abstainer  Female   40     4   1.6925899 |
17. | Pill-taker  Abstainer  Female   45     8   3.4424321 |
18. | Pill-taker  Abstainer  Female   50    16   7.0013054 |
19. | Pill-taker  Abstainer  Female   55    32  14.239432 |
20. | Pill-taker  Abstainer  Female   60    64  28.960516 |
    +------------------------------------------------+
```

[In the output above, the original pill-use coding is shown in the first column, but the second column shows the recoding of all records to abstainer status. Note that there are now 4 records at age 40 with a rate of 1.69; these are abstainer rates.]

```
. * Now treat everyone (every record) as a pill-taker
. replace pill = 1
(20 real changes made)

. predict double rate1, ir

. label var rate1 "Rates for pill-takers at each age level"

. summ rate0 rate1

    Variable |    Obs     Mean   Std. Dev.     Min      Max
---------+-------------------------------------------------
      rate0 |     20  11.06726   10.1855   1.69259  28.96052
      rate1 |     20  15.53501  14.29729  2.375873  40.65162

. * recode pill use back to the original values, so margins can compute 2
rates
. replace pill = opill
(10 real changes made)

. * use margins to produce the rates
. margins pill, predict(ir)

Predictive margins                          Number of obs   =      20
Model VCE    : OIM

Expression  : Predicted incidence rate, predict(ir)

--------------------------------------------------------------------
            |            Delta-method
            |   Margin   Std. Err.    z    P>|z|   [95% Conf. Interval]
--------+-----------------------------------------------------------
       pill |
  Abstainer | 11.06726  1.065325  10.39  0.000   8.979256   13.15525
 Pill-taker | 15.53501  1.907959   8.14  0.000   11.79548   19.27454
--------------------------------------------------------------------
```

It would be nice to compare the marginal rates with a difference regression model, but that model fails to converge using age as a continuous linear term, unless the normal family is used for the error terms. The model will converge if age levels are entered as indicators, so that model is used:

```
. glm rate i.pill i.age5 [iw=time1k], link(identity) family(poisson) nolog
note: rate1k has noninteger values
```

```
Generalized linear models                   No. of obs    =        20
Optimization    : ML                        Residual df   =        14
                                            Scale parameter =       1
Deviance    =  16.9864735                   (1/df) Deviance =  1.21332
Pearson     =  18.0258181                   (1/df) Pearson  =  1.287558

Variance function: V(u) = u                 [Poisson]
Link function     : g(u) = u                [Identity]

                                            AIC           =  4.389435
Log likelihood  = -37.89435239              BIC           = -24.95378
```

```
-----------------------------------------------------------------------
             |              OIM
      rate1k |   Coef.  Std. Err.    z P>|z|    [95% Conf. Interval]
-------------+---------------------------------------------------------
        pill |
 Pill-taker  | 1.642192  1.181987  1.39  0.165  -.6744598   3.958844
             |
        age5 |
          45 | 2.230713  1.435443  1.55  0.120  -.5827038    5.04413
          50 | 6.423323  1.850007  3.47  0.001   2.797375   10.04927
          55 | 14.25602  2.454218  5.81  0.000   9.445836   19.06619
          60 | 29.87079  3.36868   8.87  0.000   23.26829   36.47328
             |
       _cons | 1.115137  .9847943  1.13  0.257  -.8150241   3.045298
-----------------------------------------------------------------------
```

Marginal commands can display the marginal rates for pill-takers and abstainers that were used to estimate the rate difference of 1.6. The **margins** command will not accept the **predict(ir)** option after this difference model, but **predict(mu)** will calculate the mean rates:

```
. margins pill, predict(mu)

Predictive margins                          Number of obs    =        20
Model VCE    : OIM

Expression  : Predicted mean rate1k, predict(mu)

-----------------------------------------------------------------------
             |           Delta-method
             | Margin  Std. Err.     z    P>|z|   [95% Conf. Interval]
-------------+---------------------------------------------------------
```

```
      pill |
Abstainer |   11.6145  1.036412  11.21  0.000   9.583171   13.64583
Pill-taker |  13.25669 1.136964  11.66  0.000   11.02828   15.4851
------------------------------------------------------------------
```

The age-adjusted rate difference for pill-munchers from the difference regression model is 1.6, unlike the estimate of 4.5 from marginal commands after fitting a rate ratio model. With adjustment, there is no reason to expect a marginal rate difference from a ratio model will be the same as the estimate from a difference regression model. We have to choose between these two estimates. Before choosing, let us examine models adjusted for both age and sex.

21.9 FULL ADJUSTMENT FOR AGE AND SEX

We will use the robust variance for a model adjusting for sex and age:

```
. poisson bites i.pill female age5, irr exp(time1k) nolog vce(robust)
note: you are responsible for interpretation of noncount dep. variable
```

```
Poisson regression                          Number of obs    =      20
                                            Wald chi2(2)     =       .
                                            Prob > chi2      =       .
Log pseudolikelihood = -34.140781           Pseudo R2        =  0.6788
------------------------------------------------------------------
            |          Robust
      bites |   IRR Std. Err.      z    P>|z|   [95% Conf. Interval]
------------+-----------------------------------------------------
       pill |
Pill-taker |     2 1.98e-08 7.0e+07  0.000       2          2
     female |     2 1.84e-08 7.5e+07  0.000       2          2
       age5 |     2 6.16e-09 2.3e+08  0.000       2          2
      _cons |     1 1.36e-08   -0.45  0.654       1          1
 ln(time1k) |     1 (exposure)
------------------------------------------------------------------
```

```
. margins pill, predict(ir) vce(unconditional)
```

```
Predictive margins                          Number of obs    =      20
```

Expression : Predicted incidence rate, predict(ir)

```
------------------------------------------------------------------
            |        Unconditional
            |  Margin Std. Err.      z    P>|z|   [95% Conf. Interval]
------------+-----------------------------------------------------
       pill |
Abstainer |     9.3 2.102755   4.42  0.000   5.178676   13.42132
Pill-taker |    18.6  4.20551   4.42  0.000   10.35735   26.84265
------------------------------------------------------------------
```

```
. margins r.pill, predict(ir) vce(unconditional)

Contrasts of predictive margins

Expression  : Predicted incidence rate, predict(ir)
-----------------------------------
           |    df     chi2   P>chi2
-----------+-----------------------
      pill |     1    19.56   0.0000
-----------------------------------


--------------------------------------------------------------------
                          |          Unconditional
                          |  Contrast   Std. Err.   [95% Conf. Interval]
--------------------------+-----------------------------------------
                   pill   |
(Pill-taker vs Abstainer) |    9.3      2.102755    5.178676   13.42132
--------------------------------------------------------------------
```

The rate difference of 9.3 for pill-swallowers cannot be compared with an estimate from a difference regression model using the Poisson family, because difference models with both age and sex would not converge. We can get an approximately correct difference model estimate using the normal family (Lumley, Kronmal, and Ma 2006), as discussed in Chapter 10:

```
. glm rate1k i.pill female age5 [iw=time1k], /*
>      */ link(identity) family(normal) nolog vce(robust)

Generalized linear models                No. of obs      =          20
Optimization    : ML                     Residual df     =          16
                                         Scale parameter =    25.03047
Deviance       = 400.4875376             (1/df) Deviance =    25.03047
Pearson        = 400.4875376             (1/df) Pearson  =    25.03047

Variance function: V(u) = 1              [Gaussian]
Link function    : g(u) = u              [Identity]

                                         AIC             =    5.003624
Log pseudolikelihood = -46.03623629      BIC             =    352.5558

--------------------------------------------------------------------
            |             Robust
     rate1k |   Coef.   Std. Err.     z     P>|z|    [95% Conf. Interval]
------------+-------------------------------------------------------
       pill |
Pill-taker  |  8.970735  3.162014    2.84   0.005    2.773302   15.16817
     female |  8.546899  2.582953    3.31   0.001    3.484405   13.60939
       age5 |  7.501181  1.045779    7.17   0.000    5.451493    9.55087
       _cons| -11.26803  4.045761   -2.79   0.005   -19.19757   -3.33848
--------------------------------------------------------------------
```

We know from the data generation process that the ratio model is preferred. Indeed, the rate ratio estimates of 2 for pill consumption, 2 for female sex, 2 for each 5-year age increase, and 1 for the intercept are exactly those used to generate these data. Further adjustment using indicators for age or for the interaction of age and sex produced no change in the adjusted rate ratio for pill-taking. Several tests indicated that the fully adjusted rate ratio model is best. A link test rejected the rate difference model but showed no evidence to reject the ratio model. So we should probably choose the rate difference of 9.3 (95% CI 5.2, 13.4) compared with the difference of 9.0 (95% CI 2.8, 15.2). The rate differences of 9.3 and 9.0 are similar. The difference model had to deal with considerable rate heterogeneity on the additive scale, which resulted in a larger CI. In this example, the difference model was not notably inaccurate, but it was statistically inefficient, compared with the ratio model.

21.10 MARGINAL COMMANDS FOR INTERACTIONS

The rate ratio for skunk bite, comparing vitamin pill-user with abstainers, was 2.0 for men and women. Homogeneity on the ratio scale indicates heterogeneity on the difference scale, because the baseline rates for male and female abstainers differed. Marginal methods can estimate the separate pill-related rate differences for men and women and test whether these differ statistically. Having picked a rate ratio model as best, we can start by formally checking whether the rate ratio for pill-swallowing varies by sex on the multiplicative scale:

```
. poisson bites i.pill##i.female age, exp(time1k) irr nolog
(output omitted)
```

```
---------------------------------------------------------------------
        bites |    IRR  Std. Err.     z   P>|z|   [95% Conf. Interval]
--------------+------------------------------------------------------
         pill |
  Pill-taker |      2  .6433185   2.15  0.031   1.064715   3.756876
              |
       female |
       Female |      2  .5916695   2.34  0.019   1.119992   3.571453
              |
  pill#female |
Pill-taker#Female | .9999999  .3808835  -0.00  1.000   .4740141   2.109641
              |
          age | 1.148698  .0161916   9.83  0.000   1.117398   1.180876
         _cons | .0039062  .0033247  -6.52  0.000   .0007367   .0207132
   ln(time1k) |      1  (exposure)
---------------------------------------------------------------------
```

The rate ratio that compares pill-taking males to abstainer males, adjusted for age, is the estimate of 2.0 for pill-takers in the regression table, because males are the baseline category of sex (female = 1 for females, 0 for males). The interaction term between female sex and pill use is 1 (0.999 ...), so the pill-taking rate ratio for women is $2 \times 1 = 2$. The P-value for the interaction term is 1. Given these findings, we can omit the interaction term from the model and proceed with our best rate ratio model with a robust variance:

```
. poisson bites i.pill i.female age, exp(time1k) irr nolog vce(robust)
note: you are responsible for interpretation of noncount dep. variable
```

```
Poisson regression                          Number of obs   =        20
                                            Wald chi2(2)    =         .
                                            Prob > chi2     =         .
Log pseudolikelihood = -34.140781           Pseudo R2       = 0.6788
```

```
----------------------------------------------------------------------
                |             Robust
         bites |     IRR  Std. Err.      z    P>|z|   [95% Conf. Interval]
----------------+-----------------------------------------------------
          pill |
    Pill-taker |       2  1.98e-08   7.0e+07  0.000        2          2
                |
        female |
        Female |       2  1.84e-08   7.5e+07  0.000        2          2
           age | 1.148698  7.08e-10  2.3e+08  0.000   1.148698   1.148698
         _cons | .0039062  1.42e-10  -1.5e+08 0.000   .0039062   .0039063
    ln(time1k) |       1  (exposure)
----------------------------------------------------------------------
```

In this output, the SEs are all effectively zero, because there was no variation in the ratios. We will see here that the SEs for the rate differences are not zero, because there is variation on the difference scale. Marginal methods can produce the four age-adjusted rates for men and women who did and did not take the vitamin:

```
. margins pill#female, post predict(ir) vce(unconditional)
(output omitted)
```

```
---------------------------------------------------------------------
                     |             Unconditional
                     |  Margin  Std. Err.      z    P>|z|   [95% Conf. Interval]
---------------------+-----------------------------------------------
         pill#female |
      Abstainer#Male |    6.2   1.251525    4.95   0.000   3.747055   8.652945
    Abstainer#Female |   12.4   2.503051    4.95   0.000   7.494111   17.30589
     Pill-taker#Male |   12.4   2.503051    4.95   0.000   7.494111   17.30589
   Pill-taker#Female |   24.8   5.006102    4.95   0.000   14.98822   34.61178
---------------------------------------------------------------------
```

The rate differences for pill-taking versus abstaining, for both men and women, can be computed from the table above. We can use **lincom** to calculate these differences and their ancillary statistics. The age-adjusted rate difference associated with pill-use for men is:

```
. lincom _b[1.pill#0.female] - _b[0.pill#0.female]

 ( 1)  - 0bn.pill#0bn.female + 1.pill#0bn.female = 0
```

```
---------------------------------------------------------------------
                |    Coef.  Std. Err.      z    P>|z|   [95% Conf. Interval]
----------------+----------------------------------------------------
            (1) |     6.2   1.251525    4.95   0.000   3.747056   8.652945
---------------------------------------------------------------------
```

Repeat this step for women:

```
. lincom _b[1.pill#1.female] - _b[0.pill#1.female]

( 1)  - 0bn.pill#1.female + 1.pill#1.female = 0
```

```
------------------------------------------------------------
          |   Coef.   Std. Err.    z    P>|z|   [95% Conf. Interval]
----------+-------------------------------------------------
      (1) |   12.4   2.503051   4.95  0.000    7.494111   17.30589
------------------------------------------------------------
```

The sequential use of **margins** and **lincom** produced age-adjusted mortality rate differences per 1,000 person-years for women (12.4) and men (6.2), comparing pill-takers and abstainers of the same sex. The commands also provided SEs, P-values, and CIs which accounted for the variances and covariances of these statistics. One further step remains, to estimate the difference between the female and male rate differences and formally test whether they are different beyond chance. This is done next, estimating that the age-adjusted rate difference is greater for women by 6.2 deaths per 1000 person-years and this difference is statistically significant: $p < .001$ for a test of homogeneity.

```
. lincom _b[1.pill#1.female] - _b[0.pill#1.female] /*
>     */ - (_b[1.pill#0.female] - _b[0.pill#0bn.female])

( 1)  0bn.pill#0bn.female - 0bn.pill#1.female - 1.pill#0bn.female + 1.
pill#1.female = 0
```

```
------------------------------------------------------------
          |   Coef.   Std. Err.    z    P>|z|   [95% Conf. Interval]
----------+-------------------------------------------------
      (1) |   6.2    1.251525   4.95  0.000    3.747056   8.652945
------------------------------------------------------------
```

An alert reader may notice that the estimated difference of 6.2 is identical to the difference for men reported earlier. That is because of the unrealistic symmetry in these data and is not something to be generally expected.

This use of **margins** and **lincom** is a little busy, but it produces results that are easy to understand and interpret for anyone familiar with the **lincom** command. The same results can be produced by marginal commands. First fit the Poisson model again, or bring saved estimates from the model back into memory if a previous command used the **post** option to put marginal estimates into memory; the marginal commands need the regression model information, not the previously posted marginal rates:

```
. qui poisson bites i.pill i.female age, exp(time1k) irr nolog vce(robust)

. margins r.pill, at(female=(0/1)) predict(ir) vce(unconditional)

Contrasts of predictive margins

Expression  : Predicted incidence rate, predict(ir)
```

```
1._at          : female     =       0
2._at          : female     =       1


-------------------------------------------------
                         |   df    chi2    P>chi2
-------------------------+-----------------------
                 pill@_at |
(Pill-taker vs Abstainer) 1 |    1   24.54   0.0000
(Pill-taker vs Abstainer) 2 |    1   24.54   0.0000
                    Joint |    1   24.54   0.0000
-------------------------------------------------


---------------------------------------------------------------
                         |          Unconditional
                         |  Contrast  Std. Err.   [95% Conf. Interval]
-------------------------+-------------------------------------------
                 pill@_at |
(Pill-taker vs Abstainer) 1 |    6.2   1.251525   3.747056   8.652945
(Pill-taker vs Abstainer) 2 |   12.4   2.503051   7.494111   17.30589
---------------------------------------------------------------
```

This command produced the age-adjusted pill-use rate differences by sex, with the same SEs and CIs previously produced by **lincom**. We can also use marginal methods to estimate the difference in the male and female rate differences, with a test of any difference:

```
. margins r.pill, at(female=(0/1)) contrast(atcontrast(r)) predict(ir)
vce(unconditional)

Contrasts of predictive margins

Expression  : Predicted incidence rate, predict(ir)

1._at          : female     =       0
2._at          : female     =       1
-----------------------------------------
           |   df    chi2    P>chi2
--------+--------------------------
 _at#pill |    1   24.54   0.0000
-----------------------------------------

---------------------------------------------------------------
                         |          Unconditional
                         |  Contrast  Std. Err.   [95% Conf. Interval]
-------------------------+-------------------------------------------
                  _at#pill |
(2 vs 1) (Pill-taker vs Abstainer) |   6.2   1.251525   3.747056   8.652945
---------------------------------------------------------------
```

21.11 MARGINAL METHODS FOR A CONTINUOUS VARIABLE

So far, I have used marginal methods for two categorical variables, pill-use and sex. Marginal methods can be applied to a continuous variable, age in this example. For example, how do the pill-use-adjusted rates of death vary by age for men and women?

```
. quietly poisson bites i.pill i.female age, exp(time1k) irr nolog
vce(robust)

. margins female, at(age=(40(2.5)60)) predict(ir) vce(unconditional)

Predictive margins                          Number of obs  =       20

Expression  : Predicted incidence rate, predict(ir)
1._at       : age         =          40
2._at       : age         =        42.5
3._at       : age         =          45
4._at       : age         =        47.5
5._at       : age         =          50
6._at       : age         =        52.5
7._at       : age         =          55
8._at       : age         =        57.5
9._at       : age         =          60
```

	Margin	Unconditional Std. Err.	z	P>|z|	[95% Conf. Interval]	
_at#female						
1#Male	1.5	.1147079	13.08	0.000	1.275177	1.724823
1#Female	3	.2294157	13.08	0.000	2.550353	3.449647
2#Male	2.12132	.1622214	13.08	0.000	1.803372	2.439269
2#Female	4.242641	.3244428	13.08	0.000	3.606744	4.878537
3#Male	3	.2294157	13.08	0.000	2.550353	3.449647
3#Female	6	.4588315	13.08	0.000	5.100707	6.899293
4#Male	4.242641	.3244428	13.08	0.000	3.606744	4.878537
4#Female	8.485281	.6488857	13.08	0.000	7.213489	9.757074
5#Male	6	.4588315	13.08	0.000	5.100707	6.899293
5#Female	12	.9176629	13.08	0.000	10.20141	13.79859
6#Male	8.485281	.6488857	13.08	0.000	7.213489	9.757074
6#Female	16.97056	1.297771	13.08	0.000	14.42698	19.51415
7#Male	12	.9176629	13.08	0.000	10.20141	13.79859
7#Female	24	1.835326	13.08	0.000	20.40283	27.59717
8#Male	16.97056	1.297771	13.08	0.000	14.42698	19.51415

```
    8#Female |   33.94113    2.595543    13.08    0.000    28.85396    39.0283
    9#Male   |         24    1.835326    13.08    0.000    20.40283    27.59717
    9#Female |         48    3.670652    13.08    0.000    40.80566    55.19435
------------------------------------------------------------------------------
```

```
. marginsplot, xlabel(40(5)60) /*
>      */ title("") /*
>      */ plotregion(style(none)) /*
>      */ xscale(noextend) /*
>      */ yscale(noextend) /*
>      */ ytitle("Adjusted Rate per 1000 person-years") /*
>      */ saving(Fig21.1.gph, replace)
```

The **margins** and **marginsplot** commands created Figure 21.1, which shows how model predicted rates are related to age and sex, after adjustment for pill-taking. The marginal commands made predictions at every 2.5 years from age 40 to 60, even though there were no subjects with ages 42.5, 47.5, 52.5, or 57.5. The labeling of age in the plot was more parsimonious. If the log scale is used for the vertical axis, the plot shows two parallel lines (Figure 21.2) because these predicted rates are from a model that used a log link and ln(age) was treated as linear in the model. The **marginsplot** command offers many options. Continuous lines without markers can be used, CIs can be shown as areas, and the rate differences between men and women can be plotted instead of the two separate lines for each sex.

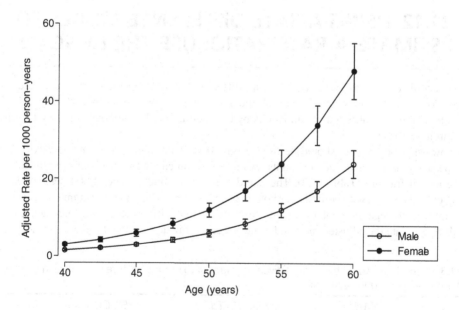

FIGURE 21.1 Predicted skunk bite rates by age and sex, adjusted for pill-taking, from a rate ratio model applied to hypothetical data described in the text. Vertical bars are pointwise 95% CIs.

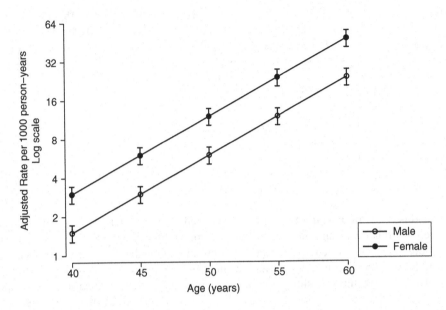

FIGURE 21.2 Predicted skunk bite rates by age and sex, adjusted for pill-taking, from the same model used for Figure 20.1. Adjusted rates are plotted on the log scale. Vertical bars are pointwise 95% CIs.

21.12 USING A RATE DIFFERENCE MODEL TO ESTIMATE A RATE RATIO: USE THE LN SCALE

An analyst could reverse this process; fit a rate difference model and then estimate a rate ratio. This should be done on the ln scale. The ln of the rate ratio should be estimated with its CIs. Then exponentiate this ln rate ratio and obtain its CIs by exponentiating the endpoints of the CI for the ln rate ratio (Cummings 2011).

To show why the ln scale should be used, I will show what happens when this advice is ignored. Consider person-year data and fracture counts for men and women who were given a treatment intended to reduce the rate of fracture (Table 21.3). The rate difference for fractures per 1,000 person-years was −4, comparing treated persons with controls, for both men and women. The female fracture rate was greater than the male rate by 5, regardless of treatment. Now use a rate difference model and then use marginal commands to estimate the adjusted rates and to incorrectly estimate statistics for the rate ratio:

TABLE 21.3 Hypothetical data for persons given a treatment to reduce fracture rates. Person-years are in units of 1,000, rates are per 1,000 person-years.

SEX	TREATED	FRACTURES	PERSON-YEARS	RATE
Male	No	5	.25	20
Male	Yes	8	.5	16
Female	No	10	.4	25
Female	Yes	21	1	21

```
. glm rate i.rx female [iweight=ptime], link(id) family(poisson) nolog
```

```
Generalized linear models                      No. of obs        =          4
Optimization    : ML                           Residual df       =          1
                                               Scale parameter =            1
Deviance        = 1.77636e-15                  (1/df) Deviance = 1.78e-15
Pearson         = 9.86076e-32                  (1/df) Pearson  = 9.86e-32

Variance function: V(u) = u                    [Poisson]
Link function     : g(u) = u                   [Identity]

                                               AIC             =   4.109157
Log likelihood  = -5.218314584                 BIC             =  -1.386294
```

rate	Coef.	OIM Std. Err.	z	P>|z|	[95% Conf. Interval]
rx					
Treated	-4	6.91638	-0.58	0.563	-17.55586 9.555856
female	5	6.215442	0.80	0.421	-7.182042 17.18204
_cons	20	6.87484	2.91	0.004	6.525561 33.47444

```
. margins rx, predict(mu) post
```

```
Predictive margins                             Number of obs   =          4
Model VCE    : OIM
```

```
Expression  : Predicted mean rate, predict(mu)
```

	Margin	Delta-method Std. Err.	z	P>|z|	[95% Conf. Interval]
rx					
Control	23.25581	5.949703	3.91	0.000	11.59461 34.91702
Treated	19.25581	3.572954	5.39	0.000	12.25295 26.25868

```
. nlcom (IRR: _b[1.rx]/_b[0.rx])
```

```
    IRR: _b[1.rx]/_b[0.rx]
```

	Coef.	Std. Err.	z	P>|z|	[95% Conf. Interval]
IRR	.828	.2607192	3.18	0.001	.3169998 1.339

According to this output, the rate ratio is 0.83 with a P-value of .001 and a 95% CI of 0.32, 1.34. Something is wrong. How can these CIs, which widely straddle 1, be correct when the P-value is so small?

The rate ratio is correct, but the P-value is not, because **nlcom** tested the null hypothesis that the rate ratio is 0, instead of testing a null hypothesis of 1. The command estimated a ratio, but it has no idea that we consider 1 to be the null value for a ratio. By default, **nlcom** thinks the null hypothesis is 0, so it constructed CIs on the difference scale. To get the correct results, fit the model and use **margins** to post the adjusted rates, but then proceed using the ln of the rate ratio:

```
. nlcom (lnrr: ln(_b[1.rx]/_b[0.rx])), post

    lnrr: ln(_b[1.rx]/_b[0.rx])
```

```
------------------------------------------------------------------------
            |     Coef.   Std. Err.      z    P>|z|    [95% Conf. Interval]
------------+-----------------------------------------------------------
      lnrr |  -.1887421   .3148783   -0.60   0.549    -.8058922    .4284079
------------------------------------------------------------------------
```

```
. display "Rate ratio = " exp(_b[lnrr]) _skip(3) /*
>     */ "95% CI = " exp(_b[lnrr] -invnormal(1-.05/2)*_se[lnrr]) /*
>     */ ", "      exp(_b[lnrr] +invnormal(1-.05/2)*_se[lnrr])

Rate ratio = .828   95% CI = .44668923, 1.534812
```

The rate ratio of 0.83 is just what we obtained earlier, but the P-value is now 0.5 and the 95% CI is 0.45, 1.53, further from 0 than the previous interval. The transform-the-endpoints method produced a CI that was symmetric around the ln rate ratio. The moral is: for ratios work on the ln scale. We can compare these results with estimates from a Poisson rate ratio model shown below. They are similar in this example:

```
. * poisson rate ratio model
. poisson fractures rx female, irr exp(ptime) nolog
```

```
Poisson regression                          Number of obs   =          4
                                            LR chi2(2)      =       0.91
                                            Prob > chi2     =     0.6333

Log likelihood = -8.2356173                 Pseudo R2       =     0.0526
```

```
------------------------------------------------------------------------
  fractures |     IRR   Std. Err.      z    P>|z|    [95% Conf. Interval]
------------+-----------------------------------------------------------
         rx |  .8273536   .2634464   -0.60   0.552    .4432523   1.544299
     female |  1.289452   .4265781    0.77   0.442    .6742327   2.466044
       _cons |  19.58785   6.680444    8.72   0.000   10.03885   38.21988
  ln(ptime) |        1  (exposure)
------------------------------------------------------------------------
```

This chapter focused mostly on obtaining rates, rate differences, and ancillary statistics after fitting a rate ratio model. Thanks to marginal methods, we can use whichever model has a better fit to the data, multiplicative or additive, and still get the estimates, rate ratios or differences, that we want. We can have our cake and eat it too. Only a few of the things that marginal commands can accomplish have been described. These commands simplify chores that were onerous in the past.

Bayesian Methods

22

The Bayesian approach requires the analyst to define a probability distribution for the quantity of interest before new data are analyzed. The choice of prior distribution may use information from previous studies, expert opinion, or values that the analyst judges to be plausible, possible, or otherwise worthy of study. A Bayesian analysis may utilize a range of prior distributions to test how sensitive the results are to the choice of the prior. The prior distribution information is then combined with the new data to generate a new, or posterior, probability distribution for the quantities of interest.

Bayesian regression can be closely approximated with modifications of ordinary maximum likelihood software. For example, Discacciati, Orsini, and Greenland (2015) created a Stata command, **penlogit**, that modifies Stata's usual logistic regression command to incorporate prior distribution information for the regression coefficients. They amended the logistic likelihood to a penalized likelihood, which pulls the size of the regression odds ratios toward the prior distribution values. Prior distribution information is provided to the software by adding records to the data, a procedure called data augmentation. Sullivan and Greenland (2013) described this approach for logistic, conditional logistic, Poisson, and Cox proportional hazards regression using SAS software. Both articles (Sullivan and Greenland 2013, Discacciati, Orsini, and Greenland 2015) used data regarding the birth outcomes of 2992 women in labor. Only 17 of the babies died, so when 14 variables were used in an ordinary logistic regression model with death as the outcome, some implausibly large odds ratios appeared due to sparse-data bias (Greenland, Mansournia, and Altman 2016). By incorporating prior information in a penalized likelihood model, the inflated estimates shrank to more realistic values.

In some respects, the Bayesian approach, compared with a frequentist analysis, reverses the order in which data are considered. The Bayesian summarizes previous studies into priors that are incorporated into an analysis of new data to produce an updated estimate. The frequentist analyzes the new data first but may then combine the new estimates with old information in a meta-analysis.

With version 14, released in 2015, Stata introduced fully Bayesian regression using Markov chain Monte Carlo simulation. Stata's Bayesian commands were described in a 270-page electronic manual, although rate regression received little attention. With the release of version 15, in 2017, Bayesian commands were expanded and the manual grew to 535 pages. This chapter provides a brief introduction to Bayesian regression for rates.

22.1 CANCER MORTALITY RATE IN ALASKA

Cancer mortality of Alaskans in 2010 was described for 11 age groups in Table 6.2. Bayesian commands can estimate the overall rate using the 11 age categories:

```
. set seed 93514

. bayesmh deaths, ///
>     likelihood(poisson, exposure(pop100k)) ///
>     prior({deaths:_cons}, flat)
```

```
Burn-in ...
Simulation ...

Model summary
- - - - - - - - - - - - - - - - - - - - - - - - - - - - - - - - - - - - - - - - - -
Likelihood:
 deaths pop100k ~ poissonreg({deaths:_cons})

Prior:
 {deaths:_cons} ~ 1 (flat)
- - - - - - - - - - - - - - - - - - - - - - - - - - - - - - - - - - - - - - -


Bayesian Poisson regression              MCMC iterations   =    12,500
Random-walk Metropolis-Hastings sampling Burn-in           =     2,500
                                         MCMC sample size  =    10,000
                                         Number of obs     =        11
                                         Acceptance rate   =     .3982
Log marginal likelihood = -1199.0747     Efficiency        =     .2294


- - - - - - - - - - - - - - - - - - - - - - - - - - - - - - - - - - - - - - - -
               |                                         Equal-tailed
   deaths |    Mean   Std. Dev.      MCSE    Median   [95% Cred. Interval]
- - - - - -+- - - - - - - - - - - - - - - - - - - - - - - - - - - - - - - - -
   _cons  | 4.823153  .033914   .000708  4.822427  4.758657  4.890828
- - - - - - - - - - - - - - - - - - - - - - - - - - - - - - - - - - - - - - -

. scalar mean  = exp(el(e(mean),1,1))

. scalar lower = exp(el(e(cri),1,1))

. scalar upper = exp(el(e(cri),2,1))

. display _newline(1) "Mean rate: " %5.3f mean _skip(3) ///
>     "95% credible interval: " %5.3f lower ", " %5.3f upper

Mean rate: 124.357  95% credible interval: 116.589, 133.064
```

The Bayesian method uses data simulation. The **set seed** command was invoked so the simulated results could be repeated. The same seed (93514 is my ZIP code) was used for all the examples in this chapter. The first line of the **bayesmh** regression command told Stata to fit a Bayesian regression model with one variable, the count of deaths in each age category. The second line declared this to be a Poisson model for the mean rate. Person-time was entered using the **exposure(pop100k)** option, with person-time in units of 100,000 person-years. The third line said that the prior distribution for the rate is flat, meaning that we claim to be ignorant about the prior distribution. Braces {} identify the mean to be estimated by this command. The simulation process started with 2500 burn-in estimates that were discarded. The next 10,000 estimates were used for the final estimate. The choice of 2500 burn-in steps followed by 10,000 iterations are Stata's default choices, but these can be changed. After fitting this model, an analyst can invoke commands that check that the model converged in the expected way. Those steps are in the Stata manuals and will be omitted here.

The regression table output is on the ln scale, with ln mean rate = 4.8, so three scalar commands were used to exponentiate the mean and its upper and lower credible bounds. We could have used another command to produce the mean rate ratio with credible intervals: **bayesstats summary (exp({deaths:_cons}))**. The **bayesstats** command produces a slightly different rate ratio: 124.428, instead of 124.357. The **bayesstats** command reports the average of the rate ratios, whereas the **scalar meanrr** command, shown above, reports the exponentiated average of the ln rates. There is little difference in this example.

The Bayesian rate was 124.4 with a 95% credible interval of 116.6, 133.1, similar to results from ordinary Poisson regression: 124.5 deaths per 100,000 person-years, 95% CI 116.5, 132.9. This example shows how Bayesian regression can be used to mimic the results of frequentist regression.

With version 15 of Stata, syntax for Bayesian estimation was greatly simplified. The Poisson model used here can now be estimated with the following command:

```
. bayes: poisson deaths, exp(pop100k) irr

Burn-in ...
Simulation ...

Model summary
- - - - - - - - - - - - - - - - - - - - - - - - - - - - - - - - - - - - - - - -
Likelihood:
  deaths ~ poisson({deaths:_cons})
Prior:
  {deaths:_cons} ~ normal(0,10000)
- - - - - - - - - - - - - - - - - - - - - - - - - - - - - - - - - - - - - - - -


Bayesian Poisson regression                 MCMC iterations    =   12,500
Random-walk Metropolis-Hastings sampling    Burn-in            =    2,500
                                            MCMC sample size   =   10,000
                                            Number of obs      =       11
                                            Acceptance rate    =    .3982
Log marginal likelihood = -1199.7744        Efficiency         =    .2288

- - - - - - - - - - - - - - - - - - - - - - - - - - - - - - - - - - - - - - -
             |                                          Equal-tailed
    deaths |      IRR   Std. Dev.    MCSE     Median  [95% Cred. Interval]
- - - - - -+- - - - - - - - - - - - - - - - - - - - - - - - - - - - - - - -
     _cons |  124.4282   4.227715   .08838  124.2663  116.5892   133.0638
- - - - - - - - - - - - - - - - - - - - - - - - - - - - - - - - - - - - - -
Note: Variable pop100k is included in the model as the exposure.
Note: Default priors are used for model parameters.
```

In this output, most statistics are almost identical to those previously given, but the command was greatly simplified. More information about the prior expectation is given and the **irr** option told the software to present the overall rate (a rate ratio compared with a rate of 1), instead of the ln(rate). While 12,500 iterations sounds a bit daunting, this command produced the final results in just 2.1 seconds on a desktop computer.

Imagine that Alaska cancer mortality was 100 in 2009. This would be a good first guess, or prior estimate, for the rate in 2010. The SE for the person-time weighted rate in 2010 (124.5) from a Poisson model (not shown) was 4.2, so the variance for the SE of the mean is about $4.2^2 = 18$. When the mean count is large, the Poisson distribution starts to look like a Normal distribution (Figure 4.2), so a

Normal prior can be used to incorporate the 2009 rate into an estimate of the 2010 rate, assuming the variance is 18 for the 2009 rate:

```
. bayesmh deaths, ///
>     likelihood(dpoisson({mean}*pop100k)) ///
>     prior({mean}, normal(100,18)) initial({mean} 100)


Burn-in ...
Simulation ...

Model summary
- - - - - - - - - - - - - - - - - - - - - - - - - - - - - - - - - - - - - - - -
Likelihood:
  deaths ~ poisson({mean}*pop100k)

Prior:
  {mean} ~ normal(100,18)
- - - - - - - - - - - - - - - - - - - - - - - - - - - - - - - - - - - - - - - -


Bayesian Poisson model                      MCMC iterations      =    12,500
Random-walk Metropolis-Hastings sampling    Burn-in              =     2,500
                                            MCMC sample size     =    10,000
                                            Number of obs        =        11
                                            Acceptance rate      =     .4512
Log marginal likelihood = -1205.7273        Efficiency           =     .2182
```

	Mean	Std. Dev.	MCSE	Median	Equal-tailed [95% Cred. Interval]	
mean	112.9817	2.775935	.059421	112.9796	107.5591	118.4521

In the command above, the likelihood used the **dpoisson** option to directly model the distribution of the rates, as opposed to the **poisson** option, which used the ln link and estimated the ln of the mean rate. You can use either approach, but **dpoisson** has the convenience of producing the mean rate, instead of the ln mean rate. The likelihood expression seems a bit strange to a frequentist, because it looks at first glance as if the quantity to be estimated is the mean count of deaths or the mean count of deaths multiplied by person-time; neither quantity is a rate. But the **bayesmh** command estimates whatever is placed in the braces ({mean}) and in this equation the goal was to estimate the count of deaths = {mean rate} x person-time, which can be rewritten as {mean rate} = deaths/person-time. Previously, using the poisson option, the software was able to figure out that we wanted to estimate the ln of mean count {deaths:_cons} with a person-time offset. But with the **dpoisson** option we have to create a variable name to indicate the mean rate; I labeled this variable {mean}, but I could have named it {mu} or {average} or {meanrate}. The 2009 prior rate information was provided by the **normal(100,18)** option. The age-specific rates varied a lot and the Bayesian convergence process could not find a good starting value. Introducing an initial value of 100 gave the convergence a shove in the right direction, but the choice of initial value made little difference; a choice of 50 produced the same results.

The use of the mortality rate in 2009 pulled the 2010 rate estimate from 124 toward 100. The SD of the rate shrank, compared with the size of the rate, because the 2009 rate contributed to the estimate of the spread of the rates. Incorporating prior information can improve precision. Similar gains in precision can arise in a meta-analysis of results from several frequentist analyses.

When dealing with the Poisson distribution, it is sometimes helpful to use a gamma distribution prior (Gelman et al. 1995, p48-51). A gamma distribution is defined by shape parameter A and scale parameter B; the A/B ratio defines the mean of the distribution and the size of B defines the tails of the distributions.

22.2 THE RATE RATIO FOR FALLING IN A TRIAL OF EXERCISE

A randomized trial of exercise for the prevention of falls was described in Chapters 12 and 13 (Tables 12.1 and 13.1). This rate ratio using Bayesian methods and a flat (noninformative) prior:

```
. bayesmh fallcnt exercise, ///
>     likelihood(poisson, exposure(time)) ///
>     prior({fallcnt:_cons} {exercise}, flat)

Burn-in ...
Simulation ...

Model summary
------------------------------------------------------------------
Likelihood:
  fallcnt time ~ poissonreg(xb_fallcnt)

Prior:
  {fallcnt:_cons exercise} ~ 1 (flat)                            (1)
------------------------------------------------------------------
(1) Parameters are elements of the linear form xb_fallcnt.
```

Bayesian Poisson regression   MCMC iterations   =   12,500
Random-walk Metropolis-Hastings sampling   Burn-in   =   2,500
                                                    MCMC sample size   =   10,000
                                                    Number of obs   =   453
                                                    Acceptance rate   =   .2176
                                                    Efficiency: min   =   .1204
                                                              avg   =   .1297
Log marginal likelihood = -1049.5628   max   =   .139

```
-------------------------------------------------------------------------
             |                                        Equal-tailed
   fallcnt   |   Mean   Std. Dev.   MCSE    Median  [95% Cred. Interval]
-------------+-----------------------------------------------------------
   exercise  | -.2824125  .0759341  .002036  -.2813908  -.4309884  -.1414757
      _cons  |  .5691735  .0500262  .001442   .5701479   .4697046   .6646675
-------------------------------------------------------------------------
```

```
. scalar meanrr = exp(el(e(mean),1,1))
. scalar lower = exp(el(e(cri),1,1))
. scalar upper = exp(el(e(cri),2,1))
```

```
. display _newline(1) "Mean rate ratio: " %5.3f meanrr _skip(3) ///
>       "95% credible interval: " %5.3f lower ", " %5.3f upper

Mean rate ratio: 0.754   95% credible interval: 0.650, 0.868
```

The Bayesian estimates are similar to the results from ordinary Poisson regression: rate ratio 0.75 (95% CI 0.64, 0.87). The main problem with both methods is that they fail to account for the overdispersion in these data; that is, the confidence and credible intervals are too narrow.

A negative binomial model can be fit using Bayesian commands, but the resulting credible intervals are arguably still too narrow, compared with results shown in Table 13.1 from robust, bootstrap, or randomization methods:

```
. gen double ltime = ln(time)
. bayesmh fallcnt, /*
>       */ likelihood(llf(lngamma((1/{alpha})+fallcnt) /*
>       */ - lngamma(fallcnt+1) /*
>       */ - lngamma(1/{alpha}) /*
>       */ + (1/{alpha})*log((1/(1+{alpha}*exp({cons} /*
>       */ + {exercise}*exercise+ltime)))) /*
>       */ + fallcnt*log(1-(1/(1+{alpha}*exp({cons}+{exercise}*exercise+
ltime))))))) /*
>       */ prior({cons=0} {exercise=0}, flat) /*
>       */ prior({alpha}, igamma(0.1,0.1)) block({alpha=1}) /*
>       */ block({cons} ) block({exercise})


Burn-in ...
note: invalid initial state
Simulation ...


Model summary
- - - - - - - - - - - - - - - - - - - - - - - - - - - - - - - - - - - - - - - -
Likelihood:
 fallcnt ~ logdensity(<expr1>)
Priors:
 {cons exercise} ~ 1 (flat)
         {alpha} ~ igamma(0.1,0.1)
Expression:
    expr1  :   lngamma((1/{alpha})+fallcnt)-lngamma(fallcnt+1)-lngamma
               (1/{alpha})+(1/{alpha})*log((1/(1+{alpha}*exp({cons}
               +{exercise}*exercise+ltime))))+fallcnt*log(1-(1/(1
               +{alpha}*exp({cons}+{exercise}*exercise+ltime)) ))
- - - - - - - - - - - - - - - - - - - - - - - - - - - - - - - - - - - - - - - -
```

```
Bayesian regression                          MCMC iterations  =    12,500
Random-walk Metropolis-Hastings sampling     Burn-in          =     2,500
                                             MCMC sample size =    10,000
                                             Number of obs    =       453
                                             Acceptance rate  =      .451
                                             Efficiency:  min =    .08407
                                                          avg =     .1352
Log marginal likelihood = -761.13452                      max =     .2362
```

	Mean	Std. Dev.	MCSE	Median	Equal-tailed [95% Cred. Interval]	
alpha	1.639595	.1777506	.003657	1.631821	1.317418	2.01058
cons	.5757118	.1020582	.003494	.5745606	.3807857	.7807979
exercise	-.2863482	.146405	.005049	-.2879719	-.5702851	.0007267

```
. scalar meanrr = exp(el(e(mean),1,3))
. scalar lower = exp(el(e(cri),1,3))
. scalar upper = exp(el(e(cri),2,3))
. display _newline(1) "Mean rate ratio: " %5.3f meanrr _skip(3) ///
>     "95% credible interval: " %5.3f lower ", " %5.3f upper

Mean rate ratio: 0.751  95% credible interval: 0.565, 1.001
```

This brief chapter shows only the most basic of rate models. To take advantage of these methods, the reader will want to study the Stata manuals and textbooks about Bayesian methods (Gelman et al. 1995, Congdon 2001).

Exact Poisson Regression

23

Confidence intervals (CI) and P-values based upon Wald, score, or likelihood ratio statistics rely upon normality assumptions. Those assumptions are reasonable when counts are sufficiently large. When rates are based upon small counts, large sample methods are no longer justified. We can turn instead to exact methods, which avoid normality assumptions. Large sample and exact methods were described and contrasted in Chapter 4. Here we discuss exact Poisson regression, which relies on describing the distribution of the data.

23.1 A SIMPLE EXAMPLE

Imagine that we have two records: (1) in a group of people followed in aggregate for 1 unit of person-time, 1 outcome event occurred and, (2) in another group also followed for 1 person-time unit, but all exposed to a risk factor for the outcome, four outcomes occurred. The rate ratio comparing those exposed to the risk factor with those not exposed is equal to 4. But what is the CI around this estimate? First try Poisson regression:

```
. poisson outcome riskfactor, exposure(ptime) irr
Iteration 0:   log likelihood = -2.6329297
Iteration 1:   log likelihood = -2.6328764
Iteration 2:   log likelihood = -2.6328764
(output omitted)
------------------------------------------------------------------------
    outcome |     IRR   Std. Err.       z    P>|z|    [95% Conf. Interval]
------------+-----------------------------------------------------------
 riskfactor |       4   4.472136     1.24   0.215    .4470826    35.78757
      _cons |       1          1     0.00   1.000    .1408635    7.099071
  ln(ptime) |       1   (exposure)
------------------------------------------------------------------------
```

Next try exact Poisson regression:

```
. expoisson outcome riskfactor, exp(ptime) irr saving(exact1, replace)
Enumerating sample-space combinations:
observation 1:   enumerations =        6
observation 2:   enumerations =        6
note: saving distribution to file exact1_riskfactor.dta

Exact Poisson regression
                                            Number of obs =        2
```

```
---------------------------------------------------------------
     outcome |    IRR       Suff.    2*Pr(Suff.)    [95% Conf. Interval]
-------------+-------------------------------------------------------
  riskfactor |     4          4        0.3750       .3958333   196.9899
   ln(ptime) |     1      (exposure)
---------------------------------------------------------------
```

Instead of reporting a convergence log, the exact command reports that it "enumerated" the "sample-space combinations" for each record. There were six enumerations for each observation. This means the software estimated the outcome distribution for the variables in the model; in this case, there is only one variable (aside from the constant term), riskfactor. A file called exact1 was saved. Stata will save a file called "exact1_variable" for each variable in the model. Since the only variable in the model was "riskfactor", a file called "exact1_riskfactor" was saved. We can call this file into memory and list the contents:

```
. use exact1_riskfactor, clear

. egen sum = sum(_w_)

. gen newwgt = _w_/sum

. list

    +------------------------------------------------+
    |                _w_   riskfa~r      sum  newwgt |
    |------------------------------------------------|
 1. | .0083333333333         0    .2666667  .03125  |
 2. | .0416666666667         1    .2666667  .15625  |
 3. | .0833333333333         2    .2666667  .3125   |
 4. | .0833333333333         3    .2666667  .3125   |
 5. | .0416666666667         4    .2666667  .15625  |
    |------------------------------------------------|
 6. | .0083333333333         5    .2666667  .03125  |
    +------------------------------------------------+
```

The software saved only two variables in the file. One of these, called riskfactor, lists the possible values for records coded as 1 for exposure to the risk factor. Those values are just counts from 0 to 5, because the total number of outcome events in the data was $1 + 4 = 5$. So given that there were five outcomes (or "conditional upon" five outcomes, in statistical jargon), the software estimated the relative weights (called "_w_" in the saved file) for each of these outcomes if someone was exposed. The weights are symmetrical around the mean count in these data, a count of 2.5. Counts of 0 and 5 both received weights of .00833, counts of 1 and 4 were assigned weights of .04166, and counts of 2 and 3 also received identical weights. (This symmetry is not always expected; for example, if the person-time for the unexposed is changed to 2, this symmetry vanishes.) I added 2 variables to these data: "sum", which is the sum of all the weights, and "newwgt", which is a normalized weight equal to each _w_ divided by 0.266, the sum of the _w_ values. The new weights add up to 1.0 and they have a probability interpretation. For example, given the observed data, the probability that 0 (or fewer) outcomes would occur among those exposed to the risk factor is .03125.

The formula for the distribution weights is described in the methods section that describes the **expoisson** command in Stata's electronic manual. The weights come from a formula which is similar to the formula for the Poisson distribution, expression 4.1. Although a permutation method describes the data distribution, the method relies upon the assumption that the counts arose from a Poisson process.

Among those exposed to the risk factor, four outcomes were observed. The probability that 4 or more outcomes would be observed in the exposed group, given the data, is .15625 + .03125 = .1875. This is a one-sided test. The probability that 4 or fewer outcomes would be observed is also a one-sided P-value: 03125 + .15625 + .3125 + .3125 + .15625 = .96875. To get the two-sided P-value for the observed 4 outcomes, we double the smaller of these P-values: 2 × .1875 = .375, which is the P-value reported for the rate ratio of 4 by **expoisson**. The regression table reports a rate ratio which is identical to the rate ratio from the **poisson** command; both commands estimated this ratio using maximum likelihood. But **expoisson** also reports the number of outcomes for the riskfactor variable, 4, which is labeled "Suff." for sufficient statistic. Finally, **expoisson** calculated the 95% CI for the rate ratio, using a method that accounted for the data distribution. Both the P-value and CI reported by the exact method were larger than those from ordinary Poisson regression.

Because counts are discrete, rather than continuous, exact P-values and CIs may be larger than desired for the given level of alpha. Because counts change in integer steps, P-values (and their corresponding CIs), change by discrete steps. If we select alpha = .05 as the acceptable frequency for a false positive test statistic, the P-value from an exact test corresponds to an alpha level of .05 or a *smaller* frequency. Similarly, the exact 95% CI covers 95% or *more* of the rate ratios we would obtain if we collected new data and reestimated the rate ratio. So when exact methods are used, the resulting test statistics may reject the null hypothesis less often than anticipated for the chosen alpha level. If this behavior is considered undesirable, one option, discussed in Chapter 4, is to use mid-P values and mid-P CIs. These statistics will correspond to the chosen level of alpha *on average*, but may be larger or smaller than desired in any particular set of data. We can obtain mid-P statistics from the **expoisson** command by using the **midp** option:

```
. expoisson outcome riskfactor, exp(ptime) irr midp
(output omitted)
```

```
-----------------------------------------------------------------------------
   outcome |    IRR      Suff.     2*Pr(Suff.)     [95% Conf. Interval]
-----------+-----------------------------------------------------------------
 riskfactor |     4          4        0.2188        .5024931    98.98019
  ln(ptime) |     1      (exposure)
-----------------------------------------------------------------------------
mid-p-value computed for the probabilities and CIs
```

As expected, both the P-value and CI are smaller compared with results without the mid-p option. Stata's **ir** command can estimate the same two-sided mid-p value, but it does not estimate the mid-p CI or the exact P-value.

23.2 A PERFECTLY PREDICTED OUTCOME

Imagine that the exposure perfectly determines the outcome. Using the same set of two records described earlier, assume that no outcomes occurred among those not exposed to riskfactor, but four outcomes occurred among those who were exposed. Now apply Poisson regression:

```
. poisson outcome riskfactor, exposure(ptime) irr nolog
(output omitted)
```

```
--------------------------------------------------------------------
   outcome |      IRR    Std. Err.       z   P>|z|  [95% Conf. Interval]
-----------+--------------------------------------------------------
riskfactor | 1.23e+08    6.81e+11     0.00   0.997          0        .
     _cons | 3.25e-08    .0001804    -0.00   0.998          0        .
 ln(ptime) |        1   (exposure)
--------------------------------------------------------------------
```

The event rate was 4 among those exposed to the risk factor and 0 otherwise. Dividing 4 by 0 resulted in a gigantic rate ratio: 1.23×10^8. An enormous P-value was produced along with CIs that are infinitely wide. Given the small counts, we should take these results with a pillar of salt. Now try exact regression:

```
. expoisson outcome riskfactor, exp(ptime) irr
Enumerating sample-space combinations:
observation 1:   enumerations =        5
observation 2:   enumerations =        5
note: CMLE estimate for riskfactor is +inf; computing MUE


Exact Poisson regression
                                              Number of obs =        2
--------------------------------------------------------------------
   outcome |      IRR     Suff.   2*Pr(Suff.)   [95% Conf. Interval]
-----------+--------------------------------------------------------
riskfactor | 5.285214*       4      0.1250      .660124        +Inf
 ln(ptime) |        1   (exposure)
--------------------------------------------------------------------
(*) median unbiased estimates (MUE)
```

Exact Poisson regression gave up on the conditional maximum likelihood method because it estimated an infinite rate ratio. The software turned instead to the median unbiased estimate (MUE). This estimate is the rate ratio that corresponds to the point on a cumulative probability curve equal to 0.5. It is the rate ratio for which the two-sided P-value function is at a maximum. Stata's electronic manuals have a nice discussion of this topic. The probability that the true rate ratio is 5.285 or greater is equal to the probability that the true rate ratio is 5.285 or less. (More correctly, it is the rate ratio at which the probability of the test statistic of 4 or more is equal to the probability of a statistic of 4 or less (Greenland and Rothman 2008a p221).) Although **expoisson** will automatically report median unbiased estimates when the conditional maximum likelihood estimate of the rate ratio is infinite, you can also obtain median unbiased estimates for any variable by adding the **mue** option to the regression command.

23.3 MEMORY PROBLEMS

To produce P-values and CIs, **expoisson** must estimate conditional distributions for the model variables. This is a trivial matter in the examples used so far, but with larger counts or several variables, the distribution information that must be generated can quickly become enormous. In Chapters 12 (Table 12.1) and 13 I described data for 453 subjects in a randomized trial with falls as the outcome. If

expoisson is used to estimate the rate ratio of falls for the intervention versus control arm, an error message is produced: "total number of events, 695, is too large for an exact poisson model." Even if the data is collapsed into two records (not a good idea, as useful information about how the falls were distributed among subjects would be lost), one for the intervention and one for the controls, the same error message appears.

Exact Poisson regression can be so computer intensive that the **expoisson** command can eat up all of a computer's memory. Using an earlier version of this command, I once generated so much data that the computer's operating system was overwhelmed and the machine froze. To prevent this, Stata puts a limit on the amount of memory that can be used and the analyst must allocate additional memory if needed. Imagine that you have the data listed here:

```
     +-------------------------------------------+
     | risk1  risk2  risk3  risk4  outcome  ptime |
     |-------------------------------------------|
  1. |    0      0      0      0        2      1  |
  2. |    0      1      0      0        4      1  |
  3. |    0      0      1      0        6      1  |
  4. |    1      0      0      0        8      2  |
  5. |    0      1      1      0       12      1  |
  6. |    1      0      1      0       12      1  |
  7. |    1      1      0      0        8      1  |
  8. |    1      1      1      0       24      1  |
     |-------------------------------------------|
  9. |    0      0      0      1        1      1  |
 10. |    0      1      0      1        4      2  |
 11. |    0      0      1      1        3      1  |
 12. |    1      0      0      1        2      1  |
 13. |    0      1      1      1        6      1  |
 14. |    1      0      1      1       12      2  |
 15. |    1      1      0      1        4      1  |
 16. |    1      1      1      1       12      1  |
     +-------------------------------------------+
```

Using ordinary Poisson regression to analyze these data, it took a desktop computer 0.6 seconds to produce this output:

```
. poisson outcome risk1 risk2 risk3 risk4, exp(ptime) irr nolog
(output omitted)
```

```
------------------------------------------------------------------------
  outcome |     IRR   Std. Err.      z    P>|z|    [95% Conf. Interval]
----------+-------------------------------------------------------------
    risk1 |       2    .39437      3.52   0.000    1.358895    2.943569
    risk2 |       2   .3775745     3.67   0.000    1.381446    2.895516
    risk3 |       3   .6141326     5.37   0.000    2.008496    4.480964
    risk4 |      .5   .094885     -3.65   0.000     .344697    .7252747
     _cons |       2   .5225312     2.65   0.008    1.198506    3.337488
 ln(ptime) |       1  (exposure)
------------------------------------------------------------------------
```

When exact Poisson regression was used with a gigabyte of memory allocated to the output files, the results here were produced after 301 seconds:

```
. expoisson outcome risk1 risk2 risk3 risk4, exp(ptime) irr saving(memory2,
replace) memory(1g)

Estimating: risk1
Enumerating sample-space combinations:
observation 1:   enumerations =        45
observation 2:   enumerations =      1035
observation 3:   enumerations =     47265
observation 4:   enumerations =    113070
observation 5:   enumerations =   1748484
observation 6:   enumerations =   2297890
observation 7:   enumerations =   3405865
(output omitted)
```

```
Exact Poisson regression

                                            Number of obs =        16
----------------------------------------------------------------------
  outcome |      IRR      Suff.   2*Pr(Suff.)    [95% Conf. Interval]
----------+-----------------------------------------------------------
    risk1 |  1.999738      82       0.0004      1.342725     3.026148
    risk2 |  2.000129      74       0.0003      1.36297      2.962323
    risk3 |  3.000016      87       0.0000      1.987315     4.627365
    risk4 |   .499945      44       0.0003       .3365712     .7346223
ln(ptime) |         1   (exposure)
----------------------------------------------------------------------
```

Only the initial output from the enumeration log is shown. For observation 7 there were 3.4 million estimates for the distribution. The total number of enumerations for all four variables was over 70 million. Both commands produced estimated rate ratios that are the same, except for rounding errors, and the other statistics were so similar that the exact approach was superfluous.

To speed up the estimation command, or make estimation feasible when it otherwise would not be, it is possible to enter just one or two variables at a time and designate the other variables as conditional. For example, to get the rate ratio for the variable risk1, adjusted for risk2, risk3, and risk4, the following command will work:

```
. expoisson outcome risk1, exp(ptime) irr saving(memory2, replace) memory
(1g) condvars(risk2 risk3 risk4)

Estimating: risk1
Enumerating sample-space combinations:
observation 1:   enumerations =        45
observation 2:   enumerations =      1035
(output omitted)

Exact Poisson regression
                                            Number of obs =        16
```

```
-----------------------------------------------------------------
 outcome |       IRR       Suff.   2*Pr(Suff.)    [95% Conf. Interval]
---------+-------------------------------------------------------
  risk1 |  1.999738          82      0.0004      1.342725    3.026148
ln(ptime) |        1  (exposure)
-----------------------------------------------------------------
```

This command took 73 seconds to run. The output for risk1 is just what it was when all four rate ratios were estimated simultaneously. This approach may make some estimates possible when the simultaneous model for all variables is not possible.

23.4 A CAVEAT

Exact regression can produce valid P-values and CIs when outcomes are too rare for estimation methods that require large samples. But the exact approach still relies upon the assumption that the counts were generated by a Poisson process with independence of events and a constant (stationary) rate. When the counts in rate numerators are small, we usually have little ability to check those assumptions. Extra caution in interpretation is therefore required when counts are small. In many situations the best solution will be to obtain more data.

Instrumental Variables

24

Instrumental variable analysis of rates can be implemented in Stata using generalized method of moments estimation. To explain why an analyst might consider this approach, I will start with a problem related to the analysis and interpretation of randomized controlled trials.

24.1 THE PROBLEM: WHAT DOES A RANDOMIZED CONTROLLED TRIAL ESTIMATE?

A randomized trial of fall rates (Shumway-Cook et al. 2007) was described in Chapters 12 and 13 (Table 12.1). Enrollment was limited to sedentary adults age 65 years or older. The 226 persons assigned to the intervention were offered 6 hours of instruction about fall prevention, plus a free exercise program 3 days per week for a year. The exercise was intended to improve strength and balance. The 227 persons assigned to the control group were simply given two brochures about fall prevention. After a year of follow-up, the fall rate was 1.33 falls/person-year in the intervention arm and 1.77 in the control arm. The rate ratio of 0.75 (95% CI 0.52–1.09) is the intention-to-treat estimate, a measure of the causal effect of recommending the experimental exercise treatment. Because assignment was random, confounding by observed and unobserved factors should not be a systematic source of bias and estimates of significance and precision are fully justified.

Despite random assignment, the intention-to-treat estimate may be biased if follow-up regarding the outcome is incomplete. In the fall-prevention study only 11 subjects failed to provide a full year of fall data. Complete data were missing for only 1.3% of the 453 person-years of planned follow-up (Table 12.1). So the intention-to-treat estimate in this trial is probably free of noteworthy bias.

The intention-to-treat rate ratio of 0.75 estimates the effect of recommending treatment, not the effect of receiving treatment. In the trial intervention arm, six subjects failed to attend any exercise classes, mean attendance for classes was 49%, and the median attendance was 58% (Figure 24.1). It is reasonable to wonder what might have been observed if those in the exercise arm had actually attended all of their exercise classes. What was the effect of treatment among those who actually received treatment?

24.2 ANALYSIS BY TREATMENT RECEIVED MAY YIELD BIASED ESTIMATES OF TREATMENT EFFECT

To create the simplest example, I will dichotomize both the exposure and the outcome.

Persons who attended two-thirds or more of their exercise classes will be designated as receiving treatment; 38% of the intervention subjects (86/226) met this definition (Figure 24.1).

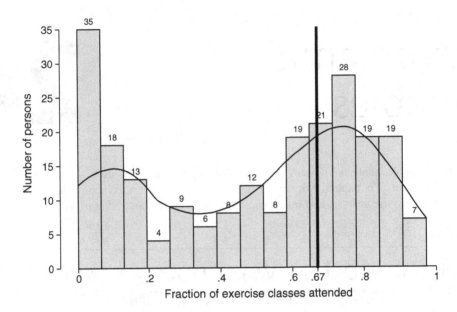

FIGURE 24.1 Histogram showing how the fraction of exercise classes attended was distributed among 226 persons assigned to the exercise arm of a trial of fall prevention. Vertical bar height corresponds to the number of study persons in each of 15 bins; counts of subjects are on the top of each bar. The curved solid line is a smoothed plot of these counts, using a kernel density smoother. The vertical line at fraction 0.67 demarcates those who attended two-thirds or more of their exercise classes from those who attended fewer.

The outcome will similarly be divided into those who had any fall during follow-up (56% = 254/453) and those who never fell. Dichotomizing exposure and outcome ignores useful information and makes unrealistic assumptions (Hollander, Sauerbrei, and Schumacher 2004, Royston, Altman, and Sauerbrei 2006). For example, a person who attended 67% of their exercise classes is considered to have received the same treatment as someone who attended 97%. But using a binary exposure and outcome simplifies this example. In addition, any possible effect of the 6 hours of instruction regarding fall prevention will be ignored. Everyone will be treated as if they were followed for 1 year and the outcome was cumulative incidence (risk) of any fall (Table 24.1). The intention-to-treat analysis of these data can be expressed as a risk difference, comparing the intervention (exercise) arm with the control subjects, of $(43 + 81)/(43 + 43 + 81 + 59) - 130/(130 + 97) = .549 - .573 = -.024.$

TABLE 24.1 Classification of persons in a trial of fall prevention according to their randomly assigned treatment and whether they had any falls in follow-up. Intervention arm is divided into those who attended two-thirds or more of their exercise classes and those who attended fewer.

TREATMENT ASSIGNED	ATTENDED TWO-THIRDS OR MORE OF EXERCISE CLASSES	NUMBER WHO FELL	NUMBER WHO DID NOT FALL	FALL RISK
Exercise	Yes	43	43	.500
	No	81	59	.579
Control		130	97	.573

We could estimate the effect of actually receiving the treatment by comparing the 86 persons who attended two-thirds or more of their exercise sessions with all the other 367 study subjects: risk difference = 43/(43 + 43) − (81 + 130)/(81 + 59 + 130 + 97) = .500 − .575 = −.075. Or we can compare the 86 who attended two-thirds or more of their classes with the 227 controls only: risk difference 43/(43 + 43) − 130/(130 + 97) = .500 − .573 = − .073. Both of these comparisons may be biased because the persons who attended two-thirds of their classes did this for reasons that may be related to their risk of falling. They might, compared with others, have been healthier, stronger, or more agile, factors that might lower their risk of falling aside from any effect of exercise. The comparison of those who received treatment with others ignores the random assignment and may therefore be biased by confounding factors.

24.3 USING AN INSTRUMENTAL VARIABLE

I now use this simple example to show how an instrumental variable analysis can be done, closely following a description in Weiss and Koepsell (2014 pp260–263,268–269). When describing instrumental variables, many authors designate treatment received as X, the outcome as Y, an unmeasured confounder as U, and the instrumental variable as Z. In this simplified fall-study example these variables are binary (0,1) with X = 1 if a subject attended two-thirds or more of their exercise classes, Y = 1 if they fell, and U is an unmeasured binary confounder. For example, U might indicate muscle strength (weak = 0, strong = 1) and those with U = 1 might be both more likely to attend exercise classes and less likely to fall because of their greater strength, regardless of the exercise program. The relationship between these variables can be depicted in a casual (directed acyclic) graph (Figure 24.2) (Morgan and Winship 2007b pp61–86, Glymour and Greenland 2008, Weiss and Koepsell 2014 pp236–245). In this example the treatment X can influence the risk of falling (Y). This relationship is confounded by U. If U is measured and used in an appropriate model, we could obtain unbiased estimates of the X–Y association. Z, an instrumental variable or instrument, affects the possibility that X = 1.

To be a valid instrument, Z must have several properties:

1. Z affects the treatment X.
2. Z influences the outcome Y only through the treatment X. The effect of Z on Y is mediated entirely through the treatment X. This is indicated in Figure 24.2 by the causal arrows from Z to X to Y. No causal arrow leads directly from Z to Y.
3. Z and Y share no common causes. There is no confounding of the Z-Y association once we have accounted for the influence of Z on treatment X. We can say that Z is independent of U.

An instrumental variable which has these three properties can be used to place limits or bounds on the values of the population average treatment effect of X on Y (Robins and

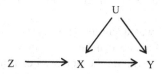

FIGURE 24.2 Causal diagram (directed acyclic graph) showing relationships between treatment (X), outcome (Y), unmeasured confounder (U), and an instrumental variable (Z). Z affects Y only by changing the probability that X = 1. Z has no direct pathway to Y. U affects both X and Y.

Greenland 1996, Angrist, Imbens, and Rubin 1996, Balke and Pearl 1997, Palmer et al. 2011). These limits are not estimates of precision, such as confidence limits, but limits on the potential size of average treatment effect given the data. To move beyond these limits and produce valid estimates of causal effects, such as risk differences or rate ratios, one of these additional properties must be true:

4A. Homogeneity. If the effect of treatment X on Y is the same (homogeneous) for all subjects, then the instrument Z can be used to estimate an average treatment effect for everyone in the study. This strong assumption is often not realistic.

4B. Homogeneity within levels of Z. When Z = 0 or Z = 1, the effect of X on Y is the same for treated and untreated subjects. This means the size of the treatment effect is the same for all levels of Z. There is no interaction between treatment effect and the instrumental variable Z. This assumption is weaker than 4A, but often not plausible.

4C. Monotonicity. This weaker assumption means that the effect of Z on X is in one direction only. Assume that when Z = 1, a subject is more likely to receive treatment (X = 1). To put this another way, when Z = 1, some subjects may ignore this value of Z and still not receive treatment, while others will be influenced by Z to change from no treatment (X = 0) to treatment (X = 1). This means that some will comply with treatment assignment while others ignore the assignment. Monotonicity means that there are no curmudgeons who will move in the opposite direction, contrary to their level of Z. No one who would have otherwise not have received treatment will obtain it because their Z value was 0. No one who otherwise would have received treatment, will avoid it because their Z-value happens to be 1. Those who behave in this contrary manner have been labeled defiers (Angrist, Imbens, and Rubin 1996).

By now you may have guessed that the random assignment to the exercise arms and control arms of the trial can serve as an instrumental variable Z. Property 1 can be checked with data. Property 1 was met because random assignment affected receipt of the exercise treatment (X = 1). In the intervention arm, 38% received treatment (meaning 2/3rds or more of their exercise classes). In the control arm, no one received any exercise classes. (I will ignore the remote possibility that some controls leaped from their recliners and joined an exercise program similar to the study intervention.) Property 2 cannot be proved, but it seems plausible that assignment to intervention or control arm would not change anyone's fall risk, aside from some effect of the exercise treatment X. (A skeptic could argue that the 6 hours of fall prevention instruction undermines Property 2.) Property 3 means that treatment assignment was unrelated to the confounder U. This is believable, as assignment was random. Finally, 4C, monotonicity, also seems likely. There was probably no one who decided to avoid exercise classes just because they were randomly assigned to the exercise group. As far as we know, no one assigned to the control arm suddenly joined a gym because they resented their assignment to the control group. In summary, property 1 is confirmed and properties 2, 3, and 4C seem credible.

An excellent discussion of the assumptions required for instrumental variable analysis is in a paper by Angrist, Imbens, and Rubin (1996); these authors have considerable enthusiasm for this method. Another fine discussion with a skeptical viewpoint is by Hernán and Robins (Hernán and Robins 2006).

Imagine now that confounder U was accurately measured, it is the only confounder of the X – Y association, and its confounding influence can be fully removed by using a dichotomous variable (weak = 0, strong = 1). We can then estimate the unbiased causal risk difference for treatment X = 1 versus X = 0, using an ordinary linear regression model (Expression 24.1), where RD means risk difference.

$$Y = \text{risk}(Y = 1) = b_0 + b_1 X + b_2 U = \text{constant} + RD_X X + RD_U U \qquad \text{(Ex.24.1)}$$

In Expression 24.1, RD_X is a valid estimate, on the risk difference scale, of the causal effect of treatment on the risk of falling during 1 year. This estimate, adjusted for strength, is free of systematic bias because U (strength) was accurately measured and accounted for in the analysis and there were no other confounders.

We now define some proportions: (1) p1 = proportion who adhered to exercise (X = 1) when assigned to exercise (Z = 1) = 86/226 = .3805, (2) p0 = proportion with (X = 1) when assigned to control arm (Z = 0) = 0/227 = 0, (3) u1 = proportion strong (U = 1) when assigned to exercise (Z = 1) = unknown, (4) u0 = proportion strong (U=1) when assigned to control (Z = 0) = unknown. So p1 and p0 are known, but u1 and u0 are not known because we lack measurements of U.

If we can estimate RD_X and RD_U, we can estimate the average fall risk for those who were assigned to the control arm (Z = 0, Expression 24.2) and those in the treatment arm (Z = 1, Expression 24.3).

$$\text{risk}_{Z0} = b_0 + RD_X \times p0 + RD_U \times u0 \qquad \text{(Ex.24.2)}$$

$$\text{risk}_{Z1} = b_0 + RD_X \times p1 + RD_U \times u1 \qquad \text{(Ex.24.3)}$$

Now let us rearrange expressions 24.2 and 24.3 to estimate the risk difference for a fall for those with Z = 1 and those with Z = 0, in expression 24.4.

$$\begin{aligned}\text{risk}_{Z1} - \text{risk}_{Z0} &= (b_0 + RD_X \times p1 + RD_U \times u1) - (b_0 + RD_X \times p0 + RD_U \times u0 \\ &= RD_X \times (p1 - p0) + RD_U \times (u1 - u0)\end{aligned} \qquad \text{(Ex.24.4)}$$

If property 3 is true for Z, there is no confounding of the Z–Y association. By definition, Z is independent of *any* variables that may influence outcome Y, after accounting for X. Given that Z was randomly assigned, this is arguably true. Therefore, the term $RD_U \times (u1 - u0)$ must be equal to 0. This term is in Expression 24.4 only to remove confounding of the association between Z (represented by $RD_x \times (p1 - p0)$) and outcome Y (represented by $\text{risk}_{z1} - \text{risk}_{z0}$). But property 3 tells us there is no confounding of the association between Z and Y. Therefore, either $RD_U = 0$ or $(u1 - u0) = 0$, or both. Because $RD_U \times (u1 - u0)$ must be equal to 0, we can rearrange expression 24.4 to estimate the unbiased causal risk difference, RD_X, using quantities that are easy to obtain (Table 24.1) and without any measurement of the potential confounder, U.

$$\begin{aligned}RD_X &= (\text{risk}_{Z1} - \text{risk}_{Z0})/(p1 - p0) \\ &= ((43 + 81)/(43 + 43 + 81 + 59) - 130/(130 + 97))/(.3805 - 0) \\ &= (.549 - .573)/.3805 = -.024/.3805 = -.063.\end{aligned} \qquad \text{(Ex.24.5)}$$

The causal risk difference estimate in this simple example has been called the ratio or Wald estimate. The numerator (−.024) of this ratio is the intention-to-treat estimate of the Z-Y association, the observed fall proportions of the exercise group minus that of the control group. The denominator (.3805) is a scaling factor equal to the Z-X association, the fraction attending 2/3rds or more of exercise classes among those assigned to exercise minus the fraction of frequent exercisers among controls.

24.4 TWO-STAGE LINEAR REGRESSION FOR INSTRUMENTAL VARIABLES

We could estimate the same Wald ratio by using two linear regression models. First estimate the Z–Y association (–.024), then estimate the Z–X association (.3805), and then divide the first estimate by the second. These two stages are carried out simultaneously in the method of two-stage least squares linear regression (Wooldridge 2008 pp506–525, Angrist and Pischke 2008 pp113–218). I will apply this venerable method to the simplified analysis of falls. In these models the outcome (Y) is contained in variable anyfall: no falls (anyfall = 0), at least one fall (anyfall = 1). The random treatment assignment (Z) is in the instrumental variable exercise and attendance at two-thirds or more of exercise classes (X) is indicated by twothird = 1. Stata's **reg3** command implements this model:

```
. reg3 (anyfall twothird) (twothird exercise), 2sls
```

Two-stage least-squares regression

Equation	Obs	Parms	RMSE	"R-sq"	F-Stat	P
anyfall	453	1	.4965493	0.0034	0.26	0.6069
twothird	453	1	.3436931	0.2354	138.83	0.0000

	Coef.	Std. Err.	t	P>|t|	[95% Conf. Interval]
anyfall						
twothird	-.0631083	.122618	-0.51	0.607	-.3037581	.1775415
_cons	.5726872	.0329571	17.38	0.000	.5080056	.6373688
twothird						
exercise	.380531	.0322963	11.78	0.000	.3171463	.4439156
_cons	-5.55e-17	.0228117	-0.00	1.000	-.0447702	.0447702

Endogenous variables: anyfall twothird
Exogenous variables: exercise

In this output, the Z–X association is .3805, as expected, and the risk difference of – .063 is the average effect of treatment on fall risk among compliers. This is the estimate shown earlier using Expression 24.5. The instrumental variable, exercise, is called an exogenous variable by the software. The confidence interval (CI) around the treatment estimate is so wide that this estimate is not terribly useful. We can obtain the same results using Stata's **ivregress** command, which is designed for instrumental variable linear regression:

```
. ivregress 2sls anyfall (twothird = exercise), vce(robust) first
```

First-stage regressions
- - - - - - - - - - - - - - - - - -
Warning: variance matrix is nonsymmetric or highly singular

		Number of obs	=	453
		F(0, 451)	=	.
		Prob > F	=	.
		R-squared	=	0.2354
		Adj R-squared	=	0.2337
		Root MSE	=	0.3437

twothird	Coef.	Robust Std. Err.	t	P>|t|	[95% Conf. Interval]
exercise	.380531	.	.	.	. .
_cons	2.78e-17	.	.	.	. .

Instrumental variables (2SLS) regressi

		Number of obs	=	453
		Wald chi2(1)	=	0.27
		Prob > chi2	=	0.6060
		R-squared	=	0.0034
		Root MSE	=	.49545

anyfall	Coef.	Robust Std. Err.	z	P>|z|	[95% Conf. Interval]
twothird	-.0631083	.1223479	-0.52	0.606	-.3029057	.1766892
_cons	.5726872	.0328336	17.44	0.000	.5083345	.6370399

Instrumented: twothird
Instruments: exercise

The output from **ivregress** shows no standard error (SE) estimate for the proportion (.3805) that attended two-thirds of their exercise classes, because these people only appeared in the exercise arm of the trial. The treatment-outcome association is again –.063 and use of a robust variance estimator did little to change the CI for the twothird treatment variable. Bootstrap methods (not shown) provided essentially the same CIs.

24.5 GENERALIZED METHOD OF MOMENTS

There are several good ways to estimate parameters of interest; least squares regression and maximum likelihood are two of these. A third approach is called generalized method of moments (GMM) (Cameron and Trivedi 2005 pp166–199, Wooldridge 2010 pp207–233). Stata implements this with a **gmm** command and we can use this for the simplified fall study analysis:

```
. gmm (anyfall - {b1}*twothird - {cons}), instruments(exercise) nolog

Final GMM criterion Q(b) = 4.78e-34
note: model is exactly identified

GMM estimation

Number of parameters =  2
Number of moments     =  2
Initial weight matrix: Unadjusted              Number of obs  =      453
GMM weight matrix:     Robust


------------------------------------------------------------------------
            |              Robust
            |    Coef.   Std. Err.      z    P>|z|     [95% Conf. Interval]
- - - - -+--------------------------------------------------------------
     /b1 |  -.0631083   .1223479   -0.52   0.606   -.3029057    .1766892
    /cons |   .5726872   .0328336   17.44   0.000    .5083345    .6370399
------------------------------------------------------------------------
Instruments for equation 1: exercise _cons
```

By default, the **gmm** command used a robust variance estimator. The estimated effect of good adherence to treatment on fall risk was again –.063, with the same SE and CI obtained by **ivregress**. In this simple example, GMM estimation offers no advantage over two-stage linear regression. The GMM method has the drawback of requiring the user to learn a new command syntax. But the GMM approach has an important feature; it can be applied to a variety of non-linear instrumental variable problems (Mullahy 1997, Winkelmann 2008 pp162–167, Wooldridge 2010 pp207–233,525–547, Cameron and Trivedi 2013a pp45–46,397–401). The **gmm** command can fit an exponential model which can use the instrumental variable method to estimate the unbiased (thanks to randomization) risk ratio for any fall, comparing those who attended two-thirds or more of the exercise classes with controls:

```
. gmm (anyfall - exp({xb:twothird}+{cons})), instruments(exercise) nolog

Final GMM criterion Q(b) = 2.72e-29
note: model is exactly identified

GMM estimation

Number of parameters  =  2
Number of moments      =  2
Initial weight matrix: Unadjusted              Number of obs  =      453
GMM weight matrix:     Robust


------------------------------------------------------------------------
            |              Robust
            |    Coef.   Std. Err.      z    P>|z|     [95% Conf. Interval]
-------+----------------------------------------------------------------
twothird |  -.1167549   .2351426   -0.50   0.620   -.5776259    .344116
------ +----------------------------------------------------------------
   /cons |  -.5574156   .0573326   -9.72   0.000   -.6697853   -.4450458
------------------------------------------------------------------------
```

```
Instruments for equation 1: exercise _cons

. lincom twothird, irr

( 1)  [xb]twothird = 0
-------------------------------------------------------------------------
            |      IRR   Std. Err.       z    P>|z|     [95% Conf. Interval]
    --------+----------------------------------------------------------------
        (1) |  .8898032   .2092306    -0.50   0.620      .5612292    1.410742
-------------------------------------------------------------------------
```

24.6 GENERALIZED METHOD OF MOMENTS FOR RATES

The **gmm** command shown earlier does not have an option for showing a regression table of exponentiated coefficients and it does not allow offsets for person-time. But Stata has an **ivpoisson gmm** command that does both these things and is well suited for an instrumental variable analysis when the outcomes are rates (Mullahy 1997, Winkelmann 2008 pp162–167, Cameron and Trivedi 2013a pp45–46,397–401).

We can now abandon the simplified binary definition of treatment adherence. The variable exfrac is the fraction of exercise classes attended by each person in the intervention arm, ranging from 0 to .97 (Figure 24.1). We can analyze these data according to treatment received, as expressed by exercise fraction as a linear term on the log scale:

```
. poisson fallcnt exfrac, exp(time) vce(robust) irr nolog

Poisson regression                              Number of obs    =       453
                                                Wald chi2(1)     =      2.68
                                                Prob > chi2      =    0.1015
Log pseudolikelihood = -1046.0894               Pseudo R2        =    0.0061


----------------------------------------------------------------------------
            |               Robust
    fallcnt |      IRR    Std. Err.       z    P>|z|     [95% Conf. Interval]
------------+---------------------------------------------------------------
     exfrac |  .6483052    .171561    -1.64   0.101      .3859456    1.089013
      _cons |  1.710964   .2210567     4.16   0.000      1.328206    2.204023
   ln(time) |         1   (exposure)
----------------------------------------------------------------------------
```

We can fit the same model using GMM. The estimates will be slightly different because the fitting methods differ:

```
. ivpoisson gmm fallcnt exfrac, exp(time) multiplicative irr nolog

Final GMM criterion Q(b) = 1.19e-33

note: model is exactly identified
```

Exponential mean model with endogenous regressors

Number of parameters = 2   Number of obs =   453
Number of moments   = 2
Initial weight matrix: Unadjusted
GMM weight matrix: Robust

```
------------------------------------------------------------------------
             |              Robust
   fallcnt   |     IRR    Std. Err.     z    P>|z|    [95% Conf. Interval]
------------------------------------------------------------------------
     exfrac  |  .6475984  .1744838   -1.61   0.107    .3819133   1.098112
      _cons  |  1.698364   .219771    4.09   0.000    1.317904   2.188656
  ln(time)   |        1   (exposure)
------------------------------------------------------------------------
```

(no endogenous regressors)

   The estimated rate ratio of 0.65 is based on treatment received; it estimates the effect of the
exercise program on fall rates, comparing someone who attended all their exercise classes with
someone who was not exposed to any exercise classes. But this estimate is probably biased, as each
intervention subject made his or her decision about exercise attendance. So we turn to an instrumental
variable analysis, using the random assignment as an instrument:

. ivpoisson gmm fallcnt (exfrac = exercise), exp(time) multiplicative irr
nolog

Final GMM criterion Q(b) = 1.09e-33

note: model is exactly identified

Exponential mean model with endogenous regressors

Number of parameters = 2   Number of obs =   453
Number of moments   = 2
Initial weight matrix: Unadjusted
GMM weight matrix: Robust

```
------------------------------------------------------------------------
             |              Robust
   fallcnt   |     IRR    Std. Err.     z    P>|z|    [95% Conf. Interval]
------------------------------------------------------------------------
     exfrac  |  .5568029  .2001504   -1.63   0.103    .2752488   1.126361
      _cons  |  1.763779  .2695879    3.71   0.000    1.307196   2.379839
  ln(time)   |        1   (exposure)
------------------------------------------------------------------------
```

Instrumented: exfrac
Instruments: exercise

   The constant term in the last model is the fall rate (1.76) among the controls, as estimated by
the GMM method. It is the same rate (not shown) a GMM model will report for the constant term
when an intention-to-treat analysis is done. The two prior models (**poisson** and **ivpoisson**) that used

treatment received as the exposure reported smaller control rates of 1.71 and 1.70 because they included some intervention subjects who never exercised in the baseline group, as if they were controls. In the last instrumental variable analysis, the estimate of complier-averaged treatment effect (0.56) was stronger than the estimate (0.65) based on treatment received. CIs were wide around both estimates.

Is this instrumental variable analysis unbiased? Even if Z fulfills all the desired properties of an instrument, this analysis assumes that exercise fraction as a linear term on the ln scale is a good expression of the biological effect of exercise. This linearity assumption may not be true in some studies (Angrist and Imbens 1995, Silverwood et al. 2014, Burgess, Small, and Thompson 2015). If we fit a Poisson regression model for the 226 intervention subjects only, with fall rate as the outcome and exercise fraction as a linear term, the fitted line falls from a rate of 1.48 falls per person-year when exercise fraction is 0 to 1.20 falls when exercise fraction is .97 (Figure 24.3). If two fractional polynomial terms are used to fit a more flexible curve, the plot shows that fall rates increase as exercise fraction increases from about 10 to 55%, and thereafter fall rates decrease. Is this plausible? Whatever the flaws of the intention-to-treat analysis, it avoided some subjective choices about how treatment participation should be measured and modeled. In trials of a vaccine or surgery, where receipt of treatment is necessarily binary, these additional issues could be avoided.

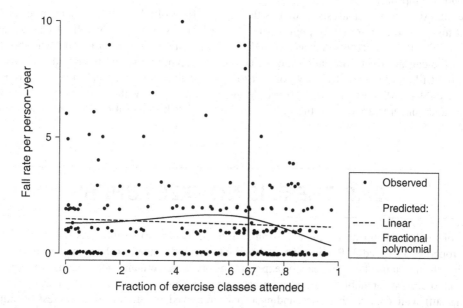

FIGURE 24.3 Scatterplot showing the observed fall rates of 226 persons assigned to the exercise trial arm, against the fraction of exercise classes they attended. The straight dashed line is from a Poisson model that used a linear term for exercise class attendance fraction. The solid curve is from a Poisson model that used two fractional polynomial terms for exercise class attendance. To make the plot more readable: (1) random jitter was added to reduce the overlap of identical rates, and (2) the vertical scale was changed by omitting two subjects with the highest rates (13 for fraction 0.64 and 11 for fraction 0.73) from the plot, but these subjects were included in the regression models. The vertical line at fraction 0.67 demarcates those who attended two-thirds or more of their exercise classes from those who attended fewer.

24.7 WHAT DOES AN INSTRUMENTAL VARIABLE ANALYSIS ESTIMATE?

The rate ratio of 0.56 is unbiased if all the instrumental analysis assumptions are true. This interpretation, however, requires some caution (Fang, Brooks, and Chrischilles 2012). This is an estimate of the rate for a person who attended all of their exercise classes, compared with the rate of someone who attended no classes. It is not an estimate of the effect of treatment for all study subjects (or people in the population like them). That would require that property 4A, homogeneity, be true. Nor is it an estimate of the effect of treatment among the treated; that would require property 4B, homogeneity of treatment effect among the treated. Both these homogeneity assumptions are implausible in many studies. If monotonicity is true (4C), a weaker assumption than 4A and 4B, the rate ratio of 0.56 estimates the effect of perfect treatment adherence among those who are good at following recommended treatment. It is the treatment effect among compliers, the goody-two-shoes who attended most of their classes. These cooperative folks are in both trial arms; there are controls who would have complied if they had been assigned to treatment. But there is typically no way to identify this group of compliers. This estimate has been called the local average treatment effect (Angrist, Imbens, and Rubin 1996), the average causal effect for compliers (Angrist, Imbens, and Rubin 1996), and the complier-averaged causal effect (Dunn, Maracy, and Tomenson 2005, Burgess, Small, and Thompson 2015).

The intention-to-treat analysis estimates the causal effect of advising treatment: rate ratio 0.75 It is an estimate for the entire study population and suggests that the rate of falling can be decreased by 25% if the trial intervention was offered to a population. The instrumental-variable analysis estimates the causal effect (rate ratio 0.56) of actually receiving all of the treatment. A conscientious person might like to know that if they commit to exercise three times a week, they may reduce their fall rate by 44%. All these interpretations should be tempered by the wide CIs around the point estimates and concerns about how the falls counts were distributed (Table 12.1), as was discussed in Chapter 12.

24.8 THERE IS NO FREE LUNCH

The use of random treatment assignment as an instrument is easy to swallow, as randomization usually fulfills properties 1, 2, and 3. But instrumental variable methods have also been applied to observational studies in which treatment assignments or exposure history were certainly not random. The goal of these analyses is to estimate an unbiased association between treatment X and outcome Y. This typically means collecting sufficient data so that confounding can be removed by stratification, regression adjustment, matching, weighting, propensity scores, or some combination of these methods. All these methods produce estimates that may be biased from the true causal effect of X on Y by residual confounding. The idea that an instrumental variable Z can eliminate confounding of the X – Y association, without using or even measuring the confounding variables, seems almost magical.

Instrumental variable analysis has its own limitations. Studies have used distance to a college or a hospital, quarter (3-month period) of birth, physician prescribing choices, and regional variations in treatment as instruments. Property 1, the association of the instrument with the treatment, can be checked in the data. But properties 2 and 3 usually rely upon reasoning which is not always convincing and cannot be verified by data. The instrumental method substitutes an assumption of no residual confounding of the Z – Y association for an assumption of no confounding of the X – Y association.

Any method of analysis of observational data may be biased by residual confounding (or other sources of systematic bias, such as measurement error or selection bias), and instrumental variable analyses share these limitations. Several articles discuss biases that may arise when using instrumental variable methods (Martens et al. 2006, Hernán and Robins 2006, Swanson and Hernán 2013, Garabedian et al. 2014, Jackson and Swanson 2015). In many instrumental variable studies, it is not hard to imagine that the instrument may have a direct effect on the outcome aside from its effect upon treatment or that the instrument and the outcome may share a common cause. Other sources of bias may be less obvious. For example, several studies have compared the effectiveness of two treatments using a variety of instruments. Superficially, these studies resemble randomized trials of two treatments. Swanson et al (Swanson et al. 2015) have shown that these instrumental variable studies may be biased if those who received a third treatment or no treatment are omitted from the comparisons. I am not suggesting that instrumental variables methods cannot be used because they may be biased. Any observational study *may* be biased, but by doing them as well as possible, we may still gain new knowledge about causal relationships. In some instances, instrumental variable methods may be deemed superior to other approaches, perhaps depending on the availability of information about potential confounders or the availability of a suitable instrument. In other situations, the use of other methods may be a better choice. Instructive comparisons of instrumental variable analyses with other methods have been published (Newhouse and McClellan 1998, Klungel et al. 2004, Huybrechts et al. 2011, Davies et al. 2013a).

Instrumental variable methods have well-known limitations. First, a suitable instrument may not be available. Second, instrumental methods require lots of data (Wooldridge 2008 pp510–514, Boef et al. 2014). These large sample methods may be biased in small samples. Instrumental variable methods typically produce large CIs; many observations are needed to achieve precision. Third, if there is even slight confounding of the Z–Y association, the resulting bias in an instrumental variable analysis can be large. If the instrument has little effect on treatment received, the Z-X association, it is called a weak instrument. Because this association is used to scale up the Z–Y association, a weak instrument is worrisome because the weak Z–X relationship may result in a uselessly wide CI and any bias in the estimated Z–Y relationship will be greatly exaggerated.

24.9 FINAL COMMENTS

Several authors have made suggestions regarding the reporting of instrumental variable analyses (Davies et al. 2013b, Swanson and Hernán 2013, Boef et al. 2013). These articles are worth reading not only for their advice about reporting, but also for insight into the problems that may arise in such an analysis.

In randomized controlled trials the intention-to-treat analysis can be supplemented by using random assignment as an instrument to estimate the effect of treatment among compliers. The trial must be sufficiently large to effectively use of these methods. This approach is superior to an analysis based upon treatment received and can provide valuable information. In observational studies, instrumental variable methods are an additional tool that can be used to combat confounding bias. As with any method, the limitations of this approach should be considered.

Hazards

25

Survival analysis is often described as a group of methods used to study the time to an event. Cox proportional hazards regression, with its variants and extensions, is the focus of several books about survival analysis (Parmar and Machin 1995, Kleinbaum 1996, Klein and Moeschberger 1997, Therneau and Grambsch 2000, Hosmer, Lemeshow, and May 2008, Cleves et al. 2010). Poisson regression can also be used for data about outcomes and time. This chapter compares Poisson regression with the Cox proportional hazards model.

25.1 DATA FOR A HYPOTHETICAL TREATMENT WITH EXPONENTIAL SURVIVAL TIMES

Data were created for an imaginary cohort of 5000 persons who were followed for 10 years. A drug treatment intended to reduce mortality was taken by 3000 cohort members. The mortality rate per person-year was 0.1 for women age 55 years who did not take the drug. Men and the elderly were more likely to take the treatment, compared with women and younger people. On a ratio scale, the true effect of the treatment was a mortality reduction of 20% (rate ratio 0.8) and the true effect of being male increased mortality (rate ratio 1.3). Mortality increased with year of age according to a quadratic curve on the log scale: $1.02 \times age + 1.005 \times age^2$. The ratio change associated with a 1-year age increment was $1.02 \times 1.005 = 1.025$. Using these quantities, the time to death for each subject was simulated by randomly selecting times from an exponential distribution. (Exponential decay was described in Expressions 2.1–2.10.) The survival times were generated as if they came from a process for a constant rate for each level of treatment, sex, and age. The simulated times were produced by a Stata program, **survsim**, written by Crowther and Lambert (Crowther and Lambert 2012, 2013), which creates survival times using a pseudo-random generator.

The survival times from one simulation had a roughly exponential distribution, with many short times and fewer longer times as follow-up continued (Figure 25.1). Survival was initially worse in the treated group because treated persons were older and more often male. The fluctuations in Figure 25.1 were largely due to changes over time in the proportion of subjects who were male or elderly.

25.2 POISSON REGRESSION AND EXPONENTIAL PROPORTIONAL HAZARDS REGRESSION

There were 3654 deaths in the simulated data. Deaths were more common among the treated (73.5%) compared with others (72.5%). Comparing these crude proportions would provide a biased estimate of treatment because treated persons were more often male and elderly (Table 25.1), characteristics associated with greater mortality. Poisson regression can estimate the adjusted association between

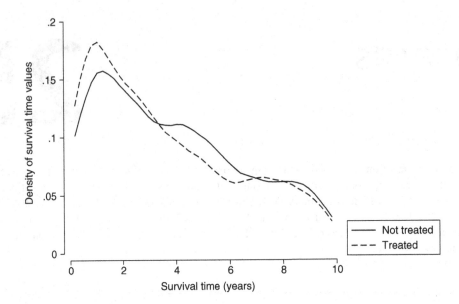

FIGURE 25.1 Density of survival times for a hypothetical comparison of 3000 treated persons with 2000 untreated persons. Survival times were randomly generated from an exponential distribution. Survival times of 10 or more years were excluded from the plot as follow-up ended at 10 years.

TABLE 25.1 Descriptive data for a hypothetical cohort study of a drug treatment.

	TREATMENT	
CHARACTERISTIC	YES (N = 3,000) N (%)	NO (N = 2,000) N (%)
Male	2,000 (67)	1,000 (50)
Age		
<50	176 (6)	787 (39)
50–54	457 (15)	705 (35)
55–59	771 (26)	415 (21)
60+	159 (53)	93 (5)
Died	2,204 (73)	1,450 (73)

treatment and death. The variables treated and male were coded 0/1, agec indicates age centered at 55 years (age in years − 55), and agec2 means agec squared:

```
. poisson died treated male agec agec2, exp(time) irr nolog
Poisson regression                        Number of obs  =      5,000
                                          LR chi2(4)     =     772.55
                                          Prob > chi2    =     0.0000
Log likelihood = -7439.6317               Pseudo R2      =     0.0494
```

```
------------------------------------------------------------------
    died |      IRR    Std. Err.      z   P>|z|     [95% Conf. Interval]
---------+--------------------------------------------------------
 treated | .7720842    .0345404   -5.78   0.000    .7072693   .8428387
    male | 1.281468    .0514376    6.18   0.000    1.184516   1.386355
    agec | 1.019533    .0033938    5.81   0.000    1.012903   1.026206
   agec2 | 1.005241      .00023   22.84   0.000    1.004791   1.005692
   _cons | .1000985    .0041737  -55.20   0.000    .0922436   .1086223
ln(time) |        1  (exposure)
------------------------------------------------------------------
```

The survival times were drawn at random, just once, from the true distribution, so the estimated associations were approximately the same as the true rate ratios in the population: treated rate ratio 0.77 (true value 0.80), male rate ratio 1.28 (true value 1.30), agec rate ratio 1.0195 (true value 1.0200), agec2 rate ratio 1.0052 (true value 1.0050), and the rate for women age 55 and untreated (the _cons term) was 0.1001 (true value 0.1000).

These data were created using an exponential distribution for survival times, so it makes sense to analyze the data using Stata's command for a parametric exponential survival model. A constant rate of mortality over time, for each covariate pattern, implies an exponential decay in survival, as discussed in Chapter 2. The **stset** command was used to tell Stata how time, the outcome, and a unique identifier for each subject (called id) were designated and then an exponential regression model was invoked by the **streg** command:

```
. stset time, failure(died) id(id)

              id:  id
   failure event:  died != 0 & died < .
obs. time interval:  (time[_n-1], time]
 exit on or before:  failure

------------------------------------------------------------------
   5000  total observations
      0  exclusions
------------------------------------------------------------------
   5000  observations remaining, representing
   5000  subjects
   3654  failures in single-failure-per-subject data
27022.926  total analysis time at risk and under observation
                                    at risk from t =         0
                                earliest observed entry t =         0
                                  last observed exit t =        10

. streg treated male agec agec2, distribution(exponential) nolog
        failure _d:  died
   analysis time _t:  time

Exponential regression - - log relative-hazard form
No. of subjects =        5,000              Number of obs   =      5,000
No. of failures =        3,654
Time at risk    =  27022.926
                                           LR chi2(4)      =     772.55
Log likelihood  =  -7439.6317              Prob > chi2     =     0.0000
```

_t	Haz. Ratio	Std. Err.	z	P>|z|	[95% Conf. Interval]
treated	.7720842	.0345404	-5.78	0.000	.7072693 .8428387
male	1.281468	.0514376	6.18	0.000	1.184516 1.386355
agec	1.019533	.0033938	5.81	0.000	1.012903 1.026206
agec2	1.005241	.00023	22.84	0.000	1.004791 1.005692
_cons	.1000985	.0041737	-55.20	0.000	.0922436 .1086223

The exponential regression results are identical to those from Poisson regression. Both models assume a constant rate over time. After using the **streg** command, we can use the **stcurve** command to plot the hazard functions for treated and untreated subjects at the mean values of age and male sex (Figure 25.2). The hazard for the untreated is the instantaneous rate of death at each point in time, which is a constant rate of .1624 deaths per person-year for the entire 10-year interval. The rate is 23% lower (close to the true value of 20%) on a ratio scale, for the treated. Both the Poisson and Cox models estimate a rate ratio that is constant (proportional) over time. I will show later that the assumptions of constant baseline rate and rate ratio over time can be relaxed.

Although the survival times came from an exponential process, these data are not from a Poisson distribution because only one death was possible for each cohort member and death was common. If a robust variance is used, the standard errors become smaller for both models.

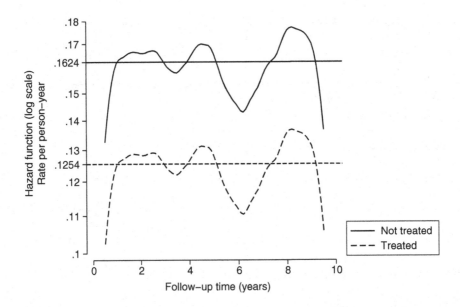

FIGURE 25.2   The two horizontal lines show the hazard functions (rates per person-year in this example) from a parametric exponential survival model for a hypothetical comparison of 3000 treated persons with 2000 untreated persons. The two fluctuating curves are the smoothed hazard functions (instantaneous rates per person-year) from a Cox proportional hazards model for the same data. Rates and hazards are plotted for the average values of sex and age in these data. The adjusted rate ratio and hazard ratio for treated compared with untreated persons were both 0.77. Survival times were from an exponential distribution.

25.3 POISSON AND COX PROPORTIONAL HAZARDS REGRESSION

Consider the output from a Cox proportional hazards model (Breslow and Day 1987, Parmar and Machin 1995, Kleinbaum 1996, Klein and Moeschberger 1997, Therneau and Grambsch 2000, Hosmer, Lemeshow, and May 2008, Cleves et al. 2010, Vittinghoff et al. 2012):

```
. stcox treated male agec agec2, nolog
        failure _d: died
  analysis time _t: time

Cox regression - - no ties

No. of subjects =        5,000              Number of obs  =      5,000
No. of failures =        3,654
Time at risk    =    27022.926
                                            LR chi2(4)     =     745.82
Log likelihood  =   -28861.929             Prob > chi2    =     0.0000

-------------------------------------------------------------------------
      _t | Haz. Ratio Std. Err.       z    P>|z|      [95% Conf. Interval]
---------+---------------------------------------------------------------
 treated |   .7723144  .0345808    -5.77   0.000      .7074261    .8431546
    male |   1.281787  .0514776     6.18   0.000      1.184762    1.386758
    agec |   1.019526  .0033986     5.80   0.000      1.012887    1.026209
   agec2 |   1.005251  .0002348    22.42   0.000       1.00479    1.005711
-------------------------------------------------------------------------
```

The Cox regression table results are close to those from the Poisson model. Differences in the rate ratio estimates appear only after three or four decimals. The Cox model chops up person-time using the time of each death, and comparisons are made using risk sets that consist of one (or more) persons who died at time t, and the remaining cohort survivors at the time of that death. In this example, the first person to die, at 0.0252 years of follow-up, was an untreated woman age 52.6 years. So at 0.252 years of follow-up, the survival of the treated and untreated subjects was compared using all 5000 subjects in the first risk set. The second to die, at 0.0260 years, was a 48-year-old untreated man; the second risk set consists of this man and the remaining 4998 persons. The follow-up time for all 4999 persons in this second risk set was from the time of the first death (0.0252 years) to the time of the second death (0.0260 years). The Cox model estimates are slightly different from the Poisson and exponential estimates because the Cox model is making slightly different comparisons in simulated data that do not *perfectly* follow an exponential distribution.

The Cox model allows the underlying rates to change over time by slicing time into discrete windows; comparisons are made at each failure time. In the jargon of survival analysis, the baseline hazard is allowed to vary over time. This variation is apparent in Figure 25.2, where the hazards (instantaneous rates) of death at each failure time have been combined into a continuous curve using a kernel smoother. The hazard rate of death fluctuates up and down around the mean (constant hazard) values from the parametric exponential survival model (Figure 25.2) The results from both the parametric and the Cox models both produced proportional hazard curves; the hazard ratio was 0.77 at each point in time. The smoothed hazard curves from the Cox model show the initial rise in rates as events start to occur. Males and older persons had a higher rate of death; after an initial die off in these groups, the proportion of the survivors who were male or old started to swing up and down. This produced the oscillation of the Cox-model hazard curves after about 3 years.

We can use Poisson regression to obtain exactly the same results produced by Cox regression, if we slice up person-time in the same way. Stata's **stsplit** command, discussed in Chapter 20, can do this for us:

```
. stsplit, at(failures) riskset(riskset)
(3654 failure times)
(11,592,315 observations (episodes) created)
```

The **stsplit** command created risk set records for each death. For the first risk set 4999 records were generated for survivors at the time of the first death; these new records had the covariate patterns of each survivor but were all assigned the same follow-up time of 0.0252 years. For the second risk set 4998 records were created, again with the same covariate patterns of the survivors, but with follow-up times equal to 0.0260–0.0252 = 0.0008 years. It took one minute for a desktop computer to create 11,592,315 records needed for each risk set. A new variable, _d, was created, coded as 1 for the record with a death, 0 otherwise. One advantage of the Cox model is that all these risk set comparisons are made quickly without creating new records.

Now estimate the Poisson model with an indicator variable for each risk set, so that the comparisons are made within risk sets. When I tried to do this, Stata balked because the default matrix size was not big enough for the 3,654 indicator variables needed for each risk set. We could increase the allowable matrix size, but Chapter 20 showed that we can condition out matching indicators by using conditional Poisson regression. We can use that trick here to save computing time and output:

```
. xtset riskset
    panel variable:  riskset (unbalanced)

. xtpoisson _d treated male agec agec2, fe exp(time) irr nolog
```

```
Conditional fixed-effects Poisson regression    Number of obs    = 11,595,969
Group variable: riskset                         Number of groups =      3,654
                                                Obs per group:
                                                             min =      1,347
                                                             avg =    3,173.5
                                                             max =      5,000
                                                Wald chi2(4)     =     911.28
Log likelihood = -28861.929                     Prob > chi2      =     0.0000
------------------------------------------------------------------------------
     died |      IRR    Std. Err.       z    P>|z|     [95% Conf. Interval]
------------------------------------------------------------------------------
  treated |  .7723144    .0345808    -5.77   0.000     .7074261     .8431546
     male |  1.281787    .0514776     6.18   0.000     1.184762     1.386758
     agec |  1.019526    .0033986     5.80   0.000     1.012887     1.026209
    agec2 |  1.005251    .0002348    22.42   0.000      1.00479     1.005711
 ln(time) |         1   (exposure)
------------------------------------------------------------------------------
```

A desktop computer took 2.5 minutes to produce these regression results. All estimates are exactly the same as those from the Cox model. The mathematical equivalence of these models, when they are parameterized in the same way, has been noted by others (Whitehead 1980, Laird and Olivier

1981, Carstensen 2005). A discussion of the mathematical equivalence of these models is presented by Royston and Lambert (Royston and Lambert 2011 pp47–62). This interchangeability of Cox and Poisson models was described in Chapter 20 (Section 20.13) with regard to matched data. A Poisson model that compares people matched on risk set, all with the same follow-up time within each risk set, is equivalent to the Cox model. The usual Poisson model compares people as if they were all in a single risk set, allows them to have different follow-up times, and makes no allowance for changes in the baseline hazard over time.

25.4 HYPOTHETICAL DATA FOR A RATE THAT CHANGES OVER TIME

When a rate is constant over time, the exponential distribution describes the survival proportion (and survival times). Expression 2.1 was given as

$$N_t = N_0 \times e^{-\text{rate} \times t} \tag{Ex.2.1}$$

The proportion still surviving at time t is often described as the survival function S(t) and for a constant rate (or hazard), this is:

$$S(t) = N_t/N_0 = e^{-\text{rate} \times t} \tag{Ex.25.1}$$

We can modify the survival function to allow the rate to vary with some power of time. The Greek letter gamma γ is often used to designate this power, and Stata uses the caret (^) symbol to indicate a power relationship, so Expression 25.1 becomes:

$$S(t) = N_t/N_0 = e^{-(\text{rate} \times t)^\wedge \gamma} = \exp(-(\text{rate} \times t)^\gamma) \tag{Ex.25.2}$$

The instantaneous rate (hazard) at time t can be described as (Royston and Lambert 2011 p95):

$$\text{hazard at time } t = \gamma \times \text{rate} \times t^{\gamma^\wedge - 1} = \gamma \times \text{rate} \times t^{(1/\gamma)} \tag{Ex.25.3}$$

If a rate changes with time in the multiplicative manner described in Expression 25.3, this is called a Weibull distribution. Under a Weibull distribution, the rate will change monotonically, meaning that it steadily increases or decreases over time. This distribution can be very different from the exponential.

For the same data described in Table 25.1, new survival times were created using two Weibull distributions that were mixed. The details of these distributions are not important here. For each of the 5000 cohort members, their values for treatment, sex, and age were identical to those used previously and the ratios for their instantaneous hazards are unchanged, but all survival times now differ. In just the first 3 years of follow-up nearly everyone died (Figure 25.3). Only a few lived beyond 4 years and by 10 years, only eight treated and four untreated persons were still alive. Now apply the Poisson model:

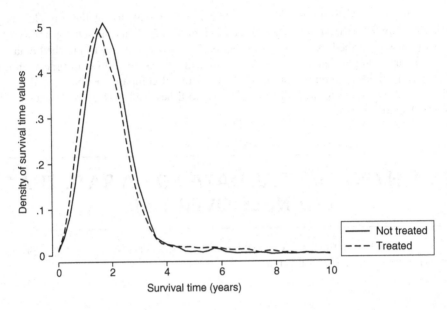

FIGURE 25.3 Density of survival times for a hypothetical comparison of 3000 treated persons with 2000 untreated persons. Survival times were randomly generated from a mixed Weibull distribution. Survival times of 10 or more years were excluded from the plot as follow-up ended at 10 years.

```
. poisson died treated male agec agec2, exp(time) irr nolog
(output omitted)
-----------------------------------------------------------------------------
       died |       IRR   Std. Err.       z   P>|z|    [95% Conf. Interval]
------------+----------------------------------------------------------------
    treated |  .8662549   .0317932    -3.91   0.000    .8061299    .9308644
       male |  1.181236   .0396349     4.96   0.000    1.106052    1.261531
       agec |  1.010287   .0029434     3.51   0.000    1.004534    1.016072
      agec2 |  1.002213   .0002109    10.50   0.000       1.0018    1.002627
      _cons |  .4380579   .0152226   -23.75   0.000    .4092155    .4689332
   ln(time) |         1   (exposure)
-----------------------------------------------------------------------------
```

In this output the rate ratios are all more biased than previously: 0.87 (versus 0.80), 1.18 (versus 1.30), 1.01 (versus 1.0200), and 1.002 (versus 1.0050). These values are further from the true values because the times to first event (death) were not generated by an exponential process and the outcomes are common. Given how different the new survival times are from a Poisson process (compare Figure 25.3 with 25.1), perhaps it is remarkable that the rate ratio estimates are not more biased. Now invoke the Cox model:

```
. stcox treated male agec agec2, nolog
(output omitted)
```

_t	Haz. Ratio	Std. Err.	z	P>|z|	[95% Conf. Interval]	
treated	.7831012	.0290762	-6.58	0.000	.7281371	.8422143
male	1.303463	.0440951	7.83	0.000	1.219841	1.392817
agec	1.0231	.002996	7.80	0.000	1.017244	1.028989
agec2	1.005113	.0002219	23.10	0.000	1.004678	1.005548

All the Cox model rate ratios are close to the true values. The model sliced time into 4988 segments and made comparisons within the risk sets for each of these intervals. The baseline hazards were allowed to vary in any manner over time; the Cox model does not care whether survival times follow an exponential, Weibull, or other distribution. We can use the Cox model to estimate the instantaneous rates (hazards) for the treated and untreated groups over time (Figure 25.4); mortality was much higher compared with Figure 25.2. Mortality among the untreated was nearly two deaths per person-year at 2 years and then fell into a pattern of oscillation similar to that in Figure 25.2.

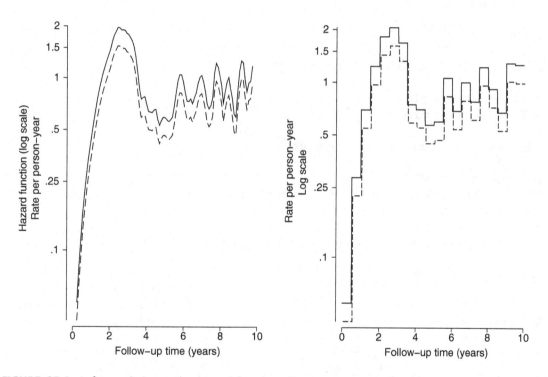

FIGURE 25.4 Left panel shows the hazard functions (instantaneous rates per person-year) from a Cox proportional hazards model for a hypothetical comparison of treated persons with those untreated; hazard ratio 0.78. Hazards are plotted for the average values of sex and age in these data. Right panel shows the same comparison from a piecewise Poisson model, adjusted for age and sex: rate ratio 0.79. The survival times were from a mixed Weibull distribution with greater mortality early in follow-up: see Figure 25.3. In both panels the untreated subjects are represented by solid lines, the treated with dashed lines.

25.5 A PIECEWISE POISSON MODEL

The Poisson and Cox models represent two extremes in their treatment of rates over time. The Poisson model treats the underlying event rate as constant over time. The Cox model slices time into many fragments, using the outcome event times as the boundaries for each time segment. The underlying rate is treated as constant within each interval but is allowed to vary in any manner from one interval to the next. The Poisson model can be modified to create something between these extremes, by dividing follow-up time into intervals and allowing the baseline rate, or hazard, to change from one interval to the next. Instead of using 3654 intervals, as the Cox model did in this example, I divided the 10 years of follow-up into 20 intervals of 0.5 years (6 months) each. If an individual is followed for the entire 10 years, they can have a different rate of death every 6 months:

```
. stsplit timecat, every(.5)
(17,396 observations (episodes) created)
```

The **stsplit** command creates new time variables that indicate the start (_t0) and end (_t) of follow-up in each risk set.

```
. gen risktime = _t - _t0

. lab var risktime "Observation time"

. gen tcat = 1 if time<=.5
(17,396 missing values generated)

. lab var tcat "6 month time intervals"

. forvalues i = 2/20 {
  2.      qui replace tcat = `i' if time<=.5*`i' & tcat==.
  3.      }

. poisson _d treated male agec agec2 i.tcat, exp(risktime) irr nolog
```

Poisson regression			Number of obs	=	22,396
			LR chi2(23)	=	4306.70
			Prob > chi2	=	0.0000
Log likelihood = -14765.579			Pseudo R2	=	0.1273

_d	IRR	Std. Err.	z	P>|z|	[95% Conf. Interval]	
treated	.7856637	.0291506	-6.50	0.000	.7305575	.8449265
male	1.303208	.044083	7.83	0.000	1.219609	1.392538
agec	1.022524	.0029955	7.60	0.000	1.01667	1.028412
agec2	1.004987	.0002211	22.61	0.000	1.004554	1.005421
tcat						
2	5.227223	.5058866	17.09	0.000	4.324067	6.319019
3	12.73362	1.185131	27.34	0.000	10.61035	15.28179

4 |	22.55504	2.099847	33.47	0.000	18.79307	27.07007
5 |	33.29901	3.159174	36.95	0.000	27.64874	40.10396
6 |	37.60266	3.757882	36.29	0.000	30.9138	45.7388
7 |	30.74397	3.464721	30.40	0.000	24.65091	38.34307
8 |	13.67738	2.09615	17.07	0.000	10.12862	18.4695
9 |	12.81197	2.180298	14.99	0.000	9.178281	17.88424
10 |	10.43173	2.070748	11.81	0.000	7.069506	15.39303
11 |	10.90877	2.284837	11.41	0.000	7.23589	16.44597
12 |	19.37168	3.562491	16.12	0.000	13.5092	27.77825
13 |	12.58144	3.103458	10.27	0.000	7.758268	20.40308
14 |	18.3283	4.245937	12.55	0.000	11.63946	28.86102
15 |	14.227	4.151014	9.10	0.000	8.030787	25.20394
16 |	22.38283	5.951478	11.69	0.000	13.29183	37.69164
17 |	16.81369	5.807823	8.17	0.000	8.54356	33.08925
18 |	12.33557	5.629153	5.51	0.000	5.043428	30.17118
19 |	23.58956	9.171253	8.13	0.000	11.00997	50.54215
20 |	23.0533	10.52181	6.87	0.000	9.423977	56.39387
|						
_cons |	.0319587	.0030476	-36.11	0.000	.0265105	.0385267
ln(risktime) |	1	(exposure)				

I could have used xtpoisson to fit the model, but there were only 20 intervals and so an indicator for each time interval was used to show the 19 rate ratios for the comparison of the baseline rate (for an untreated 55-year-old female) in each interval with the first 6-month interval. The **stsplit** command created 17,396 records instead of the millions of records previously needed to make a Poisson model identical to the Cox model. The new piecewise model rate ratio estimates for treatment, male sex, and age are now all close to the true values and close to the Cox model estimates. Notice that the offset was now risktime, the time in each ½-year interval, rather than time.

This piecewise Poisson model assumes that the rate ratio is constant (proportional) at every point in time, so the difference between the baseline and adjusted rates for treated and untreated subjects remains constant on the log scale (Figure 25.4). This constant rate ratio, or proportional hazards assumption, is superimposed on the data by all the models discussed so far in this chapter (Figures 25.2, 25.4).

When outcome events are sufficiently uncommon, many estimators of association will approximate each other. As discussed in Chapter 3, the risk ratio, rate ratio, and odds ratio all agree well when outcomes are rare. The same is true for the rate ratio and hazard ratio. In this example, splitting follow-up time into 6-month intervals made outcomes sufficiently rare within each risk set interval that the Poisson model rate ratios and Cox hazard ratios agree well.

25.6 A MORE FLEXIBLE POISSON MODEL: QUADRATIC SPLINES

The piecewise Poisson model estimated a constant baseline rate within each time interval and allowed these to change abruptly from one interval to the next (Figure 25.4). This stepwise pattern is usually not credible. The word "spline" refers to a flexible piece of wood or metal that a carpenter can use to draw a curve by anchoring it at several points (called "knots") and letting it bend between the points.

Statisticians have adopted the word to describe flexible curves. Quadratic splines (see Chapter 15) allow a curve to have one inflection (bend) between knot values. Using the data from two mixed Weibull distributions, we can split time into intervals of 0.1 years and create almost 97,000 new records so there is a risk set for each interval:

```
. stsplit timecat, every(.1)
(96,997 observations (episodes) created)

. gen risktime = _t - _t0

. lab var risktime "Observation time"
```

Now generate a new variable (midt) for the mid-point of the follow-up time (the uncensored survival times) for each subject in a risk set. If a subject survived to 6.32 years, they will appear in the risk set that covers 6.3 to nearly 6.4 years; their midt value in that risk set will be $(6.3 + 6.32)/2 = 6.31$. In the previous risk set, their midt will be $(6.2 + 6.3)/2 = 6.25$.

```
. gen double midt = (_t0 + _t)/2

. summ midt if _d==1, d
```

```
                          midt
-------------------------------------------------------------
          Percentiles      Smallest
  1%       .3193437        .0212843
  5%       .6265301        .0339947
 10%       .8243021        .0372222     Obs            4,988
 25%      1.228062         .0445355     Sum of Wgt.    4,988
 50%      1.732285                      Mean        1.945525
                          Largest       Std. Dev.   1.196237
 75%      2.324901         9.63014
 90%      3.021228         9.711858     Variance    1.430984
 95%      3.926516         9.842055     Skewness    2.467795
 99%      7.136209         9.911351     Kurtosis     12.3832
```

Selected centiles of midt values are shown for each person that died. To create a flexible curve for mid-point time, we need to pick midt values, called knots, where each quadratic curve segment joins with the next segment. Harrell has offered suggestions for knot choices (Harrell 2001 p23). The quadratic curve, or spline, segments can have one inflection point between knots, but they are constrained to join at the knots. I picked knots at 6 centiles of the midt times: 10, 25, 50, 75, 90, and 95%. The knot time values (.82, 1.23, ..., 3.93) were entered into a local macro called knotlist for convenience in writing commands. At each knot a spline (s1, s2, ..., s6) was created equal to midt minus the knot value at that knot if midt-time was greater than the knot value, otherwise 0. For example, the first spline term, s1, was equal to midt − .82 if midt >.82 and 0 otherwise. Tails of quadratic curves can have unruly behavior, so the tails were constrained to be linear on the log scale. The lower tail was made linear by omitting midt-squared from the regression model. The upper tail was made linear by subtracting the squared value of the last spline, s6, from the squared values of all the other spline terms. So spline s1 was replaced by $s1^2 - s6^2$. Further details are in a helpful paper by Greenland (Greenland 1995). The commands show the details and the Poisson model results:

```
. local knotlist ".82 1.23 1.73 2.32 3.02 3.93"

* Create 6 spline terms:
. local j = 1
. foreach i in `knotlist' {
  2.      qui gen double s`j' = midt - `i' if midt>`i'
  3.      qui replace s`j' = 0 if midt<=`i'
  4.      qui local j = 1 + `j'
  5.      }

* Square each spline and subtract the square of the last spline:
. local j = 1
. foreach i in `knotlist' {
  2.      qui replace s`j' = s`j'^2 - s6^2
  3.      qui local j = 1 + `j'
  4.      }

. poisson _d treated male agec agec2 ///
>     midt s1 - s5, irr exp(risktime) nolog
```

```
Poisson regression                          Number of obs   =   101,997
                                            LR chi2(10)     =   4193.22
                                            Prob > chi2     =    0.0000
Log likelihood = -22826.721                 Pseudo R2       =    0.0841
```

_d	IRR	Std. Err.	z	P>|z|	[95% Conf. Interval]	
treated	.7861604	.0291844	-6.48	0.000	.7309914	.8454932
male	1.297995	.0438971	7.71	0.000	1.214747	1.386947
agec	1.022566	.0029928	7.62	0.000	1.016717	1.028449
agec2	1.004986	.0002216	22.55	0.000	1.004552	1.00542
midt	17.89509	2.30253	22.42	0.000	13.90629	23.02802
s1	.1120869	.0372241	-6.59	0.000	.0584616	.2149014
s2	7.201735	4.373915	3.25	0.001	2.190114	23.6814
s3	1.112317	.5670558	0.21	0.835	.4095328	3.021124
s4	.2395179	.0946818	-3.62	0.000	.1103714	.5197797
s5	10.1147	2.64929	8.83	0.000	6.05344	16.90066
_cons	.0179459	.0019708	-36.61	0.000	.0144706	.0222557
ln(risktime)	1	(exposure)				

With 5 spline terms in the regression model, the rate ratios for treated, male, centered-age (agec), and centered-age-squared were all close to the true values. Using the regression output we can estimate the rates at each point of midt-time for an untreated (rate0) and treated (rate1) woman, age 55 years:

```
. gen rate0 = exp(_b[_cons] + _b[midt]*midt ///
>     + _b[s1]*s1 + _b[s2]*s2 + _b[s3]*s3 + _b[s4]*s4 + _b[s5]*s5)

. gen rate1 = exp(ln(rate0) + _b[treated])
```

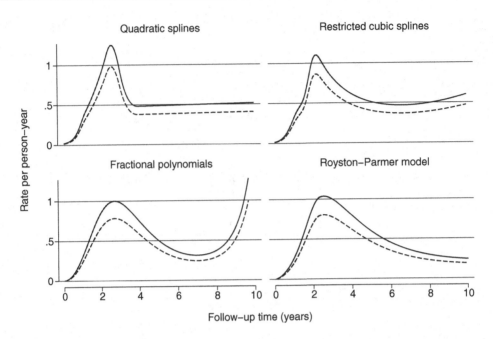

FIGURE 25.5 Adjusted rates for untreated (solid curves) and treated (dashed curves) women, age 55 years. Survival times from a mixed Weibull distribution. The smoothed curves were from Poisson models that used (1) quadratic splines with linear tails, (2) restricted cubic splines constrained to be linear beyond the boundary knots, (3) fractional polynomial terms of three dimensions, and (4) a Royston-Parmer model.

The smoothed hazards (rates) from this method (quadratic spline panel in Figure 25.5) can be compared with Figure 25.4. The rates are lower in Figure 25.5, compared with 25.4, because the curves are for baseline values: male = 0 and agec = 0. For the same reason Figure 25.5 lacks the oscillation seen in the previous figures. But the overall change in rates over time are similar in Figures 25.4 and 25.5. The curve in Figure 25.5 shows a change in direction at each knot, except at time 1.73; the corresponding regression term, s3, has a large P-value of .8. One option would be to redo the splines without using a knot at 1.73 years. In an actual analysis one could chose different knots or slice time into different segments, and compare models using Akaike or Bayesian information criteria statistics.

Unlike Figures 25.2 and 25.4, the log scale was not used for the vertical axis in Figure 25.5. Log scales are often used for multiplicative (ratio) comparisons, but the difference scale helps us to visual rate differences (Rothman, Wise, and Hatch 2011). This change regarding the vertical axis was driven partly by my desire for some variety in the figures. The log scale is often used to assess whether hazards are proportional, but Royston and Parmar (2002) suggest this visual method may not be effective.

25.7 ANOTHER FLEXIBLE POISSON MODEL: RESTRICTED CUBIC SPLINES

Cubic splines allow two inflections (changes in curve direction) between knots. This can produce curves with excessive fluctuation, beyond what is plausible, so constraints are often imposed. Not only must the curves join at the boundary knots for each interval, but the first and second derivatives of the spline functions must be the same at the knots, and the tails must be linear. The tails for these splines are the values predicted by the splines beyond the boundaries of the shortest and longest midt values. These are called restricted cubic splines (Royston and Lambert 2011 pp67–81). A user-written Stata command, **rcsgen**, can create these splines. Assuming we again split time into segments of 0.1 years and create the variables risktime and midt as shown previously, we can invoke **rcsgen**:

```
. rcsgen midt, df(5) gen(s) fw(_d) orthog
Variables s1 to s5 were created
```

The command option **df(5)** refers to the degrees of freedom. The boundary splines are at the shortest and longest midt values: 0.02 and 9.95. With five degrees of freedom, the command produced four interval splines with evenly placed knots at the 20th, 40th, 60th, and 80th centiles of midt values. Other command options allow the user to select the knots. The Poisson regression table output shows good agreement between the estimated and true rate ratios:

```
------------------------------------------------------------------------------
         _d |      IRR    Std. Err.      z    P>|z|    [95% Conf. Interval]
------------+-----------------------------------------------------------------
    treated | .7841838    .0291189    -6.55   0.000    .7291391    .8433839
       male | 1.298317    .0439276     7.72   0.000    1.215013    1.387332
       agec | 1.022468    .0029917     7.59   0.000    1.016621    1.028348
      agec2 | 1.004965    .0002216    22.45   0.000     1.00453    1.005399
         s1 |  2.26083    .0531379    34.71   0.000    2.159044    2.367414
         s2 | 2.383094    .0575534    35.96   0.000     2.27292    2.498609
         s3 | .6356739    .0165741   -17.38   0.000    .6040053     .669003
         s4 | .8857384    .0133886    -8.03   0.000    .8598822    .9123721
         s5 | .8615279    .0100603   -12.76   0.000    .8420341     .881473
       _cons | .2217466    .0093281   -35.81   0.000    .2041973    .2408043
ln(risktime) |        1  (exposure)
------------------------------------------------------------------------------
```

The hazard curves from this model (restricted cubic spline panel in Figure 25.5) are similar to those produced by quadratic splines.

25.8 FLEXIBILITY WITH FRACTIONAL POLYNOMIALS

Fractional polynomials (see Chapter 15) can also flexibly model time (Royston and Altman 1994, Royston, Ambler, and Sauerbrei 1999, Royston and Sauerbrei 2008). Proceed as before, slicing time into 0.1 year intervals, creating risktime and midt, and then fit a fractional polynomial model with three dimensions, meaning three new regression model terms for midt, each expressed using up to three polynomial terms selected from a list of eight. Stata will slog through 164 Poisson models (about 2.5 minutes on a desktop machine) and produce a table of the power terms and deviances for the best models of one, two, and three dimensions:

```
. fp <midt>, dimension(3): poisson _d treated male agec agec2 <midt>, irr
exp(risktime)
(fitting 164 models)
```

(...10%....20%....30%....40%....50%....60%....70%....80%....90%....100%)

Fractional polynomial comparisons:

```
-----------------------------------------------------------------
     midt | df  Deviance Dev. dif.   P(*)  Powers
---------+-------------------------------------------------------
  omitted |  0  49601.28 3888.191   0.000
   linear |  1  48657.94 2944.852   0.000  1
    m = 1 |  2  46366.58  653.494   0.000  -.5
    m = 2 |  4  45854.77  141.681   0.000  .5 .5
    m = 3 |  6  45713.09    0.000    - -   .5 2 2
-----------------------------------------------------------------
```

(*) P = sig. level of model with m = 3 based on chi^2 of dev. dif.
(output omitted)

. poisson, irr

```
Poisson regression                      Number of obs   =   101,997
                                        LR chi2(7)      =   4133.58
                                        Prob > chi2     =    0.0000
Log likelihood = -22856.544             Pseudo R2       =    0.0829
```

```
-------------------------------------------------------------------------
         _d |      IRR   Std. Err.      z   P>|z|    [95% Conf. Interval]
------------+------------------------------------------------------------
    treated | .7813617   .0289897   -6.65   0.000   .7265595   .8402974
       male | 1.300536   .0440209    7.76   0.000   1.217056   1.389742
       agec | 1.022383     .00299    7.57   0.000    1.01654   1.02826
      agec2 | 1.004927   .0002214   22.31   0.000   1.004493   1.005361
     midt_1 | 512.0407   82.58283   38.68   0.000   373.2684   702.4053
     midt_2 | .4606624   .0131638  -27.12   0.000   .4355711   .4871991
     midt_3 | 1.326755   .0152611   24.58   0.000   1.297179   1.357006
      _cons | .0012951    .000192  -44.86   0.000   .0009686   .0017317
ln(risktime)|        1  (exposure)
-------------------------------------------------------------------------
```

Using the rules for fractional polynomials (see Chapter 15), the term midt_1 is equal to $midt^{0.5}$, midt_2 is $midt^2$, and midt_3 is $midt^2 \times \ln(midt)$. The rate ratios are close to their true values for the regression terms of interest, so fractional polynomials have done a good job of removing bias related to changes in rates over time. A plot of the hazards for a 55-year-old woman, treated and not treated, shows an initial peak in rates around 2 years that is longer compared with the peak using splines, and a greater upward surge in rates around 10 years, compared with other approaches (Figure 25.5). If four dimensions are chosen, 494 models are fit in 8 minutes and the hazards show a rise at about 8.5 years and a fall after 9 years. The fractional polynomial model may be describing shapes in clouds for times longer than 8 years, where the data are sparse. If goal is to describe the hazard curve over time, the spline models may be better choices in this example. If the goal is to estimate unbiased rate ratios, all these methods seem to do well.

Survival times tend to be skewed; many initially, with few later on. For these methods it may be better to use the ln of midt rather than midt as a linear term (Royston 2000, Royston and Lambert 2011 pp76–78).

25.9 WHEN SHOULD A POISSON MODEL BE USED? RANDOMIZED TRIAL OF A TERRIBLE TREATMENT

When data are in grouped format, such as mortality data, the Poisson model or some variation is generally the best approach. The Cox regression model is not really an option when individual survival times are unknown. But if data about exposure, outcomes, and outcome timing are known for individuals, which model should we chose?

If the outcomes arose from a constant rate over time, survival times will follow an exponential distribution. In that case, both the Cox model and the Poisson model can estimate the same rate ratio, as illustrated by the first example in this chapter.

Using the same mixed Weibull distribution used in Section 25.4, new data were generated for a hypothetical randomized controlled trial of a new treatment; 2000 persons were assigned to treatment, 2000 served as controls. The treatment was catastrophic, as the true rate ratio for death, comparing treated persons to those not treated, was 2.0. This ratio was constant throughout follow-up, satisfying the proportional hazards assumption. Twenty-thousand sets of trial survival times were simulated and deaths, person-time, rates, and ratios of rates and hazards, were estimated after 0.3, 0.5, 1, 2, 3, 4, 6, 8, and 10 years of follow-up. After 6 years these statistics showed little further change because nearly all subjects were dead, so results in Figure 25.6 were limited to 6 years. The hazard ratios were from the Cox regression model. Poisson regression was not needed to estimate the rate ratio. Instead, at each follow-up time the count of deaths and total person-time in each trial arm were used to calculate the rate ratio.

The data were generated so that the instantaneous rate of death (the hazard) was always twice as great among the treated. The hazard ratio, which compares outcomes in risk sets of survivors at the time of each death, was 2.06 at 0.3 years, 2.02 at 0.5 years, and 2.00 thereafter (Figure 25.6, Table 25.2). The hazard ratio was slightly elevated above 2.00 initially because these are simulated data and the number of deaths at 0.3 and 0.5 years was small. The crude rate ratio was 2.06 at 0.3 years, 2.01 at 0.5 years, and 1.96 at 1 year. The risk ratio (Table 25.2) was similar to the rate ratio at these times. The finding of similar values for all three ratios during early follow-up is not surprising; this was discussed in Chapters 2 and 3. If events are sufficiently uncommon, the risk, rate, and odds ratios will be similar; the same applies to the hazard ratio. At 1 year of follow-up only 18% (362/2000) of the treated and 10% (190/2000) of the controls were dead.

Between 1 and 2 years of follow-up, 56% (1,123) of the treated subjects died. By the end of the 2nd year, 74% of treated subjects and 49% of controls were dead (Table 25.2, Figure 25.6). Although the hazard ratio remained constant, there were no longer enough survivors in the treated group to generate a count of deaths twice as great as that in the control group; the crude rates in both trial arms start to converge. After 10 years of follow-up nearly everyone is dead and the crude rate ratio was 1.42. This ratio has an interpretation: 1.42 = (deaths/person-time for the treated)/(deaths/person-time for controls) = (2000/3231)/(~2000/4580) = 4580/3231 = ratio of (time lived from start of follow-up to death for a control subject)/(time lived from start of follow-up to death by a treated subject). The ratio of 1.42 is the ratio of control survival time divided by treated-person survival time.

To summarize, if we use ordinary Poisson regression, the rate and hazard ratios will agree well if rates are more-or-less constant over time. If rates vary a lot over time, these two statistics may not agree if subjects are followed for a period of time sufficiently long that more than 10 to 20% of persons have experienced the outcome of interest. In our hypothetical trial, a safety monitoring committee would have probably stopped the trial before a year had passed; in that case, the choice between a Poisson comparison of rates and the Cox model would make little difference.

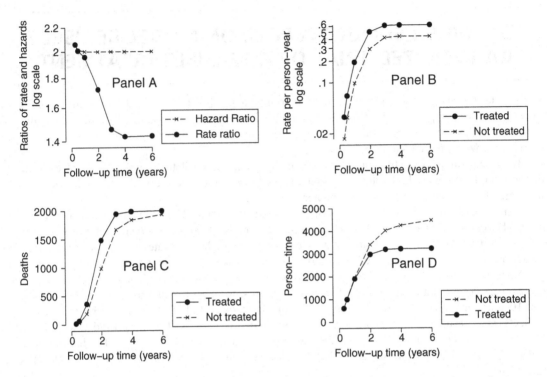

FIGURE 25.6 Data for a hypothetical randomized controlled trial. Treatment was catastrophic, as the true rate ratio for death, comparing treated persons to those not treated, was 2.0. This ratio was constant throughout follow-up. The survival times were not from a Poisson (exponential) distribution, but from a mixed Weibull distribution with survival times similar to those in Figure 25.3. The graphs show statistics after 0.3, 0.5, 1, 2, 3, 4, and 6 years of follow-up. Panel A shows the hazard ratio from a Cox model and the rate ratio was a Poisson model. For treated and control persons at each point in time, rates are in Panel B, the count of deaths in Panel C, and the sum of person-time in Panel D.

25.10 A REAL RANDOMIZED TRIAL, THE PLCO SCREENING TRIAL

The Prostate, Lung, Colorectal and Ovarian (PLCO) Cancer Screening Randomized Trial published results regarding ovarian cancer screening and mortality in 2011 (Buys et al. 2011). From November 1993 to July 2001, the study assigned 39,105 women to annual screening for ovarian cancer and 39,111 to usual care. Follow-up ended on February 28, 2010. The main analysis compared the ovarian cancer mortality of the screened patients (118 deaths, 3.1 per 10,000 person-years) with that of the controls (100 deaths, 2.6 per 10,000 person-years): rate ratio 1.18 (95% CI 0.82–1.71).

We can be confident that if the PLCO investigators had estimated the hazard ratio instead of the rate ratio, the results would have been similar. These ratios should agree well, as fewer than 0.3% of women in each trial arm had the outcome. In addition, the authors showed that deaths were distributed over time in a manner not inconsistent with either a constant hazard ratio assumption or a roughly constant rate (Buys et al. 2011). The rate of death did increase with increasing follow-up, but we expect this because the women grew older during follow-up and ovarian cancer risk increases with age. Using rates and rate ratios made the study results easy to understand. The publication also offered many

TABLE 25.2 Statistics from 20,000 simulations of data for a randomized controlled trial in which the hazard ratio for death among the treated, compared with controls, was always 2.0. A mixed Weibull distribution was used for survival times. Ratios compare treated subjects with controls.

FOLLOW-UP TIME (YEARS)	DEATHS		PERSON-TIME (YEARS)		RATE (PER PERSON-YEAR)		RISK		RATE RATIO	HAZARD RATIO	RISK RATIO
	TREATED	CONTROL	TREATED	CONTROL	TREATED	CONTROL	TREATED	CONTROL			
0.3	20.2	10.1	598	599	.034	.017	.010	.005	2.06	2.06	2.06
0.5	65.2	32.9	990	995	.066	.033	.033	.016	2.01	2.02	2.00
1	362.5	190.4	1895	1946	.191	.098	.181	.095	1.96	2.00	1.91
2	1485.5	985.8	2976	3398	.499	.290	.743	.493	1.72	2.00	1.51
3	1945.1	1668.4	3190	4019	.610	.415	.973	.834	1.47	2.00	1.17
4	1986.8	1837.8	3216	4243	.618	.433	.993	.919	1.43	2.00	1.08
6	1997.6	1931.1	3229	4463	.619	.433	.999	.966	1.43	2.00	1.03
8	1999.7	1975.3	3231	4550	.619	.434	1.000	.988	1.43	2.00	1.01
10	2000.0	1992.5	3231	4580	.619	.435	1.000	.996	1.42	2.00	1.00

details about the study design, execution, and results, and provided an even-handed discussion of the results (Cummings and Rivara 2012).

25.11 WHAT IF EVENTS ARE COMMON?

As we have seen in these examples, the usual Poisson model may not correctly estimate the hazard ratio when outcomes are common. The Cox proportional hazards model is not the only alternative. One option, shown earlier, is to split person-time into small segments and use a piecewise or flexible Poisson model that makes comparisons within risk sets. A more convenient choice may be a Royston-Parmer model. In 2002, Royston and Parmar (Royston and Parmar 2002) described how a parametric model based on the Weibull distribution, combined with the use of restricted cubic splines to model changes in the baseline hazard over time, can be used to estimate hazard ratios, including hazard ratios that may change over time (i.e., not be proportional). Royston (Royston 2001) wrote a command, **stpm** (meaning survival time parametric model), to implement this model in Stata. In 2009, Lambert and Royston (Lambert and Royston 2009) modified this command and renamed it **stpm2**. Later Royston and Lambert (Royston and Lambert 2011) published a book which describes this approach, and other methods, in detail.

After using the **stset** command, a Royston-Parmer model can be invoked to analyze the hypothetical data about treatment, age, and sex, that were used for Figure 25.5. These survival times came from a mixed Weibull distribution:

```
. stpm2 treated male agec agec2, df(4) scale(hazard) eform nolog

Log likelihood = -3620.4226                    Number of obs   =   5,000

------------------------------------------------------------------------
           |    exp(b)    Std. Err.       z    P>|z|    [95% Conf. Interval]
-----------+------------------------------------------------------------
xb         |
   treated |  .7738071    .0287084     -6.91   0.000    .7195367    .8321707
      male |  1.308399    .0442497      7.95   0.000    1.224484    1.398066
      agec |  1.023242    .0029956      7.85   0.000    1.017387    1.02913
     agec2 |  1.005105    .0002217     23.08   0.000    1.00467     1.00554
     _rcs1 |    3.8548    .0708267     73.44   0.000    3.718452    3.996148
     _rcs2 |  1.176179    .0206931      9.22   0.000    1.136313    1.217445
     _rcs3 |  1.184939    .0144288     13.94   0.000    1.156994    1.21356
     _rcs4 |  1.039859    .0065691      6.19   0.000    1.027063    1.052814
     _cons |  .3993775    .0151785    -24.15   0.000    .3707093    .4302628
------------------------------------------------------------------------
```

The degrees of freedom was set to 4 using the **df** option. This means five knots were used to create restricted cubic splines for the survival times: two outer knots at the shortest and longest survival times, with splines constrained to be linear beyond those times, and internal knots at the 25th, 50th, and 75th centiles of the uncensored survival times (the times to failure or death). The command has options to place knots in chosen locations, but Royston and colleagues (Royston and Parmar 2002, Royston and Lambert 2011) report that the choice of knots is usually not critical. My choice of 4 degrees of freedom was somewhat arbitrary, although I suspected it would work well because 5 degrees worked well earlier for a Poisson model applied to these data. In a real analysis, one could compare models with other choices. The estimated hazard ratios of interest are all close to their true values and close to the values from the Cox model shown earlier. It is easy to produce estimates of the hazards (rates) using predict commands:

```
predict haz0, hazard at(male 0 treated 0 agec 0 agec2 0)

predict haz1, hazard at(male 0 treated 1 agec 0 agec2 0)
```

These hazards are plotted in Figure 25.5. Results are similar to those from the other methods shown in the figure, except for the rates near the end of follow-up where data are sparse.

25.12 COX MODEL OR A FLEXIBLE PARAMETRIC MODEL?

The Cox proportional hazards model is the most common choice for estimating hazard ratios. The use of flexible parametric models is still uncommon, but has appeared in some studies. For example, a randomized controlled trial of screening for ovarian cancer, involving over 200 thousand women, made use of this approach for some analyses (Jacobs et al. 2016). Royston and others (Royston 2001, Royston and Parmar 2002, Carstensen 2005, Lambert and Royston 2009, Royston and Lambert 2011) suggest that a flexible parametric model, such as a Royston-Parmer model, may offer some advantages. None of these are absolute, but the following is a list of tasks that may be easier to execute with a flexible parametric approach:

1. The baseline hazard function describes the disease course over time. The smoothed hazard curve from a parametric model is more easily depicted, described, and interpreted compared with the more erratic estimates from the Cox model, which allows the baseline hazard to change at the time of each death in the data.
2. The proportional hazards assumption may not be true. It is easy to allow for this with a flexible parametric model, as interactions between time and other variables can be allowed. This will be discussed later in this chapter.
3. Multiple time-scales can be used by the parametric model, such as (1) time since study entry, (2) time since birth (age), (3) time since onset of exposure, and (4) calendar time.
4. The **stpm2** command for Royston-Parmer models easily allows for predictions of numerous statistics after fitting the model.

25.13 COLLAPSIBILITY AND SURVIVAL FUNCTIONS

The data examples used in this chapter are simplistic because they all used data with no variation in risk aside from that related to the model covariates. Chapter 8 reviewed the problem of collapsibility and showed that when variation in risk is present in data, but not accounted for in the estimating process, then hazard ratios cannot be interpreted as estimates of average causal effects. One solution to this problem is to avoid modeling of common outcomes. Some authors (Robins and Morgenstern 1987 p882, Hernán, Hernández-Diaz, and Robins 2004, Hernán 2010) suggest that when outcomes are common, survival functions (surviving proportions, survival curves) should be estimated instead of hazard ratios, because survival functions (like risks) are not afflicted by the problem of collapsibility. Survival functions, if otherwise unbiased, can be interpreted as the effect of exposure on average survival.

Survival functions can be plotted using Kaplan-Meier methods; these produce the stepped lines often used to show survival for randomized trials. Stata has a command (**sts graph**) for plotting adjusted versions of Kaplan-Meier survival plots. Adjusted survival functions can be obtained from Cox proportional hazard models (Hernán 2010); see Stata's **stcurve** command. Royston-Parmer models can create smoothed survival curves that are adjusted, directly standardized to another population distribution, or plotted for specific values of interest (Royston and Lambert 2011 pp275–282). Using the same Royston-Parmer model with 4 degrees of freedom shown earlier for Figure 25.5, commands can create smoothed survival estimates adjusted for the age and sex of the study population:

```
. predict s0, meansurv at(treated 0)
```

```
. predict s1, meansurv at(treated 1)
```

These survivor functions (survival curves or surviving proportions) can be plotted and their ratios and differences calculated (Figure 25.7). If confidence intervals (CI) are desired, these can be obtained from bootstrap or marginal methods (Royston and Lambert 2011 p282).

25.14 RELAXING THE ASSUMPTION OF PROPORTIONAL HAZARDS IN THE COX MODEL

All models considered so far in this chapter have assumed that hazards were proportional over time, meaning that the estimated rate ratios did not change with time. But we can allow for the possibility that an exposure, such as a treatment or a risk factor, might interact with time on a multiplicative scale. A rather pathological example of this was shown in Figure 3.5 and another example in Figure 5.1. A *time-varying* covariate is a variable that changes in size over time or an exposure applied intermittently as time passes. For example, an exposure which starts, then stops, then starts again. This can be accounted for in both Poisson and Cox proportional hazards regression. Here we focus on a *time-dependent* covariate, an exposure whose influence on the outcome changes with time (Royston and Lambert 2011 p168). A time-dependent exposure may be always present and not change in value, but its association with the outcome changes as time passes. To estimate a time-dependent association, the assumption of proportional hazards must be relaxed.

Imagine a randomized trial of a treatment which initially decreases the rate of death, but becomes ineffective over time. These data were generated from a Weibull distribution (Crowther and Lambert 2012). The true hazard ratio for death, comparing those treated (rx = 1) with controls (rx = 0), was exp (ln(.7) + .2 × ln(time)); so the true hazard ratio was 0.3 at the time of the first death (.015 years), 0.7 at 1 year, and 0.97 after 5 years of treatment. There were 5000 treated persons, 5000 controls, and a single simulation of these data was selected for analysis, so the estimated hazard ratios are similar to, but not exactly equal to, the true hazard ratios.

Applied to these trial data, a Poisson regression model estimated a constant rate ratio of 0.85 and the Cox proportional hazards model produced a hazard ratio of 0.83. Time is the outcome in the Cox model, so it is not immediately obvious how we can introduce an interaction that allows the hazard ratio to vary with time. Stata allows this with two options: **tvc()** and **texp()**. The first option tells the software that the variable in parenthesis is allowed to vary with time; the letters **tvc** indicate a time-varying covariate, although in this example some would call treatment a time-dependent covariate. The second

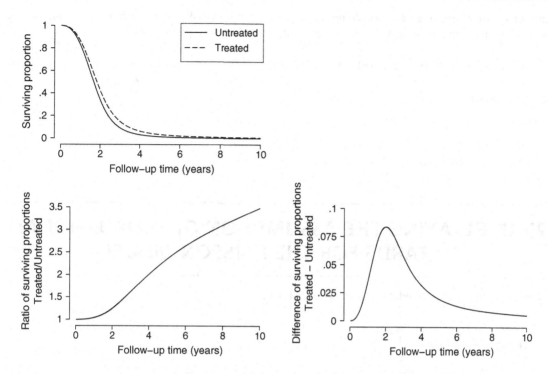

FIGURE 25.7 Surviving proportions (also called survival functions or survival curves) adjusted for age and sex, for treated and untreated persons in the mixed Weibull data (Figures 25.3–25.5). Bottom panels show ratios and differences in these proportions. Survival functions from a Royston-Parmer model.

option, **texp,** describes the expression for time that is allowed to interact with the variable in the **tvc** option. I will express time as ln(time), which mimics the data generating process:

```
. stcox rx, nolog tvc(rx) texp(ln(_t))
(output omitted)
```

```
------------------------------------------------------------------------------
         _t | Haz. Ratio  Std. Err.       z    P>|z|     [95% Conf. Interval]
------------+-----------------------------------------------------------------
main        |
         rx |   .7205583   .0281336    -8.39   0.000     .6674745    .7778638
------------+-----------------------------------------------------------------
tvc         |
         rx |   1.196362   .0433672     4.95   0.000     1.114313    1.284453
------------------------------------------------------------------------------
Note: Variables in tvc equation interacted with ln(_t).
```

The Cox model estimated a rate ratio of 0.72, comparing treated with untreated subjects at 1 year of follow-up, close to the true rate ratio of 0.70. The ln of the interaction term was ln(1.196) = 0.179, close to the true value of 0.2. A plot of the hazard ratio shows that treatment was initially helpful, but the benefit dwindled after 5 years (Figure 25.8). It took a computer 21 seconds to produce these estimates. The same results can be estimated by creating risk sets at every failure time and fitting a Cox model that included an actual interaction term. This can be done with the commands below, shown with no output. But there is a price for doing this; the expansion of risk sets at each death produced over 43 million additional records and it took a computer 11 minutes to produce the estimates:

```
stset time, failure(died=1) id(id)

stsplit, at(failures)

gen rxlnt = rx*ln(_t)

stcox rx rxlnt, nolog
```

25.15 RELAXING THE ASSUMPTION OF PROPORTIONAL HAZARDS FOR THE POISSON MODEL

Now apply the Poisson model to these same trial data:

```
. stset time, failure(died=1) id(id)
(output omitted)

. * create risk sets at every 2 hundredths of a year – about 1 week
. stsplit timecat, every(.02)
(1,762,061 observations (episodes) created)

. lab var timecat "Time cutoff"

. gen risktime = _t - _t0

. lab var risktime "Observation time"

. * collapsing the data saves estimation time
. collapse (min) _t0 (max) _t (count) n = _d (sum) risktime _d, by(rx
timecat)

. gen double midt = (_t0 + _t)/2

. gen lntime = ln(midt)

. * create restricted cubic splines (s1 s2 s3) with 4 knots for ln(time)
. rcsgen lntime, df(3) gen(s) fw(_d) orthog
Variables s1 to s3 were created

. display r(knots)
-4.605170249938965  .7080357670783997  1.226712226867676  1.609437942504883

. poisson _d rx##c.s*, irr exp(risktime) nolog
```

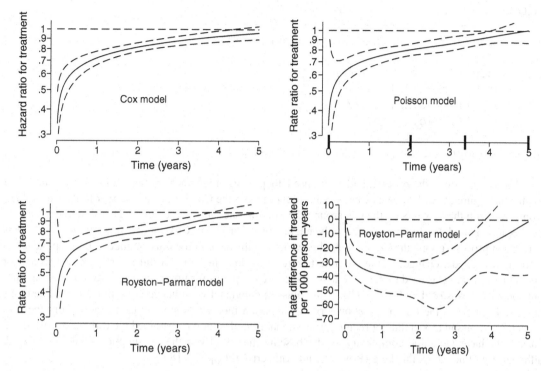

FIGURE 25.8 Hypothetical data from a randomized controlled trial in which the effect of treatment was initially helpful but faded over time. Results shown from a Cox, Poisson, and Royston-Parmar model. The horizontal axis for the Poisson model shows four thick tick-marks for the knots used to create the restricted cubic splines.

```
Poisson regression                              Number of obs   =       502
                                                LR chi2(7)      =   1493.36
                                                Prob > chi2     =    0.0000
Log likelihood = -1330.5212                     Pseudo R2       =    0.3595
------------------------------------------------------------------------------
         _d |      IRR   Std. Err.      z    P>|z|     [95% Conf. Interval]
------------+-----------------------------------------------------------------
       1.rx |  .807614   .0221357    -7.80   0.000     .7653736    .8521856
         s1 | 1.644176   .0449562    18.19   0.000     1.558383    1.734692
         s2 | .9896334   .0269948    -0.38   0.702     .9381141    1.043982
         s3 | 1.009355   .0193005     0.49   0.626     .9722271    1.047901
            |
     rx#c.s1 |
          1 | 1.186297   .0553447     3.66   0.000     1.082635    1.299885
            |
     rx#c.s2 |
          1 | .9887728   .0450028    -0.25   0.804     .9043885     1.08103
            |
     rx#c.s3 |
          1 | .9834545   .0273647    -0.60   0.549     .9312569    1.038578
            |
      _cons | .1998172   .0036354   -88.51   0.000     .1928175    .2070711
```

```
ln(risktime) |         1    (exposure)
-------------------------------------------------------------------
Note: _cons estimates baseline incidence rate.

. predictnl lrr = _b[1.rx] ///
>      + _b[1.rx#c.s1]*s1 ///
>      + _b[1.rx#c.s2]*s2 ///
>      + _b[1.rx#c.s3]*s3 ///
>      ,ci(lrr_lci lrr_uci)
note: confidence intervals calculated using Z critical values
```

The output from these commands was used to plot the time-varying rate ratios for the effect of treatment (Figure 25.8). Estimates were similar to those from the Cox model and similar to the true values. Compared with the Cox model, the CIs around the Poisson rate ratios were larger. This should not surprise us, because I used the ln(time) as the only interaction term in the Cox model; this mimicked the data generation process, giving the Cox model a better fit with the data. In the Poisson model, three spline terms were used to model changes in the baseline hazard, a flexible method that did not require us to know or guess that ln(time) was used to generate these data. Use of splines for time was effective in removing bias, but some price was paid with wider CIs. If the **poisson** command was changed to remove the spline terms and use ln(midt) as the only interaction term, the Poisson model CIs are similar to those from the Cox model. The Poisson model did not require proportional hazards, but it constrained the differences of the log hazards to have the same complexity as the baseline hazard. Even that assumption could be relaxed, although I will not show this here (Royston and Lambert 2011 pp188–189).

25.16 RELAXING PROPORTIONAL HAZARDS FOR THE ROYSTON-PARMAR MODEL

Royston-Palmer models for rates have options that easily create flexible expressions for both the baseline hazards and the time-dependent effects (Royston and Lambert 2011 pp190–225). They allow the simultaneous use of several time scales. I used a model with 5 degrees of freedom for the baseline hazard and 3 degrees of freedom for the time-varying effect of treatment in these hypothetical trial data:

```
. stset time, failure(died==1) id(id)
(output omitted)

. stpm2 rx, scale(hazard) df(5) tvc(rx) dftvc(3) nolog
(output omitted)
```

	Coef.	Std. Err.	z	P>|z|	[95% Conf. Interval]	
xb						
rx	-.2416812	.028154	-8.58	0.000	-.2968621	-.1865004
_rcs1	1.02795	.0181314	56.69	0.000	.9924126	1.063486
_rcs2	-.009847	.0151789	-0.65	0.517	-.0395971	.019903
_rcs3	.0058537	.0078495	0.75	0.456	-.009531	.0212384
_rcs4	.0036077	.003849	0.94	0.349	-.0039362	.0111517

```
    _rcs5 |  -.0038292   .0018784   -2.04   0.041   -.0075108   -.0001476
 _rcs_rx1 |   .1173925   .0298617    3.93   0.000    .0588646    .1759203
 _rcs_rx2 |  -.0020362    .025321   -0.08   0.936   -.0516645    .0475921
 _rcs_rx3 |  -.0086039   .0105821   -0.81   0.416   -.0293444    .0121366
    _cons |  -.6750783   .0189072  -35.70   0.000   -.7121356   -.6380209
----------------------------------------------------------------------
```

. range temptime 0.00001 5 200
(9,800 missing values generated)

. predict hr, hrnum(rx 1) hrdenom(rx 0) timevar(temptime) ci

The Royston-Parmar model provided a curve for the rate ratios quite similar to that from the Cox and Poisson models (Figure 25.8). The spline creation and time-varying flexibility were introduced in a single command which produced estimates in less than a second. The predict command after this model has a remarkable array of options. It was easy, for example, to predict rate differences with CIs, using just one command (Figure 25.8):

. predict hdiff, hdiff1(rx 1) hdiff2(rx 0) timevar(temptime) ci per(1000)

25.17 THE LIFE EXPECTANCY DIFFERENCE OR RATIO

For the fictional trial used in Sections 25.14–25.16, the overall hazard ratio (0.83) is arguably not the best description of the treatment effect. The change in the hazard ratio over time was modeled (Figure 25.8), but a graphical presentation is not easy to describe with words or numbers. One option is to estimate hazard or rate ratios within two or more time intervals. Another option is to use the life expectancy difference or ratio, calculated for two or more time intervals.

Because the trial data for Figure 25.8 has no censored time aside from records with the outcome, we can use Stata's **summarize** command to estimate the mean life expectancy of the treated and untreated in any time window from 0 to 5 years. But real data has censoring, people whose follow-up time was truncated for reasons other than the outcome. We need commands that can estimate mean survival time while correctly accounting for any censoring. We cannot estimate true mean survival time, because that requires us to follow everyone until they die. Doing this is unrealistic. However, we can estimate mean survival time during specific time intervals; for example, from enrollment until the end of follow-up. These are called *restricted* mean survival times. Royston has written a Stata command called **strmst** (Royston 2015). The first two letters, st, indicate this is a survival time command, and the rest of the name is an acronym for restricted mean survival time. This command fits a Royston-Parmar model to the data and extracts the restricted survival times from that model. Cronin and colleagues wrote **strmst2**, which reweights the survival times to account for any censoring (Cronin, Tian, and Uno 2016).

Using the trial data described in Section 25.14, let us estimate the restricted mean survival times for each arm of the trial, over the entire 5-year interval, using the **summarize** command:

. summ time if rx==1

```
 Variable |     Obs       Mean   Std. Dev.      Min       Max
----------+---------------------------------------------------------
     time |   5,000   3.661109   1.466398   .0153026        5
```

```
. scalar rx1time = r(mean)

. summ time if rx==0

    Variable |     Obs      Mean   Std. Dev.       Min      Max
-------------+-----------------------------------------------------
        time |   5,000   3.399843   1.560782   .0204159        5

. scalar rx0time = r(mean)

. di "Life expectancy difference = "rx1time - rx0time
Life expectancy difference = .261266

. di "Life expectancy ratio     = "rx1time/rx0time
Life expectancy ratio     = 1.0768465
```

The restricted mean survival time for control subjects was 3.4 years during the 5-year follow-up. An average control subject could say, "Looking at the next 5 years, I expect to live about 3.4 years. If I get the treatment, this may add .26 years to my life." This summary is useful but limited. Figure 25.8 suggests that most of the treatment benefit comes early. Let us use the **strmst** command to estimate the impact of treatment on survival during the first 3 years of follow-up:

```
. stset time, failure(died=1) id(id)
(output omitted)

. strmst rx, tstar(3)
(output omitted)

Using delta method for SE and CI:
-----------------------------------------------------------------------
             | Observed  Delta-meth.                    Normal-based
             |     Est.    Std. Err.      z   P>|z|   [95% Conf. Interval]
-------------+---------------------------------------------------------
       rmst1 | 2.4801517  .0113074  219.34   0.000   2.4579895  2.5023139
       rmst2 | 2.6071064  .00988412  263.77  0.000   2.587734   2.6264789
-------------+---------------------------------------------------------
       dif21 | .12695479  .01488828    8.53   0.000   .0977743   .15613529
-----------------------------------------------------------------------
```

Now the average person might reason, "In the next 3 years, I expect to live 2.61 years. If I get the treatment, this may add about .127 years to my life, or about 46 days." Now restart the follow-up clock at the 3-year point and use **strmst2** to estimate what happened in the last 2 years of follow-up:

```
. gen newtime = time-3

. drop if newtime<0
(3,649 observations deleted)

. summ newtime if rx==1

    Variable |     Obs      Mean   Std. Dev.    Min     Max
```

```
--------+-------------------------------------------------------
newtime |   3,376   1.563131   .6335567   .0000545        2
```

. summ newtime if rx==0

```
Variable |     Obs      Mean  Std. Dev.        Min     Max
--------+-------------------------------------------------------
newtime |   2,975   1.54676   .6420017   .0010575        2
```

* Since the time variable is now newtime, be sure to use stset again:
. stset newtime, failure(died=1) id(id)
(output omitted)

. strmst2 rx

Number of observations for analysis = 6351

The truncation time, tau, was not specified. Thus, the default tau (the minimum of the largest observed event time within each group), 1.999, is used.

Restricted Mean Survival Time (RMST) by arm

```
------------------------------------------------------
 Group | Estimate  Std. Err.    [95% Conf. Interval]
-------+----------------------------------------------
arm 1 |   1.563     0.011       1.541      1.584
arm 0 |   1.546     0.012       1.523      1.569
------------------------------------------------------
```

Between-group contrast (arm 1 versus arm 0)

```
-----------------------------------------------------------------
         Contrast |  Estimate    [95% Conf.    Interval]   P>|z|
-----------------+-----------------------------------------------
RMST (arm 1 - arm 0) |    0.016     -0.015       0.048     0.308
RMST (arm 1 / arm 0) |    1.011      0.990       1.031     0.308
-----------------------------------------------------------------
```

Now a patient might feel:

> I was fortunate to survive 3 years. Looking at the next 2 years, my expected survival is 1.55 years. If I get the treatment, I may live another .016 years, or 6 days. If treatment is expensive or uncomfortable or inconvenient, I may just skip it.

Several articles have useful discussions about this approach (Royston and Parmar 2011, 2013, Uno et al. 2014, Dehbi, Royston, and Hackshaw 2017, Pak et al. 2017).

25.18 RECURRENT OR MULTIPLE EVENTS

The Poisson model can be easily applied to recurrent events. When used for individual-level data, the Poisson model typically uses total follow-up time as the rate denominator for the sum of the event counts, as in the randomized trial of fall prevention discussed in Chapters 12 and 13. The timing of each event during follow-up is ignored. This method assumes the hazard for the outcome remains constant during follow-up. In particular, the hazard for each outcome is not affected by the occurrence of previous outcomes. It would, however, be easy to split the follow-up time in the falls study at each event time and allow the follow-up time clock to be reset after each fall. One could allow for the possibility that each event has some influence on the next event. If, for example, the outcome was a urinary infection, follow-time could be omitted for the period during which each infection is treated after it starts. Of course, the variance estimator should account for the clustering of events within each person.

In studies of populations, such as rates of traffic crash death by state and year, the exact timing of the deaths within each year is typically unknown. This is not really a problem for Poisson regression, as the outcomes are usually so rare that estimates would be unchanged if the Cox model were used.

The Cox model has been extended to multiple events using three methods (Therneau and Grambsch 2000 pp169–229, Hosmer, Lemeshow, and May 2008 pp287–296, Royston and Lambert 2011 pp296–304). In the first approach (Andersen and Gill 1982) the times are split so that the follow-up clock is restarted for each person at the time of each event. The shape of the hazard curve is assumed to be the same for each event. So if the outcome is a fall, no one is at risk for a second fall until they have a first fall, but after the first fall, the shape of the baseline hazard for the second fall is just the same as that for the first fall. It is as if the person had no memory of or learned nothing from their first fall. The second option (Prentice, Williams, and Peterson 1981) splits time in the same way, but the baseline hazard is allowed to vary between events. Perhaps a person who fell once would buy sensible shoes after a first fall. The last approach (Wei, Lin, and Weissfeld 1989) categorizes outcomes into specific types. For example, a study of how vision loss might cause home injuries could use three possible outcome events, such a burn related to cooking, a cut due to a cooking utensil, and a fall in the home. A person is at risk for each of these outcomes at all times during follow-up and the hazard curve can differ for each outcome. All of these methods can use a robust-type variance that allows for clustering of events within each subject. All of these methods can be implemented with the Cox model. But it may come as no surprise that the Poisson model or a Royston-Parmer model (Royston and Lambert 2011 pp297–304) can also be used.

25.19 A SHORT SUMMARY

When a rate is constant, survival times follow an exponential (Poisson) distribution and the rate ratio from a Poisson model will agree well with the hazard ratio from a Cox proportional hazards model. When a rate is not constant, outcomes times will not follow an exponential distribution, but the rate ratio and hazard ratio will still agree if outcomes are sufficiently uncommon. This will often be true for mortality data or a randomized controlled trial. But if a rate, or baseline hazard, is not constant, estimated rate ratios from Poisson and Cox proportional hazards regression will diverge as outcomes become common. In this situation, the analyst can chose the Cox model or flexible alternatives such as a Poisson model with many risk sets or a Royston-Parmer model. The use of restricted mean survival times is another option.

There are strong similarities between Poisson and Cox models; both estimate associations using rates and each can be modified to mimic the other. They represent two extremes; the Poisson model treats all survival times as if they are in the same risk set, while the Cox model estimates the rate ratio within a risk set for every survival time. An intermediate approach, modified Poisson or Royston-Parmer models, combines the parametric nature of a Poisson model with the nonparametric risk set approach of the Cox model. More details about the similarities and differences of these modeling approaches are in the excellent book by Royston and Lambert (Royston and Lambert 2011).

... So all the lovely rates lived happily ever after. THE END.

Bibliography

Agresti, A. 2002. *Categorical Data Analysis*. Hoboken, NJ: John Wiley & Sons.

Alderson, P. 2004. Absence of evidence is not evidence of absence. *BMJ* 328 (7438):476–477.

Altman, D.G. 1991. *Practical Statistics for Medical Research*. New York: Chapman & Hall.

Altman, D.G., and J.M. Bland. 1995. Absence of evidence is not evidence of absence. *BMJ* 311 (7003):485.

Altman, D.G., and J.M. Bland. 2003. Interaction revisited: The difference between two estimates. *BMJ* 326 (7382):219.

Altman, D.G., and J.M. Bland. 2004. Confidence intervals illuminate absence of evidence [letter]. *BMJ* 328 (7446):1016–1017.

Altman, D.G., J.J. Deeks, and D.L. Sackett. 1998. Odds ratios should be avoided when events are common. *BMJ* 317 (7168):1318.

Altman, D.G., and J.N. Matthews. 1996. Statistics notes. Interaction 1: Heterogeneity of effects. *BMJ* 313 (7055):486.

Altman, D.G., and J.P. Royston. 1988. The hidden effect of time. *Stat Med* 7 (6):629–637.

Altman, D.G., and P. Royston. 2000. What do we mean by validating a prognostic model? *Stat Med* 19 (4):453–473.

Andersen, P.K., and R.D. Gill. 1982. Cox's regression model for counting processes: A large sample study. *Ann Stat* 10 (4):1100–1120.

Anderson, R.N., and H.M. Rosenberg. 1998. Age standardization of death rates: Implementation of the year 2000 standard. *Natl Vital Stat Rep*, Vol 47 (3):1–16, 20. Hyattsville, MD: National Center for Health Statistics.

Andrews, D.W.K. 1988a. Chi-square diagnostic tests for econometric models: Introduction and applications. *Journal of Econometrics* 37 (1):135–156.

Andrews, D.W.K. 1988b. Chi-square diagnostic tests for econometric models: Theory. *Econometrica* 56 (6):1419–1453.

Andrews, D.W.K., and M. Buchinsky. 2000. A three-step method for choosing the number of bootstrap repetitions. *Econometrica* 68 (1):23–51.

Angrist, J.D., and G.W. Imbens. 1995. Two-stage least squares estimation of average causal effects in models with variable treatment intensity. *J Am Stat Assoc* 90 (430):431–442.

Angrist, J.D., G.W. Imbens, and D.B. Rubin. 1996. Identification of causal effects using instrumental variables (with discussion). *J Am Stat Assoc* 91 (434):444–472.

Angrist, J.D., and J.-S. Pischke. 2008. *Mostly Harmless Econometrics: An Empiricist's Companion*. Princeton, NJ: Princeton University Press.

Anonymous. 1864a. Miss Nightingale on hospitals [letter]. *Med Times Gazette* 1:211.

Anonymous. 1864b. Relative mortality in town and country hospitals. *Lancet* 83 (2113):248–250.

Anonymous. 1864c. Reviews. Notes on Hospitals. By Florence Nightingale. Third Edition. *Med Times Gazette* 1:129–130.

Anonymous. 1865. Statistics of metropolitan and provincial general hospitals for 1863. *J Stat Soc London* 28 (4):527–535.

Aranda-Ordaz, F.J. 1983. An extension of the proportional-hazards model for grouped data. *Biometrics* 39 (1):109–117.

Armitage, P., G. Berry, and J.N.S. Matthews. 2002. *Statistical Methods in Medical Research*. 4th ed. Oxford, UK: Blackwell Science.

Balke, A., and J. Pearl. 1997. Bounds on treatment effects from studies with imperfect compliance. *J Am Stat Assoc* 92 (439):1171–1176.

Barlow, W.E., R.L. Davis, J.W. Glasser, et al. 2001. The risk of seizures after receipt of whole-cell pertussis or measles, mumps, and rubella vaccine. *N Engl J Med* 345 (9):656–661.

Baron, J.A., M. Karagas, J. Barrett, et al. 1996. Basic epidemiology of fractures of the upper and lower limb among Americans over 65 years of age. *Epidemiology* 7 (6):612–618.

Bateman, H. 1910. The probability distribution of α particles. *Phil Mag J Sci* 20:704–707.

Belloco, R., and S. Algeri. 2013. Goodness-of-fit tests for categorical data. *Stata J* 13 (2):356–365.

Berkson, J. 1958. Smoking and lung cancer: Some observations on two recent reports. *J Am Stat Assoc* 58 (281):28–38.

Berkson, J. 1960. Smoking and cancer of the lung. *Staff Meet Mayo Clinic* 35 (13):367–385.

Berkson, J. 1963. Smoking and lung cancer. *Amer Statistician* 17 (4):15–22.

Berry, K.J., J.E. Johnston, and P.W. Mielke. 2014. *A Chronicle of Permutation Statistical Methods: 1920-2000, and Beyond*. New York: Springer.

Bishop, Y.M., S. Fienberg, and P.W. Holland. 1975. *Discrete Multivariate Analysis: Theory and Applications*. Springer reprint 2007 ed. Cambridge, MA: MIT Press.

Bliss, C.I., and R.A. Fisher. 1953. Fitting the negative binomial distribution to biological data. *Biometrics* 9 (2):176–200.

Blizzard, L., and D.W. Hosmer. 2006. Parameter estimation and goodness-of-fit in log binomial regression. *Biom J* 48 (1):5–22.

Boef, A.G., O.M. Dekkers, S. le Cessie, and J.P. Vandenbroucke. 2013. Reporting instrumental variable analyses [letter]. *Epidemiology* 24 (6):937–938.

Boef, A.G., O.M. Dekkers, J.P. Vandenbroucke, and S. le Cessie. 2014. Sample size importantly limits the usefulness of instrumental variable methods, depending on instrument strength and level of confounding. *J Clin Epidemiol* 67 (11):1258–1264.

Bradburn, M.J., J.J. Deeks, and D.G. Altman. 2009. Metan – A command for meta-analysis in Stata. In *Meta-Analysis in Stata: An Updated Collection from the Stata Journal*, edited by J.A.C. Sterne. College Station, TX: Stata Press.

Braem, M.G., N.C. Onland-Moret, P.A. van Den Brandt, et al. 2010. Reproductive and hormonal factors in association with ovarian cancer in the Netherlands cohort study. *Am J Epidemiol* 172 (10):1181–1189.

Breslow, N.E. 1981. Odds ratio estimators when data are sparse. *Biometrika* 68 (1):73–84.

Breslow, N.E. 1984. Elementary methods of cohort analysis. *Int J Epidemiol* 13 (1):112–115.

Breslow, N.E., and D.G. Clayton. 1993. Approximate inference in generalised linear mixed models. *J Am Stat Assoc* 88 (421):9–25.

Breslow, N.E., and N.E. Day. 1975. Indirect standardization and multiplicative models for rates, with reference to the age adjustment of cancer incidence and relative frequency data. *J Chronic Dis* 28 (5-6):289–303.

Breslow, N.E., and N.E. Day. 1980. *Statistical Methods in Cancer Research, Volume 1: the Analysis of Case-Control Studies*. Lyon, France: International Agency for Research on Cancer.

Breslow, N.E., and N.E. Day. 1987. *Statistical Methods in Cancer Research. Volume II - the Design and Analysis of Cohort Studies*. Lyon, France: International Agency for Research on Cancer.

Bristowe, J.S. 1864a. Hospital mortality. *Med Times Gazette* 1:491–492.

Bristowe, J.S. 1864b. Miss Nightingale on hospitals [letter]. *Med Times Gazette* 1:211.

Bristowe, J.S. 1864c. Mortality in hospitals [letter]. *Lancet* 83 (2120):452.

Brookes, S.T., E. Whitely, M. Egger, G.D. Smith, P.A. Mulheran, and T.J. Peters. 2004. Subgroup analyses in randomized trials: Risks of subgroup-specific analyses; power and sample size for the interaction test. *J Clin Epidemiol* 57 (3):229–236.

Buis, M.L. 2007. State tip 53: Where did my p-values go? *Stata J* 7 (4):584–586.

Burgess, S., D.S. Small, and S.G. Thompson. 2015. A review of instrumental variable estimators for Mendelian randomization. *Stat Methods Med Res* 26 (5):2333–2355.

Burnham, J.C. 2009. *Accident Prone: A History of Technology, Psychology, and Misfits of the Machine Age*. Chicago, IL: University of Chicago Press.

Buys, S.S., E. Partridge, A. Black, et al. 2011. Effect of screening on ovarian cancer mortality: The Prostate, Lung, Colorectal and Ovarian (PLCO) Cancer Screening Randomized Controlled Trial. *JAMA* 305 (22):2295–2303.

Cameron, A.C., and P.K. Trivedi. 1998. *Regression Analysis of Count Data*. New York: Cambridge University Press.

Cameron, A.C., and P.K. Trivedi. 2005. *Microeconometrics: Methods and Applications*. New York: Cambridge University Press.

Cameron, A.C., and P.K. Trivedi. 2009. *Microeconometrics Using Stata*. College Station, TX: Stata Press.

Cameron, A.C., and P.K. Trivedi. 2013a. *Regression Analysis of Count Data*. New York: Cambridge University Press.

Cameron, A.C., and P.K. Trivedi. 2013b. Regression analysis of count data, file racd03.do. http://cameron.econ.ucdavis.edu/racd2/RACD2programs.html.

Carpenter, J., and J. Bithell. 2000. Bootstrap confidence intervals: When, which, what? A practical guide for medical statisticians. *Stat Med* 19 (9):1141–1164.

Carroll, R.J., S. Wang, D.G. Simpson, A.J. Stromberg, and D. Ruppert. 1998. The Sandwich (Robust Covariance Matrix) Estimator. www.stat.tamu.edu/~carroll/ftp/sandwich.pdf.

Carstensen, B. 2005. Demography and epidemiology: Practical use of the Lexis diagram in the computer age, or who needs the Cox-model anyway? In *Annual Meeting of the Finnish Statistical Society*. Oulu, Finland.

Carter, R.E., S.R. Lipsitz, and B.C. Tilley. 2005. Quasi-likelihood estimation for relative risk regression models. *Biostatistics* 6 (1):39–44.

CDC WONDER. Compressed mortality file. CDC WONDER On-line Database. http://wonder.cdc.gov: Centers for Disease Control and Prevention, National Center for Health Statistics.

Checkoway, H., N. Pearce, and D.J. Crawford-Brown. 1989. *Research Methods in Occupational Epidemiology*. New York: Oxford University Press.

Chiang, C.L. 1961. Standard error of the age-adjusted death rate. In *Vital Statistics – Special Reports. Selected Studies. No. 9*. Washington, DC: US Department of Health, Education, and Welfare, Public Health Service, National Vital Statistics Division.

Clayton, D., and M. Hills. 1993. *Statistical Methods in Epidemiology*. New York: Oxford University Press.

Cleves, M., W. Gould, R.G. Gutierrez, and Y.V. Marchenko. 2010. *An Introduction to Survival Analysis Using Stata*. 3rd ed. College Station, TX: Stata Press.

Cochrane, W.G. 1977. *Sampling Techniques*. 3rd ed. New York: John Wiley & Sons.

Cole, S.R., H. Chu, and S. Greenland. 2014. Maximum likelihood, profile likelihood, and penalized likelihood: A primer. *Am J Epidemiol* 179 (2):252–260.

Congdon, P. 2001. *Bayesian Statistical Modeling*. West Sussex, England: John Wiley & Sons.

Cook, J.D. 2009. Notes on the negative binomial distribution. www.johndcook.com/negative_binomial.pdf.

Cook, R.D., and S. Weisberg. 1999. *Applied Regression Including Computing and Graphics*. New York: John Wiley & Sons.

Cook, R.J., and J.F. Lawless. 2007. *The Statistical Analysis of Recurrent Events*. New York: Springer.

Cornfield, J. 1951. A method of estimating comparative rates from clinical data. Applications to cancer of the lung, breast, and cervix. *J Natl Cancer Inst* 11 (6):1269–1275.

Cornfield, J., W. Haenszel, E.C. Hammond, A.M. Lilienfeld, M.B. Shimkin, and E.L. Wynder. 1959. Smoking and lung cancer: Recent evidence and a discussion of some questions. *J Natl Cancer Inst* 22 (1):173–203.

Cox, N.J. 2009. Speaking Stata: I. J. Good and quasi-Bayes smoothing of categorical frequencies. *Stata J* 9 (2):306–314.

Cronin, A., L. Tian, and H. Uno. 2016. strmst2 and strmst2pw: New commands to compare survival curves using the restricted mean survival time. *Stata J* 16 (3):702–716.

Crowther, M.J., and P.C. Lambert. 2012. Simulating complex survival data. *Stata J* 12 (4):674–687.

Crowther, M.J., and P.C. Lambert. 2013. Simulating biologically plausible complex survival data. *Stat Med* 32 (23):4118–4134.

Cummings, P. 2007a. Hip protectors and hip fracture [letter]. *JAMA* 298 (18):2139.

Cummings, P. 2007b. Policy recommendations in the discussion section of a research article (commentary). *Inj Prev* 13 (1):4–5.

Cummings, P. 2008. Propensity scores. *Arch Pediatr Adolesc Med* 162 (8):734–737.

Cummings, P. 2009a. Methods for estimating adjusted risk ratios. *Stata J* 9 (2):175–196.

Cummings, P. 2009b. The relative merits of risk ratios and odds ratios. *Arch Pediatr Adolesc Med* 163 (5):438–445.

Cummings, P. 2010. Carryover bias in crossover trials. *Arch Pediatr Adolesc Med* 164 (8):703–705.

Cummings, P. 2011. Estimating adjusted risk ratios for matched and unmatched data: An update. *Stata J* 11 (2):290–298.

Cummings, P., D.G. Grossman, F.P. Rivara, and T.D. Koepsell. 1997. State gun safe storage laws and child mortality due to firearms. *JAMA* 278 (13):1084–1086.

Cummings, P., and T.D. Koepsell. 2002. Statistical and design issues in studies of groups. *Inj Prev* 8 (1):6–7.

Cummings, P., and T.D. Koepsell. 2010. *P* values vs estimates of association with confidence intervals. *Arch Pediatr Adolesc Med* 165 (2):193–196.

Cummings, P., T.D. Koepsell, and I. Roberts. 2001. Case-control studies in injury research. In *Injury Control: A Guide to Research and Program Evaluation*, edited by F.P. Rivara, P. Cummings, T.D. Koepsell, et al. New York: Cambridge University Press.

Cummings, P., and B. McKnight. 2004. Analysis of matched cohort data. *Stata J* 4 (3):274–281.

Cummings, P., and B. McKnight. 2010. Accounting for vehicle, crash, and occupant characteristics in traffic crash studies. *Inj Prev* 16 (6):363–366.

Cummings, P., B. McKnight, and S. Greenland. 2003. Matched cohort methods in injury research. *Epidemiol Rev* 25:43–50.

Cummings, P., B. McKnight, F.P. Rivara, and D.C. Grossman. 2002. Association of driver air bags with driver fatality: A matched cohort study. *BMJ* 324 (7346):1119–1122.

Cummings, P., B. McKnight, and N.S. Weiss. 2003. Matched-pair cohort methods in traffic crash research. *Accid Anal Prev* 35 (1):131–141.

Cummings, P., B.A. Mueller, and L. Quan. 2010. Association between wearing a personal floatation device and death by drowning among recreational boaters: A matched cohort analysis of United States Coast Guard data. *Inj Prev* 17 (3):156–159.

Cummings, P., and F.P. Rivara. 2004. Car occupant death according to the restraint use of other occupants: A matched cohort study. *JAMA* 291 (3):343–349.

Cummings, P., and F.P. Rivara. 2012. Spin and boasting in research articles. *Arch Pediatr Adolesc Med* 166 (12):1099–1100.

Cummings, P., and N.S. Weiss. 2003. External hip protectors and risk of hip fracture [letter]. *JAMA* 290 (7):884; author reply 884-885.

Cummings, P., J.D. Wells, and F.P. Rivara. 2003. Estimating seat belt effectiveness using matched-pair cohort methods. *Accid Anal Prev* 35 (1):143–149.

Curfman, G.D., and J.P. Kassirer. 1999. Race, sex, and physicians' referrals for cardiac catheterization [letter]. *N Engl J Med* 341 (4):287.

Davidoff, F. 1999. Race, sex, and physicians' referrals for cardiac catheterization [letter]. *N Engl J Med* 341 (4):285–286.

Davies, N.M., G.D. Smith, F. Windmeijer, and R.M. Martin. 2013a. COX-2 selective nonsteroidal anti-inflammatory drugs and risk of gastrointestinal tract complications and myocardial infarction: An instrumental variable analysis. *Epidemiology* 24 (3):352–362.

Davies, N.M., G.D. Smith, F. Windmeijer, and R.M. Martin. 2013b. Issues in the reporting and conduct of instrumental variable studies: A systematic review. *Epidemiology* 24 (3):363–369.

Davison, A.C., and D.V. Hinkley. 1997. *Bootstrap Methods and Their Application*. New York: Cambridge University Press.

Deddens, J.A., and M.R. Petersen. 2008. Approaches for estimating prevalence ratios. *Occup Environ Med* 65 (7):501–506.

Deeks, J.J. 2002. Issues in the selection of a summary statistic for meta-analysis of clinical trials with binary outcomes. *Stat Med* 21 (11):1575–1600.

Deeks, J.J., D.G. Altman, and M.J. Bradburn. 2001. Statistical methods for examining heterogeneity and combining results from several studies in meta-analysis. In *Systematic Reviews in Health Care: Meta-Analysis in Context*, edited by M. Egger, G.D. Smith, and D.G. Altman. London: BMJ Publishing Group.

Dehbi, H.M., P. Royston, and A. Hackshaw. 2017. Life expectancy difference and life expectancy ratio: Two measures of treatment effects in randomised trials with non-proportional hazards. *BMJ* 357:j2250.

DerSimonian, R., and N. Laird. 1986. Meta-analysis in clinical trials. *Cont Clin Trials* 7 (3):177–188.

Diggle, P.J., P. Heagerty, K.-Y. Liang, and S.L. Zeger. 2002. *Analysis of Longitudinal Data*. 2nd ed. New York: Oxford University Press.

Discacciati, A., N. Orsini, and S. Greenland. 2015. Approximate Bayesian logistic regression via penalized likelihood by data augmentation. *Stata J* 15 (3):712–736.

Doll, R., and P. Cook. 1967. Summarizing indices for comparison of cancer incidence data. *Int J Cancer* 2 (3):269–279.

Doll, R., and A.B. Hill. 1950. Smoking and carcinoma of the lung: Preliminary report. *Br Med J* 2 (4682):739–748.

Doll, R., and A.B. Hill. 1956. Lung cancer and other causes of death in relation to smoking; a second report on the mortality of British doctors. *Br Med J* 2 (5001):1071–1081.

Donner, A., and N. Klar. 2000. *Design and Analysis of Cluster Randomization Trials in Health Research*. London: Arnold.

Draper, N.R., and H. Smith. 1998. *Applied Regression Analysis*. 3rd ed. New York: John Wiley & Sons.

Dunn, G., M. Maracy, and B. Tomenson. 2005. Estimating treatment effects from randomized clinical trials with noncompliance and loss to follow-up: The role of instrumental variable methods. *Stat Methods Med Res* 14 (4):369–395.

Edgington, E.S. 1995. *Randomization Tests*. 3rd ed. New York: Marcel Dekker.

Editor. 1864. Miss Nightingale's "Notes on Hospitals". *Med Times Gazette* 1:187–188.

Efron, B., and R.J. Tibshirani. 1993. *An Introduction to the Bootstrap*. New York: Chapman & Hall.

Eicker, F. 1967. Limit theorems for regressions with unequal or dependent errors. In *Proceedings of the Fifth Berkeley Symposium on Mathematical Statistics and Probability.* Berkeley, CA: University of California Press.

Eldridge, S.M., D. Ashby, C. Bennett, M. Wakelin, and G. Feder. 2008. Internal and external validity of cluster randomised trials: Systematic review of recent trials. *BMJ* 336 (7649):876–880.

Eldridge, S.M., D. Ashby, G.S. Feder, A.R. Rudnicka, and O.C. Ukoumunne. 2004. Lessons for cluster randomized trials in the twenty-first century: A systematic review of trials in primary care. *Clin Trials* 1 (1):80–90.

Eldridge, S.M., D. Ashby, and S. Kerry. 2006. Sample size for cluster randomized trials: Effect of coefficient of variation of cluster size and analysis method. *Int J Epidemiol* 35 (5):1292–1300.

Elliott, M.R. 2010. Matched cohort analysis in traffic injury epidemiology: Including adults when estimating exposure risks for children. *Inj Prev* 16 (6):367–371.

Evans, L. 1986. Double pair comparison — A new method to determine how occupant characteristics affect fatality risk in traffic crashes. *Accid Anal Prev* 18 (3):217–227.

Eyler, J.M. 2003. Understanding William Farr's 1838 article "On prognosis": Comment. *Soz Praventivmed* 48 (5):290–292.

Fang, G., J.M. Brooks, and E.A. Chrischilles. 2012. Apples and oranges? Interpretations of risk adjustment and instrumental variable estimates of intended treatment effects using observational data. *Am J Epidemiol* 175 (1):60–65.

Farcomeni, A., and L. Ventura. 2012. An overview of robust methods in medical research. *Stat Methods Med Res* 21 (2):111–133.

Farr, W. 1838. On Prognosis. *Br Med Almanack* (Supplement):199–216.

Farr, W. 1859. Letter to the registrar-general on the causes of death in England. In *Twentieth Annual Report of the Registrar-General of the Births, Deaths, and Marriages in England.* London: Printed by George E. Eyre and William Spottiswoode, for Her Majesty's Stationery Office.

Farr, W. 1863. Letter to the registrar general on the causes of death in England in 1861. In *Twenty-Fourth Annual Report of the Registrar-General of the Births, Deaths, and Marriages in England.* London: Printed by George E. Eyre and William Spottiswoode, for Her Majesty's Stationery Office.

Farr, W. 1864a. Hospital mortality [letter]. *Med Times Gazette* 1:242–243.

Farr, W. 1864b. Miss Nightingale's "Notes on Hospitals" [letter]. *Med Times Gazette* 1:186–187.

Farr, W. 1864c. Mortality in hospitals [letter]. *Lancet* 83 (2119):420–422.

Farrington, C.P. 1995. Relative incidence estimation from case series for vaccine safety evaluation. *Biometrics* 51 (1):228–235.

Farrington, C.P., J. Nash, and E. Miller. 1996. Case series analysis of adverse reactions to vaccines: A comparative evaluation. *Am J Epidemiol* 143 (11):1165–1173.

Firebaugh, G., and J. Gibbs. 1985. User's guide to ratio variables. *Am Sociol Rev* 50:713–722.

Fisher, E.S., J.A. Baron, D.J. Malenka, et al. 1991. Hip fracture incidence and mortality in New England. *Epidemiology* 2 (2):116–122.

Fisher, L.D., and G. van Belle. 1993. *Biostatistics: A Methodology for the Health Sciences.* New York: John Wiley & Sons.

Fisher, R.A. 1936. "The coefficient of racial likeness" and the future of craniometry. *J Roy Anthropol Inst Great Brit Ireland* 66:57–63.

Fisher, R.A. 1941. The negative binomial distribution. *Ann Eugenics* 11 (1):182–187.

Fisher, R.A. 1958a. Cancer and smoking [letter]. *Nature* 182 (4635):596.

Fisher, R.A. 1958b. Lung cancer and cigarettes [letter]. *Nature* 182 (4628):108.

Fitzmaurice, G.M., N.M. Laird, and J.H. Ware. 2011. *Applied Longitudinal Analysis.* 2nd ed. Hoboken, NJ: John Wiley & Sons.

Flanders, W.D., and P.H. Rhodes. 1987. Large sample confidence intervals for regression standardized risks, risk ratios, and risk differences. *J Chronic Dis* 40 (7):697–704.

Fleiss, J.L. 1993. The statistical basis of meta-analysis. *Stat Methods Med Res* 2 (2):121–145.

Fleiss, J.L., B. Levin, and M.C. Paik. 2003. *Statistical Methods for Rates and Proportions.* 3rd ed. Hoboken, NJ: John Wiley & Sons.

Forbes, C., M. Evans, N. Hastings, and B. Peacock. 2011. *Statistical Distributions.* Hoboken, NJ: John Wiley & Sons.

Ford, I., J. Norrie, and S. Ahmadi. 1995. Model inconsistency, illustrated by the Cox proportional hazards model. *Stat Med* 14 (8):735–746.

Freeman, J. 1996. Quantitative epidemiology. *Infect Control Hosp Epidemiol* 17 (4):249–255.

Frome, E.L., and H. Checkoway. 1985. Epidemiologic programs for computers and calculators. Use of Poisson regression models in estimating incidence rates and ratios. *Am J Epidemiol* 121 (2):309–323.

Gail, M.H., S.D. Mark, R.J. Carroll, S.B. Green, and D. Pee. 1996. On design considerations and randomization-based inference for community intervention trials. *Stat Med* 15 (11):1069–1092.

Garabedian, L.F., P. Chu, S. Toh, A.M. Zaslavsky, and S.B. Soumerai. 2014. Potential bias of instrumental variable analyses for observational comparative effectiveness research. *Ann Intern Med* 161 (2):131–138.

Gardiner, J.C., Z. Luo, and L.A. Roman. 2009. Fixed effects, random effects and GEE: What are the differences? *Stat Med* 28 (2):221–239.

Gardner, M.J., and D.G. Altman. 1986. Confidence intervals rather than P values: Estimation rather than hypothesis testing. *Br Med J* 292 (6522):746–750.

Gardner, W., E.P. Mulvey, and E.C. Shaw. 1995. Regression analyses of counts and rates: Poisson, overdispersed Poisson, and negative binomial models. *Psychol Bull* 118 (3):392–404.

Garthwaite, P.H., I.T. Jolliffe, and B. Jones. 2002. *Statistical Inference*. New York: Oxford University Press.

Gelman, A., J.B. Carlin, H.S. Stern, and D.B. Rubin. 1995. *Bayesian Data Analysis*. Boca Raton, FL: Chapman & Hall/CRC.

Gerstman, B.B. 2003. Comments regarding "On prognosis" by William Farr (1838), with reconstruction of his longitudinal analysis of smallpox recovery and death rates. *Soz Praventivmed* 48 (5):285–289.

Glymour, M.M., and S. Greenland. 2008. Causal diagrams. In *Modern Epidemiology*, edited by K.J. Rothman, S. Greenland, and T.L. Lash. Philadelphia, PA: Lippincott Williams & Wilkins.

Glynn, R.J., and J.E. Buring. 1996. Ways of measuring rates of recurrent events. *BMJ* 312 (7027):364–367.

Glynn, R.J., T.A. Stukel, S.M. Sharp, T.A. Bubolz, J.L. Freeman, and E.S. Fisher. 1993. Estimating the variance of standardized rates of recurrent events, with application to hospitalizations among the elderly in New England. *Am J Epidemiol* 137 (7):776–786.

Gordis, L. 2009. *Epidemiology*. 4th ed. Philadelphia, PA: Saunders.

Gould, W. 2011. Use Poisson rather than regress; tell a friend. *The Stata Blog*, http://blog.stata.com/2011/08/22/use-poisson-rather-than-regress-tell-a-friend/.

Gourieroux, C., A. Monfort, and C. Tognon. 1984a. Pseudo-maximum likelihood methods: Applications to Poisson models. *Econometrica* 52 (3):701–720.

Gourieroux, C., A. Monfort, and C. Tognon. 1984b. Pseudo-maximum likelihood methods: Theory. *Econometrica* 52 (3):681–700.

Grabowski, D.C., C.M. Campbell, and M.A. Morrisey. 2004. Elderly licensure laws and motor vehicle fatalities. *JAMA* 291 (23):2840–2846.

Green, P.J., and B.W. Silverman. 1994. *Nonparametric Regression and Generalized Linear Models. A Roughness Penalty Approach*. London: Chapman & Hall.

Greenland, S. 1987a. Bias in indirectly adjusted comparisons due to taking the total study population as the reference group. *Stat Med* 6 (2):193–195.

Greenland, S. 1987b. Interpretation and choice of effect measures in epidemiologic analyses. *Am J Epidemiol* 125 (5):761–768.

Greenland, S. 1987c. Interpreting time-related trends in effect estimates. *J Chronic Dis* 40 Suppl 2:17S-24S.

Greenland, S. 1991. Re: "Interpretation and choice of effect measures in epidemiologic analyses". The Author Replies [letter]. *Am J Epidemiol* 133 (9):964–965.

Greenland, S. 1994. Invited commentary: A critical look at some popular meta-analytic methods. *Am J Epidemiol* 140 (3):290–296.

Greenland, S. 1995. Dose-response and trend analysis in epidemiology: Alternatives to categorical analysis. *Epidemiology* 6 (4):356–365.

Greenland, S. 1996. Absence of confounding does not correspond to collapsibility of the rate ratio or rate difference. *Epidemiology* 7 (5):498–501.

Greenland, S. 2001. Ecologic versus individual-level sources of bias in ecologic estimates of contextual health effects. *Int J Epidemiol* 30 (6):1343–1350.

Greenland, S. 2002. A review of multilevel theory for ecologic analysis. *Stat Med* 21 (3):389–395.

Greenland, S. 2004. Model-based estimation of relative risks and other epidemiologic measures in studies of common outcomes and in case-control studies. *Am J Epidemiol* 160 (4):301–305.

Greenland, S. 2008a. Introduction to Bayesian statistics. In *Modern Epidemiology*, edited by K.J. Rothman, S. Greenland, and T.L. Lash. Philadelphia, PA: Lippincott Williams & Wilkins.

Greenland, S. 2008b. Introduction to regression modeling. In *Modern Epidemiology*, edited by K.J. Rothman, S. Greenland, and T.L. Lash. Philadelphia, PA: Lippincott Williams & Wilkins.

Greenland, S. 2008c. Introduction to regression models. In *Modern Epidemiology*, edited by K.J. Rothman, S. Greenland, and T.L. Lash. Philadelphia, PA: Lippincott Williams & Wilkins.

Greenland, S. 2010. Simpson's paradox from adding constants in contingency tables as an example of Bayesian noncollapsibility. *Amer Statistician* 64 (4):340–344.

Greenland, S., and L. Engelman. 1988. Re: "Inferences on odds ratios, relative risks, and risk differences based on standard regression programs". *Am J Epidemiol* 128 (2):445.

Greenland, S., and P. Holland. 1991. Estimating standardized risk differences from odds ratios. *Biometrics* 47 (1):319–322.

Greenland, S., T.L. Lash, and K.J. Rothman. 2008a. Concepts of interaction. In *Modern Epidemiology*, edited by K.J. Rothman, S. Greenland, and T.L. Lash. Philadelphia, PA: Lippincott Williams & Wilkins.

Greenland, S., M. Maclure, J.J. Schlesselman, C. Poole, and H. Morgenstern. 1991. Standardized regression coefficients: A further critique and review of some alternatives. *Epidemiology* 2 (5):387–392.

Greenland, S., M.A. Mansournia, and D.G. Altman. 2016. Sparse data bias: A problem hiding in plain sight. *BMJ* 352: i1981.

Greenland, S., and H. Morgenstern. 1990. Matching and efficiency in cohort studies. *Am J Epidemiol* 131 (1):151–159.

Greenland, S., and J.M. Robins. 1985. Estimation of a common effect parameter from sparse follow-up data. *Biometrics* 41 (1):55–68.

Greenland, S., J.M. Robins, and J. Pearl. 1999. Confounding and collapsibility in causal inference. *Stat Sci* 14 (1):29–46.

Greenland, S., and K.J. Rothman. 2008a. Fundamentals of epidemiologic data analysis. In *Modern Epidemiology*, edited by K.J. Rothman, S. Greenland, and T.L. Lash. Philadelphia, PA: Lippincott Williams & Wilkins.

Greenland, S., and K.J. Rothman. 2008b. Introduction to categorical statistics. In *Modern Epidemiology*, edited by K.J. Rothman, S. Greenland, and T.L. Lash. Philadelphia, PA: Lippincott Williams & Wilkins.

Greenland, S., and K.J. Rothman. 2008c. Introduction to stratified analysis. In *Modern Epidemiology*, edited by K.J. Rothman, S. Greenland, and T.L. Lash. Philadelphia, PA: Lippincott Williams & Wilkins.

Greenland, S., and K.J. Rothman. 2008d. Measures of occurrence. In *Modern Epidemiology*, edited by K.J. Rothman, S. Greenland, and T.L. Lash. Philadelphia, PA: Lippincott Williams & Wilkins.

Greenland, S., K.J. Rothman, and T.L. Lash. 2008. Measures of effect and measures of association. In *Modern Epidemiology*, edited by K.J. Rothman, S. Greenland, and T.L. Lash. Philadelphia, PA: Lippincott Williams & Wilkins.

Greenland, S., J.J. Schlesselman, and M.H. Criqui. 1986. The fallacy of employing standardized regression coefficients and correlations as measures of effect. *Am J Epidemiol* 123 (2):203–208.

Greenland, S., J.A. Schwartzbaum, and W.D. Finkle. 2000. Problems due to small samples and sparse data in conditional logistic regression analysis. *Am J Epidemiol* 151 (5):531–539.

Greenland, S., and D.C. Thomas. 1982. On the need for the rare disease assumption in case-control studies. *Am J Epidemiol* 116 (3):547–553.

Greenland, S., D.C. Thomas, and H. Morgenstern. 1986. The rare-disease assumption revisited. A critique of "estimators of relative risk for case-control studies". *Am J Epidemiol* 124 (6):869–883.

Greenwood, M. 1950. Accident proneness. *Biometrika* 37 (1-2):24–29.

Greenwood, M., and H.M. Woods. 1919. *The Incidence of Industrial Accidents upon Individuals with Special Reference to Multiple Accidents*. Report No. 4. London: Medical Research Committee, Industrial Fatigue Research Board, Her Majesty's Stationary Office.

Greenwood, M., and G.U. Yule. 1920. An inquiry into the nature of frequency distributions representative of multiple happenings with particular reference to the occurrence of multiple attacks of disease or of repeated accidents. *J R Stat Soc A* 83 (2):255–279.

Grima, J. 1999. Race, sex, and referral for cardiac catheterization [letter]. *N Engl J Med* 341 (26):2021.

Haight, F.A. 1967. *Handbook of the Poisson Distribution*. New York: John Wiley & Sons.

Haldane, J.B.S. 1941. The fitting of binomial distributions. *Ann Eugenics* 11 (1):179–181.

Hammond, E.C., and D. Horn. 1958a. Smoking and death rates; report on forty-four months of follow-up of 187,783 men. I. Total mortality. *J Am Med Assoc* 166 (10):1159–1172.

Hammond, E.C., and D. Horn. 1958b. Smoking and death rates; report on forty-four months of follow-up of 187,783 men. II. Death rates by cause. *J Am Med Assoc* 166 (11):1294–1308.

Hanley, J.A., A. Negassa, M.D. Edwardes, and J.E. Forrester. 2003. Statistical analysis of correlated data using generalized estimating equations: An orientation. *Am J Epidemiol* 157 (4):364–375.

Hardin, J.W., and J.M. Hilbe. 2012. *Generalized Linear Models and Extensions*. 3rd ed. College Station, TX: Stata Press.

Hardin, J.W., and J.M. Hilbe. 2013. *Generalized Estimating Equations*. 2nd ed. Boca Raton, FL: CRC Press.

Harrell, F.E., Jr. 2001. *Regression Modeling Strategies: With Applications to Linear Models, Logistic Regression, and Survival Analysis*. New York: Springer.

Harris, R.J., M.J. Bradburn, J.J. Deeks, R.M. Harbord, D.G. Altman, and J.A.C. Sterne. 2009. metan: Fixed- and random-effects meta-analysis. In *Meta-Analysis in Stata: An Updated Collection from the Stata Journal*, edited by J.A.C. Sterne. College Station, TX: Stata Press.

Hastie, T.J., and R.J. Tibshirani. 1990. *Generalized Additive Models*. London: Chapman & Hall.

Hauck, W.W., S. Anderson, and S.M. Marcus. 1998. Should we adjust for covariates in nonlinear regression analyses of randomized trials? *Control Clin Trials* 19 (3):249–256.

Hauck, W.W., J.M. Neuhaus, J.D. Kalbfleisch, and S. Anderson. 1991. A consequence of omitted covariates when estimating odds ratios. *J Clin Epidemiol* 44 (1):77–81.

Hauer, E. 2004. The harm done by tests of significance. *Accid Anal Prev* 36 (3):495–500.

Hayes, R.J., and L.H. Moulton. 2009. *Cluster Randomized Trials*. Boca Raton, FL: Chapman & Hall/CRC.

Heagerty, P.J., and S.L. Zeger. 2000. Marginalized multilevel models and likelihood inference (with discussion). *Stat Sci* 15 (1):1–26.

Hedges, L.V., and I. Olkin. 1985. *Statistical Methods for Meta-Analysis*. San Diego, CA: Academic Press.

Helft, G., S. Worthley, and S. Chokron. 1999. Race, sex, and physicians' referrals for cardiac catheterization [letter]. *N Engl J Med* 341 (4):285.

Hennekens, C.H., and J.E. Buring. 1987. *Epidemiology in Medicine*. Boston, MA: Little, Brown and Company.

Heritier, S., E. Contoni, S. Copt, and M.-P. Victoria-Feser. 2009. *Robust Methods in Biostatistics*. New York: John Wiley & Sons.

Hernán, M.A. 2010. The hazards of hazard ratios [erratum: 2011,vol 22, p134]. *Epidemiology* 21 (1):13–15.

Hernán, M.A., S. Hernández-Diaz, and J.M. Robins. 2004. A structural approach to selection bias. *Epidemiology* 15 (5):615–625.

Hernán, M.A., and J.M. Robins. 2006. Instruments for causal inference: An epidemiologist's dream? *Epidemiology* 17 (4):360–372.

Hilbe, J.M. 2010. Creating synthetic discrete-response regression models. *Stata J* 10 (1):104–124.

Hilbe, J.M. 2011. *Negative Binomial Regression*. 2nd ed. Cambridge, UK: Cambridge University Press.

Hilbe, J.M. 2014. *Modeling Count Data*. New York: Cambridge University Press.

Hill, A.B. 1965. The environment and disease: Association or causation. *Proc R Soc Med* 58 (5):295–300.

Hill, G.B. 2004. Comments on the paper "On prognosis" by William Farr: A forgotten masterpiece. In *A History of Epidemiologic Methods and Concepts*, edited by A. Morabia. Basel, Switzerland: Birkhäuser Verlag.

Hills, M., and P. Armitage. 1979. The two-period cross-over clinical trial. *Br J Clin Pharmacol* 8 (1):7–20.

Hoffmann, J.P. 2004. *Generalized Linear Models: An Applied Approach*. Boston, MA: Pearson Education.

Holcomb, R.L. 1938. Alcohol in relation to traffic accidents. *J Am Med Assoc* 111 (12):1076–1085.

Hollander, N., W. Sauerbrei, and M. Schumacher. 2004. Confidence intervals for the effect of a prognostic factor after selection of an 'optimal' cutpoint. *Stat Med* 23 (11):1701–1713.

Holmes, T. 1864a. Mortality in hospitals [letter]. *Lancet* 83 (2116):338–339.

Holmes, T. 1864b. Mortality in hospitals [letter]. *Lancet* 83 (2120):451–452.

Holmes, T. 1864c. Mortality in hospitals [letter]. *Lancet* 83 (2117):365–366.

Hosmer, D.W., Jr., S. Lemeshow, and S. May. 2008. *Applied Survival Analysis: Regression Modeling of Time to Event Data*. 2nd ed. Hoboken, NJ: John Wiley & Sons.

Hubbard, A.E., J. Ahern, N.L. Fleischer, et al. 2010. To GEE or not to GEE: Comparing population average and mixed models for estimating the associations between neighborhood risk factors and health. *Epidemiology* 21 (4):467–474.

Huber, P.J. 1967. The behavior of maximum likelihood estimates under nonstandard conditions. In *Proceedings of the Fifth Berkeley Symposium on Mathematical Statistics and Probability*. Berkeley, CA: University of California Press.

Huybrechts, K.F., M.A. Brookhart, K.J. Rothman, et al. 2011. Comparison of different approaches to confounding adjustment in a study on the association of antipsychotic medication with mortality in older nursing home patients. *Am J Epidemiol* 174 (9):1089–1099.

Hviid, A., M. Stellfeld, J. Wohlfahrt, and M. Melbye. 2003. Association between thimerosal-containing vaccine and autism. *JAMA* 290 (13):1763–1766.

Iezzoni, L.I. 1996a. 100 apples divided by 15 red herrings: A cautionary tale from the mid-19th century on comparing hospital mortality rates. *Ann Intern Med* 124 (12):1079–1085.

Iezzoni, L.I. 1996b. In defense of Farr and Nightingale: In reponse [letter]. *Ann Intern Med* 125 (12):1014.

Iezzoni, L.I. 1997. A return to Farr and Nightingale: In response [letter]. *Ann Intern Med* 127 (2):171.

Insurance Institute for Highway Safety. 1992. Crashes, fatal crashes per mile. *Status Report* 27 (11):1–7.

Jackson, J.W., and S.A. Swanson. 2015. Toward a clearer portrayal of confounding bias in instrumental variable applications. *Epidemiology* 26 (4):498–504.

Jacobs, I.J., U. Menon, A. Ryan, et al. 2016. Ovarian cancer screening and mortality in the UK Collaborative Trial of Ovarian Cancer Screening (UKCTOCS): A randomised controlled trial. *Lancet* 387 (10022):945–956.

Jensen, A., H. Sharif, K. Frederiksen, and S.K. Kjaer. 2009. Use of fertility drugs and risk of ovarian cancer: Danish Population Based Cohort Study. *BMJ* 338:b249.

Joffe, M.M., and S. Greenland. 1995. Standardized estimates from categorical regression models. *Stat Med* 14 (19):2131–2141.

Jones, B., and M.G. Kenward. 2003. *Design and Analysis of Cross-Over Trials*. 2nd ed. Boca Raton, FL: Chapman & Hall/CRC.

Kahn, H.A., and C.T. Sempos. 1989. *Statistical Methods in Epidemiology*. New York: Oxford University Press.

Keiding, N. 1987. The method of expected number of deaths, 1786-1886-1986. *Int Stat Rev* 55 (1):1–20.

Kelly, H., and B.J. Cowling. 2013. Case fatality: Rate, ratio, or risk? *Epidemiology* 24 (4):622–623.

Kelsey, J.L., W.D. Thompson, and A.S. Evans. 1986. *Methods in Observational Epidemiology*. New York: Oxford University Press.

Kelsey, J.L., A.S. Whittemore, A.S. Evans, and W.D. Thompson. 1996. *Methods in Observational Epidemiology*. 2nd ed. New York: Oxford University Press.

Keyfitz, N. 1966. Sampling variance of standardized mortality rates. *Hum Biol* 38 (3):309–317.

Keynes, J.M. *Wikiquote*, http://en.wikiquote.org/wiki/John_Maynard_Keynes.

Kilpatrick, S.J. 1963. Mortality comparisons in socio-economic groups. *J R Stat Soc. Series C (Appl Stat)* 12 (2):65–86.

Kleerekoper, M., E.L. Peterson, D.A. Nelson, et al. 1991. A randomized trial of sodium fluoride as a treatment for postmenopausal osteoporosis. *Osteoporos Int* 1 (3):155–161.

Klein, J.P., and M.L. Moeschberger. 1997. *Survival Analysis: Techniques for Censored and Truncated Data*. New York: Springer.

Klein, R.J., and C.A. Schoenborn. 2001. Age adjustment using the 2000 projected U.S. population. In *Healthy People Statistical Notes*, no. 20. Hyattsville, MD: National Center for Health Statistics.

Kleinbaum, D.G. 1996. *Survival Analysis: A Self-Learning Text*. New York: Springer.

Kleinbaum, D.G., and M. Klein. 2010. *Logistic Regression: A Self-Learning Text*. 3rd ed. New York: Springer.

Kleinbaum, D.G., L.L. Kupper, and H. Morgenstern. 1982. *Epidemiologic Research: Principles and Quantitative Methods*. New York: Van Nostrand Reinhold.

Kleinbaum, D.G., L.L. Kupper, K.E. Muller, and N. Azhar. 1998. *Applied Regression Analysis and Other Multi-variable Methods*. 3rd ed. Boston, MA: Duxbury Press.

Kleinman, L.C., and E.C. Norton. 2009. What's the risk? A simple approach for estimating adjusted risk measures from nonlinear models including logistic regression. *Health Serv Res* 44 (1):288–302.

Kluger, R. 1996. *Ashes to Ashes: America's Hundred-Year Cigarette War, the Public Health, and the Unabashed Triumph of Phillip Morris*. New York: Alfred A. Knopf.

Klungel, O.H., E.P. Martens, B.M. Psaty, et al. 2004. Methods to assess intended effects of drug treatment in observational studies are reviewed. *J Clin Epidemiol* 57 (12):1223–1231.

Knol, M.J., J.P. Vandenbroucke, P. Scott, and M. Egger. 2008. What do case-control studies estimate? Survey of methods and assumptions in published case-control research. *Am J Epidemiol* 168 (9):1073–1081.

Kochanek, K.D., J. Xu, S.L. Murphy, A.M. Miniño, and H.-C. Kung. 2012. Deaths: Final data for 2009. *National Vital Statistics Reports*. Hyattsville, MD: National Center for Health Statistics.

Koepsell, T.D. 1998. Epidemiologic issues in the design of community intervention trials. In *Applied Epidemiology: Theory to Practice*, edited by R.C. Brownson and D. Pettiti. New York: Oxford University Press.

Kraemer, H.C. 2009. Events per person-time (incidence rate): A misleading statistic? *Stat Med* 28 (6):1028–1039.

Kronmal, R.A. 1993. Spurious correlation and the fallacy of the ratio standard revisited. *J R Stat Soc A* 156 (3):379–392.

Kronmal, R.A. 1995. Author's Reply [letter]. *J R Stat Soc A* 158 (3):623–625.

Laird, N., and D. Olivier. 1981. Covariance analysis of censored survival data using log-linear analysis techniques. *J Am Stat Assoc* 76 (374):231–240.

Lambert, P.C., and P. Royston. 2009. Further developement of the flexible parametric models for survival analysis. *Stata J* 9 (2):265–290.

Lane, P.W., and J.A. Nelder. 1982. Analysis of covariance and standardization as instances of prediction. *Biometrics* 38 (3):613–621.

Lane-Claypon, J.E. 1926. *A Further Report on Cancer of the Breast, with Special Reference to Its Associated Antecedent Conditions*. London: Reports of the Ministry of Health, No. 32, His Majesty's Stationery Office.

Langmuir, A.D. 1976. William Farr: Founder of modern concepts of surveillance. *Int J Epidemiol* 5 (1):13–18.

Lawless, J.F. 1987. Regression models for Poisson process data. *J Am Stat Assoc* 82 (399):808–815.

Levene, L.S., R. Baker, M.J. Bankart, and K. Khunti. 2010. Association of features of primary health care with coronary heart disease mortality. *JAMA* 304 (18):2028–2034.

Levy, D.T., J.S. Vernick, and K.A. Howard. 1995. Relationships between driver's license renewal policies and fatal crashes involving drivers 70 years or older. *JAMA* 274 (13):1026–1030.

Liang, K.-Y., and S.L. Zeger. 1993. Regression analysis for correlated data. *Annu Rev Public Health* 14:43–68.

Lilienfeld, A.M. 1959a. Emotional and other selected characteristics of cigarette smokers and non-smokers as related to epidemiological studies of lung cancer and other diseases. *J Natl Cancer Inst* 22 (2):259–282.

Lilienfeld, A.M. 1959b. On the methodology of investigations of etiologic factors in chronic diseases: Some comments. *J Chronic Dis* 10 (1):41–46.

Lilienfeld, D.E., and P.D. Stolley. 1994. *Foundations of Epidemiology*. 3rd ed. New York: Oxford University Press.

Lindsey, J.K. 1995. *Introductory Statistics: A Modelling Approach*. Oxford, UK: Oxford University Press.

Lindsey, J.K. 1997. *Applying Generalized Linear Models*. New York: Springer.

Lindsey, J.K., and B. Jones. 1998. Choosing among generalized linear models applied to medical data. *Stat Med* 17 (1):59–68.

Lloyd, C.J. 1999. *Statistical Analysis of Categorical Data*. New York: John Wiley & Sons.

Localio, A.R., J.A. Berlin, T.R. Ten Have, and S.E. Kimmel. 2001. Adjustments for center in multicenter studies: An overview. *Ann Intern Med* 135 (2):112–123.

Localio, A.R., D.J. Margolis, and J.A. Berlin. 2007. Relative risks and confidence intervals were easily computed indirectly from multivariable logistic regression. *J Clin Epidemiol* 60 (9):874–882.

Long, J.S., and J. Freese. 2014. *Regression Models for Categorical Dependent Variables Using Stata*. 3rd ed. College Station, TX: Stata Press.

Lord, D., and B.-J. Park. Negative binomial regression models and estimation methods. www.icpsr.umich.edu/CrimeStat/files/CrimeStatAppendix.D.pdf.

Lufkin, E.G., H.W. Wahner, W.M. O'Fallon, et al. 1992. Treatment of postmenopausal osteoporosis with transdermal estrogen. *Ann Intern Med* 117 (1):1–9.

Lumley, T., P. Diehr, S. Emerson, and L. Chen. 2002. The importance of the normality assumption in large public health data sets. *Annu Rev Public Health* 23:151–169.

Lumley, T., R. Kronmal, and S. Ma. 2006. Relative risk regression in medical research: Models, contrasts, estimators, and algorithms. *UW Biostatistics Working Paper Series* (Paper 293), www.bepress.com/uwbiostat/paper293.

Lunneborg, C.E. 2000. *Data Analysis by Resampling: Concepts and Applications*. Pacific Grove, CA: Duxbury Press.

Maclure, M. 1991. The case-crossover design: A method for studying transient effects on the risk of acute events. *Am J Epidemiol* 133 (2):144–153.

Maclure, M., and M.A. Mittleman. 1997. Cautions about car telephones and collisions [editorial]. *N Engl J Med* 336 (7):501–502.

Maclure, M., and M.A. Mittleman. 2000. Should we use a case-crossover design? *Annu Rev Public Health* 21:193–221.

MacMahon, B., and D. Trichopoulos. 1996. *Epidemiology: Principles and Methods*. 2nd ed. Boston, MA: Little, Brown and Company.

Maldonado, G., and S. Greenland. 1994. A comparison of the performance of model-based confidence intervals when the correct model form is unknown: Coverage of asymptotic means. *Epidemiology* 5 (2):171–182.

Maldonado, G., and S. Greenland. 1996. Impact of model-form selection on the accuracy of rate estimation. *Epidemiology* 7 (1):46–54.

Manjón, M., and O. Martínez. 2014. The chi-squared goodness-of-fit test for count data models. *Stata J* 14 (4):798–816.

Manly, B.F.J. 2007. *Randomization, Bootstrap and Monte Carlo Methods in Biology*. 3rd ed. Boca Raton, FL: Chapman & Hall.

Mantel, N., and W. Haenszel. 1959. Statistical aspects of the analysis of data from retrospective studies. *J Natl Cancer Inst* 22 (4):719–748.

Martens, E.P., W.R. Pestman, A. de Boer, S.V. Belitser, and O.H. Klungel. 2006. Instrumental variables: Application and limitations. *Epidemiology* 17 (3):260–267.

Matthews, J.N., and D.G. Altman. 1996a. Interaction 3: How to examine heterogeneity. *BMJ* 313 (7061):862.

Matthews, J.N., and D.G. Altman. 1996b. Statistics notes. Interaction 2: Compare effect sizes not P values. *BMJ* 313 (7060):808.

Matthews, J.N.S. 2000. *An Introduction to Randomized Controlled Clinical Trials*. London: Arnold.

McCullagh, P., and J.A. Nelder. 1989. *Generalized Linear Models*. 2nd ed. New York: Chapman & Hall.

McNutt, L.-A., C. Wu, X. Xue, and J.P. Hafner. 2003. Estimating the relative risk in cohort studies and clinical trials of common outcomes. *Am J Epidemiol* 157 (10):940–943.

McShane, P. 1995. Storks, babies and linear models: A response to Kronmal [letter]. *J R Stat Soc A* 158 (3):621–623.

Michels, K.B., S. Greenland, and B.A. Rosner. 1998. Does body mass index adequately capture the relation of body composition and body size to health outcomes? *Am J Epidemiol* 147 (2):167–172.

Miettinen, O. 1976. Estimability and estimation in case-referent studies. *Am J Epidemiol* 103 (2):226–235.

Miettinen, O.S., and E.F. Cook. 1981. Confounding: Essence and detection. *Am J Epidemiol* 114 (4):593–603.

Miller, D.M. 1984. Reducing transformation bias in curve fitting. *Amer Statistician* 38 (2):124–126.

Miller, R.G., Jr. 1997. *Beyond ANOVA: Basic Applied Statistics*. Boca Raton, FL: Chapman & Hall/CRC.

Mills, E.J., A.W. Chan, P. Wu, A. Vail, G.H. Guyatt, and D.G. Altman. 2009. Design, analysis, and presentation of crossover trials. *Trials* 10:27.

Mittleman, M.A., M. Maclure, G.H. Tofler, J.B. Sherwood, R.J. Goldberg, and J.E. Muller. 1993. Triggering of acute myocardial infarction by heavy physical exertion: Protection against triggering by regular exertion. *N Engl J Med* 329 (23):1677–1683.

Mooney, C.Z., and R.D. Duval. 1993. *Bootstrapping: A Nonparametric Approach to Statistical Inference*. Newbury Park, CA: Sage Publications.

Morabia, A. 2010. Janet Lane-Claypon–Interphase epitome. *Epidemiology* 21 (4):573–576.

Morgan, S.L., and C. Winship. 2007a. The Counterfactual Model. In *Counterfactuals and Causal Inference: Methods and Principles for Social Research*. New York: Cambridge University Press.

Morgan, S.L., and C. Winship. 2007b. *Counterfactuals and Causal Inference: Methods and Principles for Social Research*. New York: Cambridge University Press.

Morgenstern, H. 1998. Ecologic Studies. In *Modern Epidemiology*, edited by K.J. Rothman and S. Greenland. Philadelphia, PA: Lippincott-Raven.

Morgenstern, H. 2008. Ecologic studies. In *Modern Epidemiology*, edited by K.J. Rothman, S. Greenland, and T. L. Lash. Philadelphia, PA: Lippincott Williams & Wilkins.

Mullahy, J. 1997. Instrumental-variable estimation of count data models: Applications to models of cigarette smoking behavior. *Rev Econ Stat* 79 (4):586–593.

Murphy, S.L., J. Xu, and K.D. Kochanek. 2013. Deaths: Final data for 2010. *National Vital Statistics Reports*. Hyattsville, MD: National Center for Health Statistics.

Murray, D.M. 1998. *Design and Analysis of Group-Randomized Trials*. New York: Oxford University Press.

Murray, D.M., P.J. Hannan, R.D. Wolfinger, W.L. Baker, and J.H. Dwyer. 1998. Analysis of data from group-randomized trials with repeat observations on the same groups. *Stat Med* 17 (14):1581–1600.

Murray, D.M., S.P. Varnell, and J.L. Blitstein. 2004. Design and analysis of group-randomized trials: A review of recent methodological developments. *Am J Public Health* 94 (3):423–432.

Nathens, A.B., G.J. Jurkovich, P. Cummings, F.P. Rivara, and R.V. Maier. 2000. The effect of organized systems of trauma care on motor vehicle crash mortality. *JAMA* 283 (15):1990–1994.

National Cancer Institute. Adjusted populations for the counties/parishes affected by Hurricanes Katrina and Rita. https://seer.cancer.gov/popdata/hurricane_adj.html.

National Highway Traffic Safety Administration. 2004. *Traffic Safety Facts 2002: A Compilation of Motor Vehicle Crash Data from the Fatality Analysis Reporting System and the General Estimates System. DOT HS 809 620*. Washington, DC: National Highway Traffic Safety Administration.

National Highway Traffic Safety Administration. 2013. *Traffic Safety Facts 2012: A Compilation of Motor Vehicle Crash Data from the Fatality Analysis Reporting System and the General Estimates System. DOT HS 812 032*. Washington, DC: National Highway Traffic Safety Administration.

Neison, F.G.P. 1844. On a method recently proposed for conducting inquires into the comparative sanatory condition of various districts, with illustrations, derived from numerous places in Great Britain at the period of the last census. *J Stat Soc London* 7 (1):40–68.

Nelder, J.A., and R.W.M. Wedderburn. 1972. Generalized linear models. *J R Stat Soc A* 135 (3):370–384.

Neter, J., W. Wasserman, and M.H. Kutner. 1990. *Applied Linear Statistical Models: Regression, Analysis of Variance, and Experimental Design.* 3rd ed. Homewood, IL: Irwin.

Nevill, A.M., and R.L. Holder. 1995. Spurious correlations and the fallacy of the ratio standard revisited [letter]. *J R Stat Soc A* 158 (3):619–621.

New York Times. 1999. Doctor bias may affect heart care, study finds. February 25.

Newbold, E.M. 1927. Practical aspects of the statistics of repeated events' particularly to industrial accidents. *J R Stat Soc* 90 (3):487–547.

Newcomb, S. 1860. Notes on the theory of probabilities. *Math Monthly* 2 (4):134–140.

Newhouse, J.P., and M. McClellan. 1998. Econometrics in outcomes research: The use of instrumental variables. *Annu Rev Public Health* 19:17–34.

Newman, S.C. 2001. *Biostatistical Methods in Epidemiology.* New York: John Wiley & Sons.

Neyman, J. 1952. On a most powerful method of discovering statistical regularities. In *Lectures and Conferences on Mathematical Statistics and Probability.* Washington, DC: US Department of Agriculture.

Nichols, A. 2010. Regression for nonnegative skewed dependent variables. www.stata.com/meeting/boston10/boston10_nichols.pdf.

Nightingale, F. 1863. *Notes on Hospitals.* 3rd ed. London: Longman, Green, Longman, Roberts, & Green.

Norvell, D.C., and P. Cummings. 2002. Association of helmet use with death in motorcycle crashes: A matched-pair cohort study. *Am J Epidemiol* 156 (5):483–487.

Nurminen, N. 1981. Asymptotic efficiency of general noniterative estimation of common relative risk. *Biometrika* 68 (2):525–530.

Olson, C.M., P. Cummings, and F.P. Rivara. 2006. Association of first- and second-generation air bags with front occupant death in car crashes: A matched cohort study. *Am J Epidemiol* 164 (2):161–169.

Page, M. 1995. Racial and ethnic discrimination in urban housing markets: Evidence from a recent audit survey. *J Urban Economics* 38 (2):183–206.

Pak, C.Y., K. Sakhaee, and J.E. Zerwekh. 1990. Effect of intermittent therapy with a slow-release fluoride preparation. *J Bone Miner Res* 5 Suppl 1:S149-1155.

Pak, K., H. Uno, D.H. Kim, et al. 2017. Interpretability of Cancer Clinical Trial results using restricted mean survival time as an alternative to the hazard ratio. *JAMA Oncol* 3 (12):1692–1696.

Palmer, T.M., R.R. Ramsahai, V. Didelez, and N.A. Sheehan. 2011. Nonparametric bounds for the causal effect in a binary instrumental-variable model. *Stata J* 11 (3):345–367.

Palmer, T.M., and J.A.C. Sterne, eds. 2015. *Meta-Analysis in Stata: An Updated Collection from the Stata Journal.* 2nd ed. College Station, TX: Stata Press.

Palmieri, G.M., J.A. Pitcock, P. Brown, J.G. Karas, and L.J. Roen. 1989. Effect of calcitonin and vitamin D in osteoporosis. *Calcif Tissue Int* 45 (3):137–141.

Paneth, N., E. Susser, and M. Susser. 2004. Origins and early development of the case-control study. In *A History of Epidemiologic Methods and Concepts*, edited by A. Morabia. Basel, Switzerland: Birkhäuser Verlag.

Parmar, M.K.B., and D. Machin. 1995. *Survival Analysis: A Practical Approach.* Chichester, UK: John Wiley & Sons.

Pearce, N. 1993. What does the odds ratio estimate in a case-control study? *Int J Epidemiol* 22 (6):1189–1192.

Pearson, K. 1897. Mathematical contributions to the theory of evolution - on a form of spurious correlation which may arise when indices are used in the measurements of organs. *Proc R Soc Lond* 60:489–498.

Peduzzi, P., J. Concato, E. Kemper, T.R. Holford, and A.R. Feinstein. 1996. A simulation study of the number of events per variable in logistic regression analysis. *J Clin Epidemiol* 49 (12):1373–1379.

Pepe, M.S. 2003. *The Statistical Evaluation of Medical Tests for Classification and Prediction.* New York: Oxford University Press.

Persaud, R. 1999. Race, sex, and referral for cardiac catheterization [letter]. *N Engl J Med* 341 (26):2021–2022.

Peto, R., and M.C. Pike. 1973. Conservatism of the approximation Σ (O-E)2 -E in the logrank test for survival data or tumor incidence data. *Biometrics* 29 (3):579–584.

Piantadosi, S. 1997. *Clinical Trials: A Methodologic Perspective.* New York: John Wiley & Sons.

Pike, M.C., A.P. Hill, and P.G. Smith. 1980. Bias and efficiency in logistic analyses of stratified case-control studies. *Int J Epidemiol* 9 (1):89–95.

Pocock, S.J. 1983. *Clinical Trials: A Practical Approach.* New York: John Wiley & Sons.

Pocock, S.J., S.E. Assmann, L.E. Enos, and L.E. Kasten. 2002. Subgroup analysis, covariate adjustment and baseline comparisons in clinical trial reporting: Current practice and problems. *Stat Med* 21 (19):2917–2930.

Poi, B.P. 2004. From the help desk: Some bootstraping techniques. *Stata J* 4 (3):312–328.

Poole, C. 1987a. Beyond the confidence interval. *Am J Public Health* 77 (2):195–199.

Poole, C. 1987b. Confidence intervals exclude nothing. *Am J Public Health* 77 (4):492–493.

Poole, C. 2010. On the origin of risk relativism. *Epidemiology* 21 (1):3–9.

Poole, C., and S. Greenland. 1999. Random-effects meta-analyses are not always conservative. *Am J Epidemiol* 150 (5):469–475.

Porta, M., ed. 2008. *A Dictionary of Epidemiology*. 5th ed. Oxford, UK: Oxford University Press.

Pregibon, D. 1980. Goodness of link tests for generalized linear models. *J R Stat Soc. Series C (Appl Stat)* 29 (1):15–24.

Prentice, R.L., and N.E. Breslow. 1978. Retrospective studies and failure time models. *Biometrika* 65 (1):153–158.

Prentice, R.L., B.J. Williams, and A.V. Peterson. 1981. On the regression analysis of multivariate failure time data. *Biometrika* 68 (2):373–379.

Press, D.J., and P. Pharoah. 2010. Risk factors for breast cancer: A reanalysis of two case-control studies from 1926 and 1931. *Epidemiology* 21 (4):566–572.

Public Health Service. 1964. *Smoking and Health: Report of the Advisory Committee of the Surgeon General of the Public Health Service*. Washington, DC: Public Health Service, U.S. Department of Health, Education, and Welfare.

Quine, M.P., and E. Seneta. 1987. Bortkiewicz's data and the law of small numbers. *Int Stat Rev* 55 (2):173–181.

Rabe-Hesketh, S., and A. Skrondal. 2012. *Multilevel and Longitudinal Modeling Using Stata*. 3rd ed. College Station, TX: Stata Press.

Redelmeier, D.A., and R.J. Tibshirani. 1997a. Association between cellular-telephone calls and motor vehicle collisions. *N Engl J Med* 336 (7):453–458.

Redelmeier, D.A., and R.J. Tibshirani. 1997b. Interpretation and bias in case-crossover studies. *J Clin Epidemiol* 50 (11):1281–1287.

Registrar General. 1863. *Twenty-Fourth Annual Report of the Registrar-General of the Births, Deaths, and Marriages in England*. London: Printed by George E. Eyre and William Spottiswoode, for Her Majesty's Stationery Office. http://books.google.com/books?id=axkoAAAAYAAJ&pg=PA355&lpg=PA355&dq=registrar-general 's+report+1861&source=bl&ots=NtVQeoGF9n&sig=uo-lv82Z97wstnUMURL6BigyXsU&hl=en&sa=X&ei= BA22UcyKAaaoywGh_IH4DQ&ved=0CCkQ6AEwADgK#v=onepage&q=registrar-general's%20report% 201861&f=false (accessed June 10, 2013).

Rice, J.A. 1995. *Mathematical Statistics and Data Analysis*. 2nd ed. Belmont, CA: Duxbury Press.

Rice, T.M., and C.L. Anderson. 2010. The inclusion of adult vehicle occupants in matched cohort studies of child restraint effectiveness: A study of potential bias. *Inj Prev* 16 (6):372–375.

Riggs, B.L., S.F. Hodgson, W.M. O'Fallon, et al. 1990. Effect of fluoride treatment on the fracture rate in postmenopausal women with osteoporosis. *N Engl J Med* 322 (12):802–809.

Riggs, B.L., E. Seeman, S.F. Hodgson, D.R. Taves, and W.M. O'Fallon. 1982. Effect of the fluoride/calcium regimen on vertebral fracture occurrence in postmenopausal osteoporosis. Comparison with conventional therapy. *N Engl J Med* 306 (8):446–450.

Ritz, J., and D. Spiegelman. 2004. Equivalence of conditional and marginal regression models for clustered and longitudinal data. *Stat Methods Med Res* 13 (4):309–323.

Rivara, F.P., P. Cummings, S. Ringold, A.B. Bergman, A. Joffe, and D.A. Christakis. 2007. A comparison of reviewers selected by editors and reviewers suggested by authors. *J Pediatr* 151 (2):202–205.

Robbins, A.S., S.Y. Chao, and V.P. Fonseca. 2002. What's the relative risk? A method to directly estimate risk ratios in cohort studies of common outcomes. *Ann Epidemiol* 12 (7):452–454.

Robins, J.M., and S. Greenland. 1996. Identification of causal effects using instrumental variables: Comment. *J Amer Stat Assoc* 91 (434):456–458.

Robins, J.M., and H. Morgenstern. 1987. The foundations of confounding in epidemiology. *Comput Math Applic* 14 (9-12):869–916.

Robinson, L.D., and N.P. Jewell. 1991. Some surprising results about covariate adjustment in logistic regression models. *Int Stat Rev* 58 (2):227–240.

Rodrigues, L., and B.R. Kirkwood. 1990. Case-control designs in the study of common diseases: Updates on the demise of the rare disease assumption and the choice of sampling scheme for controls. *Int J Epidemiol* 19 (1):205–213.

Rosenbaum, P.R. 2010. *Design of Observational Studies*. New York: Springer.

Rosenbaum, P.R., and D.B. Rubin. 1984. Difficulties with regression analyses of age-adjusted rates. *Biometrics* 40 (2):437–443.

Rosenberger, W.F., and J.M. Lachin. 2002. *Randomization in Clinical Trials: Theory and Practice*. New York: John Wiley & Sons.

Rosengart, M., P. Cummings, A.B. Nathens, P. Heagerty, R. Maier, and F. Rivara. 2005. An evaluation of state firearm regulations and homicide and suicide death rates. *Inj Prev* 11 (2):77–83.

Ross, G.J.S., and D.A. Preece. 1985. The negative binomial distribution. *J R Stat Soc D* 34 (3):323–335.

Rossing, M.A., J.R. Daling, N.S. Weiss, D.E. Moore, and S.G. Self. 1994. Ovarian tumors in a cohort of infertile women. *N Engl J Med* 331 (12):771–776.

Rothman, K.J. 1977. Epidemiologic methods in clinical trials. *Cancer* 39 (4 Suppl):1771–1775.

Rothman, K.J. 1978. A show of confidence [editorial]. *N Engl J Med* 299 (24):1362–1363.

Rothman, K.J. 1986a. *Modern Epidemiology*. 1st ed. Boston, MA: Little, Brown and Company.

Rothman, K.J. 1986b. Significance questing. *Ann Intern Med* 105 (3):445–447.

Rothman, K.J. 2012. *Epidemiology: An Introduction*. 2nd ed. New York: Oxford University Press.

Rothman, K.J., and J.D. Boice Jr. 1979. *Epidemiologic Analysis with a Programmable Calculator*. Washington, DC: National Institutes of Health.

Rothman, K.J., S. Greenland, and T.L. Lash. 2008a. Case-control studies. In *Modern Epidemiology*, edited by K.J. Rothman, S. Greenland, and T.L. Lash. Philadelphia, PA: Lippincott Williams & Wilkins.

Rothman, K.J., S. Greenland, and T.L. Lash. 2008b. Design strategies to improve study accuracy. In *Modern Epidemiology*, edited by K.J. Rothman, S. Greenland, and T.L. Lash. Philadelphia, PA: Lippincott Williams & Wilkins.

Rothman, K.J., S. Greenland, and T.L. Lash. 2008c. *Modern Epidemiology*. 3rd ed. Philadelphia, PA: Lippincott Williams & Wilkins.

Rothman, K.J., S. Greenland, and T.L. Lash. 2008d. Precision and statistics in epidemiologic studies. In *Modern Epidemiology*, edited by K.J. Rothman, S. Greenland, and T.L. Lash. Philadelphia, PA: Lippincott Williams & Wilkins.

Rothman, K.J., S. Greenland, C. Poole, and T.L. Lash. 2008. Causation and causal inference. In *Modern Epidemiology*, edited by K.J. Rothman, S. Greenland, and T.L. Lash. Philadelphia, PA: Lippincott Williams & Wilkins.

Rothman, K.J., L.A. Wise, and E.E. Hatch. 2011. Should graphs of risk or rate ratios be plotted on a log scale? *Am J Epidemiol* 174 (3):376–377.

Royall, R. 1997. *Statistical Evidence: A Likelihood Paradigm*. Boca Raton, FL: Chapman & Hall/CRC.

Royston, P. 2000. Choice of scale for cubic smoothing spline models in medical applications. *Stat Med* 19 (9):1191–1205.

Royston, P. 2001. Flexible alternatives to the Cox model, and more. *Stata J* 2001 (1):1–28.

Royston, P. 2015. Estimating the treatment effect in a clinical trial using difference in restricted mean survival time. *Stata J* 15 (4):1098–1117.

Royston, P., and D.G. Altman. 1994. Regression using fractional polynomials of continuous covariates: Parsimonious parametric modelling (with discussion). *J R Stat Soc. Series C (Appl Stat)* 43 (3):429–467.

Royston, P., D.G. Altman, and W. Sauerbrei. 2006. Dichotomizing continuous predictors in multiple regression: A bad idea. *Stat Med* 25 (1):127–141.

Royston, P., G. Ambler, and W. Sauerbrei. 1999. The use of fractional polynomials to model continuous risk variables in epidemiology. *Int J Epidemiol* 28 (5):964–974.

Royston, P., and P.C. Lambert. 2011. *Flexible Parametric Survival Analysis Using Stata: Beyond the Cox Model*. College Station, TX: Stata Press.

Royston, P., K.G. Moons, D.G. Altman, and Y. Vergouwe. 2009. Prognosis and prognostic research: Developing a prognostic model. *BMJ* 338:b604.

Royston, P., and M.K. Parmar. 2002. Flexible parametric proportional-hazards and proportional-odds models for censored survival data, with application to prognostic modelling and estimation of treatment effects. *Stat Med* 21 (15):2175–2197.

Royston, P., and M.K. Parmar. 2011. The use of restricted mean survival time to estimate the treatment effect in randomized clinical trials when the proportional hazards assumption is in doubt. *Stat Med* 30 (19):2409–2421.

Royston, P., and M.K. Parmar. 2013. Restricted mean survival time: An alternative to the hazard ratio for the design and analysis of randomized trials with a time-to-event outcome. *BMC Med Res Methodol* 13:152.

Royston, P., and W. Sauerbrei. 2008. *Multivariable Model-Building: A Pragmatic Approach to Regression Analysis Based on Fractional Polynomials for Continuous Variables*. Chichester, England: John Wiley & Sons.

Rubin, D.B. 1973. Matching to remove bias in observational studies. *Biometrics* 29 (1):159–183.

Rubin, D.B. 1997. Estimating causal effects from large data sets using propensity scores. *Ann Intern Med* 127 (8 (2)):757–763.

Rubin, D.B. 2006. *Matched Sampling for Causal Effects*. New York: Cambridge University Press.

Rutherford, E., H. Geiger, and H. Bateman. 1910. The probability variations in the distribution of α particles. *Phil Mag J Sci* 20:698–707.

Sahai, H., and A. Khurshid. 1996. *Statistics in Epidemiology: Methods, Techniques, and Applications*. Boca Raton, FL: CRC Press.

Salsburg, D. 2001. *The Lady Tasting Tea: How Statistics Revolutionized Science in the Twentieth Century*. New York: W. H. Freeman and Company.

Sankrithi, U., I. Emanuel, and G. van Belle. 1991. Comparison of linear and exponential multivariate models for explaining national infant and child mortality. *Int J Epidemiol* 20 (2):565–570.

Santos Silva, J.M.C., and S. Tenreyro. 2006. The log of gravity. *Rev Econ Stat* 88 (4):641–658.

Sartwell, P.E. 1960. "On the methodology of investigations of etiologic factors in chronic diseases"–Further comments. *J Chronic Dis* 11 (1):61–63.

Sauerbrei, W., and P. Royston. 1999. Building multivariable prognostic and diagnostic models: Transformation of the predictors by using fractional polynomials. *J R Stat Soc A* 162 (1):71–94.

Savu, A., Q. Liu, and Y. Yasui. 2010. Estimation of relative risk and prevalence ratio. *Stat Med* 29 (22):2269–2281.

Schiff, M., and P. Cummings. 2004. Comparison of reporting of seat belt use by police and crash investigators: Variation in agreement by injury severity. *Accid Anal Prev* 36 (6):961–965.

Schmidt, M., C.F. Christiansen, F. Mehnert, K.J. Rothman, and H.T. Sorensen. 2011. Non-steroidal anti-inflammatory drug use and risk of atrial fibrillation or flutter: Population based case-control study. *BMJ* 343:d3450.

Schmoor, C., and M. Schumacher. 1997. Effects of covariate omission and categorization when analysing randomized trials with the Cox model. *Stat Med* 16 (1-3):225–237.

Schrek, R., L.A. Baker, and et al. 1950. Tobacco smoking as an etiologic factor in disease; cancer. *Cancer Res* 10 (1):49–58.

Schulman, K.A., J.A. Berlin, and J.J. Escarce. 1999. Race, sex, and physician's referrals for cardiac catheterization [letter]. *N Engl J Med* 341 (4):286.

Schulman, K.A., J.A. Berlin, W. Harless, et al. 1999. The effect of race and sex on physicians' recommendations for cardiac catheterization [published erratum appears in N Engl J Med 1999 Apr8;340(14):1130]. *N Engl J Med* 340 (8):618–626.

Schwartz, L.M., S. Woloshin, and H.G. Welch. 1999. Misunderstanding about the effects of race and sex on physicians' referrals for cardiac catheterization. *N Engl J Med* 341 (4):279–283.

Schwarz, G. 1976. Estimating the dimension of a model. *Ann Stat* 6 (2):461–464.

Scribney, B. 1997. Stata 5: Goodness-of-fit chi-squared test reported by Poisson www.stata.com/gsearch.php? q=goodness+of+fit&site=stata&client=stata&proxystylesheet=stata&restrict=Default&output=xml_no_dtd.

Senn, S. 2002. *Cross-Over Trials in Clinical Research*. 2nd ed. New York: John Wiley & Sons.

Shore, R.E., B.S. Pasternack, and M.G. Curnen. 1976. Relating influenza epidemics to childhood leukemia in tumor registries without a defined population base: A critique with suggestions for improved methods. *Am J Epidemiol* 103 (6):527–535.

Shumway-Cook, A., I.F. Silver, M. Lemier, S. York, P. Cummings, and T.D. Koepsell. 2007. Effectiveness of a community-based multifactorial intervention on falls and fall risk factors in community-living older adults: A randomized, controlled trial. *J Gerontol A Biol Sci Med Sci* 62 (12):1420–1427.

Silcock, H. 1959. The comparison of occupational mortality rates. *Popul Stud* 13 (2):183–192.

Silverwood, R.J., M.V. Holmes, C.E. Dale, et al. 2014. Testing for non-linear causal effects using a binary genotype in a Mendelian randomization study: Application to alcohol and cardiovascular traits. *Int J Epidemiol* 43 (6):1781–1790.

Simonoff, J.S. 1996. *Smoothing Methods in Statistics*. New York: Springer.

Simonoff, J.S. 1998. Logistic regression, categorical predictors, and goodness-of-fit: It depends on who you ask. *Amer Statistician* 52 (1):10–14.

Siristatidis, C., T.N. Sergentanis, P. Kanavidis, et al. 2013. Controlled ovarian hyperstimulation for IVF: Impact on ovarian, endometrial and cervical cancer–A systematic review and meta-analysis. *Hum Reprod Update* 19 (2):105–123.

Sjölander, A., E. Dahlqwist, and J. Zetterqvist. 2016. A note on the noncollapsibility of rate differences and rate ratios. *Epidemiology* 27 (3):356–359.

Sjölander, A., and S. Greenland. 2013. Ignoring the matching variables in cohort studies - when is it valid and why? *Stat Med* 32 (27):4696–4708.

Skrondal, A., and S. Rabe-Hesketh. 2004. *Generalized Latent Variable Modeling: Multilevel, Longitudinal, and Structural Equation Models*. Boca Raton, FL: Chapman & Hall/CRC.

Snijders, T., and R. Bosker. 2012. *Multilevel Analysis: An Introduction to Basic and Advanced Multilevel Modeling*. 2nd ed. London: Sage Publications.

Stewart, L.M., C.D. Holman, P. Aboagye-Sarfo, J.C. Finn, D.B. Preen, and R. Hart. 2013. In vitro fertilization, endometriosis, nulliparity and ovarian cancer risk. *Gynecol Oncol* 128 (2):260–264.

Steyerberg, E.W. 2009. *Clinical Prediction Models: A Practical Approach to Development, Validation, and Updating*. New York: Springer.

Stiell, I.G. 2001. The development of clinical decision rules for injury care. In *Injury Control: A Guide to Research and Evaluation*, edited by F.P. Rivara, P. Cummings, T.D. Koepsell, et al. New York: Cambridge University Press.

Stiell, I.G., and G.A. Wells. 1999. Methodologic standards for the development of clinical decision rules in emergency medicine. *Ann Emerg Med* 33 (4):437–447.

Stigler, S.M. 1982. Poisson on the Poisson distribution. *Stat Prob Let* 1 (1):33–35.

Stigler, S.M. 1986. *The History of Statistics: The Measurement of Uncertainty before 1900*. Cambridge, MA: Harvard University Press.

Storm, T., G. Thamsborg, T. Steiniche, H.K. Genant, and O.H. Sorensen. 1990. Effect of intermittent cyclical etidronate therapy on bone mass and fracture rate in women with postmenopausal osteoporosis. *N Engl J Med* 322 (18):1265–1271.

Stukel, T.A., R.J. Glynn, E.S. Fisher, S.M. Sharp, G. Lu-Yao, and J.E. Wennberg. 1994. Standardized rates of recurrent outcomes. *Stat Med* 13 (17):1781–1791.

Subramanian, S.V., and A.J. O'Malley. 2010. Modeling neighborhood effects: The futility of comparing mixed and marginal approaches. *Epidemiology* 21 (4):475–478; discussion 479-481.

Sullivan, K.M., and D.A. Foster. 1990. Use of the confidence interval function. *Epidemiology* 1 (1):39–42.

Sullivan, S.G., and S. Greenland. 2013. Bayesian regression in SAS software. *Int J Epidemiol* 42 (1):308–317.

Susser, M., and A. Adelstein. 1975. An introduction to the work of William Farr. *Am J Epidemiol* 101 (6):469–476.

Sutton, A.J., K.R. Abrams, D.R. Jones, T.A. Sheldon, and F. Song. 2000. *Methods for Meta-Analysis in Medical Research*. Chichester, England: John Wiley & Sons.

Swanson, S.A., and M.A. Hernán. 2013. Commentary: How to report instrumental variable analyses (suggestions welcome). *Epidemiology* 24 (3):370–374.

Swanson, S.A., J.M. Robins, M. Miller, and M.A. Hernán. 2015. Selecting on treatment: A pervasive form of bias in instrumental variable analyses. *Am J Epidemiol* 181 (3):191–197.

Tang, N., J. Stein, R.Y. Hsia, J.H. Maselli, and R. Gonzales. 2010. Trends and characteristics of US emergency department visits, 1997-2007. *JAMA* 304 (6):664–670.

Tarone, R.E. 1981. On summary estimators of relative risk. *J Chronic Dis* 34 (9-10):463–468.

Tarter, M.E., and M.D. Lock. 1993. *Model-Free Curve Estimation*. New York: Chapman & Hall.

Thall, P.F. 1988. Mixed Poisson likelihood regression models for longitudinal interval count data. *Biometrics* 44 (1):197–209.

Therneau, T.M., and P.M. Grambsch. 2000. *Modeling Survival Data: Extending the Cox Model*. New York: Springer.

Tilyard, M.W., G.F. Spears, J. Thomson, and S. Dovey. 1992. Treatment of postmenopausal osteoporosis with calcitriol or calcium. *N Engl J Med* 326 (6):357–362.

U.S. Census Bureau. 2012. Methodology for the intercensal population and housing unit estimates: 2000 to 2010. www.census.gov/popest/methodology/2000-2010_Intercensal_Estimates_Methodology.pdf.

Uno, H., B. Claggett, L. Tian, et al. 2014. Moving beyond the hazard ratio in quantifying the between-group difference in survival analysis. *J Clin Oncol* 32 (22):2380–2385.

Van der Laan, M.J., A.E. Hubbard, and N.P. Jewell. 2010. Learning from data: Semiparametric models versus faith-based inference. *Epidemiology* 21 (4):479–481.

Vandenbroucke, J.P., and C.M. Vandenbroucke-Grauls. 1988. A note on the history of the calculation of hospital statistics. *Am J Epidemiol* 127 (4):699–702.

Vandenbroucke, J.P., and C.M. Vandenbroucke-Grauls. 1996. In defense of Farr and Nightingale [letter]. *Ann Intern Med* 125 (12):1014.

Vandenbroucke, J.P., and C.M. Vandenbroucke-Grauls. 1997. A return to Farr and Nightingale [letter]. *Ann Intern Med* 127 (2):170–171.

Varnell, S.P., D.M. Murray, J.B. Janega, and J.L. Blitstein. 2004. Design and analysis of group-randomized trials: A review of recent practices. *Am J Public Health* 94 (3):393–399.

Vavilala, M.S., P. Cummings, S.R. Sharar, and L. Quan. 2004. Association of hospital trauma designation with admission patterns of injured children. *J Trauma* 57 (1):119–124.

Villaveces, A., P. Cummings, V.E. Espitia, T.D. Koepsell, B. McKnight, and A.L. Kellermann. 2000. Effect of a ban on carrying firearms on homicide rates in 2 Colombian cities. *JAMA* 283 (9):1205–1209.

Vittinghoff, E., D.V. Glidden, S.C. Shiboski, and C.E. McCulloch. 2012. *Regression Methods in Biostatistics: Linear, Logistic, Survival, and Repeated Measures Models.* 2nd ed. New York: Springer.

Vittinghoff, E., and C.E. McCulloch. 2007. Relaxing the rule of ten events per variable in logistic and Cox regression. *Am J Epidemiol* 165 (6):710–718.

von Bortkewitsch, L. 1898. *Das Gesetz Der Kleinen Zahlen.* Leipzig, Germany: Druck und Verlag von B. G. Teubner.

Wacholder, S. 1991. Practical considerations in choosing between the case-cohort and nested case-control designs. *Epidemiology* 2 (2):155–158.

Wakefield, J. 2008. Ecologic studies revisited. *Annu Rev Public Health* 29:75–90.

Walker, A.M. 1982. Efficient assessment of confounder effects in matched follow-up studies. *J R Stat Soc. Series C (Appl Stat)* 31 (3):293–297.

Walker, A.M. 1985. Small sample properties of some estimators of a common hazard ratio. *J R Stat Soc. Series C (Appl Stat)* 34 (1):42–48.

Walker, A.M., H. Jick, J.R. Hunter, et al. 1981. Vasectomy and non-fatal myocardial infarction. *Lancet* 1 (8210):13–15.

Walker, A.M., H. Jick, J.R. Hunter, and J. McEvoy 3rd. 1983. Vasectomy and nonfatal myocardial infarction: Continued observation indicates no elevation of risk. *J Urol* 130 (5):936–937.

Wallenstein, S. 1988. Re: "Inferences on odds ratios, relative risks, and risk differences based on standard regression programs" [letter]. *Am J Epidemiol* 128 (2):445.

Wallenstein, S., and C. Bodian. 1987. Epidemiologic programs for computers and calculators. Inferences on odds ratios, relative risks, and risk differences based on standard regression programs. *Am J Epidemiol* 126 (2):346–355.

Watts, N.B., S.T. Harris, H.K. Genant, et al. 1990. Intermittent cyclical etidronate treatment of postmenopausal osteoporosis. *N Engl J Med* 323 (2):73–79.

Webster, D.W., J.S. Vernick, A.M. Zeoli, and J.A. Manganello. 2004. Association between youth-focused firearm laws and youth suicides. *JAMA* 292 (5):594–601.

Wei, L.J., D.Y. Lin, and L. Weissfeld. 1989. Regression analysis of multivariate incomplete failure time data by modeling marginal distributions. *J Amer Stat Assoc* 84 (408):1065–1073.

Weiss, N.S. 2001. Policy emanating from epidemiologic data: What is the proper forum? *Epidemiology* 12 (4):373–374.

Weiss, N.S. 2002. Can the "specificity" of an association be rehabilitated as a basis for supporting a causal hypothesis? *Epidemiology* 13 (1):6–8.

Weiss, N.S. 2008. Subgroup-specific associations in the face of overall null results: Should we rush in or fear to tread? *Cancer Epidemiol Biomarkers Prev* 17 (6):1297–1299.

Weiss, N.S., and T.D. Koepsell. 2014. *Epidemiologic Methods: Studying the Occurrence of Illness.* 2nd ed. New York: Oxford University Press.

West, B.T., K.B. Welch, and A.T. Galecki. 2015. *Linear Mixed Models: A Practical Guide Using Statistical Software.* 2nd ed. Boca Raton, FL: CRC Press.

Whitaker, H. 2008. The self controlled case series method. *BMJ* 337:a1069.

Whitaker, H.J., M.N. Hocine, and C.P. Farrington. 2009. The methodology of self-controlled case series studies. *Stat Methods Med Res* 18 (1):7–26.

Whitaker, H.J., C. Paddy Farrington, B. Spiessens, and P. Musonda. 2006. Tutorial in biostatistics: The self-controlled case series method. *Stat Med* 25 (10):1768–1797.

White, H. 1980. A heteroskedasticity-consistent covariance matrix estimator and a direct test for heteroskedasticity. *Econometrica* 48 (4):817–838.

White, H. 1982. Maximum likelihood estimation of misspecified models. *Econometrica* 50 (1):1–25.

Whitehead, J. 1980. Fitting Cox's regression model to survival data using GLIM. *J R Stat Soc Series C (Appl Stat)* 29 (3):268–275.

Whittemore, A.S. 1978. Collapsibility of multidimensional contingency tables. *J R Stat Soc B* 40 (3):328–340.

Wikipedia. Florence Nightingale. http://en.wikipedia.org/wiki/Florence_Nightingale.

Wikipedia. Marginal distribution. https://en.wikipedia.org/wiki/Marginal_distribution.

Wikipedia. St Thomas' Hospital. http://en.wikipedia.org/wiki/St_Thomas%27_Hospital.

Windeler, J., and S. Lange. 1995. Events per person year–A dubious concept. *BMJ* 310 (6977):454–456.

Winkelmann, R. 2008. *Econometric Analysis of Count Data*. 5th ed. Berlin, Germany: Springer.

Winsor, C.P. 1947. Quotations: "Das gesetz der kleinin zahlen". *Human Biology* 19 (3):154–161.

Wolfenden, H.H. 1923. On the methods of comparing the mortalities of two or more communities, and the standardization of death-rates. *J R Stat Soc* 86 (3):399–411.

Woloshin, S., L.M. Schwartz, and H.G. Welch. 1999. Race, sex, and referral for cardiac catheterization [letter]. *N Engl J Med* 341 (26):2022.

Wooldridge, J.M. 2008. *Introductory Econometrics: A Modern Approach*. 4th ed. Mason, OH: South-Western Cengage Learning.

Wooldridge, J.M. 2010. *Econometric Analysis of Cross Section and Panel Data*. 2nd ed. Cambridge, MA: MIT Press.

Wynder, E.L., and E.A. Graham. 1950. Tobacco smoking as a possible etiologic factor in bronchiogenic carcinoma. *J Amer Med Assoc* 143 (4):3329–3336.

Xu, Y., Y.B. Cheung, K.F. Lam, S.H. Tan, and P. Milligan. 2010. A simple approach to the estimation of incidence rate difference. *Am J Epidemiol* 172 (3):334–343.

Yates, F. 1934. The analysis of multiple classifications with unequal numbers in different classes. *J Amer Stat Assoc* 29 (185):51–66.

Yerushalmy, J., and C.E. Palmer. 1959. On the methodology of investigations of etiologic factors in chronic diseases. *J Chronic Dis* 10 (1):27–40.

Young, M.L., J.S. Preisser, B.F. Qaqish, and M. Wolfson. 2007. Comparison of subject-specific and population averaged models for count data from cluster-unit intervention trials. *Stat Methods Med Res* 16 (2):167–184.

Yule, G.U. 1910. On the distribution of deaths with age when the causes of death act cumulatively, and similar frequency distributions. *J R Stat Soc* 73 (1):26–38.

Yule, G.U. 1934. On some points relating to vital statistics, more especially statistics of occupational mortality. *J R Stat Soc* 97 (1):1–84.

Zeger, S.L., and K.Y. Liang. 1986. Longitudinal data analysis for discrete and continuous outcomes. *Biometrics* 42 (1):121–130.

Zhu, M., H. Chu, and S. Greenland. 2011. Biased standard errors from complex survey analysis: An example from applying ordinary least squares to the national hospital ambulatory medical care survey [Erratum 2012: 1(1)70]. *Ann Epidemiol* 21 (11):830–834.

Zhu, M., P. Cummings, S. Zhao, J.H. Coben, and G.S. Smith. 2015. The association of graduated driver licensing with miles driven and fatal crash rates per miles driven among adolescents. *Inj Prev* 21 (e1):e23–e27.

Zou, G. 2004. A modified Poisson regression approach to prospective studies with binary data. *Am J Epidemiol* 159 (7):702–706.

Index

Printed in the United States
by Baker & Taylor Publisher Services